Clinical Review of Oral and Maxillofacial Surgery

Clinical Review of
Oral and Maxillofacial Surgery

Shahrokh C. Bagheri, DMD, MD

Clinical Assistant Professor of Oral and Maxillofacial Surgery
Emory University School of Medicine
Division of Oral and Maxillofacial Surgery;
Private Practice
Atlanta Oral and Facial Surgery
Atlanta, Georgia

Chris Jo, DMD

Clinical Assistant Professor of Oral and Maxillofacial Surgery
Emory University School of Medicine
Division of Oral and Maxillofacial Surgery;
Private Practice
Atlanta Oral and Facial Surgery
Atlanta, Georgia

with 241 illustrations

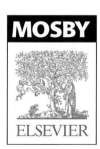

MOSBY

ELSEVIER

MOSBY
ELSEVIER

11830 Westline Industrial Drive
St. Louis, Missouri 63146

Clinical Review of Oral and Maxillofacial Surgery   978-0-323-04574-2

Notice

Knowledge and best practice in this field are constantly changing. As new research and experience broaden our knowledge, changes in practice, treatment and drug therapy may become necessary or appropriate. Readers are advised to check the most current information provided (i) on procedures featured or (ii) by the manufacturer of each product to be administered, to verify the recommended dose or formula, the method and duration of administration, and contraindications. It is the responsibility of the practitioner, relying on their own experience and knowledge of the patient, to make diagnoses, to determine dosages and the best treatment for each individual patient, and to take all appropriate safety precautions. To the fullest extent of the law, neither the Publisher nor the Authors assumes any liability for any injury and/or damage to persons or property arising out or related to any use of the material contained in this book.

The Publisher

Library of Congress Control Number 2007925886

Publisher: Linda Duncan
Senior Editor: John Dolan
Developmental Editor: Courtney Sprehe
Publishing Services Manager: Pat Joiner-Myers
Senior Project Manager: Rachel E. Dowell
Cover Design Direction: Paula Catalano
Text Designer: Paula Catalano

Printed in the United States of America

Last digit is the print number: 9   8   7   6   5   4   3   2   1

To my wife Nooshin, whose love and support gave me the energy and confidence to complete this project, and to my son, Shaheen, whose peaceful smile while falling asleep inspired me as I wrote many sections by his bedside.

To my parents, Parviz and Ladan, who have supported me for many years towards my academic and professional goals at the expense of being away from them.

To my brother, Homayoun, who at present and in my youth, has been my support and source of intellectual stimulation.

To my mentors, Dr. Robert A. Bays, Dr. Sam E. Farish, Dr. Eric J. Dierks, Dr. Bryce E. Potter, and Dr. Leon A. Assael, who through their teachings provided me the experience and tools to complete this project.

To all patients, students, and residents of oral and maxillofacial surgery.

Shahrokh C. Bagheri

To my Lord and Savior, who makes all things possible.

To my wife, Sunny, whose smile and love gives me the strength and motivation to continue in my professional, academic, and personal endeavors.

To my parents, Hae Sung and Kum Sook Jo, who taught me to pursue excellence in all things and who have tirelessly supported me during my training.

To my sister, Jenny, whose academic achievements motivated me to follow in her footsteps.

To my mentors Dr. Robert A. Bays, Dr. Vincent J. Perciaccante, Dr. Sam E. Farish, Dr. Steven M. Roser, and Dr. John E. Griffin, who gave me the training, experience, and motivation to finish this project.

To my fellow residents who were in the trenches with me during residency training: Piyush, Shahrokh, Nizar, Jennifer, Donnie, Nader, Marty, Harry, John, Mehran, Hussein, Tony, Xin, Boris, Brenda, Cang, Fernando, Deepak, Sam, Bruce, Danielle, Abtin, Jaspal, and Bill.

Chris Jo

Chapter Editors and Contributors

Chapter Editors

Shahrokh C. Bagheri, DMD, MD
Clinical Assistant Professor of Oral and Maxillofacial
  Surgery
Emory University School of Medicine
Division of Oral and Maxillofacial Surgery;
Private Practice
Atlanta Oral and Facial Surgery
Atlanta, Georgia

Deepak Kademani, DMD, MD, FACS
Assistant Professor of Surgery
Consultant, Oral and Maxillofacial Surgery
Department of Oral and Maxillofacial Surgery
Mayo Clinic
College of Medicine
Rochester, Minnesota

Husain Ali Khan, MD, DMD
Private Practice
Atlanta Oral and Facial Surgery
Cartersville, Georgia

Chris Jo, DMD
Clinical Assistant Professor of Oral and Maxillofacial
  Surgery
Emory University School of Medicine
Division of Oral and Maxillofacial Surgery;
Private Practice
Atlanta Oral and Facial Surgery
Atlanta, Georgia

Martin B. Steed, DDS
Assistant Professor and Residency Program Director
Department of Surgery
Division of Oral and Maxillofacial Surgery
Emory University
Atlanta, Georgia

Contributors

John M. Allen, DMD
Former Attending Staff
Division of Oral and Maxillofacial Surgery
Department of Surgery
School of Medicine
Emory University Hospital Center
Atlanta, Georgia

Bruce Anderson, HBSc, DDS
Resident
Department of Surgery
Division of Oral and Maxillofacial Surgery
Emory University
School of Medicine
Atlanta, Georgia

Michael L. Beckley, DDS
Department of Oral and Maxillofacial Surgery
University of the Pacific
School of Dentistry
San Francisco, California

R. Bryan Bell, DDS, MD, FACS
Clinical Assistant Professor
Department of Oral and Maxillofacial Surgery
Oregon Health and Science University;
Attending Surgeon
Oral and Maxillofacial Surgery Service
Legacy Emanuel Hospital and Health Center
Portland, Oregon

Samuel L. Bobek, DMD
Resident
Department of Oral and Maxillofacial Surgery
Oregon Health and Science University
Portland, Oregon

Gary F. Bouloux MD, DDS, MDSc, FRACDS, FRACDS(OMD)
Assistant Professor
Department of Oral and Maxillofacial Srugery
Emory University
School of Medicine
Atlanta, Georgia

Saif S. Al-Bustani, DMD
Resident
Department of Oral and Maxillofacial Surgery
Oregon Health and Science University
Portland, Oregon

Danielle Cunningham, DDS
Resident
Department of Oral and Maxillofacial Surgery
Emory University
Atlanta, Georgia

Fariba Farhidvash, MD
Board Certified Neurologist
Private Practice
Thomasville, Georgia

Sam E. Farish DMD
Assistant Professor
Department of Surgery
Division of Oral and Maxillofacial Surgery
Emory University
School of Medicine;
Chief
Department of Oral and Maxillofacial Surgery
VA Medical Center
Atlanta, Georgia

Jaspal Girn, DMD
Resident
Department of Oral and Maxillofacial Surgery
Emory University
Atlanta, Georgia

Eric P. Holmgren, MS, DMD, MD
Private Practice
Oral and Maxillofacial Surgery Associates
Bennington, Vermont and Pittsfield, Massachusetts

Anthony A. Indovina, Jr., DDS
Assistant Clinical Professor
Department of Oral and Maxillofacial Surgery
University of Minnesota
Minneapolis, Minnesota;
Private Practice
Dakota Valley Oral and Maxillofacial Surgery
Eagen, Minnesota

Jenny Jo, MD
Peachtree Women's Clinic
Atlanta Women's Health Group
Atlanta, Georgia

Matthew J. Karban, DMD
Resident
Department of Oral and Maxillofacial Surgery
Mayo Clinic
Rochester, Minnesota

Deepak G. Krishnan, BDS
Chief Resident
Division of Oral and Maxillofacial Surgery
Department of Surgery
School of Medicine
Emory University
Atlanta, Georgia

Derek H. Lamb, DMD
Resident
Department of Surgery
Division of Oral and Maxillofacial Surgery
Mayo Clinic
Rochester, Minnesota

Joyce T. Lee, DDS, MD
Clinical Assistant Professor of Surgery
Department of Oral and Maxillofacial Surgery
Emory University
Atlanta, Georgia

Mehran Mehrabi, Maj. USAF, DC
Staff Oral and Maxillofacial Surgeon
Department of Oral and Maxillofacial Surgery
Keesler Air Force Base
Biloxi, MS

Roger A. Meyer, MD, DDS, FACS
Chairman of Oral and Maxillofacial Surgery
Northside Hospital;
Private Practice
Atlanta Oral and Facial Surgery
Atlanta, Georgia

David G. Molen, DDS, MD
Private Practice, Molen Oral and Facial Surgery
Auburn, Washington

Aric Murphy, DDS
Resident
Department of Oral and Maxillofacial Surgery
Mayo Clinic
Rochester, Minnesota

Timothy M. Osborn, DDS
Resident
Department of Oral and Maxillofacial Surgery
Oregon Health and Science University
Portland, Oregon

Piyushkumar P. Patel, DDS
Private Practice
Atlanta, Georgia

Vincent J. Pericaccante, DDS
Clinical Assistant Professor
Division of Oral and Maxillofacial Surgery
Department of Surgery
Emory University
School of Medicine;
Private Practice
Atlanta, Georgia

David J.Rallis, DDS
Resident
Department of Surgery
Mayo Clinic
Rochester, Minnesota

Kevin L. Rieck, DDS, MS, MD
Instructor in Surgery
Mayo Clinic College of Medicine
Department of Surgery, Division of Oral and Maxillofacial
Surgery
Mayo Clinic
Rochester, Minnesota

Ma'Ann C. Sabino, DDS, PhD
Assistant Professor
Division of Oral and Maxillofacial Surgery
University of Minnesota
Minneapolis, Minnesota

Abtin Shahriari, DMD, MPH
Chief Resident
Division of Oral and Maxillofacial Surgery
Emory University
Atlanta, Georgia

David C. Swiderski, DDS, MD
Resident
Division of Oral and Maxillofacial Surgery
Mayo Clinic
Rochester, Minnesota

Brett A. Ueeck, DMD, MD
Assistant Professor
Department of Oral and Maxillofacial Surgery
Oregon Health and Science University;
Attending Surgeon
Cleft Lip and Palate Team
Shriners Hospital for Crippled Children
Portland, Oregon

Scott D. Van Dam, DDS, MD
Chief Resident
Department of Oral and Maxillofacial Surgery
Mayo Clinic
Rochester, Minnesota

David Verschueren, DMD, MD
Chief Resident
Department of Oral and Maxillofacial Surgery
Oregon Health and Science University
Portland, Oregon

David M. Weber, DDS, MD
Resident
Department of Oral and Maxillofacial Surgery
Mayo Clinic
Rochester, Minnesota

Lee M. Whitesides, DMD, MMSc
Private Practice
Atlanta Oral and Facial Surgery
Atlanta, Georgia

Michael S. Wilkinson, DMD
Resident
Department of Oral and Maxillofacial Surgery
Oregon Health and Science University
Portland, Oregon

Brian M. Woo, DDS, MD
Chief Resident
Department of Oral and Maxillofacial Surgery
Oregon Health and Science University
Portland, Oregon

Foreword

The purpose of all clinical didactic knowledge is to apply it towards the care of a patient: more explicitly, care that results in an improved outcome of a treatment intervention. *Clinical Review of Oral and Maxillofacial Surgery* is an idea developed by Shahrokh Bagheri during his fellowship in Portland. Along with our other Emanuel Hospital fellows and Oregon Health & Science University and University of Washington residents, Dr. Bagheri was anxious to identify pathology that requires treatment and to offer and execute treatment that works. Now in private practice in Georgia, Dr. Bagheri works with peers and residents to develop that same idea at Emory University while maintaining the practical approach of the practicing surgeon. This text is an embodiment of his thirst towards excellence in the practice of oral and maxillofacial surgery.

Clinical Review of Oral and Maxillofacial Surgery seeks to apply clinical scientific knowledge in the performance of a simulated clinical task described in the text. It applies diagnostic skills, evidence-based treatment decisions, and treatment protocols to the care of patients. Potential pitfalls and complications are described as well.

This text presents classical clinical situations in oral and maxillofacial surgery and identifies the key issues in clinical practice.

What are the key anamnestic findings in the given condition?

What are the key clinical findings in this condition?

What further imaging and laboratory tests are needed to quantify and qualify the clinical findings or to confirm a diagnosis?

What are the goals of treatment?

What clinical interventions are demonstrated to be of use?

What complications might be anticipated?

What is the evidence to support the recommended approach to a clinical problem?

The many residents who have participated in the development of this text ensure that a systematic, evidence-based approach to patient management is destined for a strong future in our specialty. It is hoped that you, the reader, will be informed and inspired to seek further knowledge and evolve your practice because of this contemporary exposition of knowledge. Clinical knowledge in oral and maxillofacial surgery has been given a new baseline to encourage new investigation and surgical technique as a result of this important contribution.

Leon A. Assael, DMD
Professor and Chairman
Oral and Maxillofacial Surgery
Oregon Health & Science University
Portland, Oregon

Preface

The purpose of *Clinical Review of Oral and Maxillofacial Surgery* is to provide the readers of oral and maxillofacial surgery with a systematic approach to the management of patients presenting with the most common surgical or pathological conditions seen in this specialty. Contrary to traditional textbooks of surgery, this book emphasizes a case-based approach to learning that is suitable for readers of oral and maxillofacial surgery at all levels of training or practice. Each chapter contains more than just patient scenarios; instead it presents carefully written *teaching cases*. Each of these cases outlines essential information pertinent to the fundamental aspects of the condition as they present in the practice of oral and maxillofacial surgery.

Experience shows that learning is enhanced by incorporating teaching around real patient scenarios. In this manner, the reader is actively engaged in the case with the intent of raising the interest and, therefore, enhancing the retention of information presented. Traditional textbooks of surgery present the material in a fashion not directly related to a patient, but instead list all the findings, pathophysiology, and treatment modalities. The intent of this book is not to replace a full-scope oral and maxillofacial surgery textbook, but instead serve as a powerful learning tool for those interested in the field.

This book provides a rapid, concise, and easily comprehensible approach to disorders that readers can encounter in their work with patients. Predoctoral students will benefit from the basic presentation of the disorders and treatment options. More advanced readers (such as residents in training or board candidates) will benefit from the more detailed material, and also become accustomed to the style of patient presentation that is reflected in clinical practice and is currently emphasized for oral and maxillofacial surgery boards and in training examinations.

ORGANIZATION

The book is divided into 14 chapters, each comprised of separate sections that present a specific topic. A total of 95 cases representing the full scope of modern practice of oral and maxillofacial surgery are included. Representative disorders or conditions have been chosen for each chapter for teaching purposes. It is not possible to encompass every disorder or condition in each chapter; therefore, the ones included are the most common, or have significant implications for modern clinical practice. The references for each case include both historic articles and recent additions to the field.

Each case illustrates the presentation, physical examination findings, laboratory and imaging studies, along with an analysis of treatment options, complications, and discussion of other relevant information.

The majority of the cases are illustrated by one or more radiographs, clinical photographs, or drawings that further enhance the reader's comprehension and retention of all content.

THE COMPANION CD-ROM

The CD-ROM included with this book features two simulated exams that allow the reader to both review the material and evaluate their test-taking skills. Each exam includes 200 multiple-choice questions, ranging in level of difficulty. Feedback is provided for each question. The questions are set up in a format similar to the current National Board and in-service examinations, including the OMSSAT.

The "test mode" exam is timed and is comprised of a randomized selection of questions pulled from a question bank of over 400 questions. Each time the reader takes this exam the questions are randomized, so it will never be the same exam twice. As the exam is timed, the reader will be able to assess their test-taking strategy and make sure they will be able to complete future exams in the time allotted.

The "study mode" exam allows the reader to pick what subject matter they want to include. For example, if the reader wants to test themselves on radiology, infection, and trauma they will simply pick those chapters, and the question will be incorporated into the exam. The exam can accommodate up to 200 questions. Using this exam, the reader will be able to review the specific material in which they are interested.

Also included on the CD-ROM is an image collection containing every image that appears in the book in full color!

NOTE FROM THE EDITORS

The last several decades have brought dramatic changes to the field of oral and maxillofacial surgery. Recent reconstructive methods; imaging technology; distraction osteogenesis; dental implants; rigid fixation; full-scope training programs; and post-residency training fellowships in cosmetic surgery, head and neck oncology, craniofacial syndromes, and trauma have rapidly reshaped this exciting specialty in the last 20 years. We hope that our readers enjoy and learn from this book as much as we did during its preparation.

Shahrokh C. Bagheri
Chris Jo

Contents

1 Oral and Maxillofacial Radiology

Shahrokh C. Bagheri, DMD, MD

This chapter addresses:
- Multilocular Radiolucent Lesion in the Pericoronal Region (Odontogenic Keratocyst)
- Unilocular Radiolucent Lesion of the Mandible (Dentigerous Cyst)
- Multilocular Radiolucent Lesion in the Periapical Region (Ameloblastoma)
- Unilocular Radiolucent Lesion in a Periapical Region (Periapical Cyst)
- Mixed Radiolucent-Radiopaque Lesion (Ossifying Fibroma)

Interpretation of radiographs is a routine part of the daily practice of oral and maxillofacial surgery. Radiographs that are commonly obtained in the office include periapical, occlusal, panoramic, and lateral cephalometric views. Computed tomography (CT) scans, although costly, are available in some offices. Knowledge of normal radiographic anatomy and recognition of pathological conditions are essential.

A complete discussion of the full spectrum of radiographic pathology is beyond the scope of this book, but here the radiographic presentation of five important and representative pathological processes is provided in case format. Included in each case is the differential diagnosis of associated conditions to guide further study.

Figure 1-1 shows the most common location of several radiographically detectable maxillofacial pathological processes.

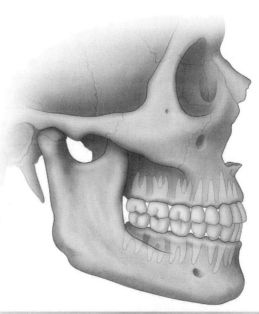

Posterior maxilla
- Pagets disease of bone

Posterior mandible
- Dentigerous cyst
- Odontogenic keratocyst
- Ameloblastoma
- Intraosseous mucoepidermoid carcinoma
- Stafne bone defect (below canal)
- Idiopathic bone marrow defect
- Calcifying epithelial odontogenic tumor (CEOT)

Anterior maxilla
- Adenomatoid odontogenic tumor (AOT)
- Nasopalatine duct cyst
- Lateral periodontal cyst (botryoid type)
- Odontoma
- Pagets disease of bone

Anterior mandible
- Periapical cemento osseous dysplasia
- Central giant cell granuloma
- Odontoma

Figure 1-1   The most common location of several radiographically detectable maxillofacial pathological processes.

Multilocular Radiolucent Lesion in the Pericoronal Region
(Odontogenic Keratocyst)

Piyushkumar P. Patel, DDS, and Chris Jo, DMD

CC

A 20-year-old man is referred for evaluation of a swelling on his right mandible.

Odontogenic Keratocysts

Odontogenic keratocysts (OKCs) show a slight predilection for males with a peak incidence between 11 and 40 years of age. Patients with larger lesions may present with pain secondary to infection of the cystic cavity. Smaller lesions are usually asymptomatic and are frequently diagnosed during routine radiographic examination.

HPI

The patient complains of a 1-month history of progressive, nonpainful swelling of his right posterior mandible (65% to 83% of OKCs occur in the mandible, most often in the posterior body and ramus region). The patient denies any history of pain to his right lower jaw, fever, purulence, or trismus. He does not report any neurosensory changes (which are generally not seen with OKCs).

PMHX/PDHX/MEDICATIONS/ALLERGIES/SH/FH

Noncontributory. There is no family history of similar presentations.

Nevoid basal cell carcinoma syndrome (NBCCS) is an autosomal dominant inherited condition with features that can include multiple basal cell carcinomas of the skin, multiple OKCs, intracranial calcifications, and rib and vertebral anomalies. Many other anomalies have been reported with this syndrome (Box 1-1). The prevalence of the NBCCS is estimated to be 1:60,000.

EXAMINATION

Maxillofacial. The patient has slight lower right facial swelling isolated to the lateral border of the mandible and not involving the area below the inferior border. The mass is hard, nonfluctuant, and nontender to palpation (large cysts may rupture and leak keratin into the surrounding tissue, provoking an intense inflammatory reaction that causes pain and swelling). There are no facial or trigeminal nerve deficits (paresthesia of the inferior alveolar nerve would be more

indicative of a malignant process). The intercanthal distance is 33 mm (normal), and there is no evidence of frontal bossing. His occipitofrontal circumference is normal (an intercanthal distance [the distance between the two medial canthus of the palpebral fissures] of greater than 36 mm is indicative of hypertelorism, and an occipitofrontal circumference greater than 55 cm is indicative of frontal bossing; both can be seen with NBCCS).

Neck. There are no palpable masses and no cervical or submandibular lymphadenopathy. Positive lymph nodes would be indicative of an infectious or a neoplastic process; a careful neck examination is paramount in the evaluation of any head and neck pathology.

Intraoral. Occlusion is stable and reproducible. The right mandibular third molar appears to be distoangularly impacted (OKCs do not typically alter the occlusion). The interincisal opening is within normal limits. There is buccal expansion of the right mandible extending from the right mandibular first molar area posteriorly toward the ascending ramus. Resorption of bone may include the cortex at the inferior border of the mandible, but this is observed at a slower rate than intermedullary bone, which is less dense. For this reason, OKCs characteristically extend anteroposteriorly than buccolingually. This pattern of expansion into less-dense bone explains why maxillary OKCs show more buccal than palatal expansion and often expand into the maxillary sinus. There is no palpable thrill or audible bruit, which are seen with arteriovenous malformations. The oral mucosa is normal in appearance with no signs of acute inflammatory processes.

Thorax-Abdomen-Extremity. The patient has no findings suggestive of NBCCS (e.g., pectus excavatum, rib abnormalities, palmar or plantar pitting, and skin lesions) (see Box 1-1).

IMAGING

A panoramic radiograph is the initial screening examination of choice for patients presenting for evaluation of intraosseous mandibular pathology (10% to 20% of OKCs are incidental radiographic findings). This provides an excellent overview of the bony architecture of the maxilla, mandible, and associated structures. Bony and soft tissue window CT scans of the mandible and neck are recommended when large lesions are found. CT scans are valuable in that they provide additional

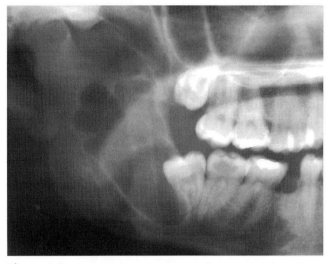

Figure 1-2 Preoperative panoramic radiograph showing a large multilocular radiolucent lesion of the right mandible body and ramus associated with an impacted third molar.

Box 1-1.	**Major Features of the Nevoid Basal Cell Carcinoma Syndrome**

50% or Greater Frequency
Multiple basal cell carcinomas
Odontogenic keratocysts
Epidermal cysts of the skin
Palmer-planter pits
Calcified falx cerebri
Enlarged head circumference
Rib anomalies (splayed, fused, partially missing, bifid)
Mild ocular hypertelorism
Spina bifida occulta of cervical or thoracic vertebrae

15% to 49% Frequency
Calcified ovarian fibromas
Short fourth metacarpals
Kyphoscoliosis or other vertebral anomalies
Pectus excavatum or carinatum
Strabismus

Less Than 15% Frequency
Medulloblastoma
Meningioma
Lymphomesenteric cysts
Cardiac fibroma
Fetal rhabdomyoma
Marfanoid build
Cleft lip and palate
Hypogonadism in males
Mental retardation

From Gorlin RJ: Nevoid basal-cell carcinoma syndrome, *Medicine* 66:98-113, 1987.

---

information such as proximity of adjacent structures (e.g., mandibular canal), integrity of cortical plates, and presence of perforations into adjacent soft tissues. CT scans provide accurate assessment of the size of the lesion and can demonstrate additional anatomic details (or lesions) that do not appear on panoramic radiographs. For evaluation of osseous structures, non–contrast-enhanced CT scans are most informative.

In addition, three-dimensional volume-reconstructed scans can be obtained. This imaging study reconstructs the bony framework of the facial skeleton and can be helpful when large intraosseous pathology is encountered. It has been demonstrated that T2-weighted magnetic resonance imaging (MRI) can detect OKCs in 85% of new cases with a readily recognizable pattern. However, the use of MRI for management of suspected OKCs is not routine.

In this patient, the panoramic radiograph reveals a large, multilocular radiolucent lesion with possible displacement of the right mandibular third molar (Figure 1-2) (70% of OKCs present as a unilocular radiolucent lesion). The multilocular appearance is more commonly seen with maxillary OKCs. There are also several carious teeth and a retained root tip of the right mandibular second bicuspid (tooth No. 29).

LABS

No laboratory tests are indicated unless dictated by the medical history.

Fine-needle aspiration (FNA) biopsy and cytokeratin-10 immunocytochemical staining have been shown to differentiate OKCs from dentigerous and other nonkeratinizing cysts. Despite their availability, these techniques are not routinely ordered.

DIFFERENTIAL DIAGNOSIS

The differential diagnosis of multilocular radiolucent lesions can be divided into lesions of cystic pathogenesis, neoplastic (benign or malignant) lesions, and vascular anomalies (which are least common). The differential diagnosis of multilocular radiolucent lesions is listed in Box 1-2 and can be further narrowed by clinical presentation. Special considerations should be given to radiolucent lesions with poorly defined or ragged borders, which have a separate differential.

BIOPSY

An incisional or excisional biopsy can be performed depending on the size of the lesion. A smaller cystic lesion can be completely excised, whereas larger lesions require an incisional biopsy to guide final therapy. It is important to aspirate the lesion before incising into the lesion (entering carefully through the cortical bone) to rule out a vascular lesion. The aspiration of bright red blood alerts the surgeon to a high-flow vascular lesion, such as an arteriovenous malformation, which could result in uncontrollable hemorrhage. In such a case, the procedure should be aborted for further radiographic and angiographic studies to characterize the vasculature of the area. The aspiration of straw-colored (or clear) fluid is characteristic of a cystic lesion, whereas the absence of any aspirate may be seen with a solid mass (tumors).

Box 1-2. Differential Diagnosis of Multilocular Radiolucent Lesions

- **Ameloblastoma**—The most common location is the posterior mandible, and its most typical radiographic appearance is that of a multilocular radiolucent lesion. This is the most frequently diagnosed odontogenic tumor.
- **Odontogenic keratocyst**—This lesion cannot be differentiated on clinical and radiographic grounds from an ameloblastoma. OKCs generally do not cause resorption of adjacent teeth. The orthokeratin variant is usually associated with an impacted tooth. OKCs are most common in the second and third decades of life.
- **Dentigerous cyst**—Large dentigerous cysts can have a multilocular appearance on a radiograph given the existence of bone trabeculae within the radiolucency. However, they are histologically a unilocular lesion. There is a high association with impacted mandibular third molars. Painless bony expansion and resorption of adjacent teeth are uncommon but can occur.
- **Ameloblastic fibroma**—Posterior mandible is also the most common site for this lesion. It is predominantly seen in the younger population, and most lesions are diagnosed within the first two decades of life. Large tumors can cause bony expansion. The lesion can manifest as a unilocular or multilocular radiolucent lesion that is often associated with an interrupted tooth. Ameloblastic fibro-odontomas are mixed radiopaque-radiolucent lesions.
- **Central giant cell tumor**—Approximately 70% of these lesions occur in the mandible; most commonly in the anterior region. Its radiographic appearance can be unilocular or multilocular. These lesions can contain large vascular spaces that can lead to substantial intraoperative bleeding. The aneurysmal bone cyst has been suggested to be a variant of the central giant cell tumor. The majority of these lesions are discovered before age 30.
- **Odontogenic myxoma**—Although myxomas are seen in any age group, the majority are discovered in patients between 20 to 40 years of age. The posterior mandible is the most common location, and its radiographic appearance can be unilocular or multilocular. At times, the radiolucent defect may contain thin, wispy trabeculae of residual bone given its "cobweb" or "soap bubble" trabecular pattern.
- **Aneurysmal bone cyst**—Lacking a true epithelial lining, these cysts most commonly occur in long bones or vertebral columns. They rarely occur in the jaws, but when they do, it is mostly in young adults. They can present as a unilocular or multilocular radiolucent lesion with marked cortical expansion that usually displaces but does not resorb teeth.
- **Traumatic bone cyst**—This lesion lacks a true epithelial lining and frequently involves the mandibular molar and premolar region in young adults. They can cause expansion and usually have a well-defined unilocular, scalloping radiolucency between the roots without resorption. The lesion always exists above the inferior alveolar canal.
- **Calcifying epithelial odontogenic tumor (CEOT)**—This is an uncommon tumor. The majority are found in the posterior mandible, mostly in patients aged 30 to 50 years. A multilocular radiolucent defect is seen more often than a unilocular radiolucency. Although it may be entirely radiolucent, calcified structures of varying sizes and density are usually seen within the defect. It can also be associated with an impacted tooth.
- **Lateral periodontal cyst (botryoid odontogenic cyst)**—Usually found in older individuals (fifth to seventh decades of life), the botryoid variant often shows a multilocular appearance. It is most commonly seen in the premolar canine areas.
- **Calcifying odontogenic cyst (COC)**—Most commonly found in the incisor canine region, this cyst is usually diagnosed in patients in the mid 30s. Although the unilocular presentation is most common, multilocular lesions have been reported. Radiopaque structures are usually present in approximately one third to one half of the lesions.
- **Intraosseous mucoepidermoid carcinoma**—This is the most common salivary gland tumor arising centrally within the jaws. Most commonly found in the mandible of middle-aged adults, radiographically they can appear as unilocular or multilocular radiolucent lesions. Association with an impacted tooth has been reported.
- **Hyperparathyroidism (Brown tumor)**—Parathyroid hormone (PTH) is normally produced by the parathyroid gland in response to decreased serum calcium levels. In primary hyperparathyroidism, there is an uncontrolled production of PTH due to hyperplasia or carcinoma of the parathyroid glands. Secondary hyperparathyroidism develops in conditions of low serum calcium levels such as renal disease, resulting in a feedback increase in PTH. Patients with hyperparathyroidism usually present with a classic triad of signs and symptoms described as "stones, bones, and abdominal groans." Patients with primary hyperparathyroidism have a marked tendency to develop renal calculi ("stones"). "Bones" refers to the variety of osseous changes that are seen, including the brown tumor of hyperparathyroidism. These lesions can appear as unilocular or multilocular radiolucent lesions most commonly affecting the mandible, clavicle, ribs, and pelvis. "Abdominal groans" refers to the tendency for the development of duodenal ulcers and associated pain. When dealing with any giant cell lesions, brown tumor of hyperparathyroidism needs to be ruled out by evaluating serum calcium (it is elevated in hyperparathyroidism). These patients will have elevated levels of PTH (confirmed by radioimmunoassay of the circulating parathyroid levels).
- **Cherubism**—In this rare developmental inherited condition, painless bilateral expansion of the posterior mandible produces cherublike facies (plump-cheeked little angels depicted in Renaissance paintings). In addition, involvement of the orbital rims and floor produces the classic "eyes upturned toward heaven." Radiographically, the lesions are usually bilateral multilocular radiolucent lesions. Although rare, unilateral involvement has been reported.
- **Intrabony vascular malformations**—Arteriovenous malformations are most often detected in patients between 10 and 20 years of age and are more commonly found in the mandible. Mobility of teeth, bleeding from the gingival sulks, an audible bruit, or a palpable thrill should alert the clinician. The radiographic appearance is variable but most commonly presents as a multilocular radiolucent lesion. The loculations may be small, giving the honeycomb appearance that produces a "soap bubble" radiographic appearance. Aspiration of all undiagnosed intrabony lesions is warranted to rule out the presence of this lesion, as fatal hemorrhage can occur after an incisional biopsy.

ASSESSMENT

Expansile multilocular radiolucent mass of the posterior right mandible associated with an impacted right mandibular third molar (25% to 40% of cases are associated with an unerupted tooth)

With this patient under intravenous anesthesia, an incisional biopsy was performed after aspiration of straw-colored fluid that showed classic histopathology for the OKC. Histological features include a thin squamous cell epithelial lining (eight cells or fewer). The basal cell layer is well defined and composed of cuboidal or columnar cells. The luminal surface exhibits a wavy or corrugated appearance. The fibrous wall is usually thin with a mixed inflammatory response. Keratinization of the lumen is not a pathognomonic finding. The fibrous wall may contain epithelial islands that show central keratinization and cyst formation; these are known as daughter-satellite cells.

TREATMENT

Controversy exists regarding the optimum treatment for OKC; discussions are centered on whether a conservative or an aggressive approach should be undertaken. Options that have been used include the following:
- Decompression by marsupialization
- Marsupialization followed by enucleation (surgical decompression of the cyst, followed by several months of daily irrigation with chlorhexidine via stents secured in the cystic cavity, followed by cystectomy)
- Enucleation with curettage alone
- Enucleation followed by chemoablation or cryotherapy
- Enucleation with peripheral ostectomy
- Enucleation with peripheral ostectomy and chemoablation or cryotherapy
- En bloc resection or mandibular segmental resection. Resection is advocated only if there have been multiple recurrences after enucleation with curettage or in large OKCs in which enucleation and curettage would result in a near continuity defect.

OKCs do not invade the epineurium; therefore, the inferior alveolar nerve can be separated and preserved. Furthermore, any perforations of the keratinized mucosa should be excised because it may contain additional epithelial rests, which can lead to recurrences. Aggressive soft tissue excision is not required, because OKCs do not usually infiltrate adjacent structures. If the cyst is removed in one unit, there is no need for curettage, unless the lining has been shred or torn. Some controversy exists regarding the optimal management (extraction versus retention) of teeth involved with an OKC. It is generally accepted that an OKC with a scalloped radiographic appearance should have the associated teeth removed because it is considered impossible to completely remove the thin-walled cystic lining. If, however, the OKC is successfully removed in one unit, the teeth may be spared without compromising recurrence. In most instances, there is no need for endodontic therapy despite surgical denerva-tion. The teeth may not become devitalized due to perfusion of the pulp via accessory canals through the periodontal ligaments.

Many surgeons advocate the application of Carnoy's solution after enucleation and curettage with methylene blue. Carnoy's solution is composed of 6 ml of absolute alcohol, 3 ml of chloroform, and 1 ml of 100% acetic acid. Carnoy's solution penetrates the bone to a depth of 1.54 mm after a 5-minute application. It does not fixate the inferior alveolar nerve, but some clinicians cover the nerve with sterile petrolatum as a caution.

The patient was treated under general anesthesia with enucleation of the lesion followed by the application of methylene blue to guide peripheral ostectomy. The patient was placed on a soft diet to reduce the risk of jaw fracture. The postoperative panoramic radiograph confirmed that the inferior border of the mandible remained intact.

The final pathology report confirmed the diagnosis of an OKC consistent with the initial incisional biopsy. He was placed on a strict recall schedule—every 6 months for the first 5 years and then yearly. The recurrence rate for OKC has been reported to range from 5% to 60%. It has been reported that most recurrences occur within 5 years, although they can recur at any time. Recurrences that occur secondary to residual cyst left in bone may be apparent within 18 months of surgery.

COMPLICATIONS

The OKC has been described as having clinical features that include potentially aggressive behavior and a high recurrence rate. Because recurrence is a major concern, clinicians vary in their surgical approach. The primary mechanism for recurrence has been postulated to be the incomplete removal of all the cystic lining or new primary cyst formation from additional activated rests.

OKCs have been reported to undergo transformation into ameloblastoma and squamous cell carcinoma, although this occurrence is rare. Other common postprocedure complications include inferior alveolar nerve paresthesia, postoperative infection, and pathological mandibular fracture in larger lesions (highest risk is at 2 weeks after enucleation).

DISCUSSION

Ever since Shear, Pindborg, and Hansen established the histological features of the OKC, many investigators have recognized that two major variants exist based on microscopic findings: a cyst with a parakeratinized epithelial lining and a cyst with an orthokeratinized epithelial lining.

Crowley and colleagues undertook a comparison of the orthokeratin and parakeratinized variants. In their review, they found that the parakeratinized variant occurred more commonly than the orthokeratinized variant (frequency of 86.2% for the parakeratinized variant compared with 12.2% for the orthokeratinized variant); 1.6% of cysts had both orthokeratin and parakeratin features.

They also found that the parakeratinized variant demonstrated a 42% recurrence rate, compared to only 2.2% for the orthokeratinized variant. In addition, the orthokeratinized variant was more frequently associated with impacted teeth. Given the different clinical behaviors of these two entities, many authors designate them as separate pathological entities. Lesions that have both orthokeratin and parakeratin features should be treated as a parakeratinized OKC.

Stimulation of residual epithelial cells is a common feature in the development of any cyst. In the case of the OKC, the epithelial cells implicated are from the rest of Serres or Malassez or from the reduced enamel epithelium. The epithelial cells proliferate into a gradually enlarging mass. With enlargement, the cells in the center are driven farther from the blood supply and eventually die, creating the lumen. The lumen subsequently becomes hypertonic, creating an osmotic gradient and resulting in an increase in hydrostatic pressure that causes bone resorption and subsequent expansion of the cyst. Additional epithelial cells are sloughed into the lumen as the cyst increases in size, and the cycle continues. The surrounding connective tissue is compressed with continued enlargement. This lining then matures, forming a basement membrane, and also contributes to enlargement of the cyst. If no treatment is rendered during the initial stages, with continual enlargement the cyst will eventually become symptomatic.

Identification of individuals who may be affected with NBCCS allows the clinician to arrange for appropriate referrals. NBCCS should be suspected when multiple lesions exist. Some abnormalities are pertinent only to the diagnosis and do not require any specific therapy. Other abnormalities may pose further risk to the patient and require the input of other specialists. Spina bifida and central nervous system tumors require referral to a neurosurgeon. In addition, genetic counseling for all patients afflicted with NBCCS is recommended. OKCs associated with this syndrome are treated in the same manner as an isolated OKC; however, these lesions have a higher rate of recurrence when associated with NBCCS (which may represent new lesions). OKCs are often associated with the follicle of a potentially functional tooth, and, when possible, marsupialization with orthodontic guidance should be considered.

Bibliography

August M, Caruso PA, Faquin WC: Report of a case: an 18-year-old man with a one-month history of nontender left mandibular swelling, *N Engl J Med* 353:2798-2805, 2005.

August M, Faquin WC, Troulis M, et al: Differentiation of odontogenic keratocysts from nonkeratinizing cysts by use of fine-needle aspiration biopsy and cytokeratin-10 staining, *J Oral Maxillofac Surg* 58:935-940, 2000.

Crowley T, Kaugras GE, Gunsolley JC: Odontogenic keratocysts: a clinical and histologic comparison of the parakeratin and orthokeratin variants, *J Oral Maxillofac Surg* 50:22-26, 1992.

Kolokythas A: OKC: to decompress or not to decompress. A comparative study between decompression and enucleation vs. resection/peripheral ostectomy, *J Oral Maxillofac Surg* 38-39, 2005.

Marx RE, Stern D: *Oral and maxillofacial pathology: A rationale for diagnosis and treatment,* Chicago, 2003, Quintessence.

Pindborg JJ, Hansen J: Studies on odontogenic cyst epithelium. Clinical and roentgenographic aspects of odontogenic keratocysts, *Acta Pathol Microbial Scand* 58:283, 1963.

Pogrel MA, Jordan RC: Marsupialization as a definitive treatment for the odontogenic keratocyst, *J Oral Maxillofac Surg* 62:651-655, 2004.

Pogrel MA, Schmidt BL: The odontogenic keratocyst, *Oral Maxillofacial Surg Clin N Am* 15, 2003.

Shear M: Primordial cysts, *J Dent Assoc S Afr* 152:1, 1960.

Unilocular Radiolucent Lesion of the Mandible (Dentigerous Cyst)

David Verschueren, DMD, MD, and Shahrokh C. Bagheri, DMD, MD

CC

A 28-year-old white man is referred for evaluation of "swelling on my right lower jaw."

Dentigerous Cyst

Dentigerous cyst (DC) has a slight male predilection, it is more common in whites, and it is most frequently seen in the age range of 10 to 30 years.

HPI

Approximately 2 months earlier, the patient noticed a nonpainful swelling of the right posterior mandible; dentigerous cysts can cause expansion but are typically nonpainful unless secondarily infected. The most common location of dentigerous cysts is the mandibular third molar region; other frequently involved teeth include the maxillary canines, maxillary third molars, and mandibular second premolars. He was seen by the referring general dentist who discovered a radiolucent lesion on a periapical radiograph. The patient denies any history of pain to his right lower jaw, fever, purulence, or trismus (inability to open the mouth due to contraction of the muscles of mastication, commonly a sign of inflammatory infiltration of the muscles secondary to infection).

PMHX/PDHX/MEDICATIONS/ALLERGIES/SH/FH

Noncontributory. There is no history of similar presentations in his family (there is no familial predisposition).

EXAMINATION

General. The patient is a well-developed and well-nourished anxious man (patients are often anxious because they fear a malignant process).

Maxillofacial. There is noticeable right lower facial swelling isolated to the lateral border of the mandible not involving the area below the inferior border. The mass is hard, nonfluctuant, and nontender to palpation, consistent with a noninflammatory process. There are no facial or trigeminal nerve deficits (paresthesia of the right inferior alveolar nerve would be indicative of a malignant process).

Neck. The patient does not have palpable masses or cervical or submandibular lymphadenopathy. Positive lymph nodes would be indicative of an infectious or neoplastic etiology, so a careful neck examination is paramount in the evaluation of any head and neck pathology.

Intraoral. The occlusion is stable and reproducible. There does not appear to be displacement of the dentition in the involved area (dentigerous cysts do not typically alter the occlusion). Interincisal opening is within normal limits. There is significant buccal expansion of the right mandible extending from the mental foramen posteriorly and ascending into the ramus (large cysts may be associated with a painless expansion of the bone, but most are asymptomatic and do not cause expansion). The patient does not have a palpable thrill or audible bruit (seen with arteriovenous malformations). The oral mucosa is normal in appearance with no signs of any acute inflammatory processes.

IMAGING

When evaluating large lesions of the mandible, the panoramic radiograph is an excellent initial study for assessment of the bony and dental anatomy. A CT scan is not essential, but it can better delineate the three-dimensional bony and regional architecture, including involvement of the cortices of the mandible (i.e., cortical perforation is seen with some tumors and locally aggressive cysts) and the position of the inferior alveolar canal.

In this patient, a panoramic radiograph (Figure 1-3) demonstrates a 7 × 3-cm well-corticated unilocular radiolucent lesion of the right posterior mandible extending from the area of the mental foramen to midway up the ramus. The right mandibular second molar (tooth No. 31) is displaced inferiorly, and the right mandibular third molar is displaced into the ascending ramus to the level of the mandibular foramen. The roots of the second molar appear to be disrupting the inferior boarder of the mandible. The left maxillary cuspid, left mandibular second and third molar, (teeth Nos. 11, 18, and 17, respectively) are also impacted.

LABS

No laboratory tests are indicated unless dictated by the medical history. If brown tumor of hyperparathyroidism is in the differential diagnosis, serum calcium levels should be obtained. This tumor is derived from primary hyperparathyroidism leading to osseous lesions with abundant hemorrhage and hemosiderin deposition within the tumor (hence giving it a brown color). Removal of the hyperplastic parathyroid tissue is necessary in this condition.

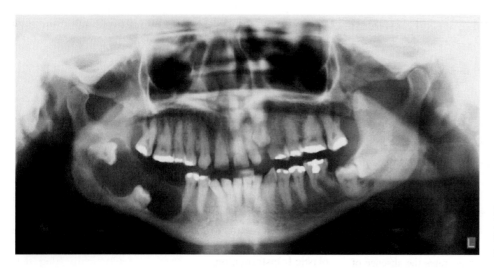

Figure 1-3 Unilocular radiolucent lesion of posterior right mandible with impacted right mandibular second and third molars.

Box 1-3.   **Differential Diagnosis of a Unilocular Radiolucency**

- **Dentigerous cyst**—This cyst is considered first on the differential given the patient's age, location, and radiographic presentation. This cannot be differentiated on clinical and radiographic grounds.
- **Odontogenic keratocyst**—This cyst can grow to a considerable size and must be distinguished from a dentigerous cyst. Frequently, large unilocular lesions that are thought to be dentigerous cysts prove to be OKCs. The orthokeratinizing odontogenic cyst can have a similar presentation.
- **Ameloblastoma**—Given the patient's radiographic presentation, unicystic variant is most likely. Ameloblastomas typically cause a painless bony expansion. This would be the most common noncystic pathology for this radiographic and clinical presentation.
- **Odontogenic myxoma**—Radiographically, this can present as a unilocular or multilocular lesion. Larger lesions tend to be multilocular with a "soap bubble" appearance.
- **Central giant cell granuloma**—This is more common in the anterior mandible. This lesion can be unilocular or multilocular and shows a female predilection.

- **Calcifying epithelial odontogenic tumor (Pindborg)**—This tumor is less likely given the patient's radiographic presentation. It usually has a mixed radiolucent-radiopaque appearance, although early lesions may be entirely radiolucent.
- **Ameloblastic fibroma**—This is an uncommon tumor that is seen usually in younger patients, during the first two decades of life.
- **Adenomatoid odontogenic tumor**—This lesion is most often seen in the anterior maxilla and in younger patients. However, it cannot be ruled out without a biopsy.
- **Arteriovenous aneurysm of bone and other vascular bone tumors**—Clinicians should always consider vascular tumors because of obvious surgical implications. Aspiration before any surgical incision is essential.
- **Carcinoma arising in a dentigerous cyst**—Although this is rare, it is well documented. Radiographically, the borders may be more irregular with ragged edges.
- **Intraosseous mucoepidermoid carcinoma**—This is also a rare condition, but should be ruled out because early diagnosis of malignant neoplasms is essential for improved survival.

DIFFERENTIAL DIAGNOSIS

The differential diagnosis can be divided into lesions of cystic pathogenesis, neoplastic (benign or malignant), and vascular anomalies (least common). Well-defined borders and the lack of a multilocular appearance are more suggestive of a cystic process, but this distinction is not predictable. The differentials found in Box 1-3 should be considered, with the first three being the most likely.

BIOPSY

An incisional biopsy would be indicated to guide final therapy for this lesion. This can be done under local, intravenous sedation or general anesthesia depending on the surgeon's preference and medical indications. It is important to obtain an aspirate of the mass before perforating the bony cortex. Bright red blood would alert the surgeon to a high flow vascular lesion that could result in uncontrollable hemorrhage. In such a case, the procedure should be aborted for further radiographic and angiographic studies to characterize the vasculature of the area. Straw-colored fluid would be characteristic of a cystic lesion, while the absence of any aspirate may be seen with tumors of the jaw.

ASSESSMENT

Expansile radiolucent mass of the posterior mandible associated with impacted right mandibular second and third molars

In this case, under intravenous anesthesia, an incisional biopsy was performed after aspiration (straw-colored fluid)

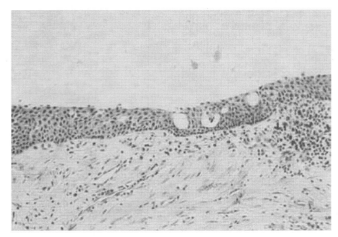

Figure 1-4 Histopathology of a dentigerous cyst with stratified squamous epithelium. This specimen demonstrates the absence of any significant inflammation.

demonstrating classic dentigerous cyst histopathology (epithelial lining of nonkeratinized stratified squamous epithelium and a loosely arranged fibrous connective tissue wall) (Figure 1-4).

TREATMENT

Complete removal of the cyst by enucleation along with removal of the unerupted tooth is the preferred treatment for dentigerous cysts. If eruption of the involved tooth into a functional position is feasible (with or without orthodontic guidance), enucleation of the cyst can be performed without removal of the tooth. The inferior alveolar neurovascular bundle is commonly displaced by the cyst and should be preserved if possible. Large cysts may be treated with marsupialization when enucleation and curettage would likely result in neurosensory dysfunction or a pathological fracture of the mandible. Postoperative maxillomandibular fixation may be prudent to allow remodeling of the bone before function, especially in larger lesions. Marsupialization permits decompression of the lesion and shrinkage of the cyst and bony defect. Definitive removal can be performed at a later date. A disadvantage of marsupialization is the need for greater patient compliance with an open cystic cavity between treatments. In addition, it does not reliably produce a reduction in the size of the cyst.

The patient was taken to the operating room and underwent enucleation and curettage via an intraoral incision. The right mandibular second and third molars were maintained due to the high risk of fracture and inferior alveolar nerve paresthesia—while this may increase the possibility of recurrence, it should be weighted against the possible complications of tooth removal. The patient was placed on a soft diet to reduce the risk of jaw fracture. The postoperative panoramic radiograph confirmed that the inferior border of the mandible remained intact.

The final pathology report confirms the diagnosis of a dentigerous cyst consistent with the initial incisional biopsy specimen.

COMPLICATIONS

Prognosis of a dentigerous cyst with adequate treatment is excellent, and recurrence is rare. The most common complications include postoperative infection, inferior alveolar nerve paresthesia, and mandibular fracture in larger cysts. Neoplastic transformation to an ameloblastoma, squamous cell carcinoma, and mucoepidermoid carcinoma has been reported in less than 2% of cases. For this reason, complete histopathological examination with enucleation may be preferable to marsupialization, which could delay the diagnosis of a neoplastic transformation.

DISCUSSION

A dentigerous cyst originates as a consequence of a build-up of fluid between the dental follicle and the crown of an unerupted tooth. It is the most common type of developmental odontogenic cyst, making up about 20% of all epithelium-lined cysts in the jaws. The pathogenesis is uncertain but is possibly related to the accumulation of fluid between the reduced enamel epithelium and the tooth crown. Dentigerous cysts most commonly involve impacted mandibular third molars but may also involve maxillary canine, maxillary third, and mandibular second molars. This cyst is most commonly discovered between ages 10 and 30 years with a slight male predilection and a higher prevalence for whites than for blacks.

Dentigerous cysts are commonly asymptomatic on presentation but can grow to a significant size, resulting in painless expansion of the bone in the involved area. Large dentigerous cysts can become secondarily infected with associated pain and swelling.

Radiographically dentigerous cysts usually show a unilocular radiolucent area that is associated with an unerupted tooth. A large dentigerous cyst may give the impression of a multilocular process because of the bony trabeculations. However, these cysts are grossly and histopathologically a unilocular process.

Bibliography

Benn A, Altini M: Dentigerous cysts of inflammatory origin: a clinicopathologic study, *Oral Surg Oral Med Oral Pathol Oral Radiol Endod* 81:203-209, 1996.

Curran AE, Damm DD, Drummond JF: Pathologically significant pericoronal lesions in adults: histopathologic evaluation, *J Oral Maxillofac Surg* 60:613-617, 2002.

Smith JL, Kellman RM: Dentigerous cysts presenting as head and neck infections, *Otolaryngol Head Neck Surg* 133:48-49, 2005.

Yasuoka T, Yonemoto K, Kato Y, et al: Squamous cell carcinoma arising in a dentigerous cyst, *J Oral Maxillofac Surg* 58:900-905, 2000.

Multilocular Radiolucent Lesion in the Periapical Region (Ameloblastoma)

Eric P. Holmgren, MS, DMD, MD, and Shahrokh C. Bagheri, DMD, MD

CC

A 34-year-old woman is referred by her general dentist complaining of a painless, swelling in the lower jaw.

Ameloblastoma

Ameloblastomas are usually diagnosed in the third to fourth decade of life, with no gender or racial predilection; however, unicystic variants tend to occur earlier in life.

HPI

For the past 2 months, the patient has noticed a progressively enlarging "hard mass" in her mandible. There have been no neurosensory changes associated with the swelling (sensory changes are particularly common in malignancies and are not usually seen in benign lesions such as ameloblastomas). On consultation, her general dentist noticed a significant buccal and lingual bony expansion adjacent to normal-appearing first and second molars on the right posterior mandible, as well as a multilocular radiolucent lesion on the panoramic radiograph (ameloblastomas occur most frequently in the posterior mandible).

PMHX/PDHX/MEDICATIONS/ALLERGIES/SH/FH

Noncontributory.

EXAMINATION

General. The patient is well developed and well nourished and appears distressed about her possible diagnosis.

    Vital Signs. Vital signs are stable and afebrile.

    Maxillofacial. There is mild right facial enlargement that is most pronounced at the angle of the mandible, with no evidence of trismus. No cervical lymphadenopathy is present. (Ameloblastomas are benign tumors and in general do not cause lymphadenopathy, which may be seen with malignant tumors.) Neurosensory testing reveals normal mandibular nerve (V3) function bilaterally and no other focal neurologic deficits (ameloblastomas generally do not invade the neurovascular bundle).

    Intraoral. There is buccal and lingual expansion of the posterior right mandible with mild tenderness but no evidence of fluctuance or purulent secretions. The mesiobuccal tip of the right mandibular third molar is partially visible. The right mandibular second molar is not mobile; however, there are periodontal pocket depths greater than 10 mm on the distal aspect.

IMAGING

The panoramic radiograph is the initial imaging study of choice for evaluation of a mandibular mass. CT scans are particularly useful to outline the three-dimensional anatomy to demonstrate the amount of expansion and areas of bony perforation. Accurate stereolithographic models can be fabricated from the CT scan and can assist in both the resection and reconstruction of the patient.

In this patient, the panoramic radiograph demonstrates a 5.0×3.5-cm multilocular, cystic-appearing lesion extending from the distal aspect of the impacted right mandibular third molar, involving the entire ramus up to the level of the sigmoid notch. The bone at the inferior border of the mandible has a normal appearance, without loss of continuity (Figure 1-5).

The CT scan shows an expansile lesion of the right posterior mandible with cortical perforation seen on axial and coronal sections at the anterior border of the ramus. There is no evidence of lymphadenopathy and no areas of abnormal enhancement (contrast-enhanced imaging provides improved delineation of soft tissue and can aid in determining any associated vascular malformations).

LABS

Baseline hemoglobin and hematocrit levels should be obtained before major maxillofacial surgical interventions. Other laboratory tests are obtained as dictated by the medical history.

DIFFERENTIAL DIAGNOSIS

The differential diagnosis of a multilocular radiolucent lesion of the posterior mandible is best categorized as lesions of cystic, neoplastic, or vascular origin, with the latter being less common. Although the above presentation is classic for an ameloblastoma (bony expansion of the posterior mandible with a multilocular or "soap bubble" appearance), this lesion cannot be distinguished on clinical and radiographic parameters. A complete differential diagnosis should be considered (see Differential Diagnosis in previous section Multilocular Radiolucent Lesion in the Pericoronal Region [Odontogenic Keratocyst]).

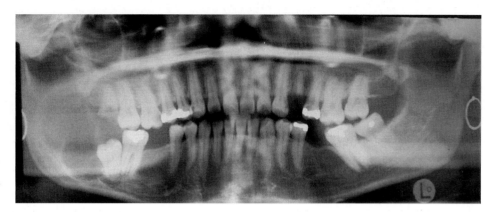

Figure 1-5 Panoramic radiograph demonstrating a multilocular radiolucent lesion of the right posterior mandible.

BIOPSY

For diagnosis of this multilocular and expansile lesion, aspiration followed by an incisional biopsy was performed with local anesthesia and intravenous sedation in the clinic. Needle aspiration was negative for blood or any clear fluids and therefore suggestive of a mass lesion. A typical buccal mucoperiosteal third molar incision was reflected (it is important to make the incision where the definitive surgical incision would ultimately be made in order to minimize dehiscence). No purulence was noted. A cystic lesion with a keratin-like substance was encountered in the large bony concavity. A large sample of the cyst lining was taken from two different locations. The wound was closed with 3-0 chromic interrupted sutures, and a specimen was sent for histopathological examination.

ASSESSMENT

Microscopic evaluation reveals islands of epithelium that resemble enamel organ in a fibrous connective tissue stroma attached to the basement membrane surrounding the islands are tall columnar cells exhibiting reversed polarity

This is consistent with the diagnosis of a multicystic, follicular ameloblastoma.

TREATMENT

The treatment of ameloblastomas has raised some controversy. In general, treatment must focus on the ability of the tumor to invade surrounding bone tissue. The average extension into surrounding bone beyond the normal tumor margin is 4.5 mm with a range of 2 to 8 mm. With this in mind, resection must be at least 10 mm beyond the bony (and radiographic) margin of the tumor for large, multicystic-type ameloblastomas. Resected tumors seldom recur, with a 95% to 98% cure rate for primary tumors compared with a high incidence of recurrence of approximately 70% for treatment of enucleation and curettage alone. Regardless of the reconstructive measure, close patient follow-up is necessary to monitor for recurrence, especially in patients who do not undergo a resection. Because ameloblastomas can recur with a variable time frame, a cure rate for an ameloblastoma does not necessarily correlate with a 5-year disease-free period compared with other neoplastic processes. Long-term follow-up is necessary.

For this patient, given the size and extensive, aggressive nature of the lesion, a segmental reconstruction was undertaken via an intraoral approach. Tumor resection was elected in this case due to the close anatomic proximity of the tumor margin at the inferior boarder, as well as cortical perforation and involvement of mucosa at the anterior border and near the sigmoid notch. Special attention was paid to the site of perforation, in which a supraperiosteal resection was performed, and the overlying mucosa and periosteum were resected with the specimen. The condyle was retained and the ramus and angle were reconstructed using a standard reconstruction plate. The inferior alveolar nerve was dissected free and preserved (ameloblastoma cells do not necessarily penetrate the nerve unless gross involvement of the inferior alveolar canal is noticed, which can theoretically allow the tumor cells to penetrate the perineural tissue).

Other reported treatment alternatives include enucleation, curettage and cryotherapy with or without bone grafting, and excision of tumor with peripheral ostectomy. Marsupialization of unicystic variants have also been reported. These treatments have not been proved to be curative, are not widely advocated, and have a higher recurrence rate compared with resection.

The mandibular defect for this patient was subsequently reconstructed using an iliac crest cancellous bone graft, performed at 4 months (to allow time for soft tissue healing), via an extraoral approach. A segmental resection with an osteotimized vascularized fibula free flap and reconstruction plate is a good alternative, especially with recurrences or large, aggressive tumors.

COMPLICATIONS

Complications associated with resection and reconstruction of this tumor include mandibular nerve anesthesia, graft failure, unacceptable facial symmetry, poor bony height and width for implant reconstruction, and donor site morbidity. Plate exposure, plate fracture, and intraoral dehiscence are possibilities. Recurrence is the most worrisome long-term complication. Recurrence can be due to persistence of the original tumor that was not resected or actual recurrence of new neoplastic cells. Aggressive surgical therapy does not necessarily eliminate the chance of tumor recurrence. All patients require long-term follow-up and imaging studies as needed.

DISCUSSION

There are seven histological types of ameloblastomas: follicular, plexiform, acanthomatous, granular cell, desmoplastic, basal cell, and unicystic variant, with the first two being the most common. Ameloblastomas can be either solid or multicystic, but they frequently demonstrate both characteristics. Although the majority of the tumors originate from within the maxilla or mandible, they can also be peripheral. The different histological variants do not significantly alter treatment considerations except for the unicystic and the peripheral types, which can typically be treated with enucleation and curettage. Unicystic ameloblastomas represent about 10% to 15% of intraosseous ameloblastomas and can be confused for a dentigerous cyst. These lesions commonly occur in younger patients and have three distinct variants (luminal, intraluminal, and mural). Luminal and intraluminal types can typically be treated with enucleation and close observation, whereas mural types should be treated more aggressively. Peripheral ameloblastomas are very uncommon, representing approximately 1% of all ameloblastomas, and are usually successfully treated with local surgical excision due to the nonaggressive behavior. Malignant ameloblastomas are extremely rare and usually metastasized to the lungs (probably from aspiration of oral tumor). The malignant variant has a poor prognosis.

Bibliography

Carlson ER, Marx RE: The ameloblastoma: primary, curative surgical management, *J Oral Maxillofac Surg* 64:484-494, 2006.

Carlson ER, Monteleone K: Analysis of inadvertent perforations of mucosa and skin concurrent with mandibular reconstruction, *J Oral Maxillofac Surg* 62:1103-1107, 2004.

Chapelle K, Stoelinga P, de Wilde P, et al: Rational approach to diagnosis and treatment of ameloblastoma and odontogenic keratocysts, *Br J Oral Maxillofac Surg* 42:381-390. 2004.

Gerzenshtein J, Zhang F, Caplan J, et al: Immediate mandibular reconstruction with microsurgical fibula flap transfer following wide resection for ameloblastoma, *Plast Reconstr Surg* 17:178-182, 2006.

Laskin DM, Giglio JA, Ferrer-Nuin LF: Multilocular lesion in the body of the mandible: clinicopathologic conference, *J Oral Maxillofac Surg* 60:1045-1048, 2002.

Nakamura N, Mitsuyasu T, Higuchi Y, et al: Growth characteristics of ameloblastoma involving the inferior alveolar nerve: a clinical and histopathologic study, *Oral Surg Oral Med Oral Pathol Oral Radiol Endod* 91:557-562, 2001.

Neville BW, Damm DD, Allen CM, et al: *Oral and maxillofacial pathology*, ed 2, New York, 2002, WB Saunders.

Sachs SA: Surgical excision with peripheral ostectomy: a definitive, yet conservative, approach to the surgical management of ameloblastoma, *J Oral Maxillofac Surg* 64:476-483, 2006.

Sampson DE, Pogrel MA: Management of mandibular ameloblastoma: the clinical basis for a treatment algorithm, *J Oral Maxillofac Surg* 57:1074-1077, 1999.

Tung-Yiu W, Jehn-Shyun H, Ching-Hung C: Epineural dissection to preserve the inferior alveolar nerve in excision of an ameloblastoma of mandible: case report, *J Oral Maxillofac Surg* 58:1159-1161, 2000.

Unilocular Radiolucent Lesion in a Periapical Region (Periapical Cyst)

Bruce Anderson, HBSc, DDS, and Shahrokh C. Bagheri, DMD, MD

CC

A 37-year-old woman is referred by her general dentist for evaluation of a periapical radiolucency associated with the right mandibular second bicuspid, which was discovered during a new patient examination.

Periapical Cyst

The periapical cyst (also called radicular or apical periodontal cyst) is the most common jaw cyst. It develops secondary to the inflammatory process associated with a nonvital tooth and is more common after the third decade of life.

HPI

The patient reports having "a cavity for a long time" with subsequent fracture approximately 6 months earlier of a portion of the crown of the right mandibular second bicuspid, which was part of a three-unit bridge. The right mandibular second molar and the right mandibular second bicuspid were treated endodontically 9 years earlier without complications. The patient denies any history of swelling or purulence in the region and is asymptomatic (periapical cysts seldom present with any clinical symptoms, but infected cysts can present with a draining fistula). The patient also denies a history of trauma in the area (periapical cysts are associated with a pulpal necrosis secondary to either caries or trauma).

PMHX/PDHX/MEDICATIONS/ALLERGIES/SH/FH

Noncontributory.

EXAMINATION

Maxillofacial. There is no discernible facial asymmetry or swelling (periapical cysts are rarely associated with any cortical expansion).

Neck. No cervical or submandibular lymphadenopathy can be detected (positive node findings could be indicative of an infectious or a neoplastic process).

Intraoral. The right mandibular second bicuspid is grossly carious and fractured at the gingival margin. There is no gingival swelling or palpation tenderness along the buccal or lingual cortices.

IMAGING

A panoramic radiograph is the initial study of choice for any intraosseous lesion as it provides an excellent overview of the bony anatomy and architecture of the maxilla and mandible and demonstrates the relationship to adjacent anatomic structures. A periapical radiograph can be obtained for small lesions, providing a more detailed outline of the borders and trabecular pattern. More extensive imaging, such as CT scanning, is seldom required for management of a periapical cyst unless the diagnosis is in question.

In this patient, a panoramic radiograph demonstrated a well-circumscribed radiolucent lesion associated with the right mandibular second bicuspid (Figure 1-6). The lesion is approximately 1 cm in diameter (periapical cysts are generally between 0.5 and 1.5 cm in diameter but may enlarge to fill an entire quadrant). There is no associated root resorption (although root resorption is uncommon in association with a periapical cyst, it can be seen, especially with larger cysts).

LABS

No routine laboratory tests are indicated for the work-up of a periapical cyst unless dictated by the medical history.

DIFFERENTIAL DIAGNOSIS

The differential diagnosis of a periapical radiolucent lesion is greatly influenced by the clinical history and vitality of the associated tooth. If the associated tooth is nonvital and there is radiographic evidence of pulpal pathology, a periapical cyst is the most likely diagnosis. However, a diagnosis based on histopathological examination is warranted because tumors, developmental cysts, metastatic disease, and early fibro-osseous lesions may also occur in a periapical location. The differential diagnosis is outlined Box 1-4.

BIOPSY

Biopsy and treatment of small periapical cysts are usually synonymous and excisional in nature and vary depending on the restorative plan of the involved tooth. If extraction is planned, then the cyst can be removed through the extraction socket. If the tooth is to be restored or the lesion is particularly large, then a periapical approach through the buccal cortex can be used.

Box 1-4.   Differential Diagnosis of Periapical Radiolucent Lesions

- **Periapical granuloma**—This lesion is radiographically indistinguishable from a periapical cyst and is treated in the same manner. Differentiation between periapical granulomas and a cyst has no clinical implication and is discussed below.
- **Residual cyst**—This is a lesion that remains following the extraction of a tooth or completion of endodontic treatment. It is radiographically and histologically identical to a periapical cyst.
- **Cemento-osseous dysplasias (early)**—The spectrum of lesions including focal, periapical, and florid cemento-osseous dysplasia can be observed in the periapical region of teeth and are most commonly seen in middle-aged women of African decent. With serial observation, these lesions will progress to mixed radiolucent-radiopaque lesions and eventually to radiopaque lesions. Associated teeth are asymptomatic and vital.
- **Idiopathic bone cavity (simple bone cyst, traumatic bone cyst)**—Most often seen in the body of the mandible of young adults, this lesion lacks an epithelial lining and has a potential for expansion. Radiographically, it is a well-demarcated radiolucent lesion that can scallop between teeth without resorption. Associated teeth are asymptomatic and vital.
- **Lingual salivary gland depressions (Stafne defect)**—This well-circumscribed radiolucent lesion is most commonly seen in the posterior mandible inferior to the mandibular canal of male patients and represents a developmental concavity of the lingual cortex containing normal salivary gland tissue. Teeth near this lesion are, of course, asymptomatic and vital as the radiolucency is in fact superimposed in the periapical location.
- **Other lesions**—Neural lesions (neurilemoma, neurofibroma) could present in a periapical location but are usually associated with the mandibular canal. Other cysts and tumors, including the lateral periodontal cysts, ameloblastomas, odontogenic keratocysts, central giant cell tumors, intraosseous mucoepidermoid carcinomas, and metastatic disease, could present in a periapical location and should be investigated. For these lesions the associated tooth is usually vital unless there is prior endodontic therapy or concomitant pathological processes.

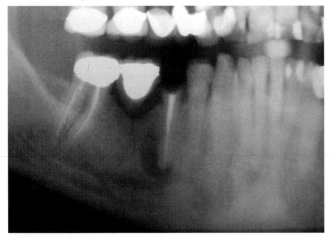

Figure 1-6 Periapical radiolucent lesion associated with endodontic treatment of the right mandibular second bicuspid, seen on a panoramic radiograph.

ASSESSMENT

Distinct periapical radiolucent lesion associated with the carious and nonvital right mandibular first molar

In this case, histopathological examination demonstrated a cystic lining of nonkeratinized stratified squamous epithelium of varying thickness with numerous curved and round hyaline bodies (Rushton bodies). The wall of the cyst showed dense fibrous connective tissue and significant mixed inflammatory infiltrate of lymphocytes, plasma cells, neutrophils, and histocytes. The central lumen was found to contain proteinaceous fluid and necrotic cellular debris. These clinical and histological findings are consistent with a periapical cyst.

TREATMENT

Periapical cysts are treated by enucleation and curettage either through an extraction socket or via a periapical surgical approach in cases where the tooth is restorable or the lesion is greater than 2 cm in diameter. If the tooth is to be preserved, endodontic treatment is necessary, if it has not been done. Some literature supports nonsurgical conservative endodontic treatment of smaller lesions, ensuring the complete removal of causative organisms, and regular radiographic follow-up to evaluate healing and monitor potential lesion enlargement. Excised cysts should always be sent for histological evaluation to rule out other possible pathologies. Recurrence is uncommon.

COMPLICATIONS

There are few complications associated with the treatment of a periapical cyst. Extraction of a tooth without removal of the cyst, or incomplete removal of the cystic lining, can result in a residual cyst. As mentioned previously, residual cysts are histologically identical to periapical cysts and treated with enucleation. Failed conservative endodontic treatment will show a persistent periapical cyst. Endodontic retreatment may be attempted before a curative surgical apicoectomy and enucleation are performed. In cases where both the buccal and lingual cortices are involved, it is possible for the area to heal with fibrous tissue (periapical scar). No treatment is necessary for periapical scars.

Complications associated with surgical removal of the cyst can be related to the regional anatomy. Neurosensory disturbances secondary to injury to the inferior alveolar nerve or branches of the mental nerve can be seen, especially with larger lesions, but these are usually temporary. Postoperative infection can occur with any surgical intervention.

DISCUSSION

The periapical cyst, or radicular cyst, results from inflammatory stimulation of the rests of Malassez within the periodontal ligament. It is relatively common, accounting for a reported 50% of all oral cysts. Its development is preceded by a periapical granuloma that forms at the tooth apex in response to pulpal bacterial infection and necrosis. A periapical granuloma consists of an outer dense fibrous tissue capsule surrounding a central area of granulation tissue. Expansion of the granuloma leads to central ischemic necrosis and development of a central lumen surrounded by an epithelial membrane. The necrotic cellular debris within the lumen creates an osmotic gradient, drawing in fluid and causing enlargement of the cyst and resorption of surrounding bone secondary to hydrostatic pressure.

There is some debate within the literature as to radiographic distinctions between periapical granulomas and cysts, but the general consensus is that they are indistinguishable. There is also a wide range of reported incidences of periapical granulomas versus cysts. The percentage of periapical radiolucent lesions that are attributed to periapical cysts is reported as close to 50%, but studies with strict histological criteria put the incidence of periapical cysts at about 15% with that of periapical granulomas at 50% to 85%. Admittedly, such debate might be considered irrelevant as the eventual treatment and prognosis of both lesions are the same.

Periapical cysts or granulomas are clearly common lesions seen by oral and maxillofacial surgeons. A careful history, clinical and radiographic presentation, and, most important, assessment of vitality of the associated tooth aid in determining the appropriate diagnosis and management of this common pathological lesion.

Bibliography

Gallego Romero D, Torres Lagares D, Garcia Calderon M, et al: Differential diagnosis and therapeutic approach to periapical cysts in daily dental practice, *Med Oral* 7:54-58, 2002.

Mass DR, Bhambhani SM: A clinical and histopathological study of radicular cysts associated with primary molars, *J Oral Pathol Med* 24:458-461, 1995.

Nair PN: New perspectives on radicular cysts: do they heal? *Int Endod J* 31:155-160, 1998.

Philipsen HP, Reichart PA, Ogawa I, et al: The inflammatory paradental cyst: a critical review of 342 cases from the literature survey, including 17 new cases from the author's file, *J Oral Pathol Med* 33:147-155, 2004.

Ramachandran Nair PN, Pajorola G, Schroeder HE: Types and incidence of human periapical lesions obtained with extracted teeth, *Oral Surg Oral Med Oral Pathol Oral Radiol Endod* 81:93-102, 1996.

Regazi JA, Sciubba JJ, Jordan RCK: *Oral pathology: clinical pathologic correlations,* ed 4, Philadelphia, 2003, WB Saunders.

Sanchis JM, Penarrocha M, Bagan JV, et al: Incidence of radicular cysts in a series of 125 chronic periapical lesions. Histopathologic study, *Rev Stomatol Chir Maxillofac* 98:354-358, 1998.

Spatafore CM, Griffin JA Jr, Keyes GG, et al: Periapical biopsy: an analysis of 10-year period, *J Endod* 16:239-241, 1990.

Stockdale CR, Chandler NP: The nature of the periapical lesion—a review of 1108 cases, *J Dent* 16:123-129, 1988.

Trope M, Pettigrew J, Petras J, et al: Differentiation of radicular cyst and granulomas using computerized tomography, *Endod Dent Traumatol* 5:69-72, 1989.

Zaiv RB, Roswati N, Ismail K: Radiographic features of periapical cysts and granulomas, *Singapore Dent J* 14:29-32, 1989.

Mixed Radiolucent-Radiopaque Lesion (Ossifying Fibroma)

Danielle Cunningham, DDS, and Chris Jo, DMD

CC

A 32-year-old woman is referred for the evaluation of a mandibular lesion, stating, "I have a tumor in my lower jaw."

Ossifying Fibroma

Ossifying fibroma most commonly occurs in the third and fourth decades of life and has a reported female predilection as high as 5:1.

HPI

Approximately 3 years earlier, the patient noticed a painless bony expansion of her anterior mandible (ossifying fibroma is much more common in the mandible than in the maxilla and rarely presents with pain or paresthesia). She states that the swelling has been slowly enlarging over the past 3 years and that she was previously scared to seek treatment. Now that the mass is so large and disfiguring she wants treatment (ossifying fibromas that are untreated can become very large). She complains of difficulty talking and chewing due to the size of the mass.

PMHX/PDHX/MEDICATIONS/ALLERGIES/SH/FH

Noncontributory.

EXAMINATION

General. The patient is well developed and well nourished and in no apparent distress.

Maxillofacial. There is an obvious enlargement of the anterior mandible. A firm, bony mass is palpable that extends from first premolar to first premolar. The mass has expanded the buccal and inferior cortices ("downward bowing" is common in large ossifying fibromas of the mandible). Sensory examination of the mental nerve distributions are intact bilaterally (perineural invasion is not seen with ossifying fibroma).

Neck. No lymphadenopathy is noted (cervical lymphadenopathy is not seen in benign neoplastic processes).

Intraoral. There is a significant amount of bony expansion of the buccal and lingual cortices in the anterior mandible, displacing the tongue posteriorly (Figure 1-7). The left and right mandibular lateral and central incisors are displaced and mobile (larger lesions may cause tooth displacement and root divergence, resorption, or both). The overlying attached gingiva and mucosa are normal in appearance (mucosal ulcerations can be a sign of a malignant process; however, traumatic ulcerations can occur within large, expansile benign lesions).

IMAGING

A panoramic radiograph is the initial screening study of choice. It provides an excellent overview of the bony anatomy and architecture of the maxilla and mandible. Osseous lesions are well characterized on a panoramic film, allowing the clinician to make a working differential diagnosis based on the lesion's location, radiodensity, locular or trabecular pattern, border demarcation, size, and effect on adjacent structures (i.e., root resorption, root divergence, scalloping, cortical expansion, cortical erosion, or destruction). CT is not always essential during the work-up or treatment of a mixed radiopaque-radiolucent lesion that is suspected to be benign. However, when there are radiographic signs of a malignant process (e.g., poorly defined radiolucency, mottled or "moth-eaten" appearance, unilateral widening of the periodontal ligament space, floating teeth, cortical perforation, or "spiked roots"), CT of the mandible and neck is required. CT provides additional information (e.g., lingual or buccal cortex thinning or perforation, location of the inferior alveolar canal) and is especially useful when the lesion is difficult to assess on plain films. A three-dimensional stereolithographic model is useful to prebend a reconstruction plate in anticipation for resection.

The radiographic appearance of ossifying fibroma varies depending on the degree of maturity of the lesion. Early ossifying fibromas are radiolucent, and as they mature they become mixed radiolucent-radiopaque and may eventually become predominantly radiopaque. Untreated, these tumors are likely to reach large proportions as they continue to grow. Expansion of the lesion is symmetric and has a spherical or egg-shaped appearance on the CT.

In this patient, the panoramic radiograph reveals a well-defined, expansile, mixed radiolucent-radiopaque mass in the anterior mandible extending from the right premolar to the left molar regions (Figure 1-8). The borders are smooth and well defined. The anterior mandibular teeth show significant displacement and root resorption. A CT scan reveals a large circular, expansile mass in the anterior mandible of a heterogeneous nature with radiopaque areas (of the same density as bone) within the lesion. There are no air- or fluid-filled spaces noted. The mass is well demarcated from surrounding structures. The stereolithographic model reconstructed from the CT illustrates the size of the lesion (Figure 1-9).

LABS

Preoperative baseline hemoglobin and hematocrit levels should be obtained before tumor resection. No other laboratory tests are indicated unless dictated by the medical history.

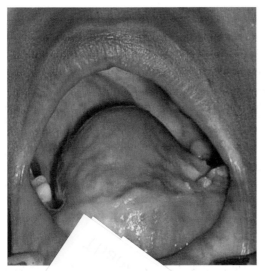

Figure 1-7   ~ving a large, expansile
lesion in the   ~r and superior displacement

DIFFERENTIAL DIAGNOSIS

The differential diagnosis of a mixed radiolucent-radiopaque mass includes odontogenic cyst, odontogenic tumor, osteogenic tumor, or process secondary to infections. Many osseous lesions can change in radiographic characteristics and radiodensity as they mature and progress from a radiolucent to a mixed or radiopaque lesion. The differential diagnosis of a mixed radiolucent-radiopaque lesion can be narrowed when radiographic findings are correlated with clinical findings. Several mixed radiolucent-radiopaque lesions other than an ossifying fibroma are listed in Box 1-5.

BIOPSY

Benign tumors of bone cannot be distinguished on clinical and radiographic information alone and require histological assessment for a definitive diagnosis. In this case, an incisional biopsy would be indicated to guide final therapy. This can be done under local, intravenous sedation or general anesthesia depending on the surgeon's preference and medical indications. In general an ossifying fibroma is well demarcated from the surrounding bone but is not encapsulated. During biopsy, it is imperative to preserve the cortical-lesional relationship.

ASSESSMENT

A large, expansile mixed radiopaque-radiolucent lesion of the mandible

In this case, histopathological examination showed a predominance of proliferative fibrous connective tissue with no

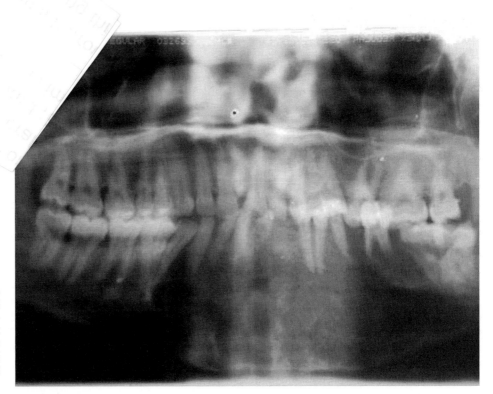

Figure 1-8 Panoramic radiograph showing a large, expansile mixed radiolucent-radiopaque lesion involving the majority of the dentate segment of the mandible. Note that there is significant root divergence, teeth displacement, root resorption, and cortical expansion.

clear capsule (ossifying fibroma can be seen with a capsule). The stroma appears avascular with some regularly shaped blood vessels (ossifying fibroma can have a mixed vascularity). A mild degree of osteoblastic activity and trabeculae of lamellar bone are also noted. Cementum-like deposits are

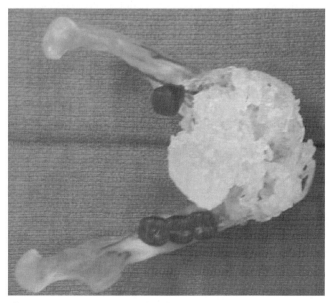

Figure 1-9 Three-dimensional stereolithographic model used to plan the resection and to prebend a reconstruction plate.

present in combination with the lamellar bone. Radiographic, clinical, history, and histopathological findings are consistent with an ossifying fibroma.

TREATMENT

Treatment varies depending on size and clinical appearance. Small tumors may be treated with enucleation and curettage with 1- to 2-mm margins, as long as they have not lost their encapsulation or the margins remain well demarcated from the surrounding bone. However, resection with 5-mm margins is recommended if:

- Tumors have reached a larger size.
- There is loss of the encapsulation (radiographically or clinically).
- Tumor is within 1 cm of the inferior border of the mandible.
- There is involvement of the maxillary sinus or nasal cavities.

If enucleation and curettage is used, the defect can be left open to heal by secondary intent or closed primarily, using resorbable packs to eliminate the dead space. Packing the defect with materials such as iodoform gauze or various bone regeneration preparations to expedite bone regeneration has not been shown to be effective. When bony reconstruction is required, various techniques (immediate or secondary cancellous marrow bone graft or immediate vascularized free

---

Box 1-5.   Mixed Radiolucent-Radiopaque Lesions

- **Fibrous dysplasia**—With higher occurrence in younger patients, this presents with a typical "ground-glass" appearance on radiographs and a "Chinese script writing" appearance on histological examination. It can affect one (monostotic) or more (polyostotic) bones in the body. Monostotic fibrous dysplasia is more common, and the jaws represent the most common site.
- **Cemento-osseous dysplasias (periapical, focal, and florid)**—Occurring in tooth-bearing areas of the jaws, these lesions are the most common type of fibro-osseous lesions. They are categorized into three groups (periapical, focal, and florid) based on clinical and radiographic features. Periapical cemento-osseous dysplasia has a 14:1 female predilection and occur mostly in blacks between the third and fifth decades of life. Focal cemento-osseous dysplasia also has a high female predilection (4:1) but is seen mostly in whites. Florid cemento-osseous dysplasias occur mostly in black women. In each case, early lesions appear radiolucent (fibroblastic proliferation stage), and in later stages, they become mixed and subsequently radiopaque as bone and cementum-like materials are deposited.
- **Paget's disease of bone (osteitis deformans)**—In general, this disease affects older patients (older than 40 years), with a 2:1 male predilection. It is characterized by haphazard and abnormal bone resorption and deposition, causing bony expansion and bone pain (most cases are polyostotic). Radiographically, it appears similar to cemento-osseous dysplasia and is described as having a "cotton-wool"

appearance (which is also seen in Gardner syndrome and gigantiform cementoma).
- **Osteomyelitis, osteoradionecrosis, and bisphosphonate-induced osteonecrosis of the jaws**—These three pathophysiologically distinct entities can have a mixed radiolucent-radiopaque appearance. Please see the respective sections for further details.
- **Osteoblastoma**—These are benign tumors of bone that typically present in second and early third decades of life, causing local expansion. The key feature of this lesion that differentiates it from an ossifying fibroma is the presence of pain. This tumor exhibits slow growth and represents a genetic alteration during osteoblastic differentiation. Radiographically, they are usually well circumscribed and can be treated by local resection with 5-mm margins. Osteoid osteoma and juvenile active ossifying fibroma may be variants of this lesion.
- **Calcifying odontogenic cyst (Gorlin cyst)**—More likely to occur in females than in males (2:1), this cyst initially appears radiolucent but, with maturation, becomes mixed radiolucent-radiopaque. It is generally asymptomatic and may cause expansion as it enlarges. It has a predilection for the maxilla but can occur in the mandible. Histological examination shows "ghost cells."
- **Other**—Adenomatoid odontogenic tumor (or cyst), calcifying epithelial odontogenic tumor, ameloblastic fibro-odontoma, odontoma, and cementoblastoma also present as well-demarcated mixed radiolucent-radiopaque lesions.

flap) can be used, depending on the clinical situation. When cancellous marrow graft is used, secondary bony reconstruction is recommended at least 3 months after the resection to allow for sufficient mucosal healing and tensile strength to prevent mucosal perforation and graft contamination.

In this patient, a partial mandibulectomy with 5-mm margins and immediate stabilization using a prebent reconstruction plate was performed. Immediate bony reconstruction cancellous–marrow bone graft is not recommended in this case because the resection involves a dentate segment that will allow for oral contaminates to penetrate the graft site. Second-stage bony reconstruction was used after 3 months of adequate soft tissue healing. While recurrence is unlikely, the patient should be followed for at least 10 years with serial panoramic radiographs due to the slow-growing nature of this lesion.

COMPLICATIONS

The prognosis of ossifying fibroma with proper treatment is excellent, and recurrence is rare. The potential complications generally are a reflection of the presenting size of the lesion. Smaller lesions can generally be treated by enucleation and curettage, without complications. Larger lesions requiring resection and reconstruction have the potential for more complex complications (wound dehiscence, wound infection, hardware failure, graft failure, facial or trigeminal nerve injury, cosmetic deformity, etc.). In particular, reconstruction of a continuity defect of the anterior mandible is challenging.

DISCUSSION

Ossifying fibroma is a slow-growing, benign lesion of bone most commonly associated with the jaws. There have been occurrences in other bones, most commonly the tibia. Many names have been used to describe this lesion (osteofibroma, fibro-osteoma, cementifying fibroma) secondary to the tumor's cell of origin. Because it is not possible to determine if the cell of origin is cementum or bone, which are both derived from mesenchymal stem cells, it has become an irrelevant point. Therefore the name ossifying fibroma is used.

Multiple studies have shown that it has a predilection for females (70%) between the second and fourth decades of life, with 58%, 23%, and 12% of ossifying fibromas occurring in whites, blacks, and Hispanics, respectively. Ossifying fibromas occur predominantly in the mandible (77%), with a greater propensity for the molar regions, followed by the premolar regions.

Juvenile ossifying fibroma is a variant of the ossifying fibroma discussed in the literature. It is an uncommon lesion of juveniles and adolescents. It is typically more aggressive than an ossifying fibroma and usually affects the paranasal sinuses and bones around the orbit. Frequent clinical features include proptosis or exophthalmos and nasal symptoms. This lesion may require more aggressive treatment, with larger margins than needed for the adult counterpart. However, it has been described that smaller lesions may be treated by enucleation and curettage. Histopathologically, the lesion may contain irregularly mineralized, cellular osteoid strands lined by plump osteoblasts. Juvenile ossifying fibromas have a reported recurrence rate between 38% and 50%.

Bibliography

Abrams AM, Melrose RJ: Fibro-osseous lesion, *J Oral Pathol* 4:158-165, 1975.

Brannon RB, Fowler CB: Benign fibro-osseous lesions: a review of current concepts, *Adv Anat Pathol* 8:126-143, 2001.

Eversole LR: Craniofacial fibrous dysplasia and ossifying fibroma, *Oral Maxillofac Surg Clin North Am* 9:625-642, 1997.

Eversole LR, Leider AS, Nelson K: Ossifying fibroma: a clinicopathologic study of sixty-four cases, *Oral Surg Oral Med Oral Pathol* 60:505-511, 1985.

Eversole LR, Merrell PW, Strub D: Radiographic characteristics of central ossifying fibroma, *Oral Surg Oral Med Oral Pathol* 59:522-527, 1985.

Eversole LR, Sabes WR, Rovin S: Fibrous dysplasia: a nosologic problem in the diagnosis of fibro-osseous lesions of the jaws, *J Oral Pathol* 1:189-220, 1972.

Fechner RE: Problematic lesions of the craniofacial bones, *Am J Surg Pathol* 13(suppl 1):17-30, 1989.

Kramer IRH, Pindborg JJ, Shear M, eds: Histological typing of odontogenic tumors. In *WHO international histological classification of tumors*, ed 2, Geneva, 1992, WHO, pp 27-29.

Marx RE, Stern D: *Oral and maxillofacial pathology: a rationale for diagnosis and treatment*, Chicago, 2003, Quintessence.

Said Al, Surwillo E: Florid osseous dysplasia of the mandible: report of a case, *Compendium* 20:1017-1030, 1999.

Sciubba JJ, Younai F: Ossifying fibroma of the mandible and maxilla: review of 18 cases, *J Oral Pathol Med* 18:315-321, 1989.

Sissons HA, Steiner GC, Dorfman HD: Calcified spherules in fibro-osseous lesions of bone, *Arch Pathol Lab Med* 117:284-290, 1993.

Su L, Weathers D, Waldron CA: Distinguishing features of focal cemento-osseous dysplasia and cemento-ossifying fibromas, II. A clinical and radiologic spectrum of 316 cases, *Oral Surg Oral Med Oral Pathol Oral Radiol Endod* 84:540-549, 1997.

Su L, Weathers SD, Waldron CA: Distinguishing features of focal cemento-osseous dysplasias and cemento-ossifying fibromas, I. A pathologic spectrum of 316 cases, *Oral Surg Oral Med Oral Pathol Oral Radiol Endod* 84:301-309, 1997.

Summerlin D, Tomich C: Focal cemento-osseous dysplasia: a clinicopathologic study of 221 cases, *Oral Surg Oral Med Oral Pathol* 78:611-620, 1994.

Waldron C: Fibro-osseous lesions of the jaws, *J Oral Maxillofac Surg* 51:828-835, 1993.

Waldron C, Giansanti J: Benign fibro-osseous lesions of the jaws: a clinical-radiologic-histologic review of sixty-five cases. Part II. Benign fibro-osseous lesions of periodontal ligament origin, *Oral Surg Oral Med Oral Pathol* 35:340-350, 1973.

Wenig B: *Atlas of head and neck pathology*, Philadelphia, 1993, WB Saunders.

2 Pharmacology

Shahrokh C. Bagheri, DMD, MD

This chapter addresses:
- Penicillin Allergy/Anaphylaxis
- Antibiotic-Associated Colitis
- Drug-Seeking Behavior
- Acute Acetaminophen Toxicity
- Opioid Side Effects
- Bisphosphonate-Related Osteonecrosis of the Jaws

The use of pharmacotherapy is an important primary or adjunctive modality of treatment in the management of the surgical patient. Antibiotics, anesthetics, and analgesics are the most commonly used medications in oral and maxillofacial surgery. Despite appropriate use of medications, side effects and complications are observed. In this chapter, we present six cases associated with the use of mediations encountered in surgery, along with discussion of related topics. A case representing the oral surgical complications associated with the use of the bisphosphonate category of medications is also presented. Cases directly related to anesthesia and anticoagulation therapy are presented separately in the anesthesia and medicine chapters, respectively. The undesired effects of medications may be the result of a single factor or a combination of factors related to the drug:

- Immunologically mediated reactions ranging from mild cutaneous manifestations to life-threatening anaphylaxis reactions

- Unwanted systemic or local (side) effects (e.g., antibiotic-associated colitis [AAC] or bisphosphonate-induced osteonecrosis of the jaws)
- Inappropriate dosing (e.g., acetaminophen overdose)
- Abuse or addictive potential leading to physiological or social complications (e.g., opioid abuse or addiction)
- Compromised or deficient metabolism and elimination capabilities of the patient, leading to toxicities (e.g., renal or hepatic failure)
- Failure of the drug to treat the intended condition, leading to exacerbation of the disease process (e.g., antibiotic resistance)
- Patient noncompliance, compromising treatment (e.g., concomitant alcohol ingestion with opioid or benzodiazepine use).

Penicillin Allergy/Anaphylaxis

Piyushkumar P. Patel, DDS, and Shahrokh C. Bagheri, DMD, MD

CC

A 21-year-old woman admitted for treatment of an open mandible body fracture complains of the sudden appearance of a rash and shortness of breath after receiving her intravenous antibiotics (anaphylaxis is more common with parenteral administration of medications).

HPI

The patient was admitted that day with a diagnosis of an open right mandibular body fracture secondary to assault. The patient did not report any known drug allergies (most frequently, patients do not have a previous history), and the admitting surgeon ordered intravenous penicillin G, morphine sulfate, and nothing-by-mouth (NPO) status in preparation for surgical treatment in the operating room. Upon arrival of the patient on the hospital ward, the nursing staff administered the first dose of intravenous aqueous penicillin G. Approximately 5 to 10 minutes later, the patient developed multiple circumscribed erythematous and raised pruritic wheals of her skin (symptoms generally develop within 5 to 60 minutes after exposure. Earlier onset is seen after parenteral introduction of the allergen). The patient also reported feeling short of breath and the onset of wheezing (secondary to bronchospasm), nausea, and cramping abdominal pain.

PMHX/PDHX/MEDICATIONS/ALLERGIES/SH/FH

The patient reports no known drug allergies. She has no history of food, environmental, or seasonal allergies (race, sex, personal or family history of atopic disease, and allergy to other drugs do not appear to be predisposing factors for penicillin allergy).

Anaphylaxis involves prior sensitization to an allergen with later reexposure, producing symptoms via an immunological mechanism. An anaphylactoid reaction produces a very similar clinical syndrome but is not immune mediated. Treatment for both conditions is similar.

EXAMINATION

General. The patient is a well-developed, well-nourished woman in moderate distress who is sitting up and leaning forward in bed.

Vital signs. Her blood pressure is 98/60 mm Hg (hypotension), heart rate 128 bpm (tachycardia), respirations 28 per minute (tachypnea), temperature 36.7°C and SaO_2 100% on 2 L of nasal cannula.

Neurological. Glasgow Coma Scale score is 15; she is alert and oriented ×3 (place, time, and person).

Maxillofacial. Examination is consistent with a mandibular body fracture.

Cardiovascular. She is tachycardic at 128 bpm. Heart is regular rate and rhythm with no murmurs, gallops, or rubs.

Pulmonary. She has bilateral wheezing. (Histamine activates H_1 and H_2 receptors. Pruritus, rhinorrhea, tachycardia, and bronchospasm are caused by activation of the H_1 receptors, whereas both H_1 and H_2 receptors mediate headache, flushing, and hypotension. Serum histamine levels correlate with the severity and persistence of cardiopulmonary manifestations.)

Abdominal. The abdomen is soft, tender to palpation (secondary to spasm of intestinal smooth muscles), and nondistended with no rebound tenderness and normal bowel sound.

Skin. The patient has urticaria (commonly known as hives, urticaria consists of circumscribed areas of raised erythema and edema of the superficial dermis).

The clinical presentation of anaphylaxis is variable and may include any combination of common signs and symptoms. Cutaneous manifestations, including urticaria and angioedema, are the most common. The respiratory system is also commonly involved, producing symptoms such as dyspnea, wheezing, and upper airway obstruction. Cardiovascular (syncope, hypotension), neurological (dizziness), and gastrointestinal (nausea, vomiting, diarrhea, and abdominal pain) manifestations affect about one third of the individuals. Headaches, rhinitis, substernal pain, pruritus without rash, and seizure occur less frequently.

IMAGING

In the acute phase of anaphylaxis, no imaging studies are indicated (any unnecessary delay may compromise other life-saving interventions). A chest radiograph and/or other studies may be indicated after the initial phase, for evaluation of possible cardiopulmonary complications.

LABS

During an acute anaphylactic episode, no laboratory tests are indicated. However, once the patient is stabilized (or if the diagnosis is in question), in addition to a complete blood cell count (CBC) and comprehensive metabolic panel (CMP), the following tests can be obtained:

Plasma histamine level. This is elevated within 5 to 10 minutes after the onset but remains elevated for only 30 to 60 minutes (histamine is released secondary to IgE-mediated mast cell degranulation).

Urinary *N*-methyl histamine. A metabolite of histamine, *N*-methyl histamine remains elevated for several hours. A 24-hour urine sample for *N*-methyl histamine may be useful.

Serum tryptase. Peaks 60 to 90 minutes after the onset of anaphylaxis and remains elevated for up to 5 hours. Tryptase is a protease specific to mast cells. It is the only protein that is concentrated selectively in the secretory granules of human mast cells.

ASSESSMENT

Acute-onset anaphylactic reaction induced by intravenously administered penicillin G

Box 2-1 outlines the differential diagnosis of anaphylactic shock.

TREATMENT

The initial management of anaphylaxis is a focused examination, involving discontinuation of the suspected medication, establishment of a stable airway (intubation if necessary), venous access (preferably two large-bore [16-gauge] peripheral intravenous catheters), and administration of epinephrine. Vital signs and the level of consciousness should also be monitored.

Immediately upon diagnosis, 0.3 to 0.5 ml of 1:1,000 epinephrine (0.3 to 0.5 mg in adults and 0.01 mg/kg in children) should be injected subcutaneously or intramuscularly, usually into the upper arm. The site can be massaged to facilitate absorption. This dose may be repeated every 10 to 15 minutes up to a total of three doses.

Patients with severe upper airway edema, bronchospasm, or significant hypotension should receive 0.5 to 1 ml of 1:10,000 epinephrine intravenously at 5- to 10-minute intervals. Alternatively, a continuous infusion of 1 to 10 µg/min epinephrine (titrated to effect) may be administered. Those receiving intravenous epinephrine require continuous cardiac monitoring because of the potential for arrhythmias and ischemia. If intravenous access cannot be established, the epinephrine can be administered via an endotracheal tube (3 to 5 ml of 1:10,000 epinephrine).

The patient should be placed in supine or Trendelenburg position. Supplemental oxygen may be administered. Persistent respiratory distress or wheezing requires additional measures. Nebulized albuterol (β_2-agonist) may be administered, and intravenous aminophylline (bronchodilator) can be considered, although its effectiveness for anaphylaxis is questionable. Large volumes of fluids may be required to treat hypotension caused by increased vascular permeability and vasodilatation. Any patients with evidence of intravascular volume depletion (e.g., hypotension, low urine output) should receive volume replacement. Additional pressors such as dopamine (5 to 20 µg/kg/min), norepinephrine (0.5 to 30 µg/kg/min), or phenylephrine (30 to 180 µg/kg/min) may be required. Antihistamines can provide dramatic relief and should be given to all patients with anaphylaxis. A combination of H_1 and H_2 blockers is superior to either agent alone. Thus, diphenhydramine (H_1-receptor blocker) 25 to 50 mg intravenously/intramuscularly every 4 to 6 hours can be used with cimetidine (H_2-receptor antagonist) 300 mg intravenously every 8 to 12 hours. Alternatively, ranitidine (H_2-receptor antagonist) 1 mg/kg intravenously can be used. Most authorities also advocate the administration of corticosteroids; their benefit is not realized for 6 to 12 hours after administration but they are probably helpful in the prevention of late-phase reactions.

Patients currently taking β-blockers pose a challenge, as they may limit the effectiveness of epinephrine. These patients may develop resistant hypotension, bradycardia, and a prolonged course. Atropine (anticholinergic) may be given for bradycardia. Some clinicians recommend administering glucagon. Glucagon exerts a positive inotropic and chronotropic effect on the heart independent of catecholamines. A 1-mg intravenous bolus followed by 1 to 5 mg every hour may improve hypotension in 1 to 5 minutes with maximal benefit at 5 to 15 minutes. All patients with anaphylaxis should be monitored for the possibility of recurrent symptoms despite initial resolution.

In the current patient, penicillin was immediately discontinued, and 0.3 mg of 1:1000 epinephrine was injected intramuscularly into her right deltoid muscle. As her airway was grossly patent, an albuterol nebulizer was ordered. Two 16-gauge peripheral intravenous lines were started at each antecubital fossa, and a bolus of normal saline was given. The patient also received the following medications intravenously: 50 mg of diphenhydramine, 300 mg of cimetidine, and 100 mg of hydrocortisone. The vital signs were continuously monitored. An additional 0.3 mg of 1:1000 epinephrine intramuscularly was given after 12 minutes. She remained stable and marked improvement was noted. She was subsequently transferred to the intensive care unit (ICU) for observation. After an uneventful overnight stay in the ICU, she was subsequently taken to the operating room the next day, where she underwent open reduction with internal fixation (ORIF) of her mandibular fracture. Upon discharge, she was thoroughly informed of her allergy and was provided with a medical alert bracelet.

COMPLICATIONS

Complications of anaphylaxis range from full recovery to anoxic brain injury and death despite adequate response and treatment. The rapidity of onset of symptoms makes this uncommon condition difficult to treat. Early recognition and treatment are essential. It is estimated that anaphylaxis causes approximately 500 to 1000 fatalities per year in the United States. Between 5% and 20% of patients experience biphasic anaphylaxis with a recurrence of symptoms 1 to 8 hours after the onset due to a late-phase reaction or protracted anaphy-

Box 2-1. Differential Diagnosis of Anaphylactic Shock

- **Other forms of shock**—Hemorrhagic/hypovolemic, cardiogenic, septic
- **Flush syndromes**—Carcinoid, postmenopausal hot flashes, red man syndrome (vancomycin), oral hypoglycemic agents with alcohol, medullary carcinoma of the thyroid, idiopathic
- **Excess endogenous production of histamine**—Systemic mastocytosis, basophilic leukemia, hydatid cyst
- **Respiratory distress**—Asthma/chronic pulmonary obstructive disease exacerbation, foreign body aspiration, vocal cord dysfunction, pulmonary embolism.
- **Nonorganic diseases**—Panic attacks, globus hystericus, Munchausen's stridor
- **Other conditions**—Ingestion of sulfites or mono sodium glutamate, hereditary angioedema, neurological (stroke or seizure), drug overdose

Box 2-2. Taking a Detailed History When Faced with a Penicillin-Allergic Patient

Taking a History of Penicillin Allergy: What to Ask

What was the patient's age at the time of the reaction?
Does the patient recall the reaction? If not, who informed them of it?
How long after beginning penicillin did the reaction begin?
What were the characteristics of the reaction?
What was the route of administration?
Why was the patient taking penicillin?
What other medications was the patient taking? Why and when were they prescribed?
What happened when the penicillin was discontinued?
Has the patient taken antibiotics similar to penicillin (for example, amoxicillin, ampicillin, cephalosporins) before or after the reaction? If yes, what was the result?

From Salkind AR, Cuddy PG, Foxworth JW: The rational clinical examination. Is this patient allergic to penicillin? An evidence-based analysis of the likelihood of penicillin allergy, *JAMA* 285:2498-2505, 2001.

laxis with persistence of symptoms for up to 48 hours despite therapy. Death most commonly results from intractable bronchospasm, asphyxiation from upper airway edema, or cardiovascular collapse.

DISCUSSION

The proportion of the population who report a history of penicillin allergy in the United States has been estimated to range from 0.7% to 10%. It has also been recognized that 80% to 90% of patients who report a penicillin allergy are not truly allergic to the drug. Of significance is that many people are falsely labeled as being penicillin allergic.

Most clinicians simply accept a diagnosis of penicillin allergy without obtaining a detailed history of the reaction. In their review, Salkind and colleagues stress the importance of a thorough history when faced with a penicillin allergic patient (Box 2-2). Penicillin is the most common cause of drug-induced anaphylaxis. It causes an estimated 75% of all anaphylactic deaths in the United States.

Allergic drug reactions are one type of adverse drug reaction (ADR). An ADR has been defined by the World Health Organization as any noxious, unintended, and undesired effect of a drug that occurs at doses used for prevention, diagnosis, or treatment. Although it has been difficult to determine the frequency of drug-induced allergic reactions specifically, it is known that they account for only a small proportion of ADRs.

An allergic drug reaction can be classified as immediate, accelerated, or late. Immediate reactions such as anaphylaxis occur within 1 hour of receiving the drug. Accelerated reactions occur 1 to 72 hours after receiving the drug and include urticaria and maculopapular rashes. Late reactions occur after 72 hours, and manifestations can range from a rash during treatment with amoxicillin to severe life-threatening conditions such as Stevens-Johnson syndrome and toxic epidermal necrolysis (TEN). Although rare, certain β-lactams can cause interstitial nephritis, hepatitis, or a vasculitis with or without signs of serum sickness. Allergic reactions can also be classified by the immune mechanism involved as described by Gell and Coombs. In this classification, type I represents an IgE-mediated response, whereas types II, III, and IV are non–IgE dependent. Type II, III, and IV reactions are classified as late reactions because they generally occur 72 hours after drug administration.

The clinical syndrome of anaphylaxis results from activation and release of mediators from mast cells and basophils (e.g., histamine). The cross-linking of mast cell–bound IgE with antigens causes the release of these mediators, with manifestations that include increases in vascular permeability (causing edema), vasodilatation (causing hypotension), respiratory smooth muscle contraction (causing bronchospasm), stimulation of the autonomic nervous system (causing tachycardia), mucus secretion, platelet aggregation, and recruitment of inflammatory cells.

Anaphylactic reactions are more common and severe when the antigen is administered parenterally compared with orally. However, it is possible (although rare) to develop anaphylaxis from airborne exposure or with contact (such as contact with latex). Certain foods may cause an anaphylactic reaction; the most common foods implicated are eggs, peanuts, cow's milk, mustard, and shellfish. Allergic reactions to food occur more frequently in children, and the incidence of anaphylaxis to most antigens is similar for males and females, although females appear to be at a greater risk for anaphylactic reactions to aspirin, latex, and neuromuscular blockers. It has been postulated that women are more sensitive to neuromuscular blockers because commercial cosmetic products often contain quaternary ammonium ions that are also found in these agents. The clinical presentation of anaphylaxis varies widely; however, cutaneous manifestations, including urticaria and angioedema, are the most common. Adult patients are more prone to anaphylactic reactions due to β-lactams.

For patients who by history appear to have an IgE-mediated response, skin testing to confirm allergy is useful if there is a compelling reason to use penicillin. Penicillin skin testing is performed by three classic methods: prick, intradermal, and patch. Skin testing itself carries a risk of fatal anaphylaxis, and the facility must be prepared to respond should a reaction occur.

Patients who are allergic to penicillin and in whom the administration of a penicillin antibiotic is very desirable or even essential can be managed by desensitizing the patient to penicillin. Desensitization is accomplished by administering increasing doses of penicillin over a period of 3 to 5 hours. The mechanism whereby clinical tolerance is achieved is not entirely clear. The most likely hypothesis is that desensitization works by making mast cells unresponsive to the specific antigen. The desensitization procedure should be undertaken in an ICU setting, where continual monitoring is available. Also, the clinician must be at the bedside or readily available.

It has been shown that desensitization is an acceptable safe approach to therapy in patients who are penicillin allergic but require β-lactams for treatment. Oral desensitization is safer than parenteral desensitization. There are no specific contraindications to desensitization. However, patients who are unable to withstand the consequences of an acute allergic reaction and its management are poor candidates.

Bibliography

Gell POH, Coombe RRA: The classification of allergic mediated underlying disease. In *Clincal Aspects of Immunology* (Coombe RRA and Gell POH, editors), Blackwell Science, 1968.

Gomez MB, Torres MJ, Mayorga C, et al: Immediate allergic reactions to beta lactams: facts and controversies, *Curr Opin Allergy Clin Immunol* 4:261, 2004.

Gruchalla R: Drug allergy, *J Allergy Clin Immunol* 111:548, 2003.

Miller EL: The penicillins: a review and update, *J Midwifery Wom Health* 47:426, 2002.

Park MA, Li JT: Diagnosis and management of penicillin allergy, *Mayo Clin Proc* 80:405, 2005.

Riedl M, Casalias A: Adverse drug reactions: types and treatment options, *Am Fam Phys* 68:1781, 2003.

Romano A, Blanca M, Torres MJ, et al: Diagnosis of nonimmediate reactions to β-lactam antibiotics, *Allergy* 59:1153, 2004.

Salkind AR, Cuddy PG, Foxworth JW: Is this patient allergic to penicillin? An evidence based analysis of the likelihood of penicillin allergy, *JAMA* 285:2498, 2001.

Tang AW: A practical guide to anaphylaxis, *Am Fam Phys* 68:1325, 2003.

Torres MJ, Blanca M, Fernandez J, et al: Diagnosis of immediate allergic reactions to beta-lactam antibiotics, *Allergy* 58:961, 2003.

Wendel GD, et al: Penicillin allergy and desensitization in serious infections during pregnancy, *N Engl J Med* 312:1229, 1985.

Antibiotic-Associated Colitis

Piyushkumar P. Patel, DDS, and Shahrokh C. Bagheri, DMD, MD

CC

A 65-year-old man status post incision and drainage (I & D) of a severe facial infection who was previously admitted to the hospital for treatment of his odontogenic infection complains of the new onset of severe "watery diarrhea."

HPI

The patient was admitted 6 days earlier and was taken to the operating room on that day, where I & D of his right submandibular/medial masticator and submental spaces, with extraction of a grossly carious right mandibular first molar, was performed. He remained intubated for 3 days and was maintained on intravenous clindamycin (900 mg every 8 hours). A previously placed nasogastric tube was also removed. The patient continued to do well and was transferred to the ward from the ICU on the fourth postoperative day with continuation of intravenous clindamycin therapy.

On hospital day 6, the patient reported lower abdominal pain and cramping of over 12 hours' duration. He also reported experiencing nausea, malaise, fever, and chills. He had several episodes of profuse watery diarrhea, which was documented by the nursing staff. There was no evidence of blood in his stool, but he has had minimal oral intake since the symptoms began.

PMHX/PDHX/MEDICATIONS/ALLERGIES/SH/FH

Allergies. The patient has a penicillin allergy (history of rash).

Current medications. He is receiving clindamycin 900 mg intravenously every 8 hours and morphine sulfate 2 mg every 4 hours as needed for pain.

EXAMINATION

General. The patient is an obese man in mild distress who is resting in bed.

Vital signs. His blood pressure is 110/68 mm Hg, heart rate 118 (tachycardia secondary to elevated temperature and gastrointestinal fluid losses), respirations 18 per minute, and temperature 38.8°C (fever secondary to release of inflammatory mediators in the gastrointestinal tract).

Maxillofacial. With decreasing facial edema, drains in the submandibular and submental space are nonproductive and are pending for removal.

Abdominal. His abdomen is soft, nontender, and nondistended with hyperactive bowel sounds in all four quadrants. There is no guarding or rebound tenderness (signs of peritonitis).

IMAGING

Plain radiographic imaging studies of the abdomen (such as kidney-ureter-bladder [KUB]) can be used to assist in the diagnosis of *Clostridium difficile*–associated diarrhea. Plain radiographs may reveal a dilated colon suggestive of ileus. Diffusely thickened or edematous colonic mucosa are often better visualized on an abdominal computed tomography (CT) scan. Thickening can sometimes be seen on abdominal plain films.

Colonoscopy or sigmoidoscopy is a more invasive diagnostic modality that is reserved for situations where rapid diagnosis is necessary or when stool samples cannot be obtained secondary to ileus. The finding of pseudomembranes is pathognomonic for *C. difficile* colitis. Due to the increased risk for intestinal perforation, endoscopy should be used sparingly in patients with suspected *C. difficile*–associated diarrhea.

As this patient is relatively stable, abdominal imaging and/or endoscopy is not indicated.

LABS

A basic metabolic panel (BMP) demonstrated an elevated sodium at 148 mEq/L and an elevated BUN and creatinine secondary to dehydration. Serial CBCs demonstrate elevation of the white blood cell (WBC) count from 12,000 to 20,000 cells/μl, with bandemia.

The patient's stool guaiac test was negative for blood. Enzyme-linked immunosorbent assay (ELISA) for *C. difficile* toxin was positive.

The gold standard for the diagnosis of *C. difficile*–mediated disease is a cytotoxin assay. Although this test is highly sensitive and specific, it is difficult to perform, and results are not available for 24 to 48 hours. In addition, it requires centers to be equipped with tissue culture capabilities. ELISA can be used to detect *C. difficile* toxin (A and/or B) in stool. This test has a sensitivity of 63% to 99% and a specificity of 93% to 100%. ELISA is rapid to perform (2 to 6 hours) and is the laboratory test most frequently used to diagnose *C. difficile* infection. Due to the wide range of specificity of this test, approximately 5% to 20% of patients will require more than one stool assay to detect the toxin (therefore most clinicians send two or three samples) (Box 2-3).

Box 2-3.	Additional Stool Laboratory Findings

- **Fecal leukocytes:** This test can be useful for distinguishing inflammatory diarrhea (bacterial colitis or inflammatory bowel disease) from noninflammatory causes (viral colitis, irrit-able bowel disease). Present in 50% to 60% of patients with *C. difficile*–associated diarrhea (not specific).
- **Occult blood:** Can be positive in some cases of *C. difficile*–associated diarrhea (not specific).
- **Fecal lactoferrin:** Lactoferrin is a marker for fecal leukocytes, and its measurement is more precise than fecal leukocyte testing. Like fecal leukocyte determination, fecal lactoferrin is not of value in patients who develop diarrhea while hospitalized, in whom testing for *C. difficile* is more likely to be helpful.
- **Stool cultures:** Most infectious causes of acute diarrhea are self-limiting. Subsequently, a consensus has not been reached on the optimal strategies for obtaining stool cultures, especially in the setting of acute diarrhea, as the necessity of documenting a pathogen is not always essential. A routine stool culture will identify *Salmonella, Campylobacter,* and *Shigella,* the three most common causes of bacterial diarrhea in the United States. When other pathogens are suspected, the laboratory needs to be notified.
- **Stool ova and parasites:** The infrequency of positive stool ova and parasites makes this test not cost effective. Indications for this test include persistent diarrhea, a community waterborne outbreak, bloody diarrhea with few or no fecal leukocytes (associated with amebiasis), and AIDS.

The average range for peripheral WBCs in patients with *C. difficile*–associated diarrhea is between 12,000 and 20,000 cells/μl, but occasionally the count is higher. An important indicator of impending fulminant colitis is a sudden rise in peripheral WBCs to between 30,000 and 50,000 cells/μl. Because progression to shock can occur even in patients who have had benign symptoms for weeks, early warning signs such as the leukocytosis can be invaluable.

ASSESSMENT

Resolving odontogenic infection now complicated by C. difficile–associated diarrhea

TREATMENT

In otherwise healthy adults, the first step is to discontinue the precipitating antibiotic and to administer fluids and electrolytes to maintain hydration. With this conservative therapy, diarrhea can be expected to resolve in 15% to 23% of patients. Specific pharmacotherapy for *C. difficile*–associated diarrhea should be initiated in older patients, patients with multiple medical problems, and patients in whom antibiotics need to be continued. Specific treatment also should be initiated if diarrhea persists despite discontinuation of the precipitating antibiotic or if there is evidence of colitis (i.e., fever, leukocytosis, characteristic findings of colitis on CT scanning or endoscopy). The use of opiates and antidiarrheal medications

should be avoided or minimized because decreased intestinal motility can exacerbate toxin-mediated disease.

For persisting symptoms, first-line therapy consists of metronidazole 500 mg orally three times daily for 10 to 14 days. Vancomycin is also an effective treatment, with a response rate of greater than 90%. If the patient is pregnant or does not respond or tolerate metronidazole, then vancomycin should be initiated at 125 to 500 mg orally four times daily for 10 to 14 days. Metronidazole is selected first because of its lower cost and to avoid the development of vancomycin-resistant enterococci (VRE). Response to therapy can be assessed by the resolution of fever, usually within the first 2 days. Diarrhea should resolve within 2 to 4 days; however, treatment is continued for 10 to 14 days. Therapeutic failure is not determined until treatment has been given for at least 5 days. The best treatment is prevention. This includes the judicious use of antibiotics, hand washing between patient contacts, rapid detection of *C. difficile* by immunoassays for toxins A and B, and isolation of patients who have *C. difficile*–associated diarrhea.

In the above case the patient was placed on contact precautions. Current guidelines from the Centers for Disease Control and Prevention (CDC) indicated that patients should be placed under contact precautions and in isolation until diarrhea has resolved. He was given a bolus of normal saline (NS) and started on maintenance fluids of D5½NS at 110 ml/hr. Clindamycin was discontinued and he was started on metronidazole 500 mg orally three times daily. His diarrhea resolved in 2 days and he was subsequently discharged. He was given non-opiate pain medication during his hospital stay and upon discharge. The patient was educated about his diagnosis and was recommended to inform other practitioners prior to initiation of antibiotic therapy.

COMPLICATIONS

Recurrence can occur and is usually due to the germination of persistent *C. difficile* spores in the colon after treatment or secondary to reinfection of the pathogen.

Approximately 3% of patients develop severe *C. difficile*–associated diarrhea. The mortality rate in these patients ranges from 30% to 85%. Treatment of severe cases must be aggressive, with intravenous metronidazole and oral vancomycin used in combination. If ileus occurs, vancomycin can be administered by nasogastric tube with intermittent clamping, retention enemas, or both. If medical therapy fails or perforation or toxic megacolon develops, surgical intervention with colectomy and ileostomy is indicated but carries a high mortality rate.

Of concern is that recent studies indicate the emergence of a new more virulent strain of *C. difficile* that is associated with more severe disease (higher rates of toxic megacolon, leukemoid reaction, shock, need for colectomy, and death). Further investigation has found that deletion of a gene in this new strain may be responsible for its greater pathogenicity. This deletion is thought to be responsible for production of 16 to 23 times more toxin A and B. This emergence underscores the importance of judicious use of antibiotics (especially cephalosporins, clindamycin, and fluoroquinolones) and the need for practitioners to be more vigilant. Strict infection control measures including contact isolation and enhanced environmental cleaning are mandatory.

DISCUSSION

C. difficile is a gram-positive, spore-forming rod that is responsible for 15% to 20% of antibiotic-related cases of diarrhea. *C. difficile* infection results in more than 300,000 cases of diarrhea in the United States and is the most common cause of nosocomial diarrhea. The case mortality rate is approximately 1% to 2.5%

Acquisition of *C. difficile* occurs primarily in the hospital setting or long-term care facilities where the organism has been cultured from bed rails, floors, windowsills, and toilets, as well as the hands of hospital workers who provide care for patients with *C. difficile* infection. The rate of *C. difficile* acquisition is estimated to be 13% in patients with hospital stays up to 2 weeks and 50% in those with hospital stays longer than 4 weeks.

The risk factors for the development of symptomatic *C. difficile*–associated diarrhea are summarized in Box 2-4.

The initiating event for *C. difficile* colitis is disruption of colonic flora with subsequent colonization. Depending on host factors, a carrier state or disease results. The disruption is usually caused by broad-spectrum antibiotics. Clindamycin and broad-spectrum penicillins and cephalosporins are most commonly implicated. *C. difficile* colitis can occur up to 8 weeks after discontinuation of antibiotics. C. difficile produces two toxins that are responsible for its pathogenesis, toxin A and B. Both toxins play a role in the pathogenesis of *C. difficile*–associated diarrhea. Toxin A is primarily an enterotoxin that causes excretion of fluid from the bowel. This fluid is profoundly inflammatory, containing neutrophils, lymphocytes, serum proteins, erythrocytes, and mucus. Toxin B is primarily cytotoxic and has little enterotoxic activity. The toxins also stimulate leukocyte chemotaxis and upregulate the production of cytokines and other inflammatory mediators. As colitis worsens, focal ulcerations occur, and the accumulation of purulent and necrotic debris forms the typical pseudomembranes.

The diagnosis of *C. difficile* colitis requires a detailed history, including use of any antibiotics over the last 3 months.

Box 2-4.	**Risk Factors for *Clostridium difficile*–Associated Diarrhea**

Admission to the ICU
Advanced age
Antibiotic therapy
Immunosuppressive therapy
Multiple and severe underlying disease
Placement of nasogastric tube
Prolonged hospital stay
Recent surgical procedure
Residing in a nursing home
Sharing a hospital room with a *C. difficile*–infected patient
Antacid use

A detailed description of the type, frequency, and consistency of diarrhea is important. The enzyme immunoassay that detects toxins A and B is the most common laboratory test for diagnosing *C. difficile*–mediated disease.

Other types of diarrhea should be considered and ruled out based on history and physical examination. These include infectious enteritis or colitis, bacterial gastroenteritis, viral gastroenteritis, amebic dysentery, inflammatory bowel disease such as Crohn's disease, ulcerative colitis, and ischemic colitis. Antibiotic intolerance manifested as diarrhea in which there is no evidence of colitis will usually resolve upon antibiotic withdrawal.

Bibliography

Bartlett JG: Antibiotic-associated diarrhea, *N Engl J Med* 346:334, 2002.

Bartlett JG, Perl TM: The new *Clostridium difficile*—what does it mean? *N Engl J Med* 353:2503-2505, 2005.

Loo VG, et al: A predominantly clonal multi-institutional outbreak of *Clostridium difficile*-associated diarrhea with high morbidity and mortality, *N Engl J Med* 353:23, 2442-2449, 2005.

McDonald LC, et al: An epidemic, toxin gene-variant strain of *Clostridium difficile, N Engl J Med* 353:23, 2433-2441, 2005.

Mylonakis E, Ryan E, Calderwood S: *Clostridium difficile*–associated diarrhea: a review, *Arch Intern Med* 161:525, 2001.

Savola KL, et al. Fecal leukocyte stain has diagnostic value for outpatients but not inpatients, *J Clin Micriobiol* 39:266, 2001.

Schroeder M: *Clostridium difficile*–associated diarrhea, *Am Fam Phys* 71:5:921, 2005.

Thomas RV: Nosocomial diarrhea due to *Clostridium difficile, Curr Opin Infect Dis* 17:323, 2004.

Drug-Seeking Behavior

Fariba Farhidvash, MD, and Chris Jo, DMD

CC

A 40-year-old man presents to your office stating, "My tooth is killing me, and I ran out of my pain meds."

HPI

The patient complains of a 3-day history of exquisite tooth pain. Upon interviewing the patient, he immediately emphasizes that he has tried everything and that only "Percocet" helps with the pain. He states that he is unable to tolerate all nonsteroidal antiinflammatory drugs (NSAIDs) due to gastric upset, and he also states that he has a "very high tolerance" for pain medications due to a history of chronic pain associated with a herniated lumbar disc. A prescription for 20 oxycodone/acetaminophen (325/5 mg) tablets was given to the patient to take as needed, and he was scheduled for surgery the next morning. On the morning of surgery, he calls to cancel his appointment due to "financial reasons" and requests more pain medication to last him through the weekend. You call his referring dentist to obtain more history and find that this patient has called several times in the past requesting opioid pain medications without compliance with the proposed treatment plans (restoration versus extraction).

PMHX/PDHX/MEDICATIONS/ALLERGIES/SH/FH

The patient has a history of back pain due to lumbar disc herniation from a fall at work (a previous history of chronic pain and narcotic analgesic use would likely cause tolerance). He also has a history of depression (this may be a consequence of chronic pain, but, in addition, patients with depression and/or anxiety are more likely to exhibit dependence or addiction).

EXAMINATION

General. The patient is a well-developed and well-nourished man that appears mildly agitated. He reports a pain level of 10/10 on the visual analog scale (VAS), although his behavior (and examination findings) do not correlate with his reported level of pain (although this is a subjective observation and its value is questionable, clinicians need to correlate subjective complaints of pain to objective clinical findings).

Intraoral. Dentition is in good general repair. His right maxillary first molar (tooth No. 3) has a small occlusal carious lesion. The patient has a dramatic painful reaction upon palpation and percussion of the tooth. There is no vestibular swelling, erythema, or any other signs of acute infection.

Pain perception is a physical sensation interpreted in the light of experience and is influenced by a great number of interacting physical, mental, biological, physiological, psychological, social, cultural, and emotional factors. Each individual learns the application of the word "pain" through experiences related to injury early in life. The response to pain is very variable subjectively, behaviorally (crying, yelling, teeth clenching, wincing), and physiologically through various individual ranges of sympathetic nervous system manifestations (hypertension, tachycardia, nausea, pupillary dilation, pallor, perspiration). A remarkable aspect of pain perception is the extreme variability of reactions that it evokes. Many factors affect the perception of pain, and therefore clinicians need to exercise caution when interpreting the patients' perception of pain.

IMAGING

A panoramic radiograph is an excellent screening tool for evaluating odontogenic sources of pain. A bite-wing and periapical radiographs provide better resolution for detection of caries.

The panoramic radiograph in the above patient showed a carious lesion on the right maxillary first molar that does not appear to involve the pulp. There is no periapical radiolucent lesion or widening of the periodontal ligament space.

LABS

No laboratory tests are needed in the work-up of acute odontogenic pain, unless dictated by the patient's medical history. For patients being admitted to the hospital for maxillofacial injuries or pathology, a urine drug screen (UDS) or blood alcohol level (BAL) can be obtained to detect recent use of illicit drugs that may influence treatment interventions. However, this may not be feasible for the patient presenting to the office.

ASSESSMENT

Carious right maxillary first molar, with subjective report of refractory odontogenic pain in the setting of other chronic pain syndromes and a history of substance abuse; patient demands to be treated for his acute dental pain with opioid medications, displaying signs of drug-seeking behavior

The picture of a patient who presents to your clinic for acute or chronic pain that is refractory to multiple pain medications, who has made multiple visits to other medical facilities to obtain medications, and who is demanding or aggressive in his attempt to receive narcotic medications is concerning for drug-seeking behavior. *Drug-seeking behavior* is a common term used among physicians and may be described as "a patient's manipulative, demanding behavior to obtain medication." Although there is no *DSM-IV (Diagnostic and Statistical Manual of Mental Disorders–Fourth Edition)* definition for drug-seeking behavior, it is related, but not synonymous, to drug abuse, dependence, and addiction.

DSM-IV criteria for abuse involves the presence of the following symptoms within a 12-month period:
- Recurrent use resulting in a failure to fulfill major obligations at work, school, or home
- Recurrent use in situations that are physically hazardous (e.g., driving while intoxicated)
- Legal problems resulting from recurrent use
- Continued use despite significant social or interpersonal problems caused by the substance use

Criteria for dependence include the following:
- Substance abuse
- Continuation of use despite related problems
- Increase in tolerance (more of the drug is needed to achieve the same effect)
- Withdrawal symptoms

Although addiction is not included in the *DSM-IV*, it is characterized by preoccupation and seeking of the drug and with continued use of the drug, leading to tolerance, physical dependence, and other adaptive changes in the brain.

TREATMENT

It is important for physicians to treat pain effectively and without fear of addiction or dependence. There are steps to effectively treat the patient's pain and curb the physician's concern. First and foremost, it is important to become familiar with the patient's medical history, especially any other pain syndromes or psychological comorbidities. It is also essential to become familiar with the different schedules of medications, dosing, adverse effects, and general pharmacokinetics. Dosing schedules and any recent changes, along with any side effects the patient may experience, should be followed closely. An interdisciplinary approach to pain and other alternatives to treatment, such as various injections or blocks or even nonmedication routes such as psychotherapy, should not be excluded. Pain should not be treated in isolation but as part of the patient's overall medical picture.

Treating acute or chronic pain should be approached in a stepwise manner. Pain management should be individualized and applied in the appropriate clinical situation; however, the World Health Organization (WHO) guidelines for the management of chronic facial pain involve a three-step ladder approach. Step 1 includes acetaminophen (drug of choice for patients with bleeding disorders, renal disease, or peptic ulcer disease), NSAIDs, and propoxyphene napsylate. Step 2 includes acetaminophen combined with various narcotic medications (codeine, hydrocodone, and oxycodone). Step 3 involves the use of anticonvulsants and tricyclic antidepressants (gabapentin, amitriptyline, tramadol, clonazepam, baclofen, imipramine), which is reserved for chronic or neuropathic pain states.

In the setting of mild to moderate acute odontogenic or postoperative pain, nonopioid analgesics (NSAIDs and acetaminophen) should be initiated. A short course of scheduled dosing of an NSAID (e.g., ibuprofen 800 mg every 8 hours for 3 days, in the absence of contraindications), along with narcotic pain medication (hydrocodone, oxycodone, meperidine, etc., with or without acetaminophen) may be prescribed for moderate to severe breakthrough pain. However, drug seekers commonly preclude the use of NSAIDs in their pain management by stating allergy or intolerance to them. If the patient has more moderate to severe pain, then higher doses of opioids with the nonopioid analgesics are used. Each medication can be increased in dose or the dosing frequency can be adjusted according to the patient's needs. In conjunction with analgesics, antibiotic therapy should be initiated when indicated. Although chronic opioid treatment has been successful and is recommended for cancer patients, controversy exists regarding the use of opioid versus nonopioid drugs in the management of chronic nonmalignant orofacial pain.

If the chronic pain is characterized as neuropathic, tricycle antidepressants or selected antiepileptics (Neurontin, Tegretol, or Lyrica) can be very effective. Other options for pain management, such as regional sympathetic blockade, steroid injections, neuroablative procedures, and the like, may have longer lasting effects without the fear of abuse. It should be noted that pain is characteristically a manifestation of an underlying problem and associated comorbidities that may include organic or psychiatric conditions that influence the perception of pain. Treatment of underlying mood or other psychiatric disorders can help relieve the subjective experience of pain.

If drug-seeking behavior is observed or if there is suspicion of dependence or abuse of prescription medication, medical intervention may be warranted. This is usually out of the realm of most specialties and is best handled by primary care physicians or psychiatrists. Various methods include pharmacological detoxification (such as supervised use of methadone) and various behavioral therapies, such as biofeedback and relaxation techniques and psychotherapy—all addressing the multiple facets of addiction and dependence.

For this case, during the course of the interview, the patient continues to focus on the tooth pain and the need for narcotic medications. He becomes more agitated, raising his voice as he explains that "nothing else has worked so far." The physician emphasizes that there are other non-narcotic alternatives and that further narcotic use will cause increased tolerance. Despite continued disagreement, the patient is emphatically informed that you will work closely with him to monitor the pain and modify treatment accordingly but will not prescribe further narcotic medication. The patient is hesitant but finally agrees to follow the strict but thorough plan for pain management.

COMPLICATIONS

Overuse of opioid analgesics, sedative-hypnotics, and stimulants is typically implicated in drug tolerance and dependence. If this problem is further escalated, it can lead to abuse, physical dependence with disruption of daily activities and functioning, and even death in the event of overdose. Beyond these effects, there are the individual adverse effects associated with each medication. The most common side effects related to narcotic or opioid drugs include nausea and vomiting, constipation, anorexia, sedation or decreased cognitive functioning, euphoria, and respiratory depression and hypotension. Although uncommon, overdose with any of the medications can cause death. These side effects may be further magnified when used in combination with other analgesic or nonanalgesic medications. These interactions may result in changes in absorption, metabolism, or excretion of either medication.

DISCUSSION

Addiction disorders can be seen in up to 15% to 30% of patients in the primary care setting and 20% to 50% of hospitalized patients. Opioid analgesics, sedative-hypnotics, and stimulants are the most commonly abused medications. Although physical dependence is rare, those with acute or chronic pain, anxiety disorders, a history of substance abuse, or attention-deficit/hyperactivity disorder are at increased risk for addiction. Identifying patients at risk is important, so obtaining past medical, psychiatric, and substance abuse his-

tories and histories of other pain disorders and psychosocial stressors is paramount.

Recognizing drug-seeking behavior can help identify patients who need close follow-up. Patients may increase the use of analgesics over time due to the increased tolerance to the drug. Patients typically focus excessively on their pain and emphasize the need for a particular drug with abuse potential. They frequently present with multiple claims that non-narcotic medications are not effective and they have several "allergies." Commonly, if one doctor does not "meet their needs" or if they wish to avoid suspicion, they will "doctor shop," a pattern difficult to identify as physicians do not have access to other physician's or hospital's charts. Patients may be involved in scams to obtain brand names or stronger medications, especially for sale on the street.

Bibliography

Longo LP, Johnson B: Addiction: Part II: identification and management of the drug-seeking patient, *Am Fam Phys* 61:2121-2128, 2000.

Mersky H, Bogduk N: Classification of chronic pain. In Mersky H, Bogduk N, eds: *Task Force on Taxonomy*, Seattle, WA, 1994, International Association for the Study of Pain, pp 209-214.

Swift JQ: Nonsteroidal anti-inflammatory drugs and opioids: safety and usage concerns in the differential treatment of postoperative orofacial pain, *J Oral Maxillofac Surg* 58(Suppl 2):8-11, 2000.

Swift JQ, Roszkowski MT: The use of opioid drugs in management of chronic orofacial pain, *J Oral Maxillofac Surg* 56:1081-1085, 1998.

Vukmir RB: Drug-seeking behavior, *Am J Drug Alcohol Abuse* 3:551-571, 2004.

Zuniga JR: The use of nonopioid drugs in management of chronic orofacial pain, *J Oral Maxillofac Surg* 56:1075-1080, 1998.

Acute Acetaminophen Toxicity

Bruce Anderson, HBSc, DDS, and Shahrokh C. Bagheri, DMD, MD

CC

A 53-year-old man is referred to your clinic with a chief complaint of severe pain associated with the left mandibular second molar. The patient also complains of generalized malaise and right upper quadrant abdominal pain.

HPI

The patient reports a 3-month history of diffuse intermittent pain of the right posterior mandible that he has treated with several over-the-counter analgesics. In the past 4 days, the pain has become constant and has progressively exacerbated. It has localized to the left mandibular second molar, causing him to repeatedly wake up during the night. Two days prior to presentation, he was seen at a walk-in dental clinic, where he was prescribed penicillin and oxycodone/acetaminophen (5/500 mg) and referred to your clinic for evaluation and extraction. Careful questioning reveals that during the past 48 hours, he has ingested the 20 prescribed tablets of oxycodone/acetaminophen and, due to continued pain, also ingested 12 additional 500-mg tablets of acetaminophen that he purchased over the counter from the local pharmacy (total ingested dose of acetaminophen in 48 hours is estimated at 16,000 mg). During the last 6 hours, he reports the onset of right upper quadrant abdominal pain and nausea.

Abdominal pain and a history of excessive acetaminophen ingestion should alert the clinician to possible hepatotoxicity and warrant immediate referral to an emergency department.

PMHX/PDHX/MEDICATIONS/ALLERGIES/SH/FH

His past medical history is significant for chronic alcohol abuse. He admits to drinking at least six cans of beer per day (suggestive of preexisting compromised liver function).

Patients with compromised liver function, as in chronic alcoholism, have a decreased ability to clear acetaminophen and are more prone to toxic injury. Conversely, acute alcohol ingestion in an otherwise healthy individual will actually induce the hepatic microsomal oxidase system and increase the removal of acetaminophen from plasma.

EXAMINATION

General. The patient is in mild distress (secondary to pain) but is cooperative. He is alert and oriented times three (altered mental status can be seen several days after ingestion of toxic doses of acetaminophen due to severe hepatotoxicity). He appears mildly cachectic (suggestive of malnutrition), slightly lethargic, and pale.

Weight. He weighs 70 kg.

Vital signs. Blood pressure is 127/83 mm Hg, heart rate 112 bpm (tachycardia due to pain), respirations 17 per minute, and temperature 37.4°C.

Intraoral. The examination is consistent with acute pulpitis of the left mandibular second molar.

Abdominal. Palpation of the right upper quadrant elicits mild pain. The liver is palpated at 6 cm inferior to the costal margin and measures over 17 cm using percussion (hepatomegaly). A normal liver margin is generally not palpable or is palpated just superior to the costal margin upon inspiration).

There are no signs of progressive hepatic encephalopathy (disturbances in consciousness, hyperreflexia, asterixis, or, rarely, seizures).

IMAGING

No immediate imaging studies are indicated in patients suspected of acute acetaminophen toxicity. The patient should be immediately transported to a local emergency department for treatment. Referral to the emergency department should not be delayed by dental radiographs or nonurgent oral surgical procedures.

In this case, a periapical and a panoramic radiograph were obtained at the walk-in dental clinic 2 days prior for evaluation of the odontogenic pathology, demonstrating pulpal caries and fractured left mandibular second molar.

LABS

Several laboratory studies are obtained in the emergency department to evaluate the extent of hepatic injury. A serum acetaminophen concentration should be immediately obtained as its result will be helpful to guide treatment and to predict the outcome of hepatotoxicity. Liver function tests (LFTs) include aspartate aminotransferase (AST), which is the best early indicator of hepatic injury. Patients with marked elevations in AST who demonstrate clinical manifestations of hepatotoxicity or failure should have expanded laboratory monitoring, including alanine aminotransferase (ALT), lactate dehydrogenase (LDH), total bilirubin, coagulation studies (PT, PTT, and INR), pH, and blood glucose. Serial laboratory testing is used to monitor the progression of hepatic injury or recovery. A CMP can also be obtained to monitor electrolyte disturbances, especially with concomitant alcohol ingestion. A BAL may also be obtained as indicated by the history.

For the above patient, the initial AST was at 1320 U/L (normal range, 5 to 40 U/L).

ASSESSMENT

Acute acetaminophen toxicity (stage II) secondary to pain caused by irreversible pulpitis of the left mandibular second molar

TREATMENT

Recognition of acetaminophen toxicity requires immediate transfer of the patient to a hospital emergency department for work-up and treatment.

Management of acetaminophen toxicity requires an understanding of its pharmacokinetics and pathophysiology. Acetaminophen (*N*-acetyl-*p*-aminophenol, or APAP) is an analgesic and antipyretic agent that is rapidly absorbed from the gastrointestinal tract, achieving peak serum concentrations between 45 minutes and 2 hours following ingestion. Peak serum concentrations following acute toxic ingestion are observed at approximately 4 hours. The elimination half-life is between 2 and 4 hours. Therapeutic doses of acetaminophen are 10 to 15 mg/kg per dose, with a daily maximum of 80 mg/kg in children and of 4 g in adults. Therapeutic serum concentrations are reported at 10 to 30 µg/ml. Toxicity is probable with single doses greater than 250 mg/kg or a daily ingestion greater than 12 g and is certain with single doses greater than 350 mg/kg.

Approximately 5% of acetaminophen is excreted unchanged in the urine. Another 75% to 90% is metabolized by the hepatic glucuronic acid pathway prior to excretion. The remaining portion is metabolized by the hepatic P450 microsomal oxidase pathway into *N*-acetyl-*p*-benzoquinoneimine (NAPQI), a toxic metabolite. At therapeutic doses, NAPQI is rapidly conjugated by hepatic glutathione and excreted, while at toxic doses glutathione stores are depleted with subsequent accumulation of NAPQI, resulting in oxidative damage and hepatocellular necrosis (Figure 2-1).

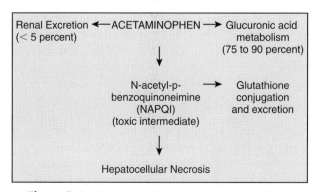

Figure 2-1 Overview of acetaminophen metabolism.

Considerations for the management of acute acetaminophen toxicity include a detailed dosing history, time of presentation, indicated laboratory studies, the presence of comorbid conditions, and clinical manifestations. The current methods of treatment include induced emesis (if diagnosed early), gastric lavage, gastrointestinal decontamination with activated charcoal (AC), and administration of *N*-acetylcysteine (NAC). Activated charcoal acts by readily absorbing acetaminophen resulting in a reduction of gastrointestinal absorption of 50% to 90%. AC is administered as a single dose of 1 g/kg and is only indicated within the first 4 hours following ingestion, as gastrointestinal absorption is complete beyond this time. NAC is a precursor of glutathione and acts to increase glutathione stores as well as combining with NAPQI directly. NAC has other beneficial effects including acting as an antiinflammatory, antioxidant, and vasodilator, thereby aiding in the preservation of multiorgan function. The standard oral regimen of NAC is a loading dose of 140 mg/kg followed by 17 doses of 70 mg/kg every 4 hours for a total of 72 hours. NAC is supplied as either a 10% or 20% oral solution (Mucomyst). Patients developing hepatic failure require a longer course of NAC therapy until clinical improvement is demonstrated and INR falls below 2.0. The efficacy of NAC treatment is significantly decreased if not administered within 8 to 10 hours of acetaminophen ingestion as cell injury may have already begun. Severe hepatotoxicity and death are rare when NAC therapy is initiated early (within 8 hours) regardless of initial serum acetaminophen concentrations. Early discontinuation of NAC therapy may be considered if the patient has become asymptomatic, has an acetaminophen concentration of less than 10 µg/ml, and has normal AST levels 36 hours postingestion. These markers demonstrate a completion of acetaminophen metabolism and safely determine that no subsequent hepatic injury will occur. The indications for initiation of NAC therapy, paired with expanded laboratory testing, are variable between acute and chronic toxic ingestions and are addressed further later.

This patient was treated in the emergency department with AC and NAC. He was admitted to a medical service, and his LFTs were normalized over 30 days. The left mandibular second molar was extracted the next day after initiation of therapy to aid in pain control. Prior to discharge, he was referred to an alcohol cessation program, and then he was to follow with a primary care provider.

COMPLICATIONS

The most feared complication associated with acute acetaminophen toxicity is severe hepatotoxicity leading to fulminant hepatic failure, hepatic encephalopathy, multiorgan failure, and death. Acute renal failure occurs in 25% and 50% of patients with significant hepatotoxicity and hepatic failure, respectively; this is primarily due to acute tubular necrosis. Hypoglycemia, lactic acidosis, hemorrhage, acute respiratory distress syndrome (ARDS), and sepsis may also occur in severe cases. Liver transplantation is indicated in patients who show a pH lower than 7.30 after hemodynamic resuscitation, a PT greater than 1.8 times the control, a creatinine greater than 3.3 mg/dl, and grade III or IV encephalopathy. Death usually occurs as a result of multiorgan failure.

The existence of comorbid conditions, including chronic alcoholism, malnutrition, and the use of drugs that influence the mixed-function oxidase pathway, may increase the risk of toxicity in some patients. Chronic alcohol abuse both depletes glutathione stores and increases P450 activity, resulting in higher production of NAPQI. Chronic alcoholic persons are reported to be at higher risk for toxicity following multiple doses of acetaminophen while not appearing to be at higher risk following single acute toxic ingestions. Malnutrition or fasting will also deplete glutathione stores in addition to adversely affecting the carbohydrate-dependent glucuronide conjugation pathway. Examples of drugs that increase P450 activity and subsequent NAPQI production include barbiturates, anticonvulsants, and antituberculosis medications.

The inability of some patients to tolerate oral NAC therapy is noteworthy and is usually successfully managed by aggressive antiemetic treatment. If this fails, intravenous administration of NAC should be considered to ensure delivery within 8 to 10 hours postingestion. Intravenous NAC, however, is associated with more adverse side effects, including anaphylactoid reactions, bronchospasm, and hypotension. Other indications for intravenous NAC include patients who have medical conditions that contraindicate oral delivery of NAC (e.g., active gastrointestinal bleed, gastrointestinal obstruction), pregnant patients (theoretical improved transplacental delivery secondary to higher serum concentrations), and patients with established fulminant hepatic failure (demonstrate little benefit from oral NAC).

DISCUSSION

Acetaminophen, which was introduced clinically in 1950, is a widely used over-the-counter analgesic that is extremely safe when used at appropriate therapeutic doses. It is present in numerous individual and combination (usually with an opioid) pharmaceuticals and is most commonly used for the treatment of pain and fever. It is also found in many over-the-counter medications in combination with sedatives, decongestants, and antihistamines. It may be this wide availability coupled with the general public's lack of knowledge of potential toxicity that has resulted in acetaminophen being responsible for the most overdoses and overdose-associated deaths yearly in the United States as reported by the American Association of Poison Control Centers. The first reported case of acetaminophen-related hepatic necrosis was in 1966; subsequently, the pharmacokinetics, risk stratification, and management of acetaminophen toxicity have been well studied and documented.

Prompt recognition of potential toxicity is vital in reducing morbidity and mortality. A detailed dosing history, including the time of last ingestion, is important. Diagnosis may be difficult to establish in cases of chronic overdose, often presenting with only mild symptoms or no symptoms at all. The clinical sequence of acetaminophen toxicity can de divided into the following four stages:

Stage I (0 to 24 hours). Hepatic injury has not yet occurred and patients are often clinically asymptomatic, giving a false sense of well-being. Some vague symptoms may be present, including nausea and vomiting, pallor, lethargy, malaise, and diaphoresis. AST levels are usually normal during this stage but may start to rise at 8 to 12 hours in severe cases.

Stage II (24 to 72 hours). It is during stage II that hepatic injury begins, coupled with its associated signs and symptoms. Patients develop abdominal right upper quadrant pain and liver enlargement but are likely to demonstrate resolution of previous symptoms evident in stage I. Laboratory markers of liver dysfunction also become evident during this stage. AST elevation is present in all patients with hepatotoxicity by 36 hours and is the most sensitive value in predicting progressive hepatic injury.

Stage III (72 to 96 hours). This is the stage of maximum hepatotoxicity, and resulting signs and symptoms vary depending on the severity of hepatic injury. Patients demonstrate nausea and vomiting, diaphoresis, jaundice, lethargy, malaise and may progress to develop fulminant hepatic failure, acute renal failure, lactic acidosis, hepatic encephalopathy, exsanguinating hemorrhage, ARDS, sepsis, and death. Pertinent laboratory findings included marked elevation of AST and ALT, elevated total bilirubin, hypoglycemia, decreased pH, and elevated PT/INR.

Stage IV (4 to 7 days). This is the recovery stage for survivors of stage III. Laboratory abnormalities normalize and symptoms resolve, but this may take weeks in severely ill patients. Histological repair of hepatic necrosis may take up to 3 months to complete, but chronic hepatic injury has not been reported in cases of acetaminophen toxicity.

Diagnosis and risk stratification of acetaminophen toxicity need to be assessed in a timely fashion. Patients presenting with suspicion of toxicity are usually divided into those with either acute or chronic overdoses with slight differences in treatment protocol. In both groups, the history and timing of ingestion, as well as the existence of any comorbid conditions, must be determined.

Patients with single acute overdoses are normally evaluated based on the Rumack-Matthew nomogram, which relates serum acetaminophen concentration to time from ingestion as a predictor of hepatotoxicity. Blood for serum acetaminophen level measurement should be drawn at 4 hours postingestion or immediately if the time of ingestion is unknown. NAC therapy is the standard of care for any patient whose serum concentration is above the line in the nomogram indicating possible risk of hepatic toxicity (Figure 2-2). Chronic overdose patients often present to emergency departments at a later stage of toxicity due to lack of early symptoms. These patients are at a high risk for hepatotoxicity if they have ingested greater than 7.5 to 10 g within 24 hours or greater than 4 g within 24 hours in the presence of comorbid conditions. Indications for the initiation of NAC therapy include

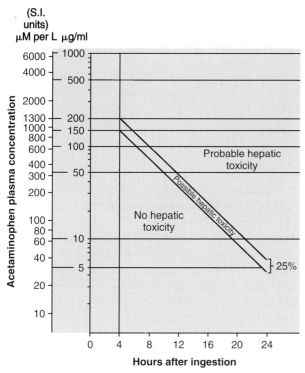

Figure 2-2 Rumack-Matthew nomogram. *(Modified from Rumack BH, Matthews H: Pediatrics 55:871, 1975.)*

acute overdose patients with serum acetaminophen concentrations above the possible risk line of the Rumack-Matthew nomogram, single ingestions greater than 7.5 g, unknown dose or time of ingestion with a serum acetaminophen concentration greater than 10 μg/ml, repeated supratherapeutic doses in the presence of comorbid conditions, and any patient with elevated AST levels or right upper quadrant abdominal pain. Most patients with toxicity recover following the standard 72-hour protocol of NAC therapy; however, in severe cases of hepatic failure, NAC therapy should continue until INR falls below 2.0, other laboratory values normalize, and clinical symptoms resolve. Low-risk patients are defined as those who are asymptomatic with acetaminophen concentrations less than 10 μg/Ml at 4 hours and normal AST levels. Low-risk patients do not require NAC therapy and can be discharged with detailed instructions and scheduled 24-hour follow-up.

Health care providers, particularly oral and maxillofacial surgeons and other clinicians who frequently prescribe acetaminophen-containing analgesic medications, should be aware of symptoms of acute acetaminophen toxicity. Patients should be carefully instructed to avoid other medications containing acetaminophen in conjunction with prescribed medications and be made aware of the risks of toxicity. Practitioners should be aware of the surgical patient presenting with a history of pain who has been self-medicating. Detailed ques-

tions to determine all ingested medications, as well as the possible existence of any comorbid conditions, are necessary. A working knowledge of the risks and symptoms of acetaminophen toxicity is vital in the early recognition and subsequent treatment of this potentially fatal condition.

Bibliography

Bagheri SC, Beckley ML, Farish SE: Acute acetaminophen toxicity: report of a case, *J California Dent Assoc* 29:687, 2001.

Bessems JG, Vermeulen NP: Paracetamol (acetaminophen)-induced toxicity: molecular and biochemical mechanisms, analogues and protective approaches, *Crit Rev Toxicol* 31:55, 2001.

Davidson DG, Eastham WN: Acute liver necrosis following overdose of paracetamol, *Br Med J* 5512:497, 1966.

Holdiness MR: Clinical pharmacokinetics of N-acetylcysteine, *Clin Pharmacokinet* 20:123, 1991.

Keays R, et al: Intravenous acetylcysteine in paracetamol induced fulminant hepatic failure: a prospective controlled study, *BMJ* 303:1026, 1991.

Litovitz TL, et al: 1997 Annual report of the American Association of Poison Control Centers Toxic Exposure Surveillance System, *Am J Emerg Med* 16:443, 1998.

Makin AJ, Wendon J, Williams R: A 7-year experience of severe acetaminophen-induced hepatotoxicity (1987-1993), *Gastroenterology* 109:1907, 1995.

Makin AJ, Williams R: The current management of paracetamol overdosage, *Br J Clin Pract* 48:144, 1994.

O'Grady JG, et al: Early indicators of prognosis in fulminant hepatic failure, *Gastroenterology* 97:439, 1989.

Prescott LF: Paracetamol overdosage: pharmacological considerations and clinical management, *Drugs* 25:290, 1983.

Prescott LF, Critchley JAJH: The treatment of acetaminophen poisoning, *Annu Rev Pharmacol Toxicol* 23:87, 1983.

Prescott LF, Proudfoot AT, Cregeen RJ: Paracetamol-induced acute renal failure in the absence of fulminant liver damage, *Br Med J* 284:421, 1982.

Rose SR, et al: Simulated acetaminophen overdose: pharmacokinetics and effectiveness of activated charcoal, *Ann Emerg Med* 20:1064, 1991.

Rumack BH: Acetaminophen hepatotoxicity: The first 35 years, *J Toxicol Clin Toxicol* 40:3, 2002.

Rumack BH, Matthew H: Acetaminophen poisoning and toxicity, *Pediatrics* 55:871, 1975.

Schiodt FV, et al: Influence of acute and chronic alcohol intake on the clinical course and outcome in acetaminophen overdose, *Aliment Pharmacol Ther* 16:707, 2002.

Singer AJ, Carracio TR, Mofenson HC: The temporal profile of increased transaminase levels in patients with acetaminophen-induced liver dysfunction, *Ann Emerg Med* 26:49, 1995.

Smilkstein MJ, et al: Efficacy of oral N-acetylcysteine in the treatment of acetaminophen poisoning, *N Engl J Med* 319:1557, 1988.

Smilkstein MJ: In Goldfrank LR, et al, eds: *Goldfrank's Toxicologic Emergencies,* Stamford, Conn, 1998, Appleton & Lange, p 541.

Smilkstein MJ: Chronic ethanol use and acute acetaminophen overdose toxicity, *J Toxicol Clin Toxicol* 36:476, 1998.

Watson WA, et al: 2003 Annual report of the American Association of Poison Control Centers Toxic Exposure Surveillance System, *Am J Emerg Med* 22:335, 2004.

Opioid Side Effects

Piyushkumar P. Patel, DDS, and Shahrokh C. Bagheri, DMD, MD

CC

A 30-year-old woman presents to the office complaining that, "the pain medication is making me feel nauseous." (Nausea is the most commonly seen adverse effect of orally administered opioids. In a large retrospective review, it was found that women have a 60% higher risk of nausea and vomiting than do men when administered opioids.)

HPI

The patient had several mandibular teeth extracted with no intraoperative complications 2 days before presentation. She was given a prescription for a combination analgesic containing hydrocodone (an opioid) and acetaminophen. She reports poor oral intake since her procedure and has been feeling nauseated with one episode of vomiting since taking the medication (opioids have a greater tendency to cause nausea and vomiting when taken on an empty stomach). She has not had any relief from pain and explains that she is now worse because she has both pain and nausea.

The term *opioid* is used to refer to all of the agonists and antagonists of the morphine-like family of compounds. This term is preferred to older terms such as *opiate* or *narcotic*. *Narcotic* refers to any drug that can cause dependence. The term is not specific for opioids (i.e., not all narcotics are opioids).

PMHX/PDHX/MEDICATIONS/ALLERGIES/SH/FH

The patient does not have any known history of narcotic abuse (risk factor for drug-seeking behavior). Current medications include hydrocodone/acetaminophen (5/325 mg tablets). She admits to have consumed four tablets in the past 6 hours with minimal oral intake.

EXAMINATION

General. The patient is a well-developed and well-nourished woman who appears her stated age and is in mild discomfort secondary to nausea. She is alert and oriented to time, place, and person (this is important to assess mental status in cases of acute opioid toxicity).

Vital signs. Her vital signs are stable and she is afebrile (AF), except for slight tachycardia at 110 bpm (caused by dehydration second to decreased oral intake).

Maxillofacial. Pupils are 3 mm, equal, round, and bilaterally reactive (pupillary constriction or miosis would be a sign of excessive opioid intake and is not affected by tolerance).

Intraoral. The examination is consistent with healing extraction sockets with no evidence of alveolar osteitis or acute infection.

Abdominal. The abdomen is soft, nontender, and nondistended; bowel sounds are present but hypoactive in all four quadrants. (Abdominal examination may not be routine in this situation, but it may demonstrate decreased bowel sounds secondary to the effect of opioids on gastrointestinal motility.)

IMAGING

No imaging studies are indicated unless the situation is compounded by other medical conditions. For patients with a suspicion of aspiration, such as those with concomitant alcohol consumption or decreased mental status secondary to excessive opioid intake, a chest radiograph may be indicated.

LABS

No laboratory studies are indicated unless dictated by preexisting medical conditions such as uncontrolled diabetes. In patients with prolonged vomiting, metabolic alkalosis and other electrolyte abnormalities may ensue. Appropriate laboratory studies should be ordered as needed.

ASSESSMENT

Acute nausea and vomiting associated with postoperative opioid analgesia, status post dentoalveolar surgery; subjective report of moderate pain that is nonresponsive to the current pharmacological regimen

It is important to distinguish acute pain, which is of recent onset and limited duration, from chronic pain, which is described as lasting for an undefined period of time, beyond that expected for the injury to heal. This distinction has both diagnostic and treatment implications. Caution should be exercised when treating chronic pain with opioids due to the development of dependence.

TREATMENT

Several different approaches can be used either alone or in combination for the management of the adverse effects of opioids; these include:

- Dose reduction of the systemic opioid
- Symptomatic management of the adverse effect
- Opioid rotation (or switching)
- Alternate routes of systemic administration

Reducing the dose of the administered opioid can result in a reduction of dose-related adverse effects. To compensate for the loss of pain control, adjunctive strategies can be used to maintain control while reducing the dose or eliminating the opioid. Common strategies include addition of a nonopioid coanalgesic or an adjuvant analgesic that is appropriate to the pain syndrome and mechanism (e.g., addition of Neurontin for the treatment of neuropathic pain). In addition, the application of therapy targeting the cause of the pain (e.g., the placement of packing material into a dry socket wound) or the application of a regional anesthetic or neuroablative intervention may be used.

Symptomatic management of the adverse effect is usually based on cumulative anecdotal experiences. In general, this involves the addition of a new medication(s). However, polypharmacy adds to medication burden, and the possibility of drug interactions needs to be considered.

Opioid rotation (also called opioid switching or substitution) requires familiarity with a range of opioid agonists and with the use of opioid dose conversion tables to find equianalgesic dosages. The objective of switching one opioid with another is to reduce the adverse effects. Alternatively, switching the route of systemic administration, such as changing from the intravenous to the oral route, has been shown to ameliorate symptoms of nausea, constipation, and drowsiness. In many acute situations, NSAIDs provide analgesia equal to the starting doses of opioids. However, unlike opioids that lack a ceiling dose, NSAIDs have a maximum dose above which no additional analgesic effect is obtained.

This patient was treated with a single dose of oral Phenergan (promethazine) at 25 mg. Her medication was switched to a nonopioid analgesic (ibuprofen 400 mg orally every 4 to 6 hours). She was also instructed to increase her oral intake, preferably with isotonic drinks. She responded well to this regimen, with resolution of her nausea and reduction of pain to an acceptable level.

COMPLICATIONS

Although opioids are well recognized as being effective for moderate to severe pain, they are frequently associated with an array of troublesome side effects (Table 2-1). Genuine allergy to opioids is rare. In most cases, patients report having an opioid allergy when they have had an opioid-related adverse effect. Opioid complications can include the following:

Nausea and vomiting. More than 30% of patients using opioids report experiencing nausea or vomiting. It is the most common and unpleasant adverse effect of opioids. Opioid receptors play an important role in the control of emesis (vomiting). They directly stimulate the chemoreceptor trigger zone, depressing the vomiting center and slowing gastrointestinal motility. Multiple medications have been used to prevent or treat nausea or vomiting. The available antiemetic agents

Table 2-1. Common Opiate-Induced Adverse Effects

Body System	Adverse Effects
Gastrointestinal	Nausea
	Vomiting
	Constipation
Autonomic	Xerostomia
	Urinary retention
	Postural hypotension
CNS	Drowsiness
	Cognitive impairment
	Hallucinations
	Delirium
	Respiratory depression
	Myoclonus
	Seizure disorder
	Hyperalgesia
Cutaneous	Itch
	Sweating

Table 2-2. Antiemetic Drugs

Pharmacological Group	Common Generic Name	Common Trade Names
Anticholinergic	Scopolamine	Scopace, Transderm Scop
Antihistamine	Cyclizine	Merezine, Migril
	Dimenhydrinate	Dimentabs, Dramamine
	Diphenhydramine	Benadryl
	Promethazine	Phenergan
Antiserotonins	Dolasetron	Anzemet
	Granisetron	Zofran
	Ondansetron	Zotran
Benzamides	Metoclopramide	Reglan, Octamide
Butyrophenones	Droperidol	Droleptan, Inapsine
	Haloperidol	Haldol
Phenothiazines	Chlorpromazine	Thorazine
Steroids	Betamethasone	Celestone
	Dexamethasone	Decadron

fall within seven different categories (Table 2-2). There is no "universal" antiemetic, and no current single antiemetic is 100% effective for all patients. The variability of clinical studies makes it difficult to recommend one of these medications over another. Some clinicians recommend the use of ondansetron for severe cases of nausea and vomiting. Ondansetron is a selective 5-hydroxytryptamine (5-HT) (serotonin) receptor antagonist (antiserotonin) that has been shown to be a powerful antiemetic in the control of chemotherapy-induced and radiation therapy–induced nausea and vomiting.

Nausea or vomiting has been shown to occur despite the use of preemptive antiemetics. Switching to an alternative opioid can reduce the severity of nausea and vomiting. In addition, it has been shown that patients who receive opioids intravenously (primarily patient-controlled analgesia pumps) exhibit more nausea and vomiting. It should also be remembered that independent of other factors, pain could be the cause of nausea or vomiting.

Constipation. This is another common adverse effect and more problematic for the patients on chronic opioid therapy. Constipation may also contribute to nausea and vomiting. It is defined by the four "too's"—stools that are too hard, too small, too difficult to expel, or too infrequent. Opioids cause constipation by binding to receptors in the gastrointestinal tract, thereby slowing peristalsis and increasing transit time. Consequently, sodium and water are reabsorbed, resulting in dry, hardened stools. Patients on long-term therapy seldom develop tolerance to this side effect and should be advised to increase fluid intake and dietary fiber to compensate for the constipation. It has been suggested that a stool softener and a large bowel stimulant (e.g., docusate sodium) be used for chronic opioid therapy. A stool softener alone should not be prescribed because opioids slow normal peristalsis and may result in an uncomfortable patient who is unable to evacuate his or her bowel. Thus, a stimulant laxative may also be prescribed. In the absence of bowel movement for 3 to 4 days, more invasive measures such as stool disimpaction or rectally administered bowel evacuants (e.g., Fleet enema) may be necessary. A single dose of an opioid can affect gastrointestinal tract motility. In addition, opioids are thought to have a role in the development of postoperative ileus (a multifactorial phenomenon).

Respiratory depression. This is the most serious and most feared adverse effect of opioid therapy. Respiratory depression to the point of apnea is dose dependent and caused by opioids acting directly on respiratory centers within the brainstem. This is characterized by a reduction in tidal volume, minute volume, respiratory rate, and the response to hypoxia and hypercapnia. Careful monitoring of the patient can prevent this adverse outcome. Equianalgesic dosages of other opioids produce the same degree of respiratory depression. Patients with impaired respiratory function or bronchial asthma are at greater risk of experiencing clinically significant respiratory depression in response to usual doses of these drugs. If respiratory depression does occur, it is often in an opioid-naive patient; other signs and symptoms such as sedation and mental clouding can also be seen. Tolerance to this effect occurs with repeated use of opioids, allowing the management of chronic pain without significant risk of respiratory depression. Naloxone (Narcan) can be used to reverse opioid-induced respiratory depression. To avoid an abrupt reversal of analgesia (which may produce a catecholamine surge resulting in tachycardia, hypertension, pulmonary edema, and arrhythmias), naloxone is administered in doses of 40 µg repeated every few minutes as necessary.

Sedation. Opioid analgesics produce sedation and drowsiness. These properties are useful in certain situations (e.g., preoperatively), but they are not desirable in ambulatory patients. The central nervous system (CNS)–depressant actions, in addition to respiratory depressant effects, are synergistic with alcohol, barbiturates, and benzodiazepines. Concurrent administration of dextromethamphetamine (2.5 to 5 mg orally twice daily) has been reported to reduce the sedative effects of opioids. However, it has also been reported that using dextromethamphetamine and similar agents can, in certain individuals, produce adverse effects such as hallucinations, delirium, psychosis, decreased appetite, tremor, and tachycardia and, thus, are contraindicated in those with psychiatric disorders and are relatively contraindicated given a history of paroxysmal tachyarrhythmia. Opioid rotation or switching the route of administration can reduce the severity of opioid sedation. Tolerance to sedative effects of opioids develops within the first several days of long-term administration. Mild cognitive impairment, delirium, and agitated confusion have also been reported in patients taking opioids. CNS effects appear to be idiosyncratic, not dose related. Meperidine was the opioid most commonly associated with adverse CNS events. After gastrointestinal effects (nausea, vomiting, and constipation), the combined CNS effects account for the second highest percentage of adverse drug events.

Pruritus. The mechanism by which opioids cause itching is not fully known, although opioid-mediated direct release of histamine from mast cells is thought to contribute to this effect (most notably with meperidine). Some opioids such as fentanyl and alfentanil do not cause histamine release but can cause mild pruritus; the mechanism of this is not clear. (Morphine, codeine, and meperidine stimulate histamine release. Fentanyl, sufentanil, and alfentanil do not.) If pruritus is accompanied by a rash, allergic reactions cannot be ruled out. In this case, an opioid from a different chemical class may be used. Options for managing itching include histamine-blocking agents such as diphenhydramine, administration of naloxone, or changing the opioid.

Urinary retention. Although urinary retention is a known side effect of opioid administration, it is uncommon when administered for a short periods of time. Opioids increase smooth muscle tone, cause bladder spasm, and increase sphincter tone, resulting in urinary retention, which occurs more frequently in the elderly. Catheterization may be required.

Cough suppression. Suppression of the cough reflex is well-known effect of opioids. In particular, codeine and derivatives are extensively used in antitussive preparations. Dextromethorphan is an over-the-counter antitussive agent that acts centrally at therapeutic doses by binding to opioid receptors. The drug is about equal to codeine in depressing the cough reflex.

Miosis. Constriction of the pupils is seen with all opioids. It is an action to which little or no tolerance develops even in chronic users. This is a valuable sign in the diagnosis of opioid overdose and toxicity (commonly used by law enforcement agents).

Truncal rigidity. An increase in the tone of large trunk muscles (stiff chest) has been seen with administration of large doses of primarily highly lipophilic opioids (e.g., fentanyl, sufentanil, alfentanil) that are administered rapidly (bolus administration). In the setting of acute respiratory distress, a rapidly acting neuromuscular agent such as succinylcholine can be administered to paralyze the muscles and allow ventilation. Alternatively, an opioid antagonist can be used, but this will also antagonize the analgesic effects.

Tolerance. Tolerance is a physiological adaptation to a drug. As a person becomes tolerant to the pharmacological effects, increasing doses are required to produce the same effect. Patients may develop tolerance to some but not all the effects of the opioid. In general, tolerance develops rapidly to the sedative, analgesic, and respiratory effects but is not commonly seen with the constipating effects or the development of miosis. The hallmark of the development of tolerance is a decrease in the duration of effective analgesia. The rate of development of tolerance varies greatly among individuals. However, a sudden increase in opioid requirement may also represent progression of the disease. Opioid rotation may be of value for patients requiring long-term treatment. In addition, combining the opioid with a nonopioid not only provides additive analgesia but also delays the development of tolerance.

Dependence. An individual is physically dependent on a drug when cessation of the drug or a rapid dose reduction initiates symptoms of withdrawal. This generally includes autonomic signs including diarrhea, rhinorrhea, piolerection, sweating, and indicators of central arousal such as sleeplessness, irritability, and psychomotor agitation. Dependence is an expected physiological phenomenon when certain drugs are used for sufficiently long periods of time and is neither a necessary nor a defining characteristic of addiction. Withdrawal can be avoided by slowly tapering the dosage.

Addiction. According to the American Society of Addiction Medicine, addiction is a primary chronic neurobiological disease that is influenced by genetic, psychosocial, and environmental factors. Characteristics of addiction include an impaired control over drug use and/or continued use despite harm and cravings. It has been shown that among persons without a history of substance abuse who are being treated for acute pain, the risk of true iatrogenic addiction is extremely low and the concerns over the development of addiction should be a minor factor in therapeutic decision-making.

Pseudoaddiction. Pseudoaddiction is an iatrogenic syndrome that mimics substance abuse. It resembles addiction but is a direct result of inadequate treatment of pain. For the treatment of acute pain (such as postsurgical pain), clinicians should attempt to provide an adequate regimen of analgesics to avoid this phenomenon.

DISCUSSION

There are three major classes of opioid receptors in the CNS, designated by the Greek letters mu (μ), kappa (κ), and delta (δ) (Table 2-3). Most of the opioids that are used work clinically by binding with relative selectivity to the mu receptors. Peripheral opioid receptors also exist and are thought to be responsible for some of the adverse events. Mu receptor agonists have no therapeutic ceiling effect. Therefore unlike nonopioid analgesics, the dose of these drugs can be adjusted until satisfactory pain control is achieved.

Most members of the opioid family are chemically similar to morphine with minor chemical modifications that change the pharmacokinetics and pharmacodynamics. Pharmacodynamics refers to the biochemical effects of drugs and their mechanism of action. Pharmacokinetics refers to the factors (absorption, distribution, biotransformation, and excretion) that determine the concentration of drug at its sites of action. Pharmacodynamics can be thought of as "what the drug does to the body," and pharmacokinetics can be thought of as "what the body does to the drug."

Individual patients could also be genetically predisposed to poor analgesia. Codeine has very little affinity for the mu receptor and may be considered a prodrug since 10% of the parent drug is converted to morphine by cytochrome P450 (CYP) 2D6. Hydrocodone and oxycodone require demethylation to hydromorphone and oxymorphone, respectively. Approximately 7% to 10% of the Caucasian population metabolizes codeine, oxycodone, and hydrocodone poorly because of inherited deficiencies of CYP2D6 and, thus, analgesia from these drugs will be less than expected.

Finally, a large number of analgesics have both nonopioid and opioid ingredients. Combinations allow a lower dosage of the opioid being used (an "opioid-sparing effect") with a decrease in opioid-related adverse effects. When prescribing these agents, it is important to be aware of the toxic dose of the nonopioid agent.

Table 2-3. Major Opioid Receptors

Receptor	Effects
Mu (μ)	
Mu1	Analgesia
Mu2	Respiratory depression, bradycardia, physical dependence, euphoria, ileus
Delta (δ)	Analgesia, modulates activity at the mu receptor. It is thought that mu and delta receptors coexist
Kappa (κ)	Analgesia, sedation, dysphoria, psychomimetic effects

Bibliography

Bates J, et al: Are peripheral opioid antagonists the solution to opioid side effects? *Anesth Analg* 98:116-122, 2004.

Cherny N, et al: Strategies to manage the adverse effects of oral morphine: an evidence based report, *J Clin Oncol* 19:2542-2554, 2001.

Cepeda MS: Side effects of opioids during short term administration: effect of age gender and race, *Clin Pharmacol Ther* 74:102-112, 2003.

Inturrisi CE: Clinical pharmacology of opioids for pain, *Clin J Pain* 18:S3-S13, 2002.

Katzung BG, ed: *Basic and clinical pharmacology,* ed 9, New York, 2004, Lang/McGraw-Hill.

Plaisance L: Opioid induced constipation. *Am J Nurs* 102:72, 2002.

Phero JC, et al: Contemporary trends in acute pain management, *Curr Opin Otolaryngol Head Neck Surg* 12:209-216, 2004.

Sachs CJ: Oral analgesics for acute nonspecific pain, *Am Fam Phys* 71:913-918, 2005.

Scuderi PE: Pharmacology of antiemetics, *Int Anesthesiol Clin* 41:41-66, 2003.

Strassels SA: Postoperative pain management: a practical review, part 1. *Am J Health Sys Pharm* 62:1904-1916, 2005.

Strassels SA: Postoperative pain management: a practical review, part 2. *Am J Health Sys Pharm* 62:2019-2025, 2005.

Swift JQ: Nonsteroidal anti-inflammatory drugs and opioids: safety and usage concerns in the differential treatment of postoperative orofacial pain, *J Oral Maxillofac Surg* 58:8-11, 2000.

Wheeler M, et al: Adverse events associated with postoperative opioid analgesia: a systematic review, *J Pain* 3:159-180, 2002.

Bisphosphonate-Related Osteonecrosis of the Jaws

Chris Jo, DMD, and Shahrokh C. Bagheri, DMD, MD

CC

A 68-year-old woman with a history of metastatic breast cancer is referred to your clinic by a general dentist for evaluation of intraoral "exposed bone" of her maxilla.

HPI

She is 4 years status post radical mastectomy of her right breast with no recurrence and has been maintained on monthly infusions of zolendronic acid (Zometa) for metastatic bone disease and associated pain and hypercalcemia. (Bisphosphonate therapy is considered the standard of care for treatment of moderate to severe hypercalcemia associated with malignancy, metastatic osteolytic lesions associated with breast cancer and multiple myeloma in conjunction with antineoplastic chemotherapeutic agents and, recently, broadened to include osteolytic lesions arising from any solid tumor.) She had tolerated her treatment well until the development of a sore spot on her left maxillary alveolar ridge approximately 6 months earlier related to her removable denture. Multiple attempts by the general dentist at conservative treatment, including relining the partial denture and minimizing denture wear, has failed to promote the formation of a granulation tissue bed. Now she is complaining of persistent pain and swelling in her left maxilla. She denies any recent history of oral trauma or dental extractions.

PMHX/PDHX/MEDICATIONS/ALLERGIES/SH/FH

The patient has a history of breast cancer and is status post radical mastectomy, receiving monthly intravenous infusions of 5 mg of zolendronic acid.

EXAMINATION

General. The patient is a cooperative, thin woman who is in mild distress.

Vital signs. Her blood pressure is 115/64 mm Hg, heart rate 85, respirations 12 per minute, and temperature 37.6°C.

Maxillofacial. There is left facial swelling with erythema and tenderness along the maxilla.

Intraoral. A 5 × 2-cm area of exposed bone is located along the buccal aspect of the left maxillary edentulous ridge (Figure 2-3). The exposed bone is sharp, irregular, discolored, and surrounded by erythematous mucosa. There is no lymphadenopathy.

Upon palpation, purulent discharge is expressed from the margins of the open wound.

The mandibular mucosa and the remaining teeth appear normal. Oral hygiene is poor.

IMAGING

The panoramic radiograph shows a 5 × 2-cm area of mottled radiolucency in the left maxilla with sharp irregularities that appear to be remnants of an unremodeled extraction socket.

Panoramic radiographs should be the first radiographic study obtained for evaluation of any involved areas. CT can be a useful adjunctive study for more accurate delineation of the lesion, sequestered segments of bone, or pathological mandibular fractures. In addition, the CT scan can be used for soft tissue evaluation and detection of areas of loculations (seen as areas of hypodensity secondary to abscess formation).

LABS

A CBC and a BMP may be necessary in select patients as dictated by the medical history. An elevated WBC count may be indicative of the systemic spread of infection. Electrolyte abnormalities may be seen in patients with compromised nutrition.

This patient presented with no abnormalities on the CBC and BMP.

ASSESSMENT

Osteonecrosis of the left maxilla secondary to bisphosphonate therapy with superimposed acute suppurative osteomyelitis

Bisphosphonate-related osteonecrosis of the jaws (BRONJ), osteonecrosis of the jaws, osteochemonecrosis, "bis-phossy jaw," and bisphosphonate-induced osteonecrosis are all terms used in the recent literature to describe this pathological process.

TREATMENT

The general consensus for the management of bisphosphonate-induced osteonecrosis in the literature appears to be very conservative in nature. This may include long-term oral antibiotics (penicillin is the antibiotic of choice), conservative local debridement, local wound care (chlorhexidine mouth rinse), biopsy, and culture of the exposed bone. Culture and

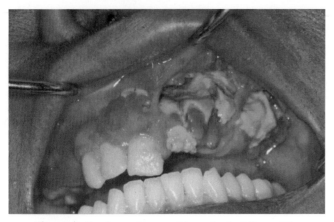

Figure 2-3 Area of exposed bone in the left maxilla.

sensitivities may be necessary to ensure that a resistant organism is not the cause of the osteomyelitis. Biopsy of the involved bone and the irregular surrounding soft tissue is prudent to rule out metastatic or a new primary disease. Local wound care should include saline and chlorhexidine mouth rinses along with systemic long-term antibiotic (penicillin for nonallergic patients). The goals of therapy are palliation and control of osteomyelitis.

In 2004, Ruggiero et al reported a series of 63 patients with bisphosphonate-induced osteonecrosis who were treated using a range of modalities from very conservative debridement to resection. The treatment was individualized based on clinical presentation and clinician's judgment. There appeared to be no clear guidelines for the extent of surgical intervention given the variation in clinical outcomes. The control of osteomyelitis is the critical goal of therapy. This is especially true in the mandible, where uncontrolled osteomyelitis may eventually progress to a pathological fracture.

The role of hyperbaric oxygen (HBO) therapy for bisphosphonate-induced ONJ is unclear. Currently, there are no studies to support or disprove any beneficial effects of HBO in this condition. HBO therapy may improve soft tissue healing and therefore it is hypothesized that is may assist in select cases of bisphosphonate-induced osteonecrosis. Bisphosphonates interfere with bone turnover, resulting in impaired healing capacity. HBO increases the tissue oxygen tension and theoretically does not affect this primary disease process. Further studies are necessary to establish the role of HBO therapy. The role of C-terminal telopeptide is being investigated as a marker of osteoclastic activity and bone turnover potential.

Management of these patients can be extremely difficult. Bisphosphonates are administered systemically, and their effects are not exclusive to the maxillomandibular region. In theory, all bones are equally affected. However, the extensive microbial flora of the oral cavity, along with frequent mucosal trauma, may be the reason this entity appears to have a predilection for the maxillomandibular region. Aggressive debridement of bone is contraindicated because it could lead to further exposure of bone and unnecessary resection. The main goal of therapy should be to control or prevent osteo-

myelitis. Surgical treatment should be reserved for patients who are symptomatic. Areas that are grossly involved and are not responsive to irrigation and antibiotic therapy should be debrided, as they may serve as a constant source of infection. No treatment modality, including cessation of bisphosphonate therapy, has been completely or uniformly effective, although discussion with the oncologist regarding possible discontinuation of bisphosphonate therapy is important.

COMPLICATIONS

ONJ is a recently identified side effect of treatment with bisphosphonates. Practitioners should be alert to identifying patients with this condition and take preventive measures to avoid adverse sequel such as osteomyelitis or pathological fractures.

The inability to definitively treat this condition can have significant quality of life implications for patients such as chronic pain, nonhealing wounds, or the inability to wear dentures.

DISCUSSION

BRONJ secondary to bisphosphonate therapy was reported in the literature by Marx in a letter to the editor of the *Journal of Oral and Maxillofacial Surgery* in 2003, warning clinicians about the alarming rise in this clinical presentation. Subsequently in 2004, Ruggiero et al reported a series of 63 patients treated with bisphosphonates with similar presentations. To this date, many similar cases have been identified.

In 2005, Marx et al published a follow-up article reviewing 119 cases of bisphosphonate-induced BRONJ, implicating Aredia, Zometa, and, to a lesser degree, Fosamax as etiological agents. The mean induction time for clinical bone exposure and symptoms for patients receiving the intravenous bisphosphonates Aredia, Zometa, or both was 14.3, 9.4, and 12.1 months, respectively. For patients receiving the oral medication Fosamax, the mean induction time was 3 years. The bisphosphonates were used in the treatment of multiple myeloma, metastatic breast or prostate cancer, and for prevention of osteoporosis. Pain was the most common finding associated with exposed bone, but about one third of patients were asymptomatic. Other presenting findings included mobile teeth and nonhealing fistulas. The condition was predominantly reported in the mandible (68%) but was also seen in the maxilla (28%) or occurring in both jaws (4%). Periodontitis, dental caries, abscessed teeth, root canal therapy, and mandibular tori were found in association with exposed bone. However, spontaneous exposure with no apparent etiology was also reported. They concluded that complete prevention of this complication in not currently possible and that preventative measures are the best option. In their series, with the use of long-term antibiotics and chlorhexidine mouth rinse, the majority of patients (90%) were able to achieve a pain-free state without resolution of the exposed bone.

The presence of osteonecrosis in the jaws may have a multifactorial etiology in the cancer patient and can be attributed to a cumulative effect of other chemotherapeutic agents and steroid therapy, which may act synergistically with bisphosphonates to promote bone necrosis. However, bisphosphonate therapy was the only common factor in all 63 patients reported by Ruggiero et al. Moreover, seven patients in this series were being treated for osteoporosis with no history of malignant disease or exposure to chemotherapeutic agents or radiation therapy. More than 3 years of oral bisphosphonate use is being considered to increase the risk of BRONJ.

Bisphosphonates are nonmetabolized analogs of pyrophosphate which localize to bone and inhibit osteoclastic function, thereby inhibiting bone resorption and decreasing bone turnover. These chemotherapeutic agents are considered the standard of care for treatment of moderate to severe hypercalcemia associated with malignancy and metastatic osteolytic lesions associated with breast cancer and multiple myeloma. Their efficacy in reducing bone pain, hypercalcemia, and skeletal complications in these patients are well documented. There are two forms of bisphosphonates. Oral bisphosphonates (alendronate, risedronate) are potent osteoclastic inhibitors, but are not efficacious in controlling malignant osteolytic disease and therefore are indicated only for treatment of osteoporosis. The intravenous preparations (pamidronate, zolendronate) are much more potent inhibitors of osteoclasts and are used in cases of metastatic disease. Both forms have been reported in the literature to be associated with ONJ, although the intravenous forms seem to be more prevalent due to its higher potency. Both the maxilla and mandible can be affected, with a slightly higher reported prevalence in the mandible. Traumatically induced and spontaneous development of this condition has been reported.

Alveolar bone appears to have a significant role in this disease process. After extraction of a tooth, the extraction socket and interdental alveolar bone are unable to regenerate new bone in the socket and remodel the sharp bony edges in the face of bisphosphonate therapy. Mucosal closure over these areas is therefore hindered. This clinical situation may progress to chronic osteomyelitis. Radical alveolectomy down to basilar bone to remove this nidus of chronic wound exposure may facilitate soft tissue healing. However, there are currently no data to support this treatment modality.

Patients presenting with pathological fractures of the mandible compromise a formidable challenge. It has been argued by some that the entire mandible is in essence dead bone and that rigid fixation is doomed to failure. Resecting the involved areas without application of an internal fixation device has been advocated, whereas others believe that locking reconstruction plates should be used with fixation screws at distant sights along the posterior border of the ramus. The optimal treatment remains to be elucidated.

The lack of any satisfactory treatment of this condition makes prevention our best treatment. A thorough dental examination and maintenance of oral health prior to and during bisphosphonate therapy are warranted. Avoidance of oral surgical procedures, unless absolutely necessary, along with reduction of denture trauma with soft tissue reliners is recommended. Root canal therapy with coronectomy should be considered in place of tooth extraction, when patients present with a history of intravenous bisphosphonate therapy. Early detection and long-term antibiotics for prevention of osteomyelitis may be prudent.

Bibliography

Athanasios ZI, Shao Z: Bisphosphonates are associated with increased risk for jaw surgery in medical claims data: is it osteonecrosis? *J Oral Maxillofac Surg* 64:917-923, 2006.

Assael LA: A time for perspectives on bisphosphonates, *J Oral Maxillofac Surg* 64:877-879, 2006.

Assael LA: New foundations in understanding osteonecrosis of the jaws, *J Oral Maxillofac Surg* 62:125-126, 2004.

Berenson JR, et al: American Society of Clinical Oncology clinical practical guidelines: the role of bisphosphonates in multiple myeloma, *J Clin Oncol* 20:3719, 2002.

Hellstein JW, Marek CL: Bisphosphonate osteochemonecrosis (bisphossy jaw): is this phossy jaw of the 21st century? *J Oral Maxillofac Surg* 63:682-689, 2005.

Hillner BE, et al: American Society of Clinical Oncology guideline on the role of bisphosphonates in breast cancer, *J Clin Oncol* 18:1378, 2000.

Marx RE: Pamidronate (Aredia) and zoledronate (Zometa) induced avascular necrosis of the jaws: a growing epidemic, *J Oral Maxillofac Surg* 61:1115-1118, 2003.

Marx RE, Sawatari Y, Fortin M, et al: Bisphosphonate-induced exposed bone (osteonecrosis/osteopetrosis) of the jaws: risk factors, recognition, prevention, and treatment, *J Oral Maxillofac Surg* 63:1567-1575, 2005.

McMahon RE, et al: Osteonecrosis: a multifactorial etiology, *J Oral Maxillofac Surg* 62:904-905, 2004.

Pogrel MA: Bisphosphonates and bone necrosis, *J Oral Maxillofac Surg* 62:391-392, 2004.

Rosenberg TJ, Ruggiero S: Osteonecrosis of the jaws associated with the use of bisphosphonates, *J Oral Maxillofac Surg* 61(Suppl 1), 2003.

Ruggiero SL, Mehrotra B, Rosenberg TJ, et al: Osteonecrosis of the jaws associated with the use of bisphosphonates: a review of 63 cases, *J Oral Maxillofac Surg* 62:527-534, 2004.

Sabino MAC, Sevcik MA, Luger NM, et al: The bisphosphonate aldendronate modulates pain, tumor growth, and skeletal remodeling in a bone cancer model, *J Oral Maxillofac Surg* 61(Suppl 1), 2003.

Schwartz HC: Osteonecrosis and bisphosphonates: correlation versus causation, *J Oral Maxillofac Surg* 62:763, 2004.

3 Anesthesia

Chris Jo, DMD

This chapter addresses:
- Laryngospasm
- Perioperative Considerations of the Pregnant Patient
- Respiratory Depression Secondary to Oversedation
- Inadequate Local Anesthesia
- Malignant Hyperthermia
- Emergent Surgical Airway

Like all things in surgery, the most important step in delivering safe and effective anesthesia is preparation. Preparation begins with a thorough knowledge and understanding of the anatomy, physiology, and pharmacology relevant to anesthesia. From this point, safe anesthetic techniques are developed and used based on the preoperative patient evaluation, practitioner's preference, and individual clinical situations. Preparation also includes exercises in avoiding and managing emergencies. Despite a thorough preoperative patient evaluation, use of safe and proven anesthetic techniques, and vigilant monitoring, emergency scenarios may arise. For these reasons, it is paramount that all practitioners continually hone their skills in the recognition and management of life-threatening emergencies in the office or operating room setting. Our

excellent safety record is evidence of training and preparation in the delivery of safe anesthesia by oral and maxillofacial surgeons.

Each of the following teaching cases deals with the management of specific clinical scenarios. The sections are structured to emphasize the key points in the preoperative evaluation and recognition of impending emergencies. Strategies in reducing the risk and the management of emergent scenarios are discussed. The highlighted clinical pearls in the preoperative patient evaluation should become incorporated into the practitioners' routine preoperative assessment.

The intent of this section is to familiarize readers with identifying risk factors and clinical signs associated with anesthetic complications (local, sedation, or general).

Laryngospasm

Michael L. Beckley, DDS, and Shahrokh C. Bagheri, DMD, MD

CC

A 17-year-old girl is undergoing extraction of four partial bony impacted wisdom teeth under intravenous general anesthesia.

HPI

After EKG, blood pressure, and pulse oximeter monitors were applied, the patient was administered 4 L of oxygen and 2 L of nitrous oxide via nasal hood. Sedation was achieved using 4 mg of midazolam and 100 µg of fentanyl titrated to effect. Prior to administration of local anesthesia, 40 mg of propofol was infused. During the incision, respiratory stridor (high-pitched inspiratory "crowing" sound) was noted. A noisy, harsh sound was heard on inspiration through the precordial stethoscope, and the patient's oxygen saturation decreased from 99% to 85%. At this point, the respiratory noises ceased. Tracheal tug and paradoxical chest wall motion were observed (signs of upper airway obstruction), and the patient began to appear cyanotic.

PMHX/PDHX/MEDICATIONS/ALLERGIES/SH/FH

Noncontributory. Recent history of upper respiratory tract infection (URI) may increase the risk of perioperative respiratory complications, especially laryngospasm. In the event of a recent URI, it may be prudent to reschedule surgery after a two-week symptom-free period.

EXAMINATION

General. A harsh inspiratory noise or "crowing" is audible on inspiration, which is best heard through the precordial stethoscope. The patient's skin color is assessed for signs of cyanosis, which is seen with severe hypoxemia.

Oropharynx. The throat pack is removed, and there is no evidence of foreign bodies. Copious amounts of mucous secretions are observed. Blood and mucus are common stimuli for airway irritation.

Neck and chest. There is evidence of tracheal tug and paradoxical chest wall motion (despite chin-lift and jaw-thrust maneuvers). This phenomenon is the result of forced inspiration against a closed glottis.

Vital signs. The patient's heart rate is 125 bpm, blood pressure 145/78 mm Hg, and respirations 0 breaths per minute.

Oxygen saturation. Oxygen saturation decreased from 99% to 85% with the onset of laryngospasm. (Continued decline in the oxygen saturation can result in respiratory acidosis.)

EKG. The patient is in sinus tachycardia. This is a common finding, but hypoxia can trigger more life-threatening cardiac arrhythmias.

IMAGING

Imaging is not relevant in the acute management of laryngospasm. This is an anesthetic emergency and is diagnosed based on the clinical presentation. Chest films can be ordered if there is suspicion of foreign body aspiration or to aid in the diagnosis of negative pressure post obstructive pulmonary edema after the acute management of the airway.

LABS

None are indicated in the acute setting.

ASSESSMENT

Intraoperative laryngospasm during surgical removal of third molars under general anesthesia

TREATMENT

Prompt recognition and treatment of laryngospasm result in a good outcome in almost all cases. Upon diagnosis, the airway should be suctioned clear of noxious stimuli and the surgical site should be packed. Any foreign bodies are removed from the oral cavity and 100% oxygen is administered. Positive pressure ventilation should be attempted, ideally with a two person technique and jaw-thrust maneuver (jaw-thrust and pressure at the angle of the mandible may also assist in breaking laryngospasms). This often "breaks" the laryngospasm. If unable to ventilate, the plane of anesthesia may be deepened with a short-acting intravenous general anesthetic. This often obviates the need for a skeletal muscle relaxant.

In rare situations, these methods are unsuccessful and it will be necessary to administer a short- and fast-acting depolarizing neuromuscular blocking agent, succinylcholine. If intravenous access is not available, succinylcholine may be administered intramuscularly at a dose of 4 mg/kg. A dose of 20 mg intravenously is usually sufficient to break the spasm (pediatric dose, 0.25 mg/kg). However, up to 60 mg can be administered if laryngospasm persists. Rapacurium, rocuronium, and mivacurium can be used for patients in whom succinylcholine is contraindicated. The longer half-life of these nondepolarizing muscle relaxants may require continuous bag-valve-mask ventilation until the spontaneous respiration resumes. Bradycardia is not uncommon after administration of succinylcholine. This usually occurs in children and in adults after repeated doses. Atropine may be administered in an effort to prevent this. Intravenous lidocaine 2 mg/kg administered before extubation was found to be effective in preventing postextubation laryngospasm in patients undergoing tonsillectomy. Other studies have found the prophylactic use of intravenous lidocaine to be ineffective.

COMPLICATIONS

Laryngospasm may produce partial or complete respiratory obstruction. Fortunately, early recognition and management allow for rapid resolution and minimal morbidity. However, with prolonged hypoxemia, the complications can be devastating. Rare complications of laryngospasm include cardiac arrhythmias, anoxic brain injury, negative pressure pulmonary edema, and death. If succinylcholine is administered, the patient may complain of general postoperative myalgia secondary to the rapid muscle depolarization. Other potential complications of succinylcholine include masticator muscle rigidity, malignant hyperthermia, and hyperkalemic cardiac arrest (secondary to the transient hyperkalemia), which can be seen in patients with undiagnosed myopathies (e.g., Duchenne's and Becker's muscular dystrophies).

DISCUSSION

Laryngospasm results in tight approximation of the true vocal cords (Figure 3-1). It is a protective reflex that is most commonly caused by a noxious stimulus to the airway during a light plane of anesthesia. The structural and functional bases of the laryngospasm reflex were described by Rex. Secretions, vomitus, blood, pungent volatile anesthetics, painful stimuli, and oral and nasal airways may elicit this protective reflex. Mediated by the vagus nerve, this reflex is designed to prevent foreign materials from entering the tracheobronchial tree. During laryngospasm, the false vocal cords and supraglottic tissues act like a "ball" valve and obstruct the laryngeal inlet during inspiration. The incidence of laryngospasm has a reported occurrence of 8.7 per 1000 patients receiving general anesthesia. It is 19 times more frequent than bronchospasm. Laryngospasm accounts for more than 50% of the cases of negative pressure/post obstructive pulmonary edema. With the use of general endotracheal intubation, laryngospasm classically occurs during extubation in a light plane of anesthesia (stage II). Children and patients experiencing recent upper respiratory tract infections are predisposed to developing laryngospasm during anesthesia.

Efforts to prevent laryngospasm include postponing surgery in patients with recent upper respiratory infections,

Front

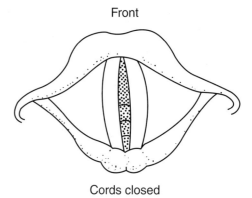

Cords closed

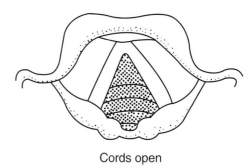

Cords open

Figure 3-1 Tight approximation of the true vocal cords as seen during laryngospasm.

maintaining a dry surgical field, and using anticholinergics and avoiding extubation during stage II of anesthesia. Laryngospasm is not uncommon in outpatient and inpatient oral and maxillofacial surgery. Recognition and early intervention are essential in preventing morbidity and mortality.

Bibliography

Baraka A: Intravenous lidocaine controls extubation laryngospasm in children, *Anesth Analg* 57:506-507, 1978.

Ciavarro C, Kelly JP: Postobstructive pulmonary edema in an obese child after an oral surgery procedure under general anesthesia: a case report, *J Oral Maxillofac Surg* 60(12):1503-1505, 2002.

Hartley M, Vaughan RS: Problems associated with tracheal extubation, *Br J Anaesth* 71:561-568, 1993.

Hurford WE, Bailin MT, Davison JK, et al: *Clinical procedures of the Massachusetts General Hospital,* ed 5, Philadelphia, 1998, Lippincott-Raven, pp 299-300, 514, 609.

Leicht P, Wisborg T, Chraemmer-Joorgensen B: Does intravenous lidocaine prevent laryngospasm after extubation in children? *Anesth Analg* 64:1193-1196, 1985.

Louis PJ, Fernandes R: Negative pressure pulmonary edema, *Oral Surg Oral Med Oral Pathol Oral Radiol Endod* 93(1):4-6, 2002.

Rex MAE: A review of the structural and functional basis of laryngospasm and a discussion of the nerve pathways involved in the reflex and its clinical significance in man and animals, *Br J Anesth* 42:891-898, 1970.

Stoelting RK, Miller RD: *Basics of anesthesia,* ed 3, New York, 1994, Churchill Livingstone, pp 85-90, 161.

Perioperative Considerations of the Pregnant Patient

Chris Jo, DMD, and Jenny Jo, MD

CC

A 29-year-old primigravida (first pregnancy) with twins at 25 weeks of gestation presents to your office for evaluation and management of an odontogenic abscess.

HPI

The patient presents complaining of a 2-week history of dental pain in the right mandible and a 2-day history of progressive swelling of her right face. She is being followed by her obstetrician and states that her pregnancy is progressing without complications. Recently, she has noted good fetal movements on two separate occasions. She denies having any vaginal bleeding or leaking of vaginal fluid (a sign that amniotic fluid may be leaking from ruptured membranes). She started having pelvic cramping just recently (cramping described by pregnant patients may actually be contractions). She has been taking acetaminophen (analgesic of choice during pregnancy) for pain and has not been able to eat adequately for the past 3 days (pregnant patients have a higher nutritional and fluid requirement). There is no history of dysphagia (difficulty swallowing), odynophagia (painful swallowing), dyspnea (difficulty breathing), or subjective fevers.

PMHX/PDHX/MEDICATIONS/ALLERGIES/SH/FH

Noncontributory.

POBHx. This is the patient's first pregnancy. Her only high-risk diagnosis is carrying twins. They are diamniotic/dichorionic (two separate sacs). The twins have had concordant growth on serial ultrasounds, and her cervical length was 4 cm (good length) at 24 weeks (a normal cervical length indicates a reduced risk for an incompetent cervix and preterm labor/delivery. Twins are at higher risk compared to singleton pregnancies).

EXAMINATION

Vital signs. The patient's blood pressure was 110/55 mm Hg, heart rate 110 to 140 bpm (tachycardic), respirations 20 per minute, and temperature 39°C (febrile).

General. She is well developed and well nourished and in no apparent distress.

Maxillofacial. There is a large right-sided facial swelling. The swelling is above the inferior border of the mandible (rules out submandibular space involvement) and below the zygomatic arch (buccal space abscess). It extends from the masseter (submasseteric space involvement) to the oral commissure. The swelling is tense, erythematous, warm, and tender to palpation. The submandibular and submental regions were normal. She has a limited opening (trismus due to involvement of the lateral masticator space) secondary to pain, limiting the intraoral examination. The right mandibular first molar is grossly decayed with adjacent vestibular swelling and purulence extravasating from the gingival sulcus. The oropharynx is not completely visible due to limited mouth opening. The floor of mouth is nonelevated (rules out sublingual space involvement). She is in no respiratory distress and is tolerating her secretions well.

Cardiovascular. The patient is tachycardic with an II/VI systolic ejection murmur (systolic ejection murmur is very common in pregnant women due to high volume of flow but is accentuated by acute tachycardia secondary to elevated temperature).

Abdominal. Examination reveals gravid uterus (pregnant uterus) appearing larger than stated gestational age (due to twins), nontender abdomen, and fetal heart rates of 190s for twin A (the lower presenting fetus in the uterus) and 180s for twin B (the heart rates are elevated above normal due to maternal temperature).

Extremities. The extremities are nontender with 1+ pitting edema at ankles bilaterally (common during pregnancy), no cords, and 2+ equal pulses. She has a negative Homen's sign (calf pain upon dorsiflexion of the foot suggestive of deep vein thrombosis [DVT]).

IMAGING

A panoramic radiograph is the initial diagnostic study of choice. When the oropharynx cannot be adequately visualized due to trismus or a deep neck space abscess is suspected, computed tomography (CT) scanning of the head and neck is necessary to rule out parapharyngeal space (lateral pharyngeal and retropharyngeal spaces) involvement. The use of intravenous contrast material is safe during pregnancy, but the lowest dosing regimen is recommended.

The effects of radiation exposure to the fetus are a potential concern. However, all necessary plain film and CT studies needed to diagnose and manage head and neck infections can be safely performed. The radiation exposure to the developing fetus is minimal and is further reduced by using shielding devices. Furthermore, the benefits outweigh the risks of exposure when dealing with acute head and neck infections. Magnetic resonance imaging (MRI) of the head and neck is also considered safe during pregnancy and can aid in imaging soft tissue pathology.

In this patient, the panoramic radiograph showed a grossly decayed right mandibular first molar with a large periradicular radiolucent lesion. CT was not indicated because the clinical suspicion of parapharyngeal space involvement was low.

LABS

A complete blood cell count (CBC) with platelets and differential is the baseline study.

In this patient, hemoglobin and hematocrit was 11.0 g/dL and 32.6%, respectively (anemia is commonly seen during pregnancy secondary to hemodilution as the increase in plasma volume is relatively larger than the increase in red blood cells; however, pregnant patients are also at risk for iron deficiency anemia). The white blood cell (WBC) count is 18,000/mm^3 with a 15% bandemia (although a slight, nonspecific elevation in WBC count can be seen during pregnancy, this patient's elevated WBC count in conjunction with bandemia and fever is indicative of an acute infection until proved otherwise).

ASSESSMENT

A 29-year-old primigravida with twins at 25 weeks of gestation with a large, right-sided buccal and submasseteric space abscess secondary to a necrotic right mandibular first molar, complicated by dehydration and potential onset of sepsis

TREATMENT

The ideal time to perform elective or semielective oral and maxillofacial surgical procedures is postpartum; otherwise, the second trimester is considered the safest period to perform nonelective surgery. However, the need for urgent or emergent surgery should not be delayed because of pregnancy, especially if procedures can be carried out under local anesthesia. Local anesthesia is the preferred method for simple procedures that can be performed in an office setting (there are no contraindications for vasoconstrictors, but aspiration to avoid intravascular injection is important). When the need arises, intravenous sedation and general anesthesia (in a hospital setting) can be safely performed without significant risk to the mother or fetus in an uncomplicated pregnancy. This is discussed later.

There should be a lower threshhold for hospital admission in the pregnant patient with a maxillofacial infection. Fever, dehydration, inability to tolerate oral intake, and potential airway compromise (risk of airway and pharyngeal edema are higher during pregnancy, especially when parapharyngeal spaces are involved) are all indications for hospital admission and initiation of supportive measures. Other obstetric concerns include risk factors for preterm contractions and preterm labor (onset of labor before 37 weeks of gestation): twins, dehydration, infection, and potential early sepsis. When a

pregnant woman is hospitalized, an obstetric consultation should be obtained. Fluid resuscitation, intravenous antibiotics, and nutritional support are extremely important. Caution should be exercised to avoid excessive fluid overload that can lead to pulmonary edema, as pregnancy and sepsis can both lead to third spacing due to increased capillary permeability. Usually, a 500-ml crystalloid bolus followed by a maintenance level of 100 to 150 ml/hr until the patient is tolerating liquids is appropriate for the average patient. Intravenous antibiotics should also be initiated (the penicillin and cephalosporin families are considered safe first-line antibiotics during pregnancy). Oral and maxillofacial infections should be aggressively treated as untreated infections and abscesses have been associated with preterm labor and maternal sepsis. If a pregnant woman is admitted into the hospital, she and the fetus should be monitored for contractions and fetal well-being with the assistance of an obstetrician. Pain management with a patient-controlled analgesia pump until the patient is tolerating oral medications is appropriate. Intravenous morphine, meperidine (Demerol), and fentanyl or orally administered hydrocodone, oxycodone, or codeine with acetaminophen combinations are all considered safe during pregnancy for necessary pain control. Routine use of nonsteroidal antiinflammatory drugs (NSAIDs) such as ibuprofen and aspirin for postoperative pain control during pregnancy is generally not recommended.

The patient was admitted to the hospital, and an obstetric consultation was obtained. Intravenous fluids and pipercillin/tazobactam 3.375 g every 6 hours were administered. The twins were evaluated for heart tones and contractions. No significant abnormalities were noted. Fetal heart rates were slightly higher than normal due to maternal temperature but were otherwise reassuring. There were no contractions noted. Her pelvic examination was unremarkable, with no evidence of cervical effacement (thinning and shortening of the cervix associated with labor) or of cervical dilatation (also a sign of labor). She was taken to the operating room for incision and drainage of the submasseteric and buccal space abscess and extraction of the right mandibular first molar. Ideally, pregnant patients need to be NPO (nothing to eat or drink, including chewing gum) for at least 8 hours before surgery. In addition to the slower gastric emptying time, pregnancy causes relaxation of the esophageal sphincter; both conditions increase the risk of aspiration associated with general anesthesia. Therefore, preoperatively, this patient received an oral antacid (to increase the pH of gastric contents), H$_2$ antagonist (to decrease gastric acid production), and metoclopramide (to accelerate gastic emptying). Due to the gestational age of the patient, the uterus was enlarged (especially with twins). Thus a roll was placed under her right hip and the table was slightly tilted to the left (this left lateral decubitus tilt of 15 degrees displaces the uterus off the aorta and inferior vena cava and prevents supine hypotensive syndrome, which is due to prolonged compression of the great vessels leading to decreased venous return and cardiac output).

After the patient was positioned, she was intubated via an awake nasal fiberoptic intubation due to her trismus (pregnant patients have edematous nasal mucosa and a potential for epistaxis, especially during a traumatic nasal intubation). The procedure was completed without complications. A thorough intraoperative examination of the oropharynx revealed no parapharyngeal involvement or edema. Her mouth opening increased to normal range after decompressing the lateral masticator (submasseteric) space. Her airway was deemed stable without risk for postoperative upper airway obstruction, and she was successfully extubated. She remained in the hospital for a total of 4 days. She received daily antenatal testing to check for fetal well-being and contractions. She was discharged home on postoperative day 4 after she had been afebrile for over 48 hours and was tolerating full liquids and a regular diet. She received intravenous antibiotics postoperatively until she was able to tolerate medications by mouth and was switched to oral antibiotics. Upon discharge, the patient had significant decrease in her facial swelling, no oral purulent discharge, normalization of her WBC count with no bandemia, and adequate pain control with opioid analgesics.

COMPLICATIONS

Complications associated with surgery under general anesthesia during pregnancy include risk of DVT, pulmonary embolism (PE), aspiration (decreased cardiac sphincter tone, decreased gastric emptying, increased gastric pressures, and hyperemesis increase the risk of regurgitation and aspiration), pulmonary edema, acute respiratory distress syndrome (ARDS), spontaneous abortion during the first trimester, and preterm labor. These are weighed against the risks of an untreated oral or maxillofacial infection, which bears a greater direct risk to both the fetus and the mother, including preterm labor and delivery with complications of a premature neonate, fetal death, eclampsia, maternal sepsis, and septic shock. All elective surgical procedures should be avoided during pregnancy, but necessary surgical interventions should not be delayed.

For the pregnant female undergoing general anesthesia, surgery should be performed in a setting where an obstetrician is available for consultation and where anesthesiologists are familiar with the physiological changes associated with pregnancy. Teratogenic and abortive agents (most important during the first trimester) should be avoided. Specific modifications may be needed as the gestational age of the fetus advances (discussed above). A consultation with an obstetrician provides the appropriate management recommendations.

Pregnancy is a hypercoaguable state (increased clotting factors V, VII, VII, X, and XII). An increase in fibrinolytic activity partially compensates for this state. Accordingly there is an increased risk of DVT (signs include leg pain, tenderness, edema, discoloration, palpable cord, and positive Homen's sign) and subsequent PE (signs include shortness of breath, tachypnea, hypoxemia, and respiratory distress). PE is the most common cause of maternal death. Early detection of DVT (using duplex Doppler ultrasound) and initiation of heparin therapy have significantly reduced maternal mortality. DVT/PE prophylaxis should be initiated upon admission (support stockings, compression devices, and/or subcutaneous heparin).

DISCUSSION

Several other anesthetic considerations are noteworthy. Propofol and thiopental (require only 35% of the normal induction dose and result in a prolonged half-life) are generally safe induction agents for the pregnant patient. There is a 20% to 40% reduction in the minimum alveolar concentration (MAC) of volatile inhalational agents (also has a faster induction rate) during pregnancy. It is important to avoid hypotension resulting in placental hypoperfusion, as has been associated with high doses of inhalational anesthetics. The use of nitrous oxide is safe in routine clinical settings. Opiates, including fentanyl and morphine, are also safe to administer. The use of local anesthesia is safe during pregnancy and is well tolerated by most pregnant patients undergoing minor oral surgical procedures. Although there is a theoretical concern for epinephrine-induced vasoconstriction leading to decreased placental blood flow, epinephrine in local anesthetics is generally considered to be safe. Despite concerns for potential teratogenic effects of benzodiazepines in the first trimester, they can be safely administered when the usual and appropriate doses are used.

For nursing mothers, it has been historically recommended that the patient "pump and dump" after a general anesthetic. With the use of current medications, nursing mothers can pump and discard breast milk for 8 to 24 hours after an intravenous sedation or general anesthetic, to err on the side of caution. Postoperative analgesics (hydrocodone, oxycodone, morphine, ketorolac [Toradol], NSAIDs) are safe to use without pumping and discarding breast milk. However, it is probably safer to "pump and dump" when meperidine is given due to its long-acting metabolite (normeperidine). Perioperative intravenous steroids to help reduce postoperative swelling can be used in pregnancy and in breastfeeding mothers if necessary.

Bibliography

Briggs GG, Freeman RK, Yaffe SJ: *Drugs in pregnancy and lactation,* ed 5, Philadelphia, 2005, Williams and Wilkins.

Cumminham FG, Leveno KJ, Bloom SL, et al: *Williams obstetrics,* ed 21, New York, 2005, McGraw-Hill Professional.

Lawrenz DR, Whitley BD, Helfrick JF: Considerations in the management of maxillofacial infections in the pregnant patient, *J Oral Maxillofac Surg* 54:474-485, 1996.

Turner M, Aziz SR: Management of the pregnant oral and maxillofacial surgery patient, *J Oral Maxillofac Surg* 60:1470-1488, 2002.

Respiratory Depression Secondary to Oversedation

Chris Jo, DMD, and Shahrokh C. Bagheri, DMD, MD

CC

A 45-year-old woman presents to your office for cosmetic eyelid surgery (blepharoplasty).

HPI

The patient is an otherwise healthy woman for whom treatment was planned for bilateral upper and lower eyelid blepharoplasties (see the section on cosmetic upper eyelid blepharoplasty in Chapter 12) with intravenous sedation. After marking the incision lines in the usual manner, EKG, blood pressure, and pulse oximeter monitors were applied. The patient was administered 4 L of oxygen and 2 L of nitrous oxide via nasal hood (nitrous oxide will decrease the amount of intravenous sedatives needed). Sedation was achieved using 5 mg of midazolam, 100 µg of fentanyl, and a propofol drip titrated to effect. Verrill's sign (50% upper eyelid ptosis indicating adequate sedation) was observed. Prior to administering local anesthesia, 40 mg of propofol was administered as a bolus (propofol may cause a 20% to 25% drop in systolic blood pressure when given as a bolus). Upon administration of local anesthesia, the patient remained motionless, and no signs of respiratory effort were seen. Apnea was attributed to the propofol bolus (combined with the respiratory depressant effects of fentanyl), which was anticipated to resolve shortly. However, the patient continued to be apneic, and her oxygen saturation decreased from 99% to 80% (pulse oximeter readings are about 30 seconds behind the real-time oxygen saturation). Tracheal tug and paradoxical chest wall motion were not observed (these would be signs of upper airway obstruction and inspiratory efforts). The patient began to appear cyanotic (bluish hue to facial skin and lips due to prolonged hypoxemia).

PMHX/PDHX/MEDICATIONS/ALLERGIES/SH/FH

A thorough medical history is important during the preoperative evaluation of any patient undergoing intravenous sedation or general anesthesia to identify potential risk factors of intraoperative or postoperative anesthetic complications.

The past medical and surgical histories are noncontributory. She is categorized as American Society of Anesthesiologist (ASA) Class I (Table 3-1). She does not use any medications and has no known drug allergies. She denies previous problems with local anesthetics (such as methemoglobinemia), intravenous sedation, or general anesthetics (problems with previous anesthesia or adverse drug reactions should alert clinicians to possible complications that may require modification of anesthetic techniques). There is no family history of complications with general anesthetics (e.g., malignant hyperthermia). She denies a history of drug or alcohol use (patients with previous drug history or alcohol abuse may require higher doses of sedatives-hypnotics), and she does not smoke (smoking decreases oxyhemoglobin concentrations and increases pulmonary secretions).

EXAMINATION

Preoperative. A thorough preoperative evaluation is important to identify potential risk factors for negative anesthetic outcomes, with an emphasis on airway anatomy.

General. The patient is a well-developed and well-nourished woman in no apparent distress who weighs 60 kg.

Airway. Maximal interincisal opening (MIO) is within normal limits (difficult intubation occurs with decreased MIO). Her oropharynx is Mallampati class I (soft palate, tonsillar pillars, and uvula completely visualized), and the thyromental distance (TMD) is three finger-breadths (there is a greater difficulty with intubation with retrognathia, a short TMD, and/or a higher Mallampati classification). The cervical spine has a full range of motion.

Cardiovascular. Heart is regular rate and rhythm without murmurs, rubs, or gallops.

Pulmonary. Lung fields are clear to auscultation bilaterally (preoperative wheezing may increase the risk of intraoperative bronchospasm).

Intraoperative. During the course of intravenous sedation (conscious sedation, deep sedation, or general anesthesia), it is important to continuously monitor the patient's level of sedation and anesthesia (to prevent oversedation and respiratory depression) and survey the ABCs (airway, breathing, and circulation [Box 3-1]).

General. The patient is sedated/unconscious and unresponsive to painful stimulus (a state of general anesthesia).

IMAGING

Preoperative and serial postoperative photoimaging is mandatory for cosmetic procedures. A preoperative chest radiograph has a limited role in healthy individuals and is not warranted unless dictated by other medical factors.

LABS

Routine laboratory tests are not indicated in healthy patients undergoing cosmetic blepharoplasty with intravenous

Table 3-1.	**The American Society of Anesthesiologist (ASA) Classification System Is Used to Stratify Patients Preoperatively by Risk**			
ASA	**Patient's Health**	**Status of Underlying Disease**	**Limitations on Activities**	**Risk of Adverse Effect**
I	Excellent; no systemic disease; excludes persons at extremes of age	None	None	Minimal
II	Disease of one body system	Well-controlled	None	Minimal
III	Disease of more than one body system or one major system	Controlled	Present but not incapacitated	No immediate danger
IV	Poor with at least one severe disease	Poorly controlled or end stage	Incapacitated	Possible
V	Very poor, moribund		Incapacitated	Imminent

Modified from American Society of Anesthesiologists: *Relative value guide,* 2003, Park Ridge, Ill, 2003, American Society of Anesthesiologists.
Note: ASA I excludes the very young and very old.

Box 3-1.   The ABCs

- **A (airway):** The upper airway is rapidly evaluated and found to be clear or any obstruction. The patient's oropharynx is clear (secretions are suctioned with a tonsillar suction), and no inspiratory or expiratory noises are heard (stridor or gurgling noises may indicate upper airway obstruction). No tracheal tug is present. Chin-tilt/jaw-thrust maneuvers are applied.
- **B (breathing):** There are no inspiratory efforts, and no chest wall or abdominal motion (apnea). Breath sounds are not heard with the precordial stethoscope (placed above the suprasternal notch), and the reservoir bag is motionless. The pulse oximetry (SpO_2) reading has been steadily falling from 99% to 80% (SpO_2 of 90% correlates with a PaO_2 of 60 mm Hg, below which corresponds to the steep portion of the oxygen-hemoglobin dissociation curve).
- **C (circulation):** Blood pressure and heart rate are stable (bradycardia and hypotension due to an extended period of hypoxemia are ominous signs of impending circulatory collapse). The electrocardiogram shows normal sinus rhythm without any ST changes (leads II and V_5 are most sensitive in detecting myocardial hypoxia).

---

sedation. Females of childbearing age who are sexually active and/or have missed their last menstrual period may require a urine pregnancy test (UPT).

ASSESSMENT

Respiratory depression secondary to oversedation during intravenous sedation for cosmetic upper and lower eyelid blepharoplasties

TREATMENT

Before the diagnosis of respiratory depression (apnea or hypopnea) as the cause of hypoxemia, possible causes of upper airway obstruction need to be rapidly ruled out by evaluating the airway, jaw position, and possibility of foreign body aspiration. Subsequently, the procedure should be stopped, any open or bleeding wounds packed, and necessary

assistance should be elicited. Attempts to arouse the patient with verbal command and painful stimulus should be made. Unresponsiveness to painful stimulus is considered to be a state of general anesthesia. Respiratory depression secondary to oversedation is a self-limiting process that requires adequate supportive measures or pharmacological interventions until spontaneous respirations resume.

Nitrous oxide is not a respiratory depressant, but it should be discontinued to allow more rapid arousal from anesthesia and to deliver 100% oxygen, with subsequent resolution of spontaneous respirations. Any anesthetic intravenous drips should be discontinued immediately. Jaw-thrust and/or tugging on the tongue anteriorly will improve the opening of the airway for more effective oxygen delivery. The anesthesia circuit should be flushed to evacuate residual nitrous oxide and to deliver a higher flow of oxygen. If these measures fail, the patient's breathing can be assisted with positive pressure ventilation (PPV), at one breath every 5 seconds (coordinated with any apparent shallow breathing). If oxygenation proves to be successful with PPV, continued ventilatory support is maintained until the sedation lightens and respiratory depression resolves. However, if ventilation is not achieved, rapid reevaluation for other etiologies (laryngospasm, bronchospasm, foreign body aspiration, chest wall rigidity) should be considered. The airway is reassessed, and chin-lift/jaw-thrust maneuvers should be optimized. Oral and/or nasal airways can be inserted if there is continued difficulty with PPV. If laryngospasm or bronchospasm is diagnosed, it should be treated promptly (see Laryngospasm earlier in this chapter). If these measures fail to reestablish ventilation, more advanced airway interventions may be necessary; this includes the use of laryngeal mask airway, endotracheal intubation, or establishment of a surgical airway (cricothyrotomy). Despite the infrequency of the latter scenario, the clinician should be prepared to establish an airway as soon as possible (see Emergent Surgical Airway later in this chapter). Once the oxygen saturation returns above 95%, the clinician can decide whether to cautiously continue with the procedure and intermittently apply PPV as needed or to abort the procedure for further evaluation.

If prolonged respiratory depression occurs, sedative effects of some agent can be pharmacologically reversed. Romazicon (flumazenil) reverses the sedative effects of benzodiazepines. It is given at 0.2 mg intravenously (or 0.01 to 0.02 mg/kg in small children) every minute up to five doses (maximum total dose of 1 mg) until reversal of sedation is accomplished (benzodiazepine overdose has a different schedule). It may be repeated every 20 minutes for resedation. Narcan (naloxone) is an opioid antagonist that reverses the sedative, respiratory depressant, and analgesic effects of opiates. Low doses are recommended (to prevent adverse effects of reversal) at 0.04 mg intravenously (or 0.001 mg/kg) every 2 to 3 minutes until reversal is accomplished (higher dosing schedule is used in narcotic overdose). Once sedation is reversed, the patient needs to be monitored for resedation, as the half-lives of naloxone and flumazenil are shorter than those of their sedative counterparts, potentially requiring redosing of the reversal agent(s). There are no reversal agents for barbiturates or propofol. Reversal of sedation from these agents relies on rapid redistribution of the drugs. It is important to remember that hypoxemia and hypercarbia can further contribute to central nervous system (CNS) depression.

In these patient, supportive measures included 100% oxygen delivered via PPV with a bag-valve-mask device. PPV was easily accomplished, and the patient's oxygen saturation steadily increased to 99%. After sufficient ventilation and oxygenation, the surgery was resumed. The propofol intravenous drip was discontinued during the apnea/hypopnea episode and was subsequently titrated down as the procedure was completed. The patient began to have spontaneous respirations and maintained an adequate oxygen saturation, and she arose from sedation shortly after completion of the procedure. Reversal agents were not required.

COMPLICATIONS

Oversedation and respiratory depression can have devastating outcomes if not promptly treated as outlined here. In most circumstances, the patient's airway and breathing can be easily supported. However, it is important to identify those patients at higher risk of difficult mask ventilation and endotracheal intubation (see Emergent Surgical Airway) before administering deep sedation. The loss of the patient's airway (cannot intubate and cannot ventilate scenario) can lead to prolonged hypoxia, which can in turn lead to cardiovascular collapse, cerebral anoxia, and death if not managed promptly.

Precipitous reversal of sedation and respiratory depression with opioid antagonists is not without adverse side effects. Naloxone (Narcan) may cause cardiac arrhythmias, pulmonary edema, severe hypotension, and cardiac arrest when given at higher doses. The analgesic effects are also reversed, which may cause the patient to experience profound surgical pain, accompanied by hypertension and tachycardia. Patients with acute or chronic opioid dependence can experience acute withdrawal symptoms. Naloxone and flumazenil have short half-lives and may require redosing every 20 to 30 minutes if resedation occurs, and thus, close patient observation is paramount.

DISCUSSION

Various levels of intravenous sedation can be administered by oral and maxillofacial surgeons. *Conscious sedation* is defined as "a controlled, pharmacologically induced, minimally depressed level of consciousness that retains the patient's ability to maintain a patent airway independently and continuously, with the ability to respond appropriately to physical stimulation and/or verbal command." *Deep sedation* is defined as "a controlled, pharmacologically induced state of depressed consciousness from which the patient is not easily aroused, and which may be accompanied by a partial loss of protective reflexes, including the ability to maintain a patent airway independently and/or respond purposefully to physical stimulation or verbal command." *General anesthesia* is defined as "an induced state of unconsciousness accompanied by partial or complete loss of protective reflexes, including the ability to independently maintain an airway and respond purposefully to physical stimulation or verbal command."

Respiratory depression from oversedation can occur during the course of a procedure or in the recovery period but is relatively uncommon when sedation is administered by an experienced oral and maxillofacial surgeon (short half-lives and lack of active metabolites are ideal properties of intravenous anesthetic agents). The short duration of action of modern intravenous anesthetics relies on rapid redistribution (alpha half-life) and/or rapid metabolism. However, repeated doses of opioids, benzodiazepines, or barbiturates for longer procedures may cause accumulation in inactive tissues (especially adipose tissue), which is later released into circulation to cause delayed emergence (beta half-life), thereby on occasion requiring a reversal agents. Naloxone is an opioid antagonist that competitively binds to mu-receptors, effectively reversing the sedative, analgesic, and respiratory-depressant effects of any given opioid (e.g., fentanyl, morphine, sufentanil, alfentanil, remifentanil, meperedine). Flumazenil is a competitive antagonist to benzodiazepines (e.g., midazolam, lorazepam, diazepam) at the central benzodiazepine receptor (alpha subunits of the GABA receptor), and it reverses all effects of benzodiazepines (e.g., sedation, respiratory depression, anxiolysis). The respiratory-depressant effects of midazolam (Versed, the most commonly used benzodiazepine) are minimal compared to those of propofol and narcotics.

Inadequate local anesthesia or insufficient time allocation for its onset may make the sedated patient appear uncooperative or undersedated. The clinician may decide to deepen the sedation to control the uncooperative patient and overcome the effects of inadequate local anesthesia. Once the painful stimulus is gone or the local anesthesia has set in, the patient may return to a deeper level of sedation or may become oversedated with respiratory depression. Risk of oversedation and respiratory depression can be minimized by using local anesthesia effectively.

Some additional precautions should be noted when administering anesthesia to pediatric and elderly patients. Small doses of benzodiazepines and opioids can cause significant respiratory depression in the elderly patient. The changes in physiology and medical comorbidities associated with aging are beyond the scope of this section, but a general precaution used by clinicians is "go low and go slow." It is important to remember that children have a lower functional residual capacity (FRC) and do not tolerate hypoventilation and hypoxemia well, which is evidenced by a more rapid drop in oxygen saturation. Differences in the pediatric airway (larger tongue, lymphyoid hypertrophy, more rostrally positioned larynx, long and floppy epiglottis, narrowest at cricoid cartilage, more compliant tracheal walls, more caudal anterior cord attachment, underdeveloped accessory muscles) are important to recognize.

Bibliography

Bennet J: Intravenous anesthesia for oral and maxillofacial office practice, *Oral Maxillofac Surg Clin N Am* 11(4):601-610, 1999.

D'Eramo EM, Bookless SJ, Howard JB: Adverse events with outpatient anesthesia in Massachusetts, *J Oral Maxillofac Surg* 61:793-800, 2003.

Dripps RD, Eckenhoff JE, Vandam LD, eds: *Introduction to anesthesia: The principles of safe practice,* ed 7, WB Saunders, 1988, Philadelphia.

Perrott DH, Yuen JP, Andresen RV, et al: Office-based ambulatory anesthesia: outcomes of clinical practice of oral and maxillofacial surgeons, *J Oral Maxillofac Surg* 61:983-995, 2003.

Rodgers SF: Safety of intravenous sedation administered by the operating oral surgeon: the first 7 years of office practice, *J Oral Maxillofac Surg* 63:1478-1483, 2005.

Winikoff SI, Rosenblum M: Anesthetic management of the pediatric patient for ambulatory surgery, *Oral Maxillofac Surg Clin N Am* 11(4):505-517, 1999.

Vezeau PJ: Anesthetic and medical management of the elderly oral and maxillofacial surgery patient, *Oral Maxillofac Surg Clin N Am* 11(4):549-559, 1999.

Inadequate Local Anesthesia

Gary F. Bouloux, MD, DDS, MDSc, FRACDS, FRACDS (OMS), and Shahrokh C. Bagheri, DMD, MD

CC

A 38-year-old man presents with left facial swelling and pain secondary to a carious left maxillary cuspid (acute infection decreases the efficacy of local anesthetics).

HPI

The patient reports a 2-month period of a toothache localized to the upper left quadrant. Two days ago, he experienced an acute exacerbation of his pain along with the development of progressively enlarging left facial swelling. He was subsequently seen by his general dental practitioner, who attempted to extract the tooth but was unsuccessful due to persistent pain despite several local anesthetic injections.

PMHX/PDHX/MEDICATIONS/ALLERGIES/SH/FH

Noncontributory. The patient has had multiple dental restorations under local anesthesia without any complications. He has no known drug allergies.

Although occasionally patients report an "allergy" to epinephrine, this is a naturally occurring catecholamine present in all individuals that plays a critical role in homeostasis and is *not* a source of allergic reactions. The transient tachycardia that may be seen with local anesthetic injections that contain epinephrine (especially with intravascular injection) is simply an adrenergic response to the epinephrine.

EXAMINATION

Maxillofacial. There is a fluctuant and tender swelling extending from the midline of the upper lip to the left cheek, consistent with left canine space abscess.

IMAGING

Panoramic radiograph reveals a carious left maxillary cuspid with an associated 1.5-cm periapical radiolucent lesion.

LABS

No routine laboratory tests are indicated unless dictated by the medical history. A WBC count may be obtained to monitor for leukocytosis.

ASSESSMENT

Left canine space infection complicated by failure to extract the left maxillary cuspid secondary to inadequate local anesthesia

TREATMENT

Management of failure to achieve adequate local anesthesia should be evaluated for any etiologic factors. Anatomical variation, accessory innervation, poor technique, inadequate volume or concentration of local anesthetic, the presence of infection, or an excessively anxious patient may all contribute to the failure to achieve adequate local anesthesia. Upon identification of potential causes, the clinician should develop a stepwise plan to address the problem. A reasonable approach may utilize supplemental anesthetic injections, regional block anesthesia (rather than infiltration), intraligamentary injections, intraosseous injections, intrapulpal injections, or addition of other medications such as nitrous oxide for anxiolysis and analgesia. With failure of all the above measures, consideration must be given to either deep sedation or general anesthesia.

In this patient, the infraorbital rim (infraorbital foramen is approximately 8 mm inferior to the rim) was palpated, and the overlying tissues was cleansed with an alcohol wipe. A total of 5 ml of 2% lidocaine with 1 : 100,000 epinephrine was injected after placing the tip of the hypodermic needle through the skin against the foramen. The tissue was gently massaged to facilitate diffusion of the local anesthetic into the foramen to anesthetize the infraorbital and anterior superior alveolar nerves. The nasopalatine and greater palatine nerves were anesthetized in the usual manner. After 10 minutes, the left maxillary cuspid was extracted without any subjective pain. No purulent drainage was obtained through the socket, and therefore a horizontal vestibular incision was made, allowing the release of approximately 10 ml of purulent drainage. A sample of the pus was sent for Gram stain, aerobic and anaerobic cultures, and antibiotic sensitivity. A drain was placed and the wound was left open to facilitate continued drainage. The patient was prescribed a 10-day course of penicillin and instructed to rinse with warm saltwater five times a day. An opioid with acetaminophen was prescribed for postoperative pain control. The patient was seen at 2 and 7 days for drain removal and follow-up with subsequent resolution of the infection.

COMPLICATIONS

Complications related to failure to achieve local anesthesia are related to the psychological impact and frustration by the patient and clinician, the added cost and time to complete a necessary procedure using a different modality, and possible toxic effects of local anesthetic due to repeat injections. The negative impact on a patient's perception of the dental profession should not be underestimated.

Complications may also be related to the progression of the disease process (such as the spread of infection) that failed to be treated due to the inadequacy of local anesthesia. Infection must be treated as soon as possible to reduce the likelihood of the patient becoming septic (disseminated infection). Furthermore, infections in close proximity to vital structures (such as the eye) may rapidly spread, causing dissemination of the infection into distant areas. This includes spread of infection into the orbit or, via communicating veins, into the cavernous sinus with the development of cavernous sinus thrombosis. The presence of significant infraorbital swelling and tenderness is a relative contraindication to the use of the extraoral infraorbital anesthetic block due to concern for the development of cavernous sinus thrombosis.

There are several strategies to overcome the inadequacy of local anesthesia in the presence of infection. A larger volume or a higher concentration of the local anesthetic solution may be used. However, care must be taken to avoid toxicity from an excessive volume of local anesthetic. Toxicity initially presents as CNS excitation, but with increasing doses, CNS depression (including respiratory depression) can be seen. Epinephrine will substantially reduce toxicity by decreasing tissue absorption. However, epinephrine can result in tachyarrhythmias and increased blood pressure, particularly with inadvertent intravascular injection.

The initial excitement and agitation seen with local anesthetic toxicity are due to the suppression of the inhibitory cortical neurons, while the more common somnolence and decreased consciousness are secondary to inhibition of excitatory cortical neurons. Treatment is purely supportive with attention to the airway, breathing, and circulation (ABCs). An increase in heart rate (beta$_1$-receptor stimulation) and blood pressure (alpha$_1$-receptor stimulation) may also follow the inadvertent intravascular administration of epinephrine containing local anesthetic. This should be considered carefully when treating patients with cardiac conditions, although local anesthetics containing epinephrine are more efficacious due to the localized vasoconstriction that reduces systemic absorption of the catecholamine. However, the pain and anxiety generated with inadequate local anesthesia may be more harmful than the administration of a local anesthetic containing epinephrine due to the release of endogenous catecholamines. Aspiration after placement of the local anesthetic needle in the tissues and prior to injection should always be performed to reduce the likelihood of intravascular injection. The toxic doses of the most commonly used anesthetics are listed in Table 3-2.

Table 3-2.	Commonly Used Local Anesthetics in Oral and Maxillofacial Surgery			
Local Anesthetic	Onset (min)	Duration of Action (min)	pK_a	Maximum Dose
Lidocaine	3 to 5	60 to 90	7.9	7 mg/kg (with vasoconstrictor) 4 mg/kg (without vasoconstrictor)
Bupivacaine	5 to 10	90 to 180	8.1	2 mg/kg*
Mepivacaine	3 to 5	45 to 90	7.8	5 mg/kg*
Articaine	3 to 5	120 to 180	7.8	7 mg/kg*

*With or without epinephrine.

DISCUSSION

Failure to achieve local anesthesia can be due to multiple factors, including the technique, anatomy, infection, and patient selection. The latter can often be predicted from the initial patient consultation and can potentially be avoided by alternate or modified surgical planning (sedation, regional block, preoperative anxiolytics). Appropriate choice of local anesthetic agent, adequate volume, and the choice of infiltration versus regional block anesthesia must be considered carefully. Anatomical variations may result in unusual neural innervation of mandibular and maxillary structures. A stepwise progression from more distal infiltration to more proximal regional block anesthesia will often overcome this difficulty. Anesthesia of maxillary structures may necessitate extraoral infraorbital anesthesia (as in the present case) or a maxillary (V$_2$) block anesthesia via the greater palatine foramen or pterygomaxillary fissure. Anesthesia of the mandibular structures may necessitate consideration of accessory neural pathways such as the nerve to mylohyoid. The use of the closed mouth (Akinosi) technique for patients with trismus should be considered. The Gow-Gates technique may also be helpful when anesthesia of the mandibular trunk is desired or in cases of failed attempts at inferior alveolar nerve block using standard technique.

The presence of infection is generally considered to reduce the effectiveness of local anesthetics due to several mechanisms. The primary mechanism is due to the altered pH of the tissue. Different local anesthetics have different dissociation constants (pK_a), which define the concentration of ionized and nonionized local anesthetic at a given pH. The nonionized form of the local anesthetic is responsible for penetrating nerve membranes and subsequently dissociating to give the ionized form, which blocks sodium channels. In the presence of infection and hence a lower tissue pH, lidocaine with a pK_a of 7.9 exists predominantly in the ionized form, which is unable to diffuse through membranes. While giving additional anesthetic is reasonable, a better choice would be to increase the concentration (percent) of the agent or to use a different agent with a lower pK_a so that more of the nonionized form is available. Additionally, the increased tissue perfusion secondary to inflammation may increase removal of the local anesthetic from the site of administration, although this plays a minor role. A more proximal regional block anesthetic injection may also suffice in the presence of infection as the local anesthetic is delivered into the uninfected tissue, and therefore problems related to a decreased tissue pH are avoided. It should be remembered, however, that chronic pain may result in both peripheral and central nervous system sensitization that may reduce the efficacy of the local anesthetic, even when given as a regional block away from the source of infection or pain.

Bibliography

Bouloux GF, Punnia-Moorthy A: Bupivacaine versus lignocaine for third molar surgery: a double blind randomized crossover study, *J Oral Maxillofac Surg* 57:510-514, 1999.

Feldman H: Toxicology of local anesthetic agents. In Rice S, Fish K, eds: *Anesthetic toxicity,* New York, 1994, Raven Press, pp 107-133.

Tofoli GR, Ramacciato JC, De Oliveira PC, et al: Comparison of effectiveness of 4% articaine associated with 1:100,000 or 1:200,000 epinephrine in inferior alveolar nerve block, *Anesth Prog* 50:164-168, 2003.

Malignant Hyperthermia

Vincent J. Perciaccante, DDS, and Shahrokh C. Bagheri, DMD, MD

CC

A 15 year-old boy (incidence of malignant hyperthermia [MH] is highest in children) is undergoing an open reduction with internal fixation (ORIF) of a left mandibular angle fracture in the operating room. He had presented to the emergency department complaining of pain, swelling, and malocclusion.

HPI

While playing ball, the patient sustained an accidental blow to the left side of the jaw from an opponent's elbow. He was diagnosed with a fractured mandible and subsequently was admitted to the hospital for treatment of his injury under general anesthesia. The patient was induced with propofol, given succinylcholine, and nasotracheally intubated without difficulty. He was maintained on sevoflurane (halogenated inhaled anesthetic) and intravenous agents. The patient had a smooth anesthetic course for the first 20 minutes of the procedure before the onset of unexplained tachycardia and elevation in his end-tidal CO_2 (earliest signs of MH). The diagnosis of MH was considered.

PMHX/PDHX/MEDICATIONS/ALLERGIES/SH/FH

He underwent tonsillectomy and adenoidectomy at age 6 under general anesthesia without any surgical or anesthetic complications (MH can be triggered in a susceptible patient who previously underwent an uneventful anesthetic). His family history is negative for MH (MH is an autosomal dominant inherited disorder. However, many patients present with MH without any prior documented FH).

EXAMINATION

MH is a life-threatening hypermetabolic state that can be recognized by a variety of signs and symptoms, most commonly while the patient is under general anesthesia.

General. Muscle rigidity (commonly seen in the masseters) and skin mottling are present.

Vital signs. His heart rate is 130 bpm (unexplained tachycardia is one of the early signs), temperature 39.2°C (hyperthermia is regarded as a hallmark feature, but it may be a late finding), and respirations 34 per minute (tachypnea).

Adjunctive monitors. His end-tidal CO_2 is 57 mm Hg and rising (hypercapnia) (end-tidal CO_2 can rise to 2 to 3 times normal at a constant minute ventilation).

EKG. He has sinus tachycardia at 130 bpm (supraventricular and ventricular arrhythmias, including cardiac arrest, can be observed).

IMAGING

No imaging studies are indicated in the acute management of MH. A chest radiograph is obtained after the initial treatment to evaluate the position of the endotracheal tube if the patient remains intubated and for evaluation of the lung fields.

LABS

Upon diagnosis of MH, a full set of serum electrolytes, liver function tests, urinalysis, and arterial blood gases should be ordered to aid in the correction and diagnosis of electrolyte and acid-base disturbances.

The laboratory findings would characteristically reflect the following metabolic conditions:

- Acidemia (elevated Pco_2 and metabolic [lactic] acidosis)
- Hyperkalemia (secondary to acidosis)
- Hypercalcemia (secondary to reduced uptake of Ca^{2+} from the sarcoplasmic reticulum of skeletal muscles)
- Elevated serum transaminases and creatinine kinase (CK) and subsequent rhabdomyolysis causing myoglobinuria (secondary to hypermetabolic skeletal muscle activity)

ASSESSMENT

Acute onset of malignant hyperthermia during ORIF of a mandible fracture

TREATMENT

The successful treatment of MH constitutes early administration of dantrolene and removal of the triggering agent. Box 3-2 details the steps that should be followed when treating MH.

Arrhythmias usually respond to correction of acidosis and hyperkalemia. Antiarrhythmic agents, excluding calcium channel blockers, may be used for arrhythmias that do not respond to correction of acidosis and hyperkalemia.

COMPLICATIONS

The mortality rate of untreated MH has been reported to be as high as nearly 70%. Approximately 25% of persons with

Box 3-2.	Steps for Treating Malignant Hyperthermia

- Activate EMS, if not within a hospital.
- Discontinue the surgical procedure as quickly as possible.
- Discontinue the triggering agents.
- Hyperventilate with 100% O_2 at 3 to 4 times the normal minute ventilation.
- Give dantrolene sodium 2.5 mg/kg intravenously, repeated every 5 to 10 minutes based on ongoing signs of MH.
  - 36 Vials should be on hand (20 mg/vial)
  - Add 60 ml of sterile water without bacteriostatic agent to each vial of dantrolene to reconstitute the drug
  - Shake vigorously to reconstitute (until clear)
  - Use IV spike transfer pins to reconstitute
  - Once mixed, protect from direct light
  - 2.5 mg/kg body weight given initially, repeated every 5 to 10 minutes
  - Continue administration until signs of MH abate
- Obtain ABGs, treat hyperkalemia (glucose, insulin, and calcium) and acidosis (bicarbonate 1 to 2 mEq/kg).
- In case of hyperthermia: Cooling measures should be instituted with cold IV fluids (normal saline), external ice packs to groin and axilla, and gastric lavage with cold solutions.
- Call the MH hotline for immediate consultation at 1-800-MH-HYPER.

MH relapse within the first 24 hours. Following an MH episode, the patient should be transferred to an intensive care unit until all vital signs have returned to normal. Dantrolene treatment should be continued during this period; the usual dose is 1 mg/kg intravenously every 4 to 6 hours.

DISCUSSION

The incidence of MH may be as high as 1:5000 to 1:65,000 in children. Triggering agents, such as succinylcholine and volatile anesthetic agents, in a genetically predisposed patient release calcium from the sarcoplasmic reticulum, leading to elevated concentrations of calcium in the muscle cells. This increased metabolism causes the muscles to contract and become rigid. The increased metabolism leads to the elevated end-tidal CO_2 and acidosis. Rhabdomyolysis leads to hyperkalemia and potential arrhythmias, as well as myoglobinuria and potential renal failure.

The routine use of succinylcholine has fallen out of favor. Many anesthesiologists use nondepolarizing agents such as rapacuronium or rocuronium when possible. However, none of these drugs have replaced succinylcholine for rapid sequence intubation or the reversal of laryngospasm. Dantolene sodium should be available in all facilities at which any triggering agents are routinely used.

In preparation for an anesthetic procedure with a known MH-susceptible patient, anesthetic vaporizers are removed or taped in the off position. The carbon dioxide absorbent (soda lime or baralyme) is changed. Oxygen at 10 L/m is flushed through the circuit via the ventilator for at least 20 minutes. During this time, a disposable, unused breathing bag should be attached to the Y-piece of the circle system and the ventilator set to inflate the bag periodically. The use of a new or disposable breathing circuit is recommended.

Bibliography

Ball SP, Johnson KJ: The genetics of malignant hyperthermia, *J Med Genet* 30:89, 1993.

Collins CP, Beirne OR: Concepts in the prevention and management of malignant hyperthermia, *J Oral Maxillofac Surg* 61(11):1340-1345, 2003.

Davison JK, Eckhardt WF, Perese DA: *Clinical anesthesia procedures of the Massachusetts General Hospital,* Boston, 2003, Little, Brown.

Malignant Hyperthermia Association of the United States: Managing MH: clinical update September 2002. Available at: http://www.mhaus.org/index.cfm/fuseaction/OnlineBrochures.Display/BrochurePK/3FFCBC12-9479-49C3-8A9E0B304EF08746.cfm. Accessed June 2006.

Rosenberg H, Fletcher JE : An update on the malignant hyperthermia syndrome, *Ann Acad Med Singapore* 23:84, 1994.

Emergent Surgical Airway

John M. Allen, DMD, and Chris Jo, DMD

CC

A 48-year-old man presents to the emergency department complaining of difficulty breathing and inability to swallow.

HPI

The patient has a 2-month history of intermittent swelling of his right mandible associated with a carious right mandibular first molar. For the past 3 days, he has developed rapidly increasing swelling of the right floor of the mouth (sublingual space) and submandibular triangle (submandibular space) that has spread to the contralateral side, consistent with Ludwig's angina (see Chapter 4, the section on Ludwig's angina). During the past 24 hours, he has been sitting upright in the sniffing position (unable to lay supine because of a choking sensation), has been unable to control his secretions, has had difficulty swallowing (dysphagia), and has been unable to open his mouth (trismus). His tongue has protruded forward (glossoptosis), and he is having difficulty talking (dysphonia). His level of anxiety has increased with the onset of progressive dyspnea (difficulty breathing), and he is now unable to clear his airway, making gurgling noises and a faint high-pitched crowing sound (signs of upper airway obstruction).

PMHX/PDHX/MEDICATIONS/ALLERGIES/SH/FH

His past medical history is significant for well-controlled type 2 diabetes and morbid obesity.

EXAMINATION

General. The patient is a well-developed moderately obese male in severe respiratory distress (obesity increases the difficulty of endotracheal intubation).

Vitals signs. His blood pressure is 168/94 mm Hg (hypertension), heart rate 120 bpm (tachycardia), respirations 25 per minute (tachypnea), and temperature 39.4°C, with oxygen saturation of 96% on 5-L oxygen via nasal cannula.

Maxillofacial. He has bilateral submandibular and submental brawny cellulitis that is tender to palpation, warm, and erythematous. The neck is moderately sized, but the trachea and larynx are easily palpable. The trachea is midline (deviated trachea increases the difficulty of intubation). The cervical spine has full range of motion (neck extension facilitates intubation or securing a surgical airway).

Intraoral. Oral examination is limited due to decreased mouth opening. He is unable to handle his secretions (dysphagia, evidenced by drooling of saliva). The floor of the mouth is elevated, tender, and edematous. The tongue is large and protruding forward. The uvula and soft palate are not visible (Mallampati Class IV). The right mandibular first molar is grossly carious. Further airway evaluation can be performed with fiberoptic nasopharygoscopy (to visualize the hyopharynx, base of tongue, pharyngeal walls, epiglottis, and vocal cords) to determine airway patency and the amount of airway edema.

Figure 3-2 is a diagrammatic representation of the surgical landmarks related to the airway; these include the thyroid notch, cricothyroid membrane, cricoid cartilage, and suprasternal notch.

IMAGING

In the setting of impending airway embarrassment, any attempts to obtain imaging studies should be delayed until a secure airway is established. Loss of an airway in the radiology suite where anesthesia staff and an experienced surgeon are not immediately available can be devastating. Therefore, upon evaluation of the patient, the surgeon needs to rapidly make a decision to either progress directly to the operating room, where optimal personnel and equipment for advanced airway interventions are available, or, in more emergent settings, proceed to establish a surgical airway in the emergency department (this should be avoided if possible).

If the patient is deemed to be stable, with no immediate threat to airway obstruction, a panoramic radiograph (to evaluate possible odontogenic sources of infection), and a CT scan with contrast (to localize loculated areas of abscess formation and to assist in airway evaluation) can be obtained. A lateral cephalometric radiograph is a readily available study that can be obtained at bedside. It can provide some information regarding the posterior airway space (prevertebral soft tissue should be less than 7 mm and 20 mm at the level of C3 and C7, respectively); with the advent of fiberoptic nasopharyngoscopy and CT, it is infrequently used.

In this patient, no radiographic studies were ordered due to airway instability, and the patient was taken directly to the operating room.

LABS

Laboratory studies should not delay the establishment of a secure airway. When possible, a CBC with differential and a basic metabolic panel are indicated for evaluation of the sys-

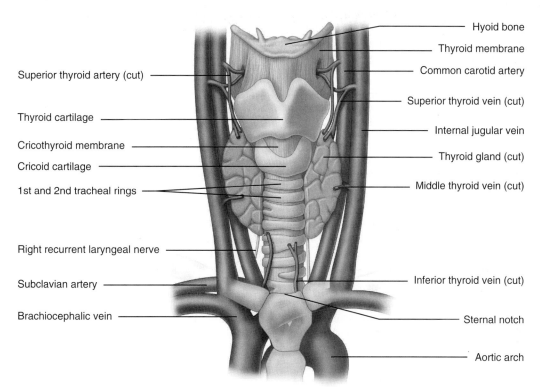

Hyoid bone

Thyroid membrane

Common carotid artery

Superior thyroid vein (cut)

Internal jugular vein

Thyroid gland (cut)

Middle thyroid vein (cut)

Inferior thyroid vein (cut)

Sternal notch

Aortic arch

Superior thyroid artery (cut)

Thyroid cartilage

Cricothyroid membrane

Cricoid cartilage

1st and 2nd tracheal rings

Right recurrent laryngeal nerve

Subclavian artery

Brachiocephalic vein

Figure 3-2   Surgical landmarks of the neck in relation to the airway.

temic response and metabolic derangements associated with severe odontogenic fascial space infections. Arterial blood gas analysis can be used to determine the adequacy of ventilation. Other laboratory values are ordered based on pertinent medical information.

A STAT laboratory study obtained by the emergency physician demonstrated a WBC count of 18,000 cells/mm³ and a blood glucose concentration of 310 mg/dl.

ASSESSMENT

A 46-year-old man with Ludwig's angina now complicated by an impending loss of airway

TREATMENT

Upon suspicion or diagnosis of impending airway embarrassment, the anesthesia team and operating room–emergency department staff needs to be notified immediately. The surgeon and anesthesiologist (if available) need to decide the safest means of rapidly obtaining a secure airway. Patients with potential difficult airways (difficult mask ventilation and difficult intubations) need to be identified in anticipation for advanced airway interventions (identified risk factors include obesity, short neck, rigid neck, small mouth opening, retrognathia, Mallampati Class III and IV, and prominent upper incisors).

Patients that are deemed difficult to intubate are potential candidates for awake fiberoptic nasal intubation or an elective awake tracheotomy in a controlled operating room setting.

However, it is possible for a "routine" intubation procedure to convert into a difficult airway during an otherwise unanticipated presentation. During the course of a difficult laryngoscopy, the anesthetist or anesthesiologist may not be able to intubate or adequately ventilate the patient, requiring an emergent surgical airway (fortunately this is uncommon). For emergent intervention of a comprised airway in the adult patient, a cricothyroidotomy is the procedure of choice. Tracheostomy is used for emergency surgical airways in the pediatric population younger than 10 to 12 years. The small size of the cricothyroid membrane (3 mm) and the poorly defined anatomic landmarks make performing a cricothyroidotomy extremely difficult in children. There is also an increased risk of laryngeal and vocal cord injury with cricothyroidotomy in this age group.

Needle cricothyroidotomy with jet insufflation can also be performed by skilled anesthesia personnel (providing temporary oxygenation but not ventilation). The patient can be oxygenated while the surgeon establishes a definitive surgical airway (tracheotomy or cricothyroidotomy). If a surgical cricothyroidotomy is performed, conversion into a formal tracheotomy should be considered, primarily depending on the anticipated duration for the surgical airway (patients requiring prolonged ventilatory support should be converted to a tracheotomy). The techniques for each are described below.

Needle cricothyroidotomy with jet insufflation. Ideally, the patient should be supine or semisupine with a shoulder bolster to hyperextend the neck. The cricothyroid membrane (slight depression between the thyroid cartilage and cricoid cartilage) is palpated, and the larynx is stabilized using the thumb and forefinger. In a thin neck with prominent landmarks, an incision is not needed and direct puncture through skin and cricothyroid membrane can be accomplished. It may be necessary to make a small incision through skin over the identified region of the cricothyroid membrane. Using a 3-ml syringe attached to a 14-gauge angiocatheter, the needle is inserted through the cricothyroid membrane, directing the needle at a 45-degree angle caudally while applying negative pressure to the syringe and aspirating as the needle is advanced (aspiration of air indicates entry into the tracheal lumen). The 14-gauge needle is removed from the angiocatheter, leaving the angiocatheter within the trachea. Once in place, the catheter can be insufflated with oxygen with commercially available kits or with clinical ingenuity. A small hole can be cut in the oxygen tubing near its attachment to the 3-ml syringe (can also be attached to a 7.5 endotracheal tube connector). The hole is occluded for 1 second and left open for 4 seconds, forcing oxygen into the trachea and allowing for some passive exhalation (if any). Adequate oxygenation can be maintained for 30 to 45 minutes, but hypercarbia will result from inadequate ventilation. Preparations should be made to convert the airway to a tracheotomy or for another attempt at endotracheal intubation, at the surgeon's and anesthesiologist's discretion.

Surgical cricothyroidotomy. The nondominant hand is used to stabilize the laryngeal cartilage, and a vertical skin incision is made using a No. 15 or 11 (or any available) blade over the cricothyroid membrane (providing the option of superior-inferior extension of the incision as needed). The incision is carried through the skin and superficial fat layer, immediately over the cricothryoid membrane, which is vertically incised with the blade. Subsequently, the blade handle is inserted into the incision site and rotated 90 degrees to provide access into the tracheal lumen. The lumen is further dilated with finger dissection or with the use of a Trousseau dilator. A small cuffed endotracheal, or tracheotomy tube, is inserted and the patient is ventilated. A positive return of carbon dioxide is the best modality to confirm correct tube placement. The tube is secured, and the chest is auscultated for bilateral breath sounds.

In this patient, an emergent surgical cricothyroidotomy was performed after the airway was lost during an unsuccessful attempt at an awake fiberoptic nasal intubation. Due to the severity of infection, difficulty of airway, and prolonged anticipation of cannulation, the cricothyroidotomy was subsequently converted to a formal tracheotomy.

COMPLICATIONS

The most feared complication involved with performing a needle cricothyroidotomy procedure is inadequate oxygenation and ventilation leading to anoxic brain injury and cardiovascular collapse. Proper placement of the insufflating needle is paramount for a successful outcome. Complications associated with the emergent nature of this procedure are associated with the placement and manipulation of the 14-gauge needle. Laceration of adjacent structures, including the thyroid, the posterior tracheal wall, and the esophagus, can occur leading to severe hemorrhage, which can cause embarrassment of the already compromised airway. Hematoma formation and aspiration of blood can contribute to a negative outcome. Improper placement of the needle can also result in subcutaneous or mediastinal emphysema.

Complications associated with surgical cricothyroidotomy include all the acute events discussed with the needle cricothyroidotomy procedure, as well as chronic complications associated with the surgical intervention. Creation of a false passage into the surrounding connective tissue and damage to the larynx and vocal cords can result from improper or forced introduction of the endotracheal tube. Subsequent laryngeal stenosis or vocal cord paralysis may occur, resulting in permanent damage.

DISCUSSION

The various possible etiologies of airway embarrassment (loss of airway) secondary to upper airway obstruction (severe maxillofacial trauma, infections, tumors, congenital or developmental deformities, laryngospasm, foreign body, or edema) can be differentiated based on chronology, presentation, and physical and radiographic findings. A true loss of airway is defined as the inability to ventilate (with bag-mask-valve, laryngeal mask airway, or Combitube) and inability to intubate an unconscious patient (a surgical emergency). Although it is usually progressive, it may have a sudden onset based on etiology and can occur prior to arrival to the operating room, during an attempted intubation, after extubation, or in an office setting during intravenous sedation. This is distinguished from loss of protective airway reflexes, in which the patient has an upper airway obstruction that is easily managed with chin-lift/jaw-thrust, oral or nasal airways, and positive pressure mask ventilation (see Chapter 3, the section on respiratory depression secondary to oversedation).

There are numerous situations where an oral and maxillofacial surgeon may encounter patients with difficult airways and/or acute airway embarrassment. The surgeon and anesthesia team should communicate to anticipate the likelihood of a difficult intubation (requiring awake fiberoptic nasal intubation) or possible loss of airway (requiring emergent surgical intervention). The surgeon should take charge once the airway is lost (cannot intubate, cannot ventilate scenario) and rapidly secure a surgical airway, as described earlier. The operating room staff should be prepared to assist for an emergent cricothyroidotomy (in the adult) or tracheotomy (in the pediatric patient).

Recognition of a compromised airway represents the most difficult and crucial step in airway management. A compromised airway may be classified as sudden and complete, insidious and partial, or progressive. Assessment and frequent reassessment of airway patency and adequacy of ventilation are crucial. A patient's refusal to lie down may be an indicator that the patient is unable to maintain the airway or handle secretions. Tachypnea is generally related to pain and anxiety but may also be an early indicator of airway or ventilatory collapse. Compromised ventilatory efforts may occur in unconscious patients with alcohol or drug abuse or neck, thoracic, or intracranial injuries. These patients often require endotracheal intubation to establish and maintain a definitive airway and to protect against pulmonary aspiration.

Objective signs of airway obstruction may be revealed with visual assessment to determine whether the patient is agitated or obtunded. Agitation may suggest hypoxia, whereas an obtunded patient may reflect hypercarbia. The abusive patient may be hypoxic and should not be presumed to be intoxicated. Cyanosis related to hypoxemia is manifest by the presence of a blue hue within the perioral tissues and the nail beds. Visualization of chest retractions and the use of accessory muscles provide further evidence of airway compromise. The chest should be evaluated by auscultation. Noisy breath sounds, snoring, gurgling, and crowing sounds (stridor) may be associated with partial upper airway obstruction. Hoarseness (dysphonia) may indicate laryngeal obstruction or edema. The trachea should be palpated to determine its position.

A definitive airway involves the presence of an endotracheal tube within the trachea, connected to an oxygen source. There are three forms of definitive airways:

- Orotracheal tube
- Nasotracheal tube
- Surgical airway (cricothyroidotomy or tracheotomy).

Initial attempts should be directed toward placement of an orotracheal or a nasotracheal tube. If edema or severe oropharyngeal hemorrhage obstructs the airway preventing endotracheal tube placement, then a surgical airway must be performed. Depending on the experience of the surgeon, a surgical cricothyroidotomy is preferred to a tracheotomy in the emergent setting, because it is easier to perform, is asso-ciated with less bleeding, and requires less time. An awake tracheotomy is more appropriate in the difficult airway without the acute loss of airway.

Bibliography

Altman KW, Waltonen JD, Kern RC: Urgent airway intervention: a 3 year county hospital experience, *Laryngoscope* 115:2101-2104, 2005.

American College of Surgeons Committee on Trauma: *Advanced trauma life support for doctors,* 2004.

Bernard AC, Kenady DE: Conventional surgical tracheostomy as the preferred method of airway management, *J Oral Maxillofac Surg* 57(3):310-315, 1999.

Lewis RJ: Tracheostomies: indications, timing and complications, *Clin Chest Med* 13(1):137-149, 1992.

Paw HG, Sharma S: Cricothyroidotomy: a short-term measure for elective ventilation in a patient with challenging neck anatomy, *Anesth Intensive Care* 34(3):384-387, 2006.

Salvino CK, Dries D, Gamelli R, et al: Emergency cricothyroidotomy in trauma victims, *J Trauma* 34(4):503-505, 1993.

Spitalnic SJ, Sucov A: Ludwig's angina: a case report and review, *J Emerg Med* 13:499, 1995.

Standley TDA, Smith HL: Emergency tracheal catheterization for jet ventilation: a role for the ENT surgeon, *J Laryngotology* 119:235-236, 2005.

Stauffer JL, Olsen DE, Petty TL: Complications and consequences of endotracheal intubation and tracheostomy, *Am J Med* 70:65, 1981.

Stock CR: What is past is prologue: a short history of the development of tracheostomy, *Throat* 66(4):166-169, 1987.

Taicher S, Givol N, Peleg M, et al: Changing indications for tracheostomy in maxillofacial trauma, *J Oral Maxillofac Surg* 54(3):292-295, 1996.

Walts PA, Murphy SC, DeCamp NM: Techniques of surgical tracheostomy, *Clin Chest Med* 24(3):413-427, 2003.

Wood DE: Tracheostomy, *Chest Surg Clin N Am* 6(4):749-764, 1996.

4 Oral and Maxillofacial Infections

Shahrokh C. Bagheri, DMD, MD

This chapter addresses:
- Ludwig's Angina
- Buccal Space Abscess
- Vestibular Space Infection
- Lateral Pharyngeal and Masticator Space Infection
- Osteomyelitis

Odontogenic and nonodontogenic maxillofacial infections are some of the oldest disease processes treated by oral and maxillofacial surgeons. These patients commonly present to the office or, in severe cases, to the hospital emergency department. Although the majority of infections can be treated in a nonemergent fashion, early recognition and correct management of severe infections can be life saving. Knowledge of the surgical anatomy and path of spread of infections in the head and neck is fundamental in providing correct diagnosis and treatment. The ability of severe infections of the sublingual, submandibular, and parapharyngeal spaces to cause airway compromise, cavernous sinus thrombosis, and possibility or mediastinal spread of infection has resulted in complications and death, especially in the medically compromised patient who presents late in the disease process.

Despite the availability of a wide spectrum of antimicrobial agents and increasing knowledge of microbiology, the treatment of odontogenic infections remains primarily surgical. Removal of the source of infection and establishment of adequate drainage for elimination of the purulent material provide the mainstay treatment. Adequate antibiotic coverage is, however, important and should not be overlooked.

The response to treatment can be monitored by several clinical (swelling, erythema, pain, interincisal opening) and laboratory (white blood cell [WBC] count, C-reactive protein) parameters. The measurement of temperature is an ancient method of monitoring the response to an infectious process. Fever occurs secondary to the production of endogenous pyrogens (e.g., cytokines, interleukins, tumor necrosis factor) that affect the hypothalamus and medulla to increase the temperature set point. The definition of *fever* is arbitrary, and there is considerable variability in "normal temperature" for a population of healthy adults. A range of definitions are acceptable (between 37.5°C to 38.5°C) depending on how sensitive an indicator the surgeon wants to use. The lower the temperature used to define *fever,* the more sensitive the indicator is for detecting an infectious process but the less specific it will be. Normal body temperature is generally considered to be 37.0°C and varies according to circadian rhythm and menstrual cycle. Many different variables can influence temperature, such as exercise and environmental factors.

Chills occur in response to the elevation in temperature setpoint during the initiation of fever. This is often accompanied by the need for increased insulation and decreased exposure of exposed skin. Shivering is also seen, contributing to the increase in temperature.

The differential is a ratio of the different types of WBCs present (polymorphonuclear neutrophils [PMNs], lymphocytes, monocytes, eosinophils, or basophils). With a rise in WBC count, as seen during an acute infection, the predominant increase occurs in the PMNs. Chemotactic factors contribute to the recruitment of PMNs to the site of infection (or injury) with a subsequent increase in production of neutrophils by the bone marrow. The increased precursor forms of the PMNs (myelocytes and promyelocytes) are released into the circulating blood. The movement toward circulation of immature forms is termed a shift to the left and is usually seen during acute infections.

In this chapter, we present four teaching cases of infections that have an odontogenic etiology. We also present a case of osteomyelitis of the mandible.

Ludwig's Angina

Jaspal Girn, DMD, and Chris Jo, DMD

CC

A 34-year-old otherwise healthy man presents to the emergency department stating, "My neck and tongue are swollen, and it all started with a toothache."

Ludwig's angina is predominantly seen in young adults with as much as a 3:1 male predilection.

HPI

The patient presented to the emergency department with a 3-day history of progressive swelling and pain in his neck. He reports a 3-week history of severe, intermittent pain in his lower right third molar. Ten days ago, his general dentist prescribed him amoxicillin for a periapical abscess and pericoronitis associated with his right mandibular third molar, which was partially impacted and decayed. Despite compliance with antibiotics, he progressively developed persistent swelling and a foul-tasting drainage around the tooth. He began to have swelling under the right side of his tongue (right sublingual space), which spread to the contralateral side (no anatomical barrier between right and left sublingual spaces). Simultaneous to the floor of the mouth swelling, the neck began to swell on the right side, which then spread to the other side. He reports having subjective fevers and chills (signs of systemic inflammatory involvement), as well as dysphagia (difficulty swallowing) and odynophagia (painful swallowing). He states that he has not been able to eat or drink in the past 48 hours (causing dehydration). He denies dysphonia (difficulty speaking, seen with edema of the vocal cords and upper airway) or any chest discomfort (seen with advanced mediastinal involvement).

PMHX/PDHX/MEDICATIONS/ALLERGIES/SH/FH

This patient is otherwise healthy. Diabetes mellitus and other immunocompromised states are risk factors for poor outcome and death (see Complications later).

EXAMINATION

General. The patient is sitting upright, appears very restless, and is unable to tolerate his oral secretions (evidenced by constant use of a Yankauer suction and drooling of saliva). He appears to be in mild respiratory distress, but there is no evidence of stridor (high-pitched crowing noise due to partial upper airway obstruction).

Airway. The airway is stable on examination. The trachea is difficult to palpate due to edema but appears to be midline. Fiberoptic nasopharyngoscopy can be performed to further evaluate the patency of the upper airway and the amount of edema of the surrounding soft tissue (see chapter 3, section on emergent surgical airway). Alternatively, computed tomography (CT) scans of the neck can delineate neck and airway swelling.

Vital signs. The patient's blood pressure is 138/89 mm Hg, heart rate 110 bpm (tachycardia), respirations 28 per minute (tachypnea), and temperature 40.0°C (febrile), with oxygen saturation 96% on room air.

Maxillofacial. There is obvious moderate to severe facial swelling over the lower third of the face. Brawny and painful induration of the submandibular and submental spaces is noted bilaterally (Figure 4-1). There is erythema over the anterior neck extending down to the clavicles. However, subcutaneous crepitus (indicative of subcutaneous air from gas producing organisms) is not present. No cervical lymphadenopathy or fluctuance was palpated (lymphadenopathy would be difficult to assess in the presence of neck edema or induration).

Intraoral. The patient's mouth opening is limited with a maximal interincisal opening of 20 mm (trismus indicates masticator space involvement or guarding secondary to pain). The floor of the mouth and tongue are elevated and edematous (sublingual space). The oropharynx is not clearly visualized due to the limited mouth opening and elevated tongue (positive predictors of difficult laryngoscopy and endotracheal intubation).

Cardiovascular. The patient is tachycardic without rubs, murmurs, or gallops (tachycardia and friction rubs can be indicative of mediastinitis). He is negative for Hamon's sign (crepitus heard with a stethoscope during systole indicative of mediastinitis).

Pulmonary. Lung fields are clear to auscultation bilaterally without rales, bronchi, or wheezes (aspiration of saliva or exudates can be seen with advanced cases).

IMAGING

Before obtaining any imaging studies, the surgeon needs to decide on the urgency of the infectious process compromising the airway. If the airway is deemed stable, imaging studies should be obtained to guide surgical treatment. However, any possibility of acute airway embarrassment should not delay direct transfer to the operating room for advanced airway interventions. Once the airway is stabilized, imaging studies can be safely obtained.

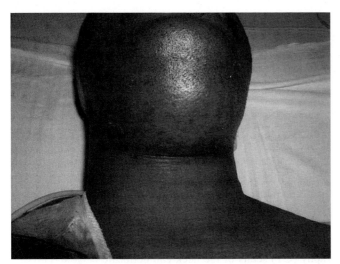

Figure 4-1 Brawny cellulitis and erythema of the bilateral submandibular and submental spaces.

A panoramic radiograph is the initial screening study of choice. It provides an excellent overview of the dentition, identifying any odontogenic sources of the infection. CT scans of the neck with contrast material is indicated when dealing with deep neck space infections (chest CT should be included if there is a suspicion of descending mediastinitis). This study can help determine the anatomical spaces involved, localize any fluid collections (loculations of purulence), and determine if the airway is deviated or compromised. CT is also helpful in surgical planning for incision and drainage. When a chest CT is deemed unnecessary, chest radiographs (posteroanterior and lateral views) can be an important screening tool to detect a widened mediastinum, which may be indicative of descending mediastinitis.

In this patient, the panoramic radiograph revealed a carious right mandibular third molar, with a large periapical radiolucent lesion. The CT scan of the patient's neck reveals a rim-enhancing fluid collection involving the bilateral submandibular, submental, and right sublingual spaces (Figure 4-2). In addition, there is diffuse soft tissue edema consistent with cellulitis in the involved spaces. No subcutaneous emphysema is seen in the cervical tissues (subcutaneous gas collection is considered a hallmark sign of cervical necrotizing fasciitis and is seen in up to 46% to 67% of cases). The patient's airway is patent and midline. A chest CT was ordered due to the erythema tracking down the anterior neck. No mediastinal involvement was observed.

LABS

A complete blood count (CBC) and complete metabolic panel (CMP) are indicated during the work-up of severe odontogenic infections. The presenting WBC count is a marker of the severity of infection and should be followed during the course of treatment. C-reactive protein (CRP) is an acute-phase reactant that is released in response to inflammation, and it can be used to monitor the response to therapy. Studies have also suggested that a very high CRP level at the time of admission is a predictor of a complicated hospital course. Electrolyte disturbances (sodium, potassium, magnesium, calcium) are common among patients with severe head and neck infections, especially when the patient is not able to tolerate oral intake due to swelling or pain. Blood urea nitrogen (BUN) and creatinine levels are useful to evaluate for prerenal azotemia due to hypovolemia. Blood cultures are indicated in the patient with persistent fever. An electrocardiogram (EKG) should be obtained with suspicion of mediastinitis. An arterial blood gas (ABG) measurement is warranted in the critically ill patient presenting with septic shock.

This patient presented with the following lab values: WBC of 21,000 cells/mm^3 with a 35% bandemia, BUN of 30 mg/dl (normal range, 7 to 18 mg/dl), and creatinine of 1.2 mg/dl (normal range, 0.6 to 1.2 mg/dl). The BUN/creatinine ratio was 25 (ratio greater than 20 is indicative of prerenal azotemia). The remainder of his electrolyte values were within normal limits.

ASSESSMENT

Ludwig's angina secondary to carious right mandibular third molar (odontogenic source of infection accounts for 70% to 90% of cases, the vast majority arising from second or third molars)

Ludwig's angina was first described by Karl Friedrich Wilhelm von Ludwig in 1836 as a rapidly progressing gangrenous cellulitis originating in the region of the submandibular area that extends without any tendency to form abscesses. Ludwig's angina is now known as an aggressively spreading cellulitis that simultaneously affects the bilateral submandibular, sublingual, and submental spaces. Although Ludwig's angina is classically described as a cellulitis, progression to abscess formation within the involved spaces is most often the case, and to this date, clinicians still use the term "Ludwig's angina" when describing a bilateral submandibular, sublingual, and submental space infection. Grodinsky and Holyoke's criteria for Ludwig's angina may no longer have any useful clinical application. The term "angina" is a misleading term, because any chest discomfort seen with this is from descending mediastinitis and is not related to ischemic heart disease.

TREATMENT

Treatment begins with evaluation of the patient's airway and appropriate management to prevent acute airway embarrassment (see Chapter 3, the section on emergent surgical airway). The airway is first evaluated by the general appearance of the patient (a distressed patient with stridorous respirations is assumed to have an airway compromise until proved otherwise). The oral cavity should be examined to evaluate the amount of tongue, floor of mouth, soft palate, and pharyngeal wall edema (many times an oral examination is very limited due to the patient's inability to open). A fiberoptic nasopharyngoscopy can be performed in the emergency

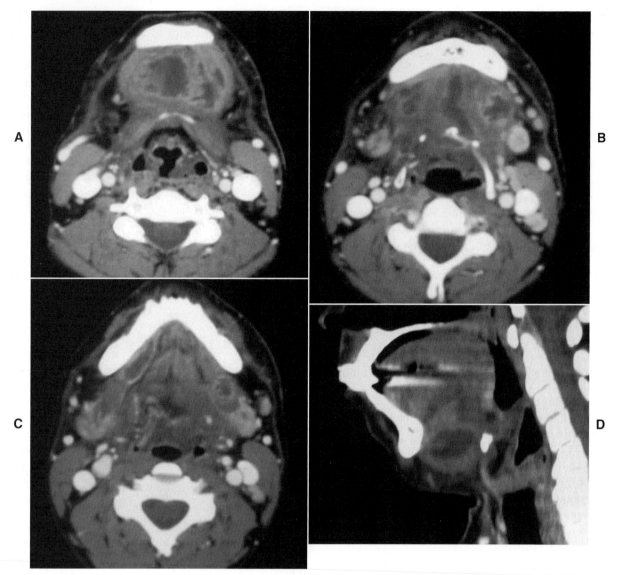

Figure 4-2 **A,** Axial view, soft tissue CT neck scan with contrast showing an enhancing fluid collection in the submental space. **B,** Axial view, soft tissue CT neck scan with contrast showing enhancing fluid collections in the submental and bilateral submandibular spaces. **C,** Axial view, soft tissue CT neck scan with contrast showing an enhancing fluid collection in the right sublingual space. Note that Wharton's duct seen on this view confirms that this abscess is above the mylohyoid muscle. **D,** Sagittal reconstruction, soft tissue CT neck scan with contrast showing a large submandibular space abscess extending from the inferior border of the anterior mandible to the hyoid bone.

department to further assess the airway, including the vocal cords. Intravenous dexamethasone can be given to reduce the airway edema in patients with impending upper respiratory obstruction. An emergent cricothyroidotomy should be performed if the patient loses the airway before arrival to the operating room. An awake tracheotomy or an awake fiberoptic nasal intubation can be performed in the operating room if the situation is less acute (oral intubation by direct laryngoscopy may also be possible in less severe cases). There is support in the current literature that a tracheotomy

may be indicated in patients with Ludwig's angina (see Complications).

Supportive measures should be initiated while arrangements are made with the operating room. This should include fluid resuscitation and initiation of broad-spectrum empiric antibiotic therapy. Fluid resuscitation is commonly needed because patients present with hypovolemia due to the lack of oral intake (insensible losses are accelerated by fever) and/or some degree of sepsis or septic shock. Adequacy of fluid resuscitation should be continuously monitored (heart rate, blood pressure, urine output, and BUN/creatinine). Vasopressive therapy may be indicated in patients presenting with septic shock. Tight glycemic control (blood glucose 90 to 110 mg/dl) is desirable, especially in the critically ill patient.

Empiric antimicrobial therapy should be promptly initiated to cover the mixed aerobic-anaerobic polymicrobial organisms (gram-positive, gram-negative, aerobic, and anaerobic) commonly involved in these infections. The combination of penicillin G with an adult dose of 4 to 30 million units per day, divided every 4 to 6 hours in combination with metronidazole, is an appropriate regimen. Other recommendations include clindamycin 900 mg intravenously every 8 hours, ticarcillin clavulanate 3.1 g intravenously every 6 hours, ampicillin sulbactam 3 g intravenously every 6 hours, or piperacillin tazobactam 3.375 g intravenously every 6 hours. Chow in 1992 recommended high-dose intravenous penicillin G combined with clindamycin, metronidazole, or cefoxitin. When available, the antibiotic regimen should be guided by cultures and sensitivity studies. CRP has been shown to be an excellent marker for severity of the infection and the patient's response to surgical and antibiotic therapy.

Aggressive surgical drainage and debridement, along with elimination of the source of infection, are necessary for definitive treatment. Delay in taking the patient to the operating room for surgical treatment is associated with a worse outcome. Cultures should be taken either via aspiration techniques or with a culturette swab. Most cases of Ludwig's angina can be managed using small incisions in the submandibular and submental regions (larger cervical hockey stick or apron incisions may be indicated when complicated by necrotizing fasciitis). Blunt dissection is carried out to explore all the involved spaces. Subperiosteal dissection and debridement are important in the area around the source of infection, and any offending teeth should be extracted. The intraoral and extraoral dissections can be dissected to freely communicate, allowing for dependent extraoral drainage. Therefore the abscess is decompressed, the necrotic debris is debrided, and the wounds are copiously irrigated. Red rubber catheters and/or Penrose drains can be used to facilitate postoperative wound irrigation and to allow dependent drainage. Drains can be slowly advanced out of the wound postoperatively or removed when purulent drainage ceases. Repeat drainage and lavage procedures in the operating room should be considered, especially in more severe infections that are refractory to treatment.

The patient was given 16 mg of dexamethasone intravenously in the emergency department, intravenous fluid resuscitation was initiated, and empiric intravenous antibiotics were administered. Antibiotic therapy consisted of ampicillin-sulbactam (Unasyn) 3.0 g every 6 hours and clindamycin 900 mg every 8 hours. The patient was urgently taken to the operating room for incision and drainage of the involved anatomical spaces of the neck and extraction of the right mandibular third molar. The patient was intubated successfully via an awake nasal fiberoptic endotracheal intubation. An 18-gauge needle was used to aspirate purulent exudate from the submandibular space, which was sent for Gram stain, aerobic and anaerobic cultures, and antibiotic sensitivity studies. The surgical drainage consisted of three incisions of 1.5 to 2 cm in length, 2 cm below the inferior border at the angle of the mandible bilaterally and anteriorly in the submental area. Blunt dissection with a hemostat and a Kelly clamp was carried out to explore all involved spaces. Copious amounts of purulence and necrotic tissue were expressed from the surgical sites. The right mandibular third molar was elevated and extracted. The gingival cuff was elevated, and subperiosteal dissection was carried out along the lingual plate to enter into the sublingual and submandibular spaces. All the incisions were connected to each other in the subplatysmal and subperiosteal planes. Irrigation drains were placed in both submandibular, sublingual, and the submental spaces. All drains were irrigated with copious amounts of antibiotic irrigation. The patient was left intubated for 3 days postoperatively due to surgical and airway edema. After significant resolution of the infection and edema, he had a positive cuff leak test and was extubated over an Eschmann tube, which was left in place for several hours. He did not experience any postextubation airway compromise and was transferred to the ward the following day.

COMPLICATIONS

The most feared complication associated with Ludwig's angina is death due to airway compromise. Loss of airway from upper airway obstruction can occur at any time during the perioperative period, before arrival at the operating room, during an attempted intubation, after an accidental or self-extubation in the intensive care unit (ICU), or after a planned extubation (see Chapter 3, the section on emergent surgical airway). Potter and colleagues in 2002 reported a 3% incidence of loss of airway for patients who received a tracheotomy versus 6% for patients maintained with endotracheal intubation. They reported two deaths (4% mortality rate) secondary to loss of airway, and both deaths occurred in the endotracheal intubation group (one occurred after a planned extubation and the other occurred after an unplanned extubation). The tracheotomy group had shorter ICU stay (1.1 versus 3.1 days) and shorter overall hospital stay (4.9 versus 5.9 days). Har-El and associates reported that patients with Ludwig's angina or a retropharyngeal space abscess had a significant need for tracheotomy. Their review of 110 patients showed that 4 of 8 patients meeting their criteria for severe infection who did not receive a tracheostomy developed upper airway obstruction necessitating an emergent surgical airway (50% incidence of airway loss in the endotracheal intubation group). They concluded that tracheotomy is indicated in patients with Ludwig's angina. Loughnan and colleagues report successful endotracheal intubation in 9 of 10 patients with Ludwig's angina using an inhalational induction technique and direct laryngoscopy, but they do not report on

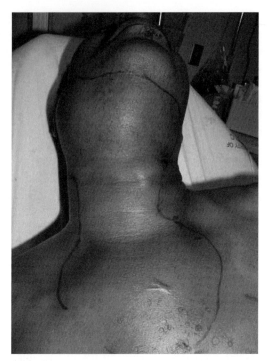

Figure 4-3 Another patient with Ludwig's angina and descending mediastinitis via the anterior paratracheal spaces and bilateral carotid spaces. Note the soft tissue edema and erythema of the anterior neck tracking down to the sternum.

Other potential complications include aspiration, ventilator-acquired pneumonia, septic shock, and acute renal failure.

DISCUSSION

Ludwig's angina is defined by the involvement of specific anatomical spaces (bilateral submandibular, sublingual, and submental spaces). The sublingual space(s) is bounded anteriorly and laterally by the mandible, superiorly by the floor of the mouth and tongue, and inferiorly by the mylohyoid muscle. There is no anatomical barrier between the left and right sublingual spaces. The submandibular space is separated from the sublingual space by the mylohyoid muscle, thus forming the roof of the submandibular space. The hyoglossus and styloglossus muscles form the medial border, and the body of the mandible forms the lateral border. The skin, superficial fascia, platysma, and superficial layer of the deep cervical fascia form the superficial boundary. The anterior bellies of the digastric muscles form the lateral borders of the submental space. The roof is formed by the mylohyoid muscle. The symphysis of the mandible and the hyoid bone form its anterior and posterior borders, respectively. The sublingual and submandibular spaces posteriorly communicate freely with each other and with the medial masticator and lateral pharyngeal spaces, which in turn is contiguous with the retropharyngeal space. Extension of the infection along the carotid sheath (contained within the posterior compartment of the lateral pharyngeal space [LPS]) or retropharyngeal space can lead to descent into the superior mediastinum. The alar fascia separates the retropharyngeal space from the "danger space" (space 4 of Grodinksy and Holyoke), which extends to the diaphragm and the posterior mediastinum. The anterior paratracheal spaces provide anterior access to the superior mediastinum (Figure 4-4).

Ludwig's angina most commonly has an odontogenic etiology (70% to 90%). A periapical abscess from the second or third mandibular molars is the most common cause. The roots of these teeth are commonly below the attachment level of the mylohyoid muscle to the internal oblique ridge. The periapical abscess perforates the lingual cortex, with spread into the sublingual (if the root is above the mylohyoid attachment) or submandibular space (if the root is below the mylohyoid attachment). The infection can then rapidly spread to adjacent continuous or contiguous spaces. Other causes include peritonsillar or parapharyngeal abscesses, oral lacerations, mandibular fractures, and submandibular sialadenitis.

The bacteriological profile of Ludwig's angina is usually polymicrobial, and it includes anerobes and ananerobes. The most common organisms are *Streptococcus viridans*, β-hemolytic streptococci, staphylococci, *Klebsiella pneumoniae,* anaerobic Bacteroides, and *Peptostreptococcus. S. viridans* is one of the most commonly isolated organisms. This is consistent with previous reports associating this organism with odontogenic infections. *K. pneumoniae* is another commonly isolated organism, with a higher incidence in patients with diabetes mellitus.

the postoperative morbidity and mortality. If postoperative endotracheal intubation is planned, adequate sedation, four-point restraints, and a secured tube (taped around the head or wired to the teeth) are paramount to prevent unanticipated self or iatrogenic extubation. Upon extubation, a cuff-leak test should be performed and an Eschmann tube should be left in place to facilitate reintubation if needed (postextubation laryngeal edema may cause loss of airway despite having a good cuff-leak test).

Before the advent of antibiotics, the mortality rate from Ludwig's angina was greater than 50%. Fortunately, the prevalence and mortality rates have significantly decreased due to better access to dental care and antibiotic therapy. When complicated by descending mediastinitis and thoracic empyema, the mortality rates remains as high as 38% to 60%, despite antibiotic therapy (Figure 4-3). When complicated by cervical necrotizing fasciitis, the more recent reported mortality rates are 18% to 22% (any delay in surgical treatment increases mortality). Tung-Yiu and colleagues reported that an immunocompromised state (e.g., diabetes mellitus) increases the risk of an odontogenic infection developing into cervical necrotizing fasciitis. Of their series of 11 cases, seven patients were immunocompromised (four with diabetes mellitus), which accounted for all major complications including two deaths. Others have reported a mortality rate as high as 67% with severe odontogenic infections associated with diabetes mellitus. Currently there is no evidence to suggest that HIV/AIDS status increases the risk of developing Ludwig's angina and its associated complications.

Sagittal section through neck

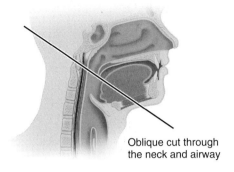

Oblique cut through
the neck and airway

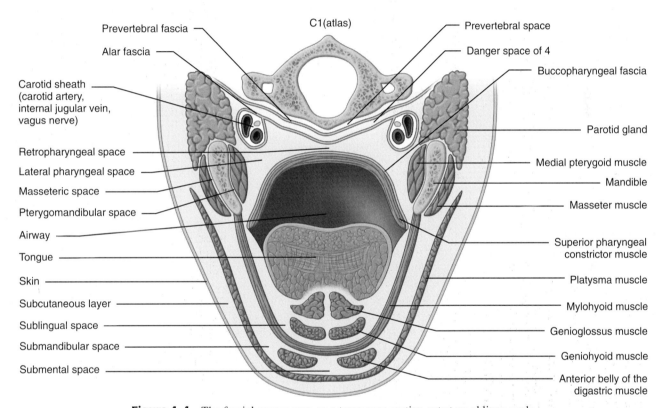

Figure 4-4 The fascial spaces seen as a transverse section cut at an oblique angle.

Bibliography

Allen D, Loughnan TE, Ord RA: A re-evaluation of the role of tracheostomy in Ludwig's angina, *J Oral Maxillofac Surg* 43:436-439, 1985.

Barsamian JG, Scheffer RB: Spontaneous pneumothorax: an unusual occurrence in a patient with Ludwig's angina, *J Oral Maxillofac Surg* 45:161-168, 1987.

Chidzonga MM: Necrotizing fasciitis of the cervical region in an AIDS patient: report of a case, *J Oral Maxillofac Surg* 63:855-859, 2005.

Chow AW: Life-threatening infections of the head and neck, *Clin Infect Dis* 14:991, 1992.

Dugan MJ, Lazow SK, Berger JR: Thoracic empyema resulting from direct extension of Ludwig's angina: a case report, *J Oral Maxillofac Surg* 56:968-971, 1998.

Fischmann GE, Graham BS: Ludwig's angina resulting from infection of an oral malignancy, *J Oral Maxillofac Surg* 43:795-796, 1985.

Loughnan TE, Allen DE: Ludwig's angina. The anaesthetic management of nine cases, *Anaesthesia* 40:295-297, 1985.

Mihos P, Potaris K, Gakidis I, et al: Management of descending necrotizing mediastinitis, *J Oral Maxillofac Surg* 62:966-972, 2004.

Potter JK, Herford AS, Ellis E: Tracheotomy versus endotracheal intubation for airway management in deep neck space infections, *J Oral Maxillofac Surg* 60:349-354, 2002.

Steiner M, Gau MJ, Wilson DL, et al: Odontogenic infection leading to cervical emphysema and fatal mediastinitis, *J Oral Maxillofac Surg* 40:600-604, 1982.

Sugata T, Fujita Y, Myoken Y, et al: Cervical cellulitis with mediastinitis from an odontogenic infection complicated by diabetes mellitus: report of a case, *J Oral Maxillofac Surg* 55:864-869, 1997.

Tsuji T, Shimono M, Yamane G, et al: Ludwig's angina as a complication of ameloblastoma of the mandible, *J Oral Maxillofac Surg* 42:815-819, 1984.

Tsunoda R, Suda S, Fukaya T, et al: Descending necrotizing mediastinitis caused by an odontogenic infection: a case report, *J Oral Maxillofac Surg* 58:240-242, 2000.

Tung-Yiu W, Jehn-Shyun H, Ching-Hung C, et al: Cervical necrotizing fasciitis of odontogenic origin: a report of 11 cases, *J Oral Maxillofac Surg* 58:1347-1352, 2000.

Ylijoki S, Suuronen R, Jousimies-Somer H, et al: Differences between patients with or without the need for intensive care due to severe odontogenic infections, *J Oral Maxillofac Surg* 59:867-872, 2001.

Zachariades N, Mezitis M, Stavrinidis P, et al: Mediastinitis, thoracic empyema, and pericarditis as complications of a dental abscess: report of a case, *J Oral Maxillofac Surg* 46:493-495, 1988.

Buccal Space Abscess

Abtin Shahriari, DMD, MPH, and Shahrokh C. Bagheri, DMD, MD

CC

A 34-year-old woman presents to the urgent care clinic complaining of pain and progressively enlarging swelling of her right cheek.

HPI

The patient has not received any dental care for the past several years (risk factor for odontogenic infections). Six months earlier, she noticed that a segment of a restoration broke off the right maxillary second molar. At the time, there was no associated pain, and she elected to neglect the tooth. Two days before presentation, she developed acute onset of right-side swelling of the cheek associated with mild pain and discomfort that have progressively exacerbated. There is no history of dysphasia, swelling of the floor of the mouth, or difficulty breathing (would be indicative of parapharyngeal or sublingual infections and are not seen with pure buccal space involvement).

PMHX/PDHX/MEDICATIONS/ALLERGIES/SH/FH

Noncontributory.

Severe odontogenic infections are most commonly seen in patients with a history of dental neglect. When infections are seen in patients with compromised immunity (AIDS, diabetes, chemotherapy), the infectious process may prove more resistant to treatment.

EXAMINATION

General. The patient was a well-developed and well-nourished woman in mild distress (patients with buccal space infections are frequently very concerned due to the extent of swelling and pain).

Vital signs. Vital signs were stable and afebrile (an elevated temperature is not always seen, especially in well-localized infections, unless there is surrounding cellulitis or systemic dissemination of the infection).

Maxillofacial. Significant right-side facial edema extended from the inferior border of the mandible superiorly to the level of the zygoma (Figure 4-5). The swelling is soft and fluctuant and with no apparent intraoral or extraoral drainage (untreated buccal space infections may spontaneously drain providing some relief or spread into other fascial spaces). There is tender right submandibular lymphadenopathy (due to active infection).

Intraoral. The maximal interincisal opening is 35 mm (trismus is not seen with buccal space infections because it does not involve the muscles of mastication). Bimanual examination of the right cheek reveals fluctuance extending to the depth of the maxillary and mandibular vestibules. The right maxillary second molar (tooth No. 2) is grossly carious. The floor of the mouth is soft and not elevated (it is important to assess the airway for patency), the oropharynx is clear, and the uvula is midline (deviation is seen with lateral pharyngeal space [LPS] infections).

A key clinical finding of buccal space infections is the general lack of extension of swelling below the inferior border of the mandible. Infections can spread in a subcutaneous plane to the neck or the periorbital tissue, but extension beyond the buccal area implies tissue involvement beyond this space. The buccal space does not compromise the airway.

IMAGING

The panoramic radiograph is the imaging study of choice for the evaluation of suspected buccal space infections and is frequently the only imaging study that is necessary. It allows a general screening of the bony anatomy of the maxillofacial region, as well as identification of potential odontogenic sources of infection (most commonly, the maxillary or mandibular first or second molars). A CT scan with intravenous contrast material can be obtained if there is clinical suspicion of orbital, parapharyngeal, or submandibular space involvement.

For this patient, the panoramic radiograph demonstrated a severely carious right maxillary second molar, with a well-demarcated periapical radiolucent lesion.

LABS

No routine laboratory tests are indicated for the evaluation and treatment of buccal space infections. A CBC can be obtained to assess for leukocytosis (elevated WBC count). This test may be valuable in cases that are refractory to treatment or in the presence of other medical comorbidities. The WBC count may not be elevated with isolated buccal space infections.

Routine use of culture and sensitivity studies for all buccal space infections is not indicated. However, in patients with multiple comorbidities or infections that are resistant to conventional therapy, culture and sensitivity studies may be useful to guide antimicrobial therapy.

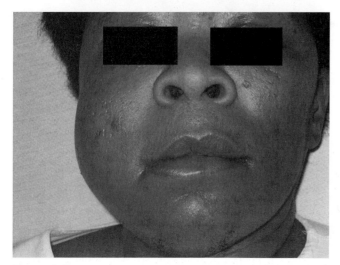

Figure 4-5 Swelling of the right face secondary to a buccal space abscess.

ASSESSMENT

Right buccal space abscess secondary to carious right maxillary second molar

TREATMENT

Surgical establishment of drainage along with removal of the source of infection is the most important treatment for buccal space infections. Antibiotic therapy is recommended and should be initiated to aid in resolution of the infection.

In cases of odontogenic etiology, tooth extraction or endodontic therapy eliminates the source of infection. When possible, extraction is more effective because it also allows spontaneous drainage of the infection. Drainage allows removal of purulent material, increases tissue perfusion, and therefore enhances the delivery of both oxygen and antibiotics. Incision and drainage is one of the oldest and most effective surgical procedures. Ideally, abscesses should be drained when fluctuant, before spontaneous rupture and drainage.

Several basic principles should be applied when draining an infection:
- The incision is best placed in healthy mucosa or skin when possible
- Camouflage of the incision in an aesthetic area such as inside the mouth or in the crease of the neck
- Anatomical placement of an incision that allows drainage by gravity
- Placement of a drain for open communication, with subsequent removal once drainage has ceased

The incision is frequently placed intraorally through the mucosa in a transverse orientation (although transcutaneous incisions may be necessary in select cases). The buccinator muscle is bluntly penetrated using a hemostat, entering into the buccal space. Culture and sensitivity studies should be obtained when indicated (see earlier). Frequent irrigation of the wound can be helpful. Other supportive measures such as intravenous fluid therapy (hydration), good oral hygiene, and nutritional support are prescribed as necessary.

For this case, with the patient under intravenous sedation anesthesia, needle aspiration of the buccal space was accomplished releasing 5 ml of brown purulent material that was sent for culture and sensitivity studies. Subsequently, a small transverse incision was placed intraorally about 1 cm superior to the depth of the mandibular vestibule, allowing drainage of another 8 ml of pus. The right maxillary second molar was extracted without any complication. The buccal space and the extraction socket were copiously irrigated, and a Penrose drain was placed and secured with a 2-0 silk suture. The patient was prescribed a 10-day course of penicillin (penicillin remains the empiric antibiotic of choice for outpatient odontogenic infections). The patient was seen in the office the next day and 3 days after demonstrating progressive resolution of her condition.

COMPLICATIONS

Complications of buccal space infections are related to:
- Delay in the diagnosis leading to systemic or local spread of the infection
- Surgical interventions resulting in inadequate drainage
- Compromised host immunity leading to failure of therapy
- Antibiotic-resistant organisms or inadequate pharmacotherapy
- Damage to vital structures due to surgical interventions

Rapid recognition of the above complications will improve the outcome.

Infection in the buccal space can spread to the cavernous sinus via the transverse facial vein (uncommon), periorbital space through the subcutaneous plane, submandibular space via inferior or posterior extensions, and superficial temporal and infratemporal spaces via the buccal fat pad. Injury to adjacent structures is usually avoided by careful attention to the regional anatomy. The buccal fat pad, Stensen's (parotid) duct, and facial artery should be avoided. However, altered anatomy due to regional edema may alter the surgical anatomy.

By far the most common etiology of buccal space infections is odontogenic. However, recurrent buccal space infections can be seen as a complication of Crohn's disease. Granulomatous lesions and ulcerations of the buccal mucosa can develop into true buccal space infections. Treatment of buccal space infections of odontogenic etiology in a patient with Crohn's or granulomatous disease may prove to be more challenging.

DISCUSSION

Dense sheets of connective tissue called fascia encompass muscles, glands, vascular, and neural structures, facilitating movement during function. Bacterial infections that penetrate the fascial spaces can therefore spread via the anatomical confines of these "potential" spaces. Bacterial infections spread via hydrostatic pressure and follow the path of least resistance, which is the loose, areolar connective tissue that surrounds the muscles enclosed by the fascial layers. Certain bacteria that produce enzymes that aid in the destruction of tissue (e.g., hyaluronidases and collagenases) are more virulent (the relative pathogenicity or the relative ability to do damage to the host). Such bacteria more easily invade the potential spaces surrounding the muscles.

The buccal space (included in the primary fascial spaces) is confined anatomically by the subcutaneous skin layer superficially and medially by the buccinator muscle. Anteriorly, it ends at the modiolus (aponeurotic junction of the buccinator and orbicularis oris muscles just posterior to the oral commissure). Posteriorly and just medial to the ascending ramus, the buccinator muscle is attached to the superior pharyngeal constrictor muscle at the pterygomandibular raphe. This formation leads to important anatomical pathways for the spread of infection into other spaces. Laterally, it creates a communication with the masseteric space (space between the masseter muscle and the lateral body of the ramus). Posteriorly and medially, the space communicates with the pterygomandibular, lateral pharyngeal, and infratemporal spaces superiorly. Extension of the buccal fat pad can allow buccal space infections to enter the superficial temporal space, extending via the transverse facial vein and pterygoid plexus into the infratemporal space. Rarely, it can erode into the transverse facial vein or pterygoid plexus and follow a posterior route to the cavernous sinus.

Infections that spread to the subcutaneous plane have no superficial anatomical barriers and can therefore spread to adjacent anatomical areas along this plane. Clinical inspection of the overlying skin can frequently aid in identification of subcutaneous spread of the infection. Demarcation of the areas of erythema with a skin-marking pen can be used to monitor the progression of the infectious process.

Odontogenic infections (such as buccal space infections) are mixed infections. A large proportion (over half) are composed of anaerobes, mostly gram-negative rods (Fusobacterium, Bacteroides). Gram-positive cocci (streptococci and peptostreptococci) are also seen in large numbers (over 25%).

Noncomplicated buccal space infections can be frequently treated in the office using intravenous sedation and close outpatient follow-up. However, the presence of systemic involvement (fever, sepsis, leukocytosis), dehydration, medical comorbidities, noncompliant patients, compromised immune status (diabetes, AIDS, chemotherapy, malnutrition), or infections that involve other deep fascial spaces may warrant hospital admission for intravenous antibiotics and medical evaluation.

In 2006, Flynn and associates conducted a prospective study to predict the length of hospital stay and the failure to respond to penicillin in severe odontogenic infections. They reported a failure of over 20% with penicillin therapy. This finding suggests a correlation between infection severity and penicillin resistance and is the basis for the recommendation of clindamycin as the empiric antibiotic of choice in odontogenic infections serious enough to require hospitalization. For outpatient treatment, penicillin resistance has not been shown to be a significant problem; therefore, penicillin remains the empiric antibiotic of choice for outpatient odontogenic infections.

Bibliography

Flynn RT, Shanti MR, Levi HM, et al: Severe odontogenic infections, part 1: prospective report, *J Oral Maxillofac Surg* 64:1093, 2006.

Flynn RT, Halpern RL: Antibiotic selection in head and neck infections, *Oral Maxillofacial Surg Clin N Am* 15:17, 2003.

Grodinsky M, Holyoke EA: The fasciae and fascial spaces of head, neck, and adjacent regions, *Am J Anat* 63:367, 1938.

Hollinshead WH: *Anatomy for surgeons: The head and neck*, ed 2, Hagerstown, MD, 1968, Harper and Row.

Laskin DM: Anatomic considerations in diagnosis and treatment of odontogenic infections, *J Am Dent Assoc* 69:308, 1964.

Vestibular Space Infection

Piyushkumar P. Patel, DDS, and Shahrokh C. Bagheri, DMD, MD

CC

A 33-year-old man presents to the clinic with the chief complaint of "my jaw is swollen and painful."

HPI

Approximately 1 week prior to presentation, the patient began to experience acute pain localized to the right posterior mandibular molars, with subsequent development of progressively increasing swelling in his right buccal vestibule over the course of 3 days. He denies any dysphagia (difficulty swallowing), dyspnea (difficulty breathing), or globus (sensation of a lump in the throat). There is no history of any fever or chills.

PMHX/PDHX/MEDICATIONS/ ALLERGIES/SH/FH

Noncontributory.

The most important risk factor for the development of a vestibular space infection is poor oral hygiene and dental neglect. Medical comorbidities that compromise the immune system and/or wound healing (smoking, malnutrition, HIV/AIDS, diabetes, chemotherapy) may complicate the treatment of this infection.

EXAMINATION

General. The patient is a well-developed and well-nourished man in no apparent distress.

Vital signs. His vital signs are stable and he is afebrile (vestibular space infections generally do not cause fever in an otherwise healthy individual).

Maxillofacial. There is slight edema of the right posterior mandible secondary to swelling of the right mandibular vestibule.

Intraoral. The floor of mouth is soft and nontender (sublingual space not involved). He is able to protrude his tongue past the vermillion-cutaneous border of the lower lip. He has no restriction of mouth opening (trismus is indicative of masticator space involvement and is not seen with vestibular space infections). There is a significant fluctuant swelling of the mandibular right posterior buccal vestibule, with no obvious purulent discharge (Figure 4-6). The right mandibular first molar has a large restoration that is painful to palpation, with open carious distal margins. The remaining teeth are asymptomatic.

IMAGING

The panoramic radiograph provides the best overall survey of the entire mandible and maxilla and serves as a screening tool for evaluation of the dentition. An intraoral periapical radiograph can be used for greater degree of detail, but this radiograph may be difficult to obtain in patients with acute pain. The development of a vestibular abscess requires the perforation of the buccal cortex or the presence of severe periodontal disease and therefore radiographic evidence of a periapical radiolucent lesion or periodontal disease is common. Caries or large restorations are frequently seen with the associated tooth.

For this patient, a panoramic radiograph demonstrates caries on the distal aspect of the right mandibular first molar that appears to extend to the pulp chamber. There is a 4 × 5-mm periapical radiolucent lesion associated with the distal root apex.

LABS

No routine laboratory testing is indicated in the management of vestibular space infections unless dictated by the medical history. Assessment of the WBC count is not necessary unless there is suspicion of systemic spread or infection (fever, malaise, sepsis). Culture and sensitivity studies are not mandatory for the initial management of vestibular space infections. However, for cases that do not respond to the initial therapy, causing spread of the infection beyond the vestibular space, Gram stain, cultures, and antibiotic sensitivity studies may be obtained to guide treatment. Despite adequate samples, it is frequently difficult for microbiology laboratories to isolate a specific organism (due to the polymicrobial nature of the infection), and therefore antibiotic sensitivity studies can be difficult to obtain.

ASSESSMENT

Buccal vestibular space abscess secondary to carious right mandibular first molar

TREATMENT

Infections that are limited to buccal vestibular space are considered low risk and can be managed conservatively on an outpatient basis with close follow-up. Successful treatment of odontogenic infections is mainly surgical and consists of the following:

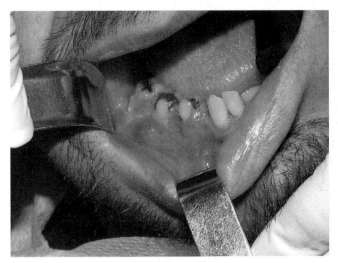

Figure 4-6 Right vestibular abscess secondary to carious right mandibular first molar.

- Elimination of the source of infection (tooth extraction or endodontic therapy)
- Establishment of drainage to aid in removal of the causative microorganisms, reducing the bacterial load to a level that can be managed by normal defense mechanisms
- Appropriate antibiotic coverage

Although antibiotic coverage is routinely used for treatment of vestibular infections, the elimination of the source of infection along with adequate drainage will successfully treat the majority of these infections.

Both aerobic and anaerobic gram-positive cocci, along with anaerobic gram-negative rods, are the most common causative organisms in odontogenic infections. For vestibular infections in an otherwise healthy individual, penicillin is still considered to be an effective empirical drug of choice and is routinely prescribed without obtaining cultures and sensitivity data.

This patient was treated by extraction of the right mandibular first molar, and a vestibular incision allowing drainage with subsequent placement of a Penrose drain (Figure 4-7). Blunt dissection was carried to the buccal mandibular cortex, identifying an area of perforation adjacent to the tooth. He was also placed on an oral dose of penicillin and discharged to home care with a follow-up appointment in 48 hours. The drain was removed at that time, with progressive resolution of his condition.

COMPLICATIONS

Complications in the treatment of vestibular infections are uncommon but mostly related to injury to adjacent anatomical structures, failure to remove the offending source of infection, antibiotic resistance, compromised host defenses, or spread to other fascial spaces. Vestibular infections can pass around the levator anguli oris muscle to enter the infraorbital space or between the buccinator and depressor anguli oris to enter the subcutaneous or buccal space.

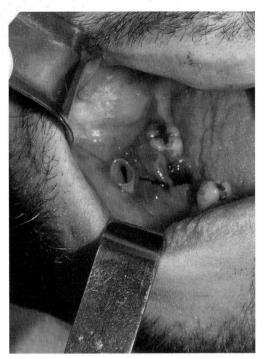

Figure 4-7 Extracted right mandibular first molar with placement of a Penrose drain in the right vestibule.

The vestibular space primarily contains areolar connective tissue, but it is crossed by the parotid duct and the long buccal and mental nerves. Incisions should be made to avoid Stensen's duct in the posterior maxillary vestibule, the mental nerve in the apical region of the mandibular premolars, the infraorbital nerve in the apical region of the maxillary cuspids, and the greater palatine neurovascular bundle in cases of palatal infections.

In infections that do not appropriately respond to treatment, consideration should be given to inadequate drainage or resistant bacterial strains. Culture and sensitivity studies should then be obtained to guide antimicrobial therapy.

DISCUSSION

Carious exposure and subsequent bacterial invasion of the pulp lead to necrosis of the pulpal tissues. The inflammatory process then spreads to the surrounding periodontal ligament and bone. The first pathological change in the area is apical periodontitis. This results in an inflammatory and immunologically mediated process that causes bone resorption and results in a localized abscess. If the process is allowed to continue, the inflammatory process will spread peripherally until cortical bone is destroyed and a subperiosteal abscess is formed. Eventually the periosteum is perforated as the infection spreads via the "path of least resistance." The severity of the abscess depends on factors such as virulence of the microorganism and the anatomical arrangement of adjacent muscles and fascia. Vestibular space infections are caused by perforation of the abscess through the buccal cortex superior to the attachment of the buccinator muscle in the mandible and inferior to the attachment of the buccinator muscle in the maxillary posterior region. The vestibular abscess is far more common than a palatal infection due to the thicker bone of the palate.

The vestibular space is the potential space between the vestibular mucosa and the underlying muscles of facial expression. The posterior boundary is bounded by the buccinator in either jaw, and the anterior boundary is made up by the intrinsic muscles of the lips and the orbicularis oris. In the anterior mandible, the abscess is confined to the vestibular space by the attachment of the mentalis muscle.

Bibliography

Flynn TR: Surgical management of orofacial infection, *Atlas Oral Maxillofac Surg Clin* 8:77-99, 2000.

Jone JL, Candelaria LM: Head and neck infections. In Fonscea RJ, ed: *Oral and maxillofacial surgery,* vol 5, Philadelphia, 2000, WB Saunders.

Mathews DC, et al: Emergency management of acute apical abscesses in the permanent dentition: a systematic review of the literature, *J Can Dent Assoc* 69:660, 2003.

Mittal N, et al: Management of extra oral sinus cases: a clinical dilemma, *J Endod* 30:541-547; 2004.

Lateral Pharyngeal and Masticator Space Infection

Piyushkumar P. Patel, DDS, and Shahrokh C. Bagheri, DMD, MD

CC

A 25-year-old man presents to the emergency department with the complaint that "my throat is swollen and I cannot swallow."

HPI

Approximately 1 week earlier, the patient began to experience acute pain localized to the posterior mandibular molars, with subsequent development of edema in his left posterior oropharynx 3 days later. He reports the onset of progressively worsening dysphagia (difficulty swallowing) and globus (sensation of a lump in the throat) that eventually prompted him to seek care. He has difficulty swallowing his secretions, either drooling or spitting them out (this is an important clinical note because it denotes significant life-threatening oropharyngeal edema). He explains that he has had minimal oral intake with the onset of fevers and chills. At this time he does not report any difficulty with breathing, but he feels more comfortable when sitting up (important clinical sign of dangerous oropharyngeal edema). The patient has a muffled "hot potato" voice (secondary to supraglottic edema).

Dental infections have become the most common etiology of deep neck infections in the Western world, involving the masticator, parapharyngeal, and submandibular spaces. More than 50% of patients presenting with infection involving these spaces have an odontogenic etiology, placing oral and maxillofacial surgeons as a preferred provider of surgical care for this group.

PMHX/PDHX/MEDICATIONS/ALLERGIES/SH/FH

The past medical and dental histories are unremarkable. The patient lives in a shelter and does not currently hold a job (although masticator space infections can be seen in individuals of all socioeconomic strata, the condition is far more predominant in the population with less access to health care, including frequent dental examinations).

Despite the lack of coexisting medical diseases in this patient, it is important to consider any conditions that impair the immune system such as AIDS, diabetes mellitus, chronic corticosteroid therapy, or chemotherapy. Patients should be questioned regarding risk factors for HIV infection and appropriately tested as needed. Masticator space infections can have very aggressive behavior in the face of immunosuppression.

EXAMINATION

General. The patient is a thin and unkempt-appearing man with a noticeable pungent odor (indicative of neglect to health and hygiene). The patient is not in respiratory distress (important to assess the need for advanced airway intervention immediately upon examination). He appears anxious, sitting up holding an emesis basin to catch his secretions as they drool from his mouth (difficulty maintaining secretions).

Vital signs. His blood pressure is 104/68 mm Hg (hypotension secondary to dehydration), heart rate 116 (tachycardia secondary to hypotension and fever), respirations 20 per minute, and temperature 39.2°C (febrile), with oxygen saturation of 98% on room air.

Maxillofacial. There is significant swelling and induration of the left side extending from the level of hyoid bone anterior to the sternocleidomastoid to the zygomatic arch. Cranial nerves II through XII are grossly intact. The pupils are equal, round, and reactive to light and accommodation (PERRLA) with no proptosis or ptosis of the eyelid (would be suggestive of cavernous sinus involvement).

Intraoral. Maximal interincisal opening is 17 mm (trismus) (Figure 4-8, *A*). The floor of mouth is soft (sublingual space not involved). The patient is able to protrude his tongue past the vermillion-cutaneous border of the lower lip. There is significant fluctuant swelling of the left oropharynx toward the right tonsillar area, with the tip of the uvula touching the right pharyngeal wall (Figure 4-8, *B*). The operculum overlying the partially bony impacted left mandibular third molar is edematous, erythematous, and tender to palpation with no obvious purulent discharge (mandibular third molars are a common cause of lateral pharyngeal infections). Mucous membranes of the buccal mucosa are dry (secondary to dehydration).

IMAGING

Before any further diagnostic imaging, the treating surgeon must decide if the patient (and the airway) is stable enough to obtain further studies or arrangements should be made to proceed directly to the operating room and establish a secure airway (endotracheal or nasotracheal intubation, tracheostomy, cricothyrotomy). Any possibility of acute respiratory obstruction should preclude the surgeon to directly proceed to the operating room. Imaging studies can be safely obtained to guide further treatment at a later time.

When available, a panoramic radiograph is an important imaging study for evaluation of suspected odontogenic

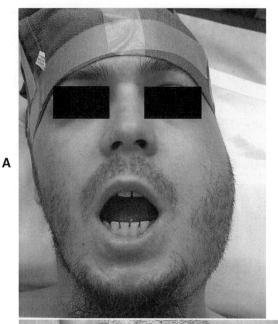

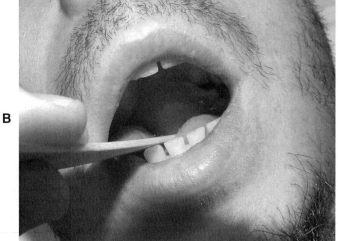

Figure 4-8 **A,** Significant swelling of the left face and maximal interincisal opening of 17 mm. **B,** Large fluctuant swelling of the posterior oropharynx partially obstructing the airway.

infections. It provides an excellent overview of the mandible and maxilla and serves as a screening tool for evaluation of the dentition. Also, in patients with trismus, other dental radiographs may be difficult to obtain. Because mandibular third molars are the most common odontogenic cause for parapharyngeal space infections, this radiograph becomes necessary to evaluate the third molars. In addition, it delineates the relationship to adjacent structures such as the inferior alveolar canal and other possible bony pathology.

The combination of contrast-enhanced CT scans and clinical examination has the highest sensitivity and specificity in the diagnosis of deep neck infections. The use of contrast improves the ability to identify the hyperemic capsule of a longstanding abscess (abscesses are seen as discrete, hypodense areas, which show an enhancing peripheral rim

with use of intravenous contrast material). In general, most radiologists interpret hypodense areas without ring enhancement to represent cellulitis or edema. However, studies have shown that, when drained, approximately 45% of hypodense areas without ring enhancement yield pus. In a study by William and associates, a hypodense area of greater than 2 ml without ring enhancement yielded purulence at the time of surgery. In the same study, CT scans were able to correctly differentiate cellulitis from an abscess in 85% of deep neck space (lateral and retropharyngeal) infections.

CT also provides important information regarding the details of adjacent anatomical structures such as integrity of the airway, tracheal deviation, and proximity of vascular structures (the carotid sheath). Airway deviation and possible risk of rupture of the pharyngeal abscess during intubation are important factors in determining the choice of securing the airway.

Magnetic resonance imaging (MRI) is also a useful imaging modality for soft tissue evaluation. Compared with CT, advantages of MRI include superior anatomical multiplanar display, high soft tissue contrast, fewer artifacts from dental amalgam, and lack of ionizing radiation. However, MRI is difficult and slower to perform on an emergency basis and is more costly, and claustrophobia may preclude examination in some patients. When possible, MRI has been shown to be superior in the assessment of deep neck infections.

Ultrasonography has shown some benefit in differentiating cellulitis from an abscess in superficial locations, but the use of this modality as a sole imaging technique for deep neck infection is in its infancy. The ultrasound probe can be placed intraorally, although in the setting of an acute infection and trismus, this can be difficult. An abscess is seen as an echo-free cavity with an irregular, well-defined circumference.

For the patient described above, the airway appeared clinically stable and a panoramic radiograph demonstrated carious and partially bony impacted left mandibular third molar. A CT scan with contrast demonstrated a significant swelling of the lateral pharyngeal area and deviation of the airway (Figure 4-9). Large rim-enhancing hypodense areas consistent with pus are seen on the left lateral masticator and lateral pharyngeal (anterior compartment) spaces.

LABS

A CBC and a basic metabolic panel should be obtained during the initial evaluation of deep neck space infections. The WBC count is an indicator of the severity of systemic response to the infection and can be obtained periodically to monitor the progression of infection (caution should be exercised in interpretation of this value in a patient who is at high risk for undiagnosed AIDS because the WBC count may appear within the normal range secondary to the inability to mount an adequate immune response).

Serum creatinine and BUN levels should be obtained before using contrast material for imaging. Contrast material has been known to cause contrast-associated nephropathy.

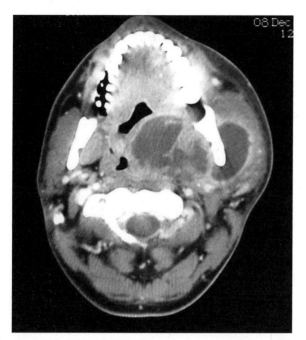

Figure 4-9 Axial cut, contrast-enhanced CT scan demonstrating large areas of rim-enhanced hypodensities (loculations) both medial and lateral to the left mandible with significant deviation of the airway.

Box 4-1.	**Risk Factors for Contrast-Associated Nephropathy**

Preexisting renal disease
Diabetes
Volume of contrast dye used
Dehydration
Congestive heart failure
Advanced age
Presence of nephrotoxic drugs (NSAIDs, ACE-Is)

From Soma VR: Contrast-associated nephropathy, *Heart Dis* 4:372-379, 2002.
ACE-Is, Angiotensin-converting enzyme inhibitors; *NSAIDs,* nonsteroidal antiinflammatory drugs.

This is the third most common cause of hospital-acquired acute renal failure and is seen following the administration of contrast material in the absence of other identifiable causes. The condition is defined as an increase in serum creatinine of greater than 25% from baseline or a rise greater than 0.5 mg/dl within 48 hours of contrast exposure in the absence of other causes. Risk factors for the development of contrast-associated nephropathy are summarized in Box 4-1. In the presence of risk factors, renal function should be carefully monitored, and a baseline serum creatinine obtained before and within 48 to 72 hours after the procedure.

The WBC count for this patient was 18.5 cell/mm³; the differential included 80% polymorphonucleocytes with a shift to the left (indicative of an acute inflammatory process).

Serum chemistries showed sodium of 150 mEq/dl (hypovolemic hypernatremia due to dehydration), BUN of 48 mg/dl, and creatinine of 1.1 mg/dl (prerenal azotemia consistent with dehydration).

ASSESSMENT

Deep neck infection involving the anterior compartment of the left LPS with significant upper airway deviation and edema, and left medial and lateral masticator space infections secondary to an impacted mandibular third molar, complicated by dehydration and potential onset of sepsis

TREATMENT

Successful treatment of fascial space infections should include the following:
- Surgical drainage of an abscess or, in select cases, drainage of cellulites
- Identification and removal of the source of infection (the tooth in cases of odontogenic etiology)
- Administration of antibiotics (guided by culture and sensitivity when possible)
- Optimization of host nutritional and immune status.

Antimicrobial therapy can abort abscess formation if administered at an early stage of infection. However, once an abscess is formed, antimicrobial therapy is more effective in conjunction with adequate surgical drainage.

Impending airway obstruction may require immediate airway management (see Chapter 3, the section on emergent surgical airway, and Ludwig's angina earlier in this chapter). Maintaining spontaneous ventilation and airway patency is critical in patients with a compromised airway. Even a small dose of a respiratory depressant may change an apparently controlled situation into an emergent one, especially in the presence of a fatiguing patient. Morbidity or death due to the loss of an airway is still reported. Available options include endotracheal intubation versus establishment of a surgical airway. The advantages and disadvantages of these methods are summarized in Table 4-1. Consideration should be given to endotracheal intubation using an awake fiberoptic technique. This requires a skilled anesthesiologist and patient cooperation and can be time consuming.

Regardless of the airway technique used, caution should be exercised to prevent rupture of the abscess during intubation, which can result in aspiration of purulent material and is associated with significant morbidity (aspiration pneumonitis, pneumonia, lung abscess, acute respiratory distress syndrome) and mortality. One useful technique is to aspirate the LPS before to any intubation attempts. This can be done in the operating room under local anesthesia. The abscess can be decompressed significantly, thereby reducing the risk of aspiration during intubation.

The anterior compartment can be approached intraorally via an incision over the pterygomandibular raphe with blunt dissection around the medial side to enter the LPS. The extraoral approach is accomplished by making a 1- to 2-cm incision approximately 2 finger-breadths inferior to the mandible; dissection is then carried through the platysma to the

Table 4-1.	Intubation Versus Surgical Airway	

Procedure	Advantages	Disadvantages
Intubation	Potentially fast method Nonsurgical procedure	Nonsecured airway Patient discomfort is required for extended periods Difficult to perform with upper airway edema Risk of rupture of abscess with subsequent aspiration Requires mechanical ventilation during period of intubation Laryngotracheal stenosis
Tracheotomy	Airway security Patient comfort Less need for ventilation and sedation Earlier transfer from unit to floor	Surgical procedure Bleeding Scarring Pneumothorax

From Potter JK: Tracheotomy versus endotracheal intubation for airway management in deep neck space infections, *J Oral Maxillofac Surg* 60:349-354; 2002.

superficial layer of the deep cervical fascia. Sufficient fascia is exposed to identify the submandibular gland and the posterior belly of the digastric muscle. Dissection is then carried just posterior to the posterior belly of the digastric muscle in a superior, medial, and posterior direction into the LPS. If finger dissection is also used, the surgeon will be able to palpate the endotracheal tube medially and the carotid sheath posterolaterally. Through-and-through intraoral-extraoral drainage can be obtained by combining the intraoral approach with the extraoral approach. If old clots are found or if any signs of carotid sheath involvement are present, then vertical extension of the incision can be made along the anterior border of the sternocleidomastoid muscle. This extension allows the carotid artery to be pulled anteriorly and controlled as necessary.

The extraoral incision should parallel the lines of relaxed skin tension and lie in a cosmetically acceptable site whenever possible. The incision should also be supported by healthy underlying dermis and subcutaneous tissue. Placement of drains should allow for gravity-dependent drainage. A rigid drain should not be placed into the LPS because of the potential for erosion into the carotid sheath.

Supportive care to ensure adequate hydration, caloric intake, and analgesia is also important. It is reported that minimum daily fluid requirements increase by 300 ml per degree of fever (°C) per day. Caloric requirements also increase by approximately 5% to 8% per degree of fever per day.

Studies have shown that gram-positive cocci and gram-negative rods have the greatest growth percentage in cultures from deep neck space infections of odontogenic origin. Penicillin is still considered to be an effective empirical drug of choice for odontogenic infections. Due to rising incidence of penicillin resistance and failure of penicillin therapy, many clinicians advocate the empiric use of clindamycin or a combination β-lactam with penicillinase inhibitor (e.g., ampicillin sulbactam) for deep neck space infections of odontogenic origin until an antibiogram is obtained. Clindamycin has the disadvantage of not covering *Eikenella corrodens*.

This patient was given a bolus of normal saline and was taken urgently to the operating room. The anesthesiologist

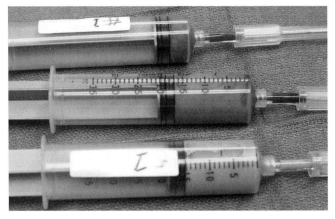

Figure 4-10 Samples of the aspirate to be sent for Gram stain and aerobic and anaerobic culture and sensitivity studies.

was informed about the parapharyngeal space involvement, and a plan for airway management was agreed on between the anesthesiologist and the surgeon. Before any attempts at intubation, 6 ml of lidocaine was injected on the mucosa of the oropharynx superficially; subsequently, 35 ml of purulent material was evacuated, allowing decompression of the swelling (Figure 4-10). Subsequently, the patient was placed in the supine position, and anatomical landmarks were marked on the neck for a tracheotomy or cricothyroidotomy. The surgeon and operating room personnel were positioned and prepared for an emergent surgical airway should the need arise. The anesthesiologist successfully intubated the patient using an awake fiberoptic nasal intubation technique. With a large-bore needle, the LPS was further aspirated and the material was sent for culture and sensitivity. The left mandibular third molar was extracted. The left medial and lateral masticator and the LPS were explored and drained via an intraoral and extraoral approach. A red rubber catheter was secured into the medial and lateral masticator spaces, and a Penrose drain was secured in the LPS. The patient was started on ampicillin-sulbactam 3 g intravenously every 6 hours. He remained intubated postoperatively and was transferred to the ICU. On the night of his surgery, he was weaned to minimal ventilator settings. He was awake and alert and in no apparent distress with a Glasgow Coma Scale score of 11T. Wound care regimen also included meticulous irrigation of the drains. On postoperative day 1, the patient's WBC count decreased to 13,000 cells/mm³ (it is not uncommon for WBC count to increase immediately after surgery due to demargination), and there was a notable decrease in pharyngeal and facial edema (it is not uncommon for surgical edema and fluid resuscitation to worsen the preexisting edema). A Gram stain revealed the presence of gram-positive cocci in pairs and chains (*Streptococcus* species) and gram-negative rods (mixed infection). On the second postoperative day, his WBC count decreased to 10,200 cells/mm³ with a significant decrease in edema with return of the uvula to midline. All sedative medications were discontinued, and the patient was extubated after passing a "cuff-leak" test. He was subsequently transferred to the ward and discharged to home care with oral antibiotics after 5 days of wound care and intravenous medications. At discharge, there was no significant drainage, and therefore all drains were removed. He was given instructions for jaw range-of-motion exercises and a follow-up appointment.

COMPLICATIONS

Complications of masticator space infections are partially dependent on the severity of the presenting infection, status of the host immune system, the virulence and resistance patterns of the infecting bacteria, and the time of presentation. Complications can be major, ranging from death from airway embarrassment to unsightly scars from incisions for drainage or tracheostomy.

Infections that have gained entry into the LPS may erode into the carotid sheath or impair any of the nerves found in the posterior compartment. Signs that indicate possible carotid sheath involvement include the following:

- Ipsilateral Horner's syndrome (ptosis, miosis, anhydrous)
- Unexplained palsies of cranial nerves IX through XII
- Recurrent small hemorrhages from the nose, mouth, or ear (herald bleeds)
- Hematoma in the surrounding tissue
- Persistent peritonsillar swelling despite adequate drainage
- Protracted clinical course
- Onset of shock

Any signs of carotid sheath involvement warrant immediate radiological evaluation, CT, or CT angiography. Surgical exploration and control of the great vessels may be required.

Involvement of the cranial nerves (vagus and glossopharyngeal nerves) can result in sudden death from bradycardia, asystole, and cardiac arrhythmia. The LPS is also subject to infection from nonodontogenic sources, including the parapharyngeal sinuses or other masticator spaces. Involvement of the retropharyngeal space can lead to descending infection involving the mediastinum. Erythema over the upper chest is suggestive of descending infection and may require cardiothoracic consultation.

Of particular concern are infections that do not appropriately respond to treatment. Consideration should be given to inadequate drainage or resistant bacterial strains. Culture and sensitivity studies can be obtained on purulent aspirates to guide antimicrobial therapy.

DISCUSSION

The LPS has the shape of an inverted pyramid or cone, the base of which is the sphenoid and the apex at the hyoid bone. The boundaries of this space are summarized in Table 4-2.

The LPS is divided by the styloid process and its muscles into an anterior and a posterior compartment. The anterior compartment contains only fat, connective tissue, and lymph nodes. The posterior compartment contains the glossopharyngeal, spinal accessory, and hypoglossal nerves. It also contains the carotid sheath (the carotid artery, internal jugular vein, and vagus nerve; the cervical sympathetic trunk lies posterior and medial to the carotid sheath). A strong fascial plane, the stylopharyngeal aponeurosis of Zuckerkandel and Testut, separates the anterior and posterior compartments. It is a barrier that helps prevent the spread of infection from the anterior to the posterior compartment.

Lateral pharyngeal infections could be caused by tonsillitis, otitis media, mastoiditis, parotitis, and, most commonly, secondary to an odontogenic etiology. Involvement of the LPS can also occur via spread through lymphatic vessels and subsequent rupture of a node. Lymphatic drainage from the nose and paranasal sinuses, ear, or oral cavity can involve this area. Infection can also spread from retropharyngeal, sublingual, submandibular, or masticator space infections. Peritonsillar abscesses that rupture through the superior constrictor muscle can also cause entry and infection of the LPS directly.

Symptoms of LPS involvement vary according to whether the anterior or posterior compartment is involved. The four most common signs of involvement of the anterior compartment are

1. Trismus
2. Induration or swelling at the angle of the jaw
3. Pharyngeal bulging with or without deviation of the uvula
4. Fever

Table 4-2.	Boundaries of the Lateral Pharyngeal Space
Space	**Boundary**
Anterior	Pterygomandibular raphe (junction of buccinator and superior constrictor muscles)
Posterior	Prevertebral fascia that communicates with the retropharyngeal space
Medial	Buccopharyngeal fascia on lateral surface of the superior constrictor muscle
Lateral	Fascia over the medial masticator, the parotid gland, and mandible

Deviation of the uvula with bulging or the pharyngeal wall can also be seen with peritonsillar abscesses; however, trismus is usually absent. With LPS infections, trismus is seen secondary to involvement of the adjacent medial pterygoid muscle. It can be difficult to differentiate a pterygomandibular space abscess from an LPS infection, but this distinction may be of academic interest only because treatment would be similar. Involvement of the posterior compartment may show posterior tonsillar deviation and retropharyngeal bulging. In this scenario, palsies of cranial nerves IX through XII may be seen, as well as ipsilateral Horner's syndrome (ipsilateral blepharoptosis, pupillary miosis, and facial anhidrosis). A common sign of LPS involvement is the presence of swelling of the lateral neck just above the hyoid and just anterior to the sternocleidomastoid muscle. This is the point at which the LPS is closest to the skin and where dependent edema or exudate is constrained by binding of the fascial layers to the hyoid bone.

Significant upper airway edema may require the patient to remain in an upright position, because assuming the supine position may lead to airway obstruction. Also, depending on the severity of the obstruction, patients may present with breathing with their mouth open or in the "sniffing position" with extension of the neck, stridor, labored breathing, intercostal retractions, tracheal tug, sore throat, or globus. Changes in voice also provide a clue to the location of airway involvement. A muffled or "hot potato" voice usually signifies a supraglottic process, while hoarseness is a sign of vocal cord involvement.

Bibliography

Brook I: Microbiology and management of peritonsillar, retropharyngeal and parapharyngeal abscesses, *J Oral Maxillofac Surg* 62:1545-1550, 2004.

Dzyak W, Zide MF: Diagnosis and treatment of lateral pharyngeal space infections, *J Oral Maxillofac Surg* 42:243-249, 1984.

Flynn TR: Surgical management of orofacial infection, *Atlas Oral Maxillofac Surg Clin* 8:77-99, 2000.

Hollinshead W: *Anatomy for surgeons,* vol 1. *The head and neck,* Philadelphia, 1982, Lippincott-Raven.

Munoz A: Acute neck infection: Prospective comparison between CT and MRI in 47 patients, *J Comput Assist Tomogr* 25:733-741, 2001.

O'Grady NP, et al: Practice parameters for evaluating new fever in critically ill adult patients. Task Force of the American College of Critical Care Medicine of the Society of Critical Care Medicine in collaboration with the Infectious Disease Society of America, 26:392-408, 1998.

Potter JK: Tracheotomy versus endotracheal intubation for airway management in deep neck space infections, *J Oral Maxillofac Surg* 60:349-354, 2002.

Rega AJ: Microbiology and antibiotic sensitivities of deep neck space infections, *J Oral Maxillofac Surg* 62:25-26, 2004.

Soma VR: Contrast-associated nephropathy, *Heart Dis* 4:372-379, 2002.

Storoe W: The changing face of odontogenic infections, *J Oral Maxillofac Surg* 59:739-748, 2001.

Styer TE: Peritonsillar abscess: diagnosis and treatment, *Am Fam Phys* 65:95, 2002.

William M: A prospective blinded comparison of clinical examination and computed tomography in deep neck infections, *Laryngoscope* 109:1873-1879, 1999.

Osteomyelitis

Jaspal Girn, DMD, and Chris Jo, DMD

CC

A 49-year-old man returns to your office 3 months after extraction of his mandibular third molars complaining that, "I still have some swelling and drainage from my mouth." (Osteomyelitis is more common in the mandible than in the maxilla due to the relatively lower blood supply.)

HPI

The patient presents with a history of persistent pain and swelling on the left side of his face, which has increased during the past month. He had four full bony impacted third molars removed 3 months ago without any acute complications. He returned 2 weeks after surgery for follow-up with a complaint of tenderness of the lower left extraction socket. The socket was noted to be filled with debris but without purulence and was irrigated clear. Instructions for follow-up were given, but the patient did not return for reevaluation. He now returns 3 months later due to the increasing pain, swelling, and some drainage from the left lower socket. He has not seen any other doctors and has not been on any antibiotics. He denies having fevers or chills, difficulty swallowing (dysphagia), or difficulty talking (dysphonia).

PMHX/MEDICATIONS/ALLERGIES/SH/FH

Noncontributory. The patient has no risk factors for osteomyelitis.

Although osteomyelitis has a higher incidence in patients who are immunocompromised (diabetes, HIV/AIDS, chemotherapy), intravenous drug users, patients with compromised splenic function (or splenectomy), patient undergoing radiation therapy, or patients who use tobacco, it can occur in patients with no risk factors.

The macrophages within the reticuloendothelial system of the spleen are involved in sequestration of encapsulated organisms (e.g., *H. influenza*, *S. pneumonia*, and *Salmonella* and *Klebsiella* species); therefore, an absent spleen or a compromised splenic function is a risk factor for osteomyelitis secondary to these organisms. Patients with sickle cell anemia are at risk because during a sickle cell crisis the splenic reticuloendothelial system is overwhelmed and becomes "clogged" by sickled red blood cells, leading to compromised splenic function and eventual "autosplenectomy." A history of bisphosphonate use should also be noted, to rule out possible osteonecrosis of the jaws.

EXAMINATION

General. The patient is a well-developed and well-nourished man in no apparent distress.

Vital signs. His blood pressure is 132/81 mm Hg, heart rate 80, respirations 16 per minute, and temperature 37.1°C (afebrile).

Maxillofacial. There is mild left facial swelling, erythema, and tenderness at the inferior border of the mandible. No fistulous tract is present (*Actinomyces israelii* infections commonly cause cutaneous fistulas). The lymph nodes were palpable in the left submandibular area (secondary to chronic infection). The inferior alveolar nerve is intact bilaterally (altered sensation can be commonly seen in osteomyelitis of the mandible).

Intraoral: The maximal interincisal opening is 25 mm (decreased due to guarding secondary to pain). The left retromolar pad is tender to palpation with moderate erythema and swelling. There is a small draining fistula distal to the left mandibular second molar in the attached gingiva. The oropharynx is clear, the uvula is midline, and the floor of the mouth is soft and nonelevated. The dentition is in good repair. There appear to be no changes in his occlusion (occlusal change would be suggestive of a pathological fracture).

IMAGING

Several imaging modalities are available for the evaluation of suspected osteomyelitis. A panoramic radiograph is the initial diagnostic study of choice when dealing with postextraction complications (e.g., retained tooth fragments, local wound infections, mandibular fractures, foreign bodies, bony sequestra, and pathology of adjacent teeth) or osteomyelitis. The destructive process of osteomyelitis must extend at least 1 cm and demonstrate 30% to 50% bone demineralization before it becomes radiographically apparent. The radiograph would show a loss of definition and lytic changes within the trabecular patterns of the involved bone. Eventually, radiopaque sequestra (fragments of bone that have become devitalized) may become visible, demonstrating a "mottled" radiolucent appearance.

Two-dimensional CT with contrast material is useful for visualizing soft tissue abnormalities such as the presence of an abscess and for assessing bony integrity or cortical disruptions. MRI can be useful for the evaluation of osteomyelitis due to the superior imaging of soft tissue, defining the extent and location of osteomyelitis. Nuclear medicine imaging

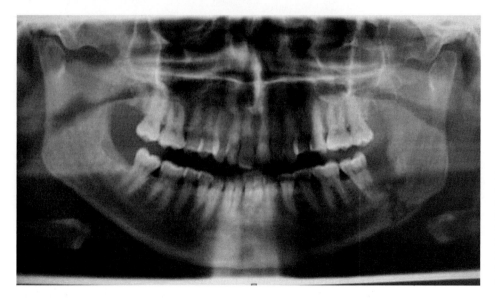

Figure 4-11 Panoramic radiograph showing mottled radiolucency at the extraction socket extending down to the inferior border. Extracortical reactive bone formation is seen at the inferior border. The proximal segment is not rotated or telescoped, suggesting that a pathological fracture has not occurred.

modalities can detect osteomyelitis 10 to 14 days earlier than conventional radiographic imaging. Scintigraphy with technetium 99m scanning is very sensitive in detecting increased bone turnover, and its specificity in detecting osteomyelitis is improved with the use of gallium 67 or indium 111.

In this patient, a panoramic radiograph (Figure 4-11) reveals a mottled radiolucent appearance in the area of the extracted left mandibular third molar, which extends to the inferior border of the mandible. There is evidence of reactive extracortical bone formation at the inferior border of the mandible. The proximal segment is not rotated superiorly (a rotated proximal segment would indicate a pathological fracture).

LABS

A CBC is necessary to evaluate the initial WBC count and to monitor the response to surgical and antibiotic therapy (WBC count may be elevated in acute or subacute osteomyelitis). This patient had a WBC count of 15,000 cells/mm^3 (elevated).

ASSESSMENT

Acute suppurative osteomyelitis of the left mandible

Although a 3-month duration may indicate a chronic state, acute suppurative osteomyelitis is the corrected diagnosis based on the fact that this disease process has not yet been managed either medically or surgically. Suppuration indicates that the body has mounted an immune response to the infection.

Several classification systems have been proposed, but no one scheme has gained acceptance. In the simplest form, osteomyelitis can be classified as acute or chronic. It is further characterized as suppurative or nonsuppurative. Waldvogel and associates proposed the staging of osteomyelitis into three separate groups based on the etiology: osteomyelitis related to a hematogenous source, secondary to a contiguous focus of infection, or associated with vascular insufficiency. The Cierny-Mader staging system is the most commonly used classification system for long-bone osteomyelitis. It divides the disease into four stages of osseous involvement and then combines it with three physiological host categories to give 12 discrete clinical stages. In addition, chronic diffuse sclerosing osteomyelitis is a unique form of osteomyelitis that is described as a painful disease state that occurs only in the mandible and is more often seen in younger female patients.

TREATMENT

Osteomyelitis is treated with a combination of surgical and medical interventions. Nonsurgical management of true osteomyelitis is futile and only allows for exacerbation of the existing condition and delay of more extensive surgical interventions.

If feasible, empiric antibiotic therapy should not be initiated until cultures are taken (purulent exudate and/or bone cultures) to accurately identify the causative organism(s). A bone culture is preferable for identification of the causative organism(s). Osteomyelitis caused by a contiguous focus of infection is often polymicrobial and, therefore, empiric broad-spectrum antibiotic(s) is initiated. Once culture and sensitivity results are available, antibiotic regimens should be adjusted to target the causative organism(s). The course and route (intravenous or oral) of antibiotic therapy are debatable and are frequently determined by clinical judgment. It has been generally accepted that a 4-week course of intravenous antibiotics is necessary, especially when dealing with chronic or refractory osteomyelitis. However, earlier stages of osteomyelitis may require only a short course of intravenous antibiotics (if needed), followed by a 1- to 2-week course of oral antibiotics based on serial clinical examinations.

Penicillin remains the empirical antibiotic of choice for osteomyelitis of tooth-bearing bone. However, many organisms responsible for osteomyelitis of the jaws are penicillin resistant, including *Prevotella, Porphyromonas, Staphylo-*

coccus, and *Fusobacterium.* Therefore it may be prudent to use a penicillin combined with a β-lactamase inhibitor (clavulanate) in combination with metronidazole (Flagyl) to improve anaerobic coverage. In patients who are allergic to β-lactam antibiotics, clindamycin is recommended due to its effectiveness against penicillinase-producing staphylococci, streptococci, and anaerobic bacteria. However, clindamycin is ineffective against *Eikenella corrodens* (common organism in osteomyelitis and odontogenic infections) and additional coverage is required. It is important to recognize that anaerobic organisms are difficult to culture, resulting in frequent false-negative anaerobic growth (therefore empiric anaerobic coverage may be prudent despite a negative anaerobic culture).

Surgical management of osteomyelitis should be planned in conjunction with medical treatment. In the early stages, surgical interventions should be limited to extraction of grossly loose teeth, debridement of fragments of bone, and incision and drainage of fluctuant areas. If the infection persists, further surgical procedures such as sequestrectomy, saucerization, decortication, or resection followed by reconstruction should be considered.

Sequestra are devitalized pieces of bone, which act as a nidus of infection. Sequestra are eventually resorbed, removed, or spontaneously expelled through the mucosa or skin, but they may persist and propagate a host response. Due to the avascular nature of necrotic sequestra, they are poorly penetrated by antibiotics and should be removed with minimal trauma, either intraorally, and/or transcutaneously. Saucerization is the "unroofing" of bone to expose the medullary cavity. The buccal cortex of the mandible is removed until bleeding bone is encountered at all margins of the surgical defect, thus producing a saucer-like defect. The purpose of this is to decompress the bone to allow extrusion of pus, debris, and any bony sequestra. The defect can be packed with a medicated dressing, changed several times over subsequent days, and irrigated daily to ensure no fragments of necrotic bone are left behind as the wound heals by secondary intention (or simply left open for irrigation). The lingual aspect of the mandible rarely requires reduction because it has a rich blood supply from the mylohyoid muscle. In the maxilla, saucerization is rarely needed because the cortex is thin and formed sequestra can be easily removed. Decortication of the mandible refers to the removal of chronically infected cortical bone, which is usually extended 1 to 2 cm beyond the affected area. Corticocancellous bone grafting of osteomyelitis has traditionally not been advocated, but there is some recent evidence suggesting the feasibility of immediate bone grafting along with stabilization of the mandible.

Refractory cases may require resection of the diseased bone and immediate stabilization with a reconstruction plate (in conjunction with a vascularized free flap or a pectoralis major flap). In cases of pathological fractures of the mandible (Figure 4-12), the diseased bone is debrided or resected, and the mandible is stabilized (using rigid internal fixation or a Joe Hall Morris biphasic external fixator), and reconstructed using several available techniques. Hyperbaric oxygen has been shown to be effective in treating osteomyelitis and should be considered in severe or refractory cases.

This patient underwent a bone culture (antibiotic therapy was not initiated until cultures were obtained) and local debridement via an intraoral approach. Intraoperatively, it was noted that the buccal and lingual cortices were intact. There were multiple loose fragments of devitalized bone (sequestra) and abundant granulation tissue tracking down to the inferior border of the mandible. After the wound was debrided, a round bur was used to remove the surrounding affected bone until normal-appearing, bleeding bone was encountered. The patient was started on empiric intravenous antibiotics (ampicillin-sulbactam and metronidazole) and remained hospitalized until the initial culture and sensitivity results were available. Cultures demonstrated growth of *Streptococcus anginosis* that was pansensitive, with negative anaerobic cultures. He was discharged home on oral amoxicillin with clavulanic acid and metronidazole, as well as chlorhexidine mouthwash. He was kept on a liquid diet until soft tissue healing occurred to prevent retention of food debris into the wound. He was subsequently switched to a soft diet for 8 weeks after surgery to prevent a postoperative pathological fracture. Final cultures did not grow any additional organisms, and therefore the antibiotic regimen was not changed during the course of his treatment. He healed without any complications.

COMPLICATIONS

Osteomyelitis is a complication of various oral and maxillofacial surgical procedures, and its incidence is related to both host factors and virulence of the infecting organisms. Treatment of osteomyelitis can itself be compounded by further complications. These include a persistent refractory infection of the bone, pathological fractures (at presentation, intraoperatively or postoperatively), necessity for resection of chronically infected bone, disfigurement, neurosensory impairment, and systemic spread of the infection.

Antibiotic therapy is associated with side effects such as diarrhea and *Clostridium difficile* pseudomembranous colitis, as well as the emergence of resistant microorganisms. Methicillin-resistant *Staphylococcus aureus* (MRSA) has become a very common community acquired organism in many communities. MRSA osteomyelitis requires intravenous vancomycin until sensitivity profiles (antibiogram) are available. If the organism is sensitive to only vancomycin, a peripherally inserted central catheter line can be used to allow delivery of intravenous antibiotics at home.

Uncontrolled diabetes mellitus presents as a special challenge. Tight glycemic control (blood glucose 90 to 110 mg/dl) is paramount for recovery from any infection. Noncompliant patients may require extended hospitalization to achieve glycemic control and delivery of intravenous antibiotics. Some patients may require an insulin pump, and critically ill patients may require an insulin drip. Sliding scale insulin is generally not regarded as adequate treatment because it designed to treat hyperglycemia rather than to prevent it (therefore it is always one step behind the hyperglycemia). Baseline insulin

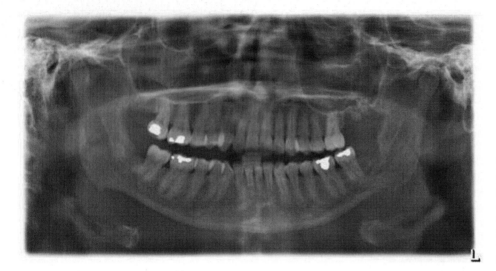

Figure 4-12 Panoramic radiograph of another patient with osteomyelitis of the left mandible after extraction of a third molar. Note that there is a pathological fracture of the left mandible with the proximal segment telescoped with the distal segment and rotated superiorly.

regimens need to be adjusted to prevent hyperglycemic episodes.

Pathological fractures of the mandible (see Figure 4-12) occur with sufficient destruction of cortical bone, primarily due to osteolytic changes associated with osteomyelitis and/or the result of periosteal stripping during an aggressive debridement (at 2 to 3 weeks postdebridement, the mandible is at greatest risk of fracture due to the critical phase of remodeling/resorption). Maxillomandibular fixation (6 to 8 weeks) should be considered for patients at higher risk for postoperative pathological fractures. A liquid or soft diet is prudent for those at moderate risk.

DISCUSSION

Osteomyelitis is an inflammatory condition involving the medullary cavity of bone that begins as a bacterial infection and can cause significant bony destruction. The microorganisms cause host tissue injury from direct cellular attack and through enzymatic degradation. The host responds by recruiting neutrophils to the area to digest the pathogens via release of enzymes and phagocytosis. When purulence (composed of necrotic tissue, dead bacteria, and WBCs) accumulates, it causes an increase in the intramedullary pressure, causing collapse of the vessels, venous stasis, and congestion. Vessels within the haversian system and Volkmann's canals of the cortical bone may undergo thrombosis or experience stasis and congestion, resulting in the surrounding bone becoming ischemic and thereby permitting the extension of osteomyelitis. If purulence continues to accumulate, the periosteum is penetrated and mucosal or cutaneous fistulas develop.

The establishment of an infection within bone is related to the compromise in the bone's vascular supply, but other factors, such as the virulence of the organism and the integrity of the host defenses, are also important. Host factors include systemic diseases with a microvascular component (e.g., diabetes), blood dyscrasias (e.g., sickle cell disease), immunosuppression (e.g., HIV infection), and collagen vascular disorders or bone dysplasias (e.g., osteopetrosis).

Initially, *Staphylococcus aureus* and *Staphylococcus epidermidis* accounted for 80% to 90% of osteomyelitis of the jaws. However, the frequency of *S. aureus* involvement in osteomyelitis has decreased due to the improved culture methods used to identify organisms, especially anaerobes. Anaerobes are frequently associated with aerobic organisms in osteomyelitis. Currently, osteomyelitis is recognized as a disease commonly caused by streptococci (α-hemolytic) and oral anaerobes such as *Peptostreptococcus, Fusobacterium,* and *Prevotella.*

Bibliography

Adekeye EO, Cornah J: Osteomyelitis of the jaws: a review of 141 cases, *Br J Oral Maxillo Surg* 23:24-35, 1985.

Benson PD, Marshall MK, Engelstad ME, et al: The use of immediate bone grafting in reconstruction of clinically infected mandibular fractures: bone grafts in the presence of pus, *J Oral Maxillofac Surg* 64:122-126, 2006.

Cieny G, Mader JT, Pennick H: A clinical staging system of adult osteomyelitis, *Contemp Orthop* 10:17-37, 1985.

Cohen MA, Embil JM, Canosa T: Osteomyelitis of the maxilla caused by methicillin-resistant *Staphylococcus aureus, J Oral Maxillofac Surg* 61:387-390, 2003.

Flynn TR: Anatomy and surgery of deep space infections of the head and neck. In *Knowledge updates, American Association of Oral and Maxillofacial Surgerons,* Rosemont, Ill, 1993.

Lew DP, Waldvogel FA: Osteomyelitis, *N Engl J Med* 336:999-1007, 1997.

Marx RE: Chronic osteomyelitis of the jaws, *Oral Maxillofac Clin North Am* 3:367-381, 1991.

Marx RE, Carlson EC, Smith BR, et al: Isolation of *Actinomyces species* and *Eikenella corrodens* from patients with chronic diffuse sclerosing osteomyelitis, *J Oral Maxillofac Surg* 52:26-33, 1994.

Mercuri LG: Acute osteomyelitis, *Oral Maxillofac Clin North Am* 3:355, 1991.

Paluska S: Osteomyelitis, *Clin Fam Pract* 6:127-156, 2004.

Peterson LJ: Microbiology of head and neck infections, *Oral Maxillofac Clin North Am* 3:247, 1991.

Vibhagool A, Calhoun J, Mader JP, et al: Therapy of bone and joint infections, *Hosp Formul* 28:63, 1993.

Waldvogel FA, Medoff G, Swartz MN: Osteomyelitis: a review of clinical features, therapeutic considerations and unusual aspects, *N Engl J Med* 282:316-322, 1970.

5 Dentoalveolar Surgery

Shahrokh C. Bagheri, DMD, MD, and Husain Ali Khan, MD, DMD

This chapter addresses:
- Third Molar Odontectomy
- Alveolar Osteitis (Dry Socket)
- Surgical Exposure of an Impacted Maxillary Canine
- Lingual Nerve Injury
- Displaced Root Fragments During Dentoalveolar Surgery

Dentoalveolar surgery is the most commonly performed surgical procedure by oral and maxillofacial surgeons. This refers to the surgical procedures associated with the dentate segment of the maxilla or mandible, termed the alveolar ridge. They include a variety of procedures ranging from simple tooth extractions, alveoplasty (recontouring of the alveolar bone), removal of tori, exposure of impacted teeth for orthodontic treatment, and extraction of impacted third molars. The origins and the current practice of oral and maxillofacial surgery are heavily based on dentoalveolar surgery. Over 50% of the practice of oral and maxillofacial surgeons worldwide compromises dentoalveolar procedures. Placement of dental implants has been added to the rehabilitative and reconstructive options of the maxillofacial region, replacing the more traditional preprosthetic procedures.

Since its establishment in 1918, the American Association of Oral and Maxillofacial Surgeons (AAOMS) has gone through extensive change, reflecting progressive changes in the specialty. Initially called the American Society of Exodontists, it was originally formed by a group of oral surgeons in Chicago after the National Dental Association meeting. As the association has grown, it has gone through several name changes, each reflecting the expansion of the specialty. Despite the wide scope of training of graduating oral and maxillofacial surgeons as evidenced by the sections in this book, dentoalveolar surgery remains the foundation of the specialty.

In this chapter we present five teaching cases representing some of the important aspects of this branch of oral and maxillofacial surgery. Three cases focus on complications of dentoalveolar surgery (dry socket, lingual nerve injury, and displacement of a tooth fragment during surgery), and two discuss the current issues in the treatment of impacted canines and third molars.

Third Molar Odontectomy

Shahrokh C. Bagheri, DMD, MD, and Husain Ali Khan, MD, DMD

CC

A 17-year-old boy is referred to your clinic for consultation regarding his third molars.

HPI

The patient has recently completed his orthodontic therapy. For the past few weeks, he has experienced increasing discomfort in the posterior mandible and was subsequently referred by his orthodontist for evaluation. He denies any fever, swelling, or drainage from the area.

PMHX/PDHX/MEDICATIONS/ALLERGIES/SH/FH

Non-contributory . He does not report any symptoms suggestive of temporomandibular joint (TMJ) dysfunction (TMD) and does not take any medications. He smokes approximately one pack of cigarettes per day (risk factor for the development of dry sockets).

EXAMINATION

General. The patient is a well-developed and well-nourished man in no apparent distress (higher levels of anxiety may require a deeper level of sedation/anesthesia).

Maxillofacial. There is no soft tissue abnormality with no lymphadenopathy (LAD). He has a good range of mandibular motion with an maximal interincisal opening (MIO) of 45 mm. Examination of the TMJ reveals no abnormalities (clicks or pain upon palpation). The muscles of mastication are nontender to palpation (important to detect preexisting symptoms of TMD).

Intraoral. Oral soft tissue is free of any lesions with no evidence of acute infection. The mandibular third molars are partially erupted with approximately 20% of the crown visible in the oral cavity with insufficient room for functional eruption. The overlying operculum appears slightly inflamed with evidence of food debris, and periodontal pockets of greater than 6 mm on the distal of the left and right mandibular second molars. The right and left maxillary third molars are partially erupted. Oral hygiene is fair.

IMAGING

A panoramic radiograph is the minimum imaging modality necessary for the evaluation and treatment of impacted third molars. Computed tomography (CT) scans are not necessary for the routine evaluation, but they may be used in select cases of suspected maxillofacial pathology or for accurate determination of the inferior alveolar nerve anatomy.

In this patient, the panoramic radiograph reveals a partial lack of space to accommodate the eruption of the mildly mesioangularly impacted mandibular molars with 75% root development (Figure 5-1). The roots are not fused and do not extend below the level of the neurovascular bundle. The outlines of mandibular canals are easily discerned on the radiograph. There is no diversion of the inferior alveolar canal, darkening of the third molar root, and interruption of the cortical white line (risk factors associated with inferior alveolar nerve injury) (Box 5-1). The maxillary third molars are vertically positioned with partial bony impaction. The maxillary sinuses and the remainder of the radiograph are within normal limits.

LABS

No routine laboratory tests are indicated for the routine evaluation of impacted third molars unless dictated by underlying medical conditions.

ASSESSMENT

Partial bony impaction of the right and left maxillary and mandibular third molars with insufficient room for eruption; localized gingivitis and early periodontal pocketing noted around the left and right mandibular third molars

TREATMENT

Two major professional organizations have made contradictory recommendations towards the prophylactic removal of impacted third molars. The AAOMS Third Molar Clinical Trials published several scientific articles that link third molars to future health problems in adults. In light of these findings, in 2005, the AAOMS suggested that removal of the third molars during young adulthood may be the most prudent option. In contrast, the National Health Service (NHS) of Great Britain and its associated arm, the National Institute of Clinical Excellence (NICE), published a series of guidelines recommending that "the practice of prophylactic removal of pathology-free impacted third molars should be discontinued in the NHS." These guidelines, made public in 2000, did acknowledge the ongoing AAOMS Third Molar Clinical

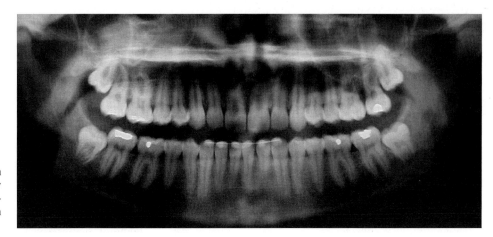

Figure 5-1 Panoramic radiograph demonstrating impacted maxillary and mandibular third molars (orthodontic retainer appliance is noted in the mandibular anterior incisors).

Box 5-1. **Rood's Radiographic Predictors of Potential Tooth Proximity to the Inferior Alveolar Canal**

- Darkening of root
- Deflection of the root
- Narrowing of the root
- Dark and birid root apex
- Interruption of the white line of the canal
- Diversion of the canal
- Narrowing of the canal

In Miloro M, ed: *Peterson's principles of oral and maxillofacial surgery,* ed 2. London, 2004, BC Decker, Table 41-1, p 820.

Trials, but as of this writing, their recommendations remain to be revised to account for more recently published evidence.

While in some regions of the world, socioeconomic and available resources play a major role in the determination of guidelines for third molar extractions, current scientific evidence remains unchanged. The cumulative financial costs of treating the health complications of retained third molars in the older population should be considered. While it is clear that the extraction of third molars poses some risks to the patient, determination of extraction versus nonextraction of asymptomatic third molars must compare the cost and risks of surgical extraction with the lifetime health and cost benefits from prevention and elimination of any pathological processes associated with retention of the third molars.

The effectiveness, safety, and relatively minimal cost incurred by extraction of third molars using outpatient office-based anesthesia, along with the currently available scientific evidence linking asymptomatic third molars to multiple health hazards, overwhelmingly support the extraction of asymptomatic third molars in young adults.

The patient described here was seen in the clinic for extraction of his teeth under intravenous sedation. Monitors (pulse oximeter, blood pressure, and a three-lead electrocardiography) are placed, and oxygen is delivered via a nasal mask at 4 L/min followed by nitrous oxide. A steroid was slowly infused intravenously (decreases incidence of postoperative swelling and discomfort). Midazolam and fentanyl were slowly titrated until a comfortable state of conscious sedation was achieved. Local anesthesia with epinephrine was injected, and adequate time was allowed for the local anesthetic block. A bite block was place for TMJ stabilization. An oral screen with loosely packed moist gauze was placed to protect the airway from accidental aspiration. A full mucoperiosteal flap was elevated using a buccal envelope incision with a distal hockey-stick extension for the mandibular third molars. Special consideration was given to not traumatize the lingual tissue. A buccal trough was made using a high-speed instrument, and the teeth were elevated and extracted. Careful attention is given to not violate the lingual cortex. The neurovascular bundle was not visualized, and there was no excessive hemorrhage from the socket (both associated with increased risk of inferior alveolar nerve injury). The wound was irrigated with normal saline, and the flaps where closed with chromic suture with careful attention to suture only the superficial lingual mucosa, to avoid lingual nerve injury. The upper third molars were removed through an envelope mucoperiosteal flap. Care was taken to avoid the roots of maxillary second molars (a possible complication). There was no evidence of an oral antral communication. The tooth follicles were removed and the sites were irrigated. Gauze was placed between the teeth to promote hemostasis, and the patient was monitored in the recovery room until he was fully awake and alert.

COMPLICATIONS

Third molar extraction is the most commonly performed surgical procedure by oral and maxillofacial surgeons. A well-planned surgical approach with the goal of prevention is the best way to minimize complications. Despite our best efforts, complications are expected, and it is best to counsel patients preoperatively for potential risks. Clinicians need to be aware of the risk factors associated with an increased risk of complications, especially for this commonly performed procedure.

Sensory nerve injury is well documented. Injury to the inferior alveolar nerve can lead to a range of symptoms in its distribution (anesthesia, hypoesthesia, dysesthesia, or paresthesia). A review of the literature demonstrates an incidence of nerve injury between 0.4% and 5%. In one large study with 367,170 patients, the incidence of nerve injury was 0.4% (22% of whom had symptoms lasting longer than 12 months). The incidence of inferior alveolar nerve injury is slightly more common than for the lingual nerve. However, the inferior alveolar nerves have a higher incidence of spontaneous recovery (due to its position in the bony canal allowing greater possibility of the nerve endings to reapproximate). Injury to the long buccal nerve is also possible, but it is less concerning, causing minimal to no subjective disability. Patients with severed inferior alveolar nerve or lingual nerve should be referred to a microneurosurgeon for prompt evaluation and potential surgical intervention (decompression, neurolysis, or neurorrhaphy). Complications from local anesthesia are also reported probably due to direct needle trauma to the inferior alveolar nerve. The reported incidence ranges between 1:400,000 to 1:750,000.

Not unlike any other procedures, infections are commonly associated with third molar removal both preoperatively and postoperatively. This appears to by more common after removal of partial and full bony impactions. Infections can occur as early as within several days of the procedure or may present late (within several weeks) and can be localized to the area of the third molar or occasionally spread to adjacent facial spaces to cause severe life-threatening infections. Most infections are easily managed with local measures and the use of antibiotics. The incidence of postoperative infection is approximately 3%.

Localized osteitis (dry socket) is a well-known complication of teeth extractions and is discussed in detail elsewhere in this text (see Alveolar Osteitis [Dry Socket] later in this chapter). Other complications associated with third molar surgery include periodontal complications, maxillary sinus involvement (oral antral communications, displacement of a fragment into the sinus), breaking of instruments, aspiration or swallowing of foreign objects, TMJ pain, maxillary tuberosity fractures, root fracture, injury to adjacent teeth, hemorrhage/hematoma, wound dehiscence, mandible fracture, and soft tissue emphysema.

DISCUSSION

Indications for the removal of third molars are variable and determined by many factors. Insufficient room for adequate eruption of the teeth can create a noncleanable environment for both the surrounding soft tissue and adjacent teeth. The increased difficulty and risks of third molar removal with increasing age, inadequate oral hygiene, and tooth position, as well as periodontal health and orthodontic considerations, should be taken into account. Erupted or partially erupted third molars have been shown to have a negative impact on the periodontal health. In a study by Dodson, attachment levels and probing depths improved after third molar removal.

However, the relationship between third molars and periodontal disease pathogenesis requires further study. There is no clear consensus on the ability of mandibular third molars to cause crowding of the anterior teeth. Although some investigators have shown a statistical association of third molars and late anterior crowding, this association is not strong. The majority of the literature does not support this hypothesis.

Offenbacher and colleagues published a study looking at periodontal disease and the risk of preterm delivery. They looked at 1020 pregnant women who received antepartum and postpartum periodontal examinations. The conclusions clearly demonstrate that maternal periodontal disease increases the relative risk of preterm or spontaneous preterm births. The mothers with third molar periodontal pathology had elevated serum markers of systemic inflammation (C-reactive protein, isoprostanes). Periodontal disease was also a predictor of more severe adverse pregnancy outcomes.

For extraction of third molars, there are a wide range of choices of anesthetic and surgical techniques related to the surgeon's training and experience. As the common dictum proclaims, "There is more than one way to do it." Many different surgical flaps and instruments have been developed over the years. A variation of the buccal hockey-stick incision appears to be the most commonly used and has the lowest incidence of permanent neurosensory injury. Similarly, the choice of anesthesia can vary from local anesthesia to intravenous sedation using a variety of medications, to general anesthesia with endotracheal intubation. This is influenced by many factors, including patient preference, available resources, operator training, and practice patterns within the region.

The anatomy of the inferior alveolar nerve is variable, but the canal is usually located inferior and buccal to the impacted mandibular third molars. In the largest cadaveric study of lingual nerve anatomy, by Behnia and associates, 669 nerves from 430 fresh cadavers were examined. In 94 cases (14%) the nerve was above the lingual crest, and in one case the nerve was in the retromolar pad region. In the remaining 574 cases (86%) the mean horizontal and vertical distances of the nerve to the lingual plate and the lingual crest were 2.1 mm and 3.0 mm, respectively. In 149 cases (22.3%) the nerve was in direct contact with the lingual plate of the alveolar process. This unpredictable anatomy of the lingual nerve in relation to the mandibular third molar lends itself susceptible to injury.

Bibliography

Alling CC: Dysesthesia of the lingual and inferior alveolar nerves following third molar surgery, *J Oral Maxillofac Surg* 44:454, 1986.

Alling C, Helfrick J, Alling R: *Impacted teeth,* Philadelphia, 1993, WB Saunders.

American Association of Oral and Maxillofacial Surgeons News Release: Research study links wisdom teeth to health problems in young adults, September 20, 2005.

Bagheri SC, Khan HA: Extraction versus non-extraction management of third molars. In Perciaccante VJ, ed: Management of impacted third molars, *Oral Maxillofac Surg Clin North Am,* February 2007.

Behnia H, Kheradvar A, Shahrokhi M: An anatomic study of the lingual nerve in the third molar region, *J Oral Maxillofac Surg* 58(6):649-651; discussion 652-653, 2000.

Blaeser BF, August MA, Donoff RB, et al: Panoramic radiographic risk factors for inferior alveolar nerve injury after third molar extraction, *J Oral Maxillofac Surg* 61(4):417-421, 2003.

Blakey GH, Jacks MT, Offenbacher S, et al: Progression of periodontal disease in the second/third molar region in subjects with asymptomatic third molars, *J Oral Maxillofac Surg* 64(2):189-193, 2006.

Blakey GH, Marciani RD, Haug RH, et al: Periodontal pathology associated with asymptomatic third molars, *J Oral Maxillofac Surg* 60(11):1227-1233, 2002.

Dodson TB: Management of mandibular third molar extraction sites to prevent periodontal defects, *J Oral Maxillofac Surg* 62(10):1213-1224, 2004.

Elter JR, Cuomo CJ, Offenbacher S, White RP Jr: Third molars associated with periodontal pathology in the Third National Health and Nutrition Examination Survey, *J Oral Maxillofac Surg* 62(4):440-445, 2004.

Hall HD, Bildman BS, Hand CD: Prevention of dry socket with local application of tetracycline, *J Oral Surg* 29:35, 1971.

Herpy AK, Goupil MT: A monitoring and evaluation study of third molar surgery complications at a major medical center, *Milit Med* 156:1, 1991.

Kiesselbach JE, Chamberlain JG: Clinical and anatomic observations on the relationship of the lingual nerve to the mandibular third molar, *J Oral Surg* 42:565, 1984.

National Institute for Clinical Excellence: Guidance on the extraction of wisdom teeth. Available at: http://www.nice.org.uk/pdf/wisdomteethguidance.pdf. Accessed March 9, 2006.

Offrenbacher S, Boggess KA, Murtha AP, et al: Progressive periodontal disease and risk of very preterm delivery, *Obstet Gynecol* 107(1):29-36, 2006.

Osborn TP, Frederickson G, Small IA, et al: A prospective study of complications related to mandibular third molar surgery, *J Oral Maxillofac Surg* 43:767-771, 1985.

Pogrel MA: Complications of third molar surgery. In Kaban LB, Pogrel MA, Perrott DH, eds: *Complications of Oral and Maxillofacial Surgery,* Philadelphia, 1997, WB Saunders.

Rood JP, Shehab AAN: The radiological predictors of inferior alveolar nerve injury during third molar surgery, *Br J Oral Maxillofac Surg* 28:20, 1990.

Sweet JB, Butler DP: Predisposing and operative factors, effect on the incidence of localized osteitis in mandibular third molar surgery, *J Oral Surg* 46:206, 1978.

White RP Jr, Madianos PN, Offenbacher S, et al: Microbial complexes detected in the second/third molar region in patients with asymptomatic third molars, *J Oral Maxillofac Surg* 60(11):1234-1240, 2002.

Alveolar Osteitis (Dry Socket)

Eric P. Holmgren, MS, MD, DMD, and Shahrokh C. Bagheri, DMD, MD

CC

A 19-year-old woman presents to your clinic 5 days after removal of four impacted third molars with a complaint of increasing pain that is difficult to control with prescription pain medications.

HPI

The patient underwent removal of four difficult full bony impactions. Postoperatively, she was given a prescription for an opioid/acetaminophen combination medication for pain control. On the fifth postoperative day, she describes a dull, aching pain that radiates to her left ear. She complains of a bad odor (halitosis) and taste within her mouth emanating from her lower jaw. She reports to have adhered closely to the postoperative instructions.

PMHX/PDHX/MEDICATIONS/ALLERGIES/SH/FH

The patient uses birth control pills and smokes one pack of cigarettes per day (both risk factors for the development of alveolar osteitis) (Box 5-2).

EXAMINATION

General. The patient appears to be in mild distress secondary to pain. The accompanying parent is very concerned.

Vital signs. Her vital signs are within normal limits (dry sockets do not cause fever).

Maxillofacial. There is bilateral edema of the lower face consistent with her surgery. There are no cranial nerve deficits.

Intraoral. The extraction sockets of the maxillary third molars and the right mandibular third molar appear to be healing adequately with no evidence of exposed alveolar bone. The extraction socket of the left mandibular third molar shows evidence of exposed bone, food debris, and sensitivity upon irrigation. There is no purulence (alveolar osteitis is not an infection).

IMAGING

A panoramic radiograph is not routinely indicated for the evaluation of alveolar osteitis, unless there is suspicion of a retained bony or tooth fragments within the sockets. Non-resorbable dry socket packs must contain a radiopaque material to ensure removal of any packing material upon subsequent visits, which can be confirmed with radiographs.

The preoperative panoramic radiograph should be evaluated for the proximity of the inferior alveolar nerve before the application of eugenol-based medicaments, due to the possible neurotoxic effects of this medication.

LABS

No laboratory tests are indicated for the routine management of alveolar osteitis.

ASSESSMENT

Alveolar osteitis (dry socket) of the extraction socket of the left mandibular third molar

TREATMENT

The primary goal of treatment is relief of pain through this phase of delayed healing. Medicaments such as eugenol and lidocaine jelly have been advocated for packing of the socket. Packings can be changed every day or every other day for approximately 3 to 6 days until the pain is resolved. It is imperative to avoid the use of a eugenol-based packings if one suspects close proximity of the inferior alveolar nerve due to eugenol's neurotoxic properties. It is important to evaluate the preoperative panoramic radiograph and the operative note for evidence of close proximity or exposure of the inferior alveolar nerve to the roots and/or socket of the third molars. In such instances, alternatives such as lidocaine jelly soaked in $1/4$-inch gauze strips may be used. Once the pain has subsided, the packing should be removed to avoid the development of a foreign body reaction. Previously it was thought that curettage of the socket can induce bleeding and therefore healing. This has not been shown to promote healing. Aggressive curettage of the socket is unnecessary and contraindicated. There is no indication for the use of antibiotics for treatment of dry sockets.

In this patient, gentle irrigation with warm saline (without curettage) and an iodoform/eugenol-based packing placed into the socket, along with prescription antiinflammatory medication, were used. She had improvement of her pain within minutes and subsequently returned 48 hours later with marked reduction of pain. The packing was removed and the socket was gently irrigated. She was instructed to maintain good oral hygiene and rinse with a warm saline until the socket no longer collects debris.

| Box 5-2. | Factors That Are Suggested to Influence the Incidence of Alveolar Osteitis |

Increased Risk With
- Smoking
- Birth control pills
- History of pericoronitis
- Increased age
- Traumatic extraction (inexperienced surgeon)
- Inadequate irrigation

Decreased Risk With
- Prerinsing with chlorhexidine
- Maintenance of good oral hygiene perioperatively
- Thorough intraoperative lavage

COMPLICATIONS

The vast majority of cases of alveolar osteitis heal despite any intervention. Most medicaments (which usually contain eugenol) that are placed in the socket are palliative and may not necessarily expedite recovery. However, one must identify chronic nonhealing extraction sockets, especially in patients at risk for the development of osteomyelitis (diabetes or chronic steroid use) and osteoradionecrosis (history of radiation therapy to the surgical site). Patients who do not respond to routine care of diagnosed alveolar osteitis must undergo further evaluation for other pathological processes.

DISCUSSION

The onset of alveolar osteitis is variable but commonly occurs between 3 and 7 days postextraction. The etiology, prevention, and treatment of alveolar osteitis are up for debate. The most prevailing theory of the pathogenesis of alveolar osteitis is the destruction of the initial clot by fibrinolytic activity, impairing the formation of granulation tissue that promotes the initial fibrillar bone and ultimately mature bone formation. Bacteria may play an important but not clearly defined role. The incidence of alveolar osteitis is between 1% and 3% of all extraction sockets but has been reported as high as 20% of impacted mandibular third molars. The next most commonly involved teeth are the mandibular premolars, followed by the maxillary premolars, molars, canines, and incisors.

It is well known that smoking, oral contraceptive pills, a history of existing pericoronitis, traumatic extractions (correlating with the surgeon's experience), older age, and inadequate irrigation at the time of surgery are highly associated with the development of alveolar osteitis. Based on several studies, preoperative rinsing with chlorhexidine and thorough intraoperative lavage using physiological saline reduce the incidence of alveolar osteitis by up to 50%. Studies on the efficacy of topical/intraalveolar antibiotics and its benefits are debatable. Recent studies have not demonstrated any benefits.

Similarly, the use of systemic perioperative antibiotics has not been shown to be of any benefit. At present, the literature does not support the use of perioperative antibiotics in reducing the incidence of alveolar osteitis.

Despite current thinking, factors such as vasoconstrictive use, seasonal affects, the degree of bacterial load within the socket, flap design, and negative pressure dislodging the clot (use of a straw or spitting). have *not* been shown to increase the incidence of dry sockets. As mentioned, there is evidence that the use of oral contraceptives is a risk factor but female gender alone is not.

Bibliography

Alexander RE: Dental extraction wound management: a case against medicating postextraction sockets, *J Oral Maxillofac Surg* 58(5): 538-551, 2000.

Betts NJ, Makowski G, Shen YH, Hersh EV: Evaluation of topical viscous 2% lidocaine jelly as an adjunct during the management of alveolar osteitis, *J Oral Maxillofac Surg* 53(10):1140-1144, 1995.

Caso A, Hung LK, Beirne OR: Prevention of alveolar osteitis with chlorhexidine: a meta-analytic review, *Oral Surg Oral Med Oral Pathol Oral Radiol Endod* 99(2):155-159, 2005.

Hermesch CB, Hilton TJ, Biesbrock AR, et al: Perioperative use of 0.12% chlorhexidine gluconate for the prevention of alveolar osteitis: efficacy and risk factor analysis, *Oral Surg Oral Med Oral Pathol Oral Radiol Endod* 85(4):381-387, 1998.

Garcia AG, Grana PM, Sampedro FG, et al: Does oral contraceptive use affect the incidence of complications after extraction of a mandibular third molar? *Br Dent J* 194(8):453-5, Apr 26, 2003.

Larsen PE: Alveolar osteitis after surgical removal of impacted mandibular third molars. Identification of the patient at risk, *Oral Surg Oral Med Oral Pathol* 73(4):393-397, 1992.

Poeschl PW, Eckel D, Poeschl E: Postoperative prophylactic antibiotic treatment in third molar surgery—a necessity? *J Oral Maxillofac Surg* 61(1):3-8, 2004.

Rood JP, Shehab BA: The radiological prediction of inferior alveolar nerve injury during third molar surgery, *Br J Oral Maxillofac Surg* 28(1):20-25, 1990.

Sanchis JM, Sáez U, Peñarrocha M, Gay C: Tetracycline compound placement to prevent dry socket: a postoperative study of 200 impacted mandibular third molars, *J Oral Maxillofac Surg* 62(5):587-591, 2004.

Surgical Exposure of an Impacted Maxillary Canine

Bruce Anderson, HBSc, DDS, and Chris Jo, DMD

CC

A 14-year-old boy is referred to your office by his orthodontist for exposure and bracketing of an impacted left maxillary canine (normally erupting between ages 11 and 12).

The maxillary canines are the second most commonly impacted teeth (the most common are the third molars).

HPI

The patient has a history of premature loss of the primary left maxillary canine secondary to trauma (premature loss of teeth with subsequent arch length reduction is one of the many causes of impaction). Orthodontic treatment has begun and sufficient arch space has been accommodated for the guided eruption of the impacted canine. The patient has no history of any other impacted or congenitally missing teeth and presents with an otherwise full dentition.

PMHX/PDHX/MEDICATIONS/ALLERGIES/SH/FH

Noncontributory.

EXAMINATION

General. The patient is a well-developed and well-nourished boy in no apparent distress.

Maxillofacial. He has a symmetrical facial appearance with no obvious skeletal abnormalities.

Intraoral. Orthodontic bands, brackets, and arch wires are in place. A well-healed edentulous space is present in the area of the left maxillary cuspid with an adequate alveolar ridge. A small, painless, palpable bony buccal protuberance can be noted in the area of the left maxillary cuspid, consistent with the crown of the impacted canine (clinical evaluation to determine palatal or buccal impaction is important and often sufficient to determine the approach for access to the tooth). The gingival and palatal tissue appear healthy with no notable periodontal defects.

IMAGING

A panoramic radiograph is the initial screening study of choice for evaluating impacted teeth. It provides an excellent overview of the dentition, associated dentoalveolar structures, and location of impacted teeth. Periapical "shift shots" can help determine if the tooth is buccal/labial or palatal/lingual (the SLOB rule: Same Lingual, Opposite Buccal, is frequently used to determine the position of the tooth as the cone of the x-ray machine is moved anteriorly or posteriorly to observe the position of the tooth on the subsequent film). Occlusal films, lateral cephalometric films, or CT scans can be used for precisely locating the position and orientation of impacted teeth.

In this patient, the panoramic radiograph shows a fully formed impacted left maxillary cuspid with a mesioangular orientation. Figure 5-2 demonstrates the position of the impacted canine before the initiation of orthodontic therapy. The crown of the canine appears to have a pericoronal radiolucent lesion consistent with a hyperplastic dental follicle (although a dentigerous cyst or other pathological processes are also possible). No crestal bone loss is noted in the surrounding region. The full bony impacted third molars are also noted.

LABS

No laboratory studies are indicated for routine exposure and orthodontic bracket placement of impacted teeth unless dictated by the medical history.

ASSESSMENT

Full bony mesioangular labially impacted left maxillary canine

TREATMENT

Current popular treatments of impacted canines can be divided into open and closed surgical techniques, differing slightly in regard to palatal versus labial impactions. Autotransplantation and extraction with implant replacement are less commonly used techniques and are described with other historical techniques below.

Open techniques. These surgical techniques are indicated when the crown of the impacted canine is in an appropriate location near the alveolar process, allowing exposure and access for orthodontic bracket placement. For palatal impactions, the excision of overlying soft tissue may be performed with a surgical blade or electrocautery. Bone removal may be performed with a rotary instrument, rongeurs, or hand instruments to expose the crown to the level of the cervical margin. Complete exposure of the crown may not be feasible in cases where the crown is in close proximity to incisor roots. Any dental follicle remnants should be excised at this time, and gentle luxation of the tooth may be performed to rule out

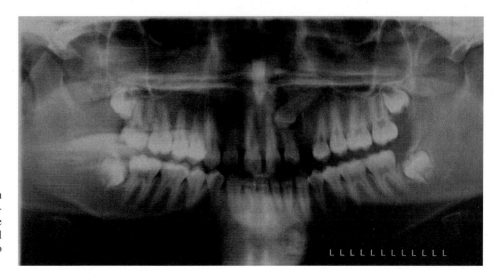

Figure 5-2 Panoramic radiograph demonstrating the horizontal impaction of the left maxillary canine before orthodontic therapy. The full bony impacted third molars are also noted.

ankylosis. An orthodontic bracket with gold chain may be etched and bonded to the crown with the chain attached passively to existing orthodontic arch wires. The wound may be left open or packed with a periodontal dressing for a period of 4 to 5 days. It is generally accepted that a period of 6 to 8 weeks be observed in both palatal and labial impactions to allow for spontaneous eruption prior to the application of orthodontic forces. The apically repositioned flap is the open technique of choice for labially impacted canines. Electrocautery, or a "window" excision of overlying soft tissue, should be avoided with labial impactions as it usually results in a lack of attached gingiva following eruption with a possible need for a secondary graft procedure. A full-thickness mucoperiosteal flap with vertical incisions is raised to the level of the vestibular sulcus, followed by bone removal, follicle removal, and crown exposure as previously described. The distal aspect of the flap is positioned apically and sutured with chromic gut at the level of the cervical margin, thus placing attached gingiva at the level of the cementoenamel junction. Again, the bracket with chain may be bonded at this time.

Closed techniques. These surgical techniques are indicated when the crown is not near the alveolar process or is in a position that inhibits the apical repositioning of a flap. In both palatal and labial impactions, a full-thickness mucoperiosteal flap is raised, allowing subsequent crown exposure, gentle luxation, and bonding of the orthodontic bracket with chain. At this point, the chain may be brought through the distal aspect of the flap, or through a stab incision within the body of the flap, and then the full flap is repositioned and sutured. In closed techniques, orthodontic forces may be applied after 1 week to allow for soft tissue healing.

COMPLICATIONS

The most prevalent complication associated with surgical exposure of impacted canines is failure of the orthodontic bracket bond or fracture of the chain. This is of higher consequence in closed techniques as it requires surgical reexposure of the crown before replacement of the bracket. Moisture

in the surgical field during bracket bonding may be the likely cause of this complication. Reexposure will also be required with the low occurrence of gingival overgrowth in open techniques.

Periodontal defects may occur as a result of inappropriate flap design and/or bone loss adjacent to the surgical site. Damage to the erupting tooth and adjacent tooth roots, including root resorption, may occur secondary to difficulty controlling the path of eruption.

Ankylosis of the impacted tooth should be considered if no movement is observed following a sufficient application of orthodontic forces and time. Intrusion of the anchoring dentition may be observed in this situation. Some suggest that the act of gently luxating the tooth at the time of exposure may cause ankylosis as a result of bleeding and inflammation.

DISCUSSION

Excluding third molars, canines are the most commonly treated impactions by the oral and maxillofacial surgeon. Bass reported the frequency of impacted canines as 2%, with palatal impactions occurring more frequently than labial. Chaushu and associates in 2005 reviewed the surgical exposure and bracketing of 60 patients with 71 non–third molar impactions (57 canines, 14 central incisors). In their study, palatal impactions occurred most frequently (2:1), and they found that the use of a closed technique for palatal impactions had a statistically significant improvement in mean recovery time. Most impacted canines have an unknown etiology; however, numerous etiologies have been attributed to canine impactions, including mechanical obstruction by adjacent teeth or pathology, arch length discrepancy (more prevalent in labial impactions), premature loss of deciduous teeth, associated syndromes, questionable genetic predispositions, and endocrine abnormalities such as hypothyroidism and hypopituitarism.

Historical treatments of impacted canines include the placement of crown forms or cervical wires. Adapted aluminum or plastic crown forms were commonly placed following exposure with a closed technique with resulting erosion of overlying soft tissue secondary to a foreign body reaction. Once visible in the oral cavity, the crown form was removed and orthodontic brackets were placed. Wires secured around the cervical neck of the canine were also popularly used, but this was a more technically demanding procedure, sometimes requiring excessive manipulation of the tooth, and erosion of the canine at the cervical neck has been reported with this technique.

Additional surgical options include autotransplantation, segmental osteotomy, and extraction with subsequent implant placement. Autotransplantation may be indicated in circumstances of deep impactions and involves the creation of a bony socket for the extracted and transplanted canine. Survival rates have been reported at 70%, and as high as 94% when the periodontal membrane is intact at time of transplantation. This technique, however, is not commonly used as it is less predictable, with several reported cases of external root resorption. Segmental osteotomy is seldom performed and carries the risks of a more technical procedure. The incidence of extraction and replacement with osseointegrated implants has increased in recent years, but the use of implants in growing children is still controversial. Implants have been shown to migrate and may become submerged as growth continues vertically. The latter complication may be avoided by placement of the implant after vertical growth of the alveolus is completed. Despite these concerns, successful restoration using implants has been demonstrated in numerous studies and warrants further investigation.

The decision between using an open versus a closed technique is often left up to the practitioner and may be one of personal choice. As mentioned previously, there are certain physical location factors of the involved impacted tooth that may dictate one technique over another, but the trend in the literature seems to show a smaller overall complication rate associated with open techniques. Studies have reported a 2-fold rate of complication in closed compared to open techniques, with the primary complication in closed cases being bond or wire failure and the primary complication in open cases being soft tissue overgrowth. Bond failure in open techniques is a minor complication, and some suggest delaying bracket placement until after the observational period, allowing greater control of moisture in the surgical field. No significant differences in subsequent periodontal complications have been reported between the two groups. The consensus appears to be that both techniques are acceptable and provide predictable results for the treatment of impacted canines.

Bibliography

Bass T: Observation on the misplaced upper canine tooth, *Dent Pract Dent Rec* 18:25-33, 1967.

Caminiti MF, et al: Outcomes of the surgical exposure, bonding and eruption of 82 impacted maxillary canines, *J Can Dent Assoc* 64(8):572-579, 1998.

Chaushu S, Becker A, Zelster R, et al: Patient's perception of recovery after exposure of impacted teeth: a comparison of closed- versus open-eruption techniques, *J Oral Maxillofac Surg* 63:323-329, 2005.

Felsenfeld AL, Aghaloo T: Surgical exposure of impacted teeth, *Oral Maxillofac Surg Clin N Am* 14:187-199, 2002.

Ferguson JW, Parvizi F: Eruption of palatal canines following surgical exposure: a review of outcomes in a series of consecutively treated cases, *Br J Orthod* 24(3):203-207, 1997.

Jacobs SG: The impacted maxillary canine. Further observations on aetiology, radiographic localization, prevention/interception of impaction, and when to suspect impaction, *Aust Dent J* 41(15):310-316, 1996.

Johnson W: Treatment of palatally impacted canine teeth, *Am J Orthod* 56(6):589-596, 1969.

Moss JP: Autogenous transplantation of maxillary canines, *Br J Oral Surg* 26:775, 1968.

Pearson MH, et al: Management of palatally impacted canines: the findings of a collaborative study, *Eur J Orthod* 19(5):511-515, 1997.

Pogrel MA: Evaluation of over 400 autogenous tooth transplants, *J Oral Maxillofac Surg* 45:205-211, 1987.

Tiwanna PS, Kushner GM: Management of impacted teeth in children, *Oral Maxillofac Surg Clin N Am* 17:365-373, 2005.

Lingual Nerve Injury

Shahrokh C. Bagheri, DMD, MD, and Roger A. Meyer, MD, DDS, FACS

CC

A 26-year-old woman is referred to a microneurosurgeon for evaluation of anesthesia of the left tongue (absence of perception of any stimulation of the mucosa).

HPI

The patient had all four third molars extracted by an oral and maxillofacial surgeon 11 weeks before presentation. Upon follow-up at 7 days with the referring surgeon, the patient complained of persistent anesthesia on the left tongue and altered taste sensation. No neurosensory testing was done at that time. Six weeks after surgery, the patient continued to report profound numbness of the right tongue and no improvement in taste perception. All surgical wounds were healed. Neurosensory testing of the tongue (pinprick and light touch) demonstrated total anesthesia of the anterior two thirds of the left tongue, floor of mouth, and lingual gingiva. Photographic documentation of the affected area of the tongue was made. The patient was appointed for reevaluation in 4 weeks. At follow-up (10 weeks postsurgery), repeat neurosensory testing revealed no change (persistent total anesthesia) from the previous examination. The patient was subsequently referred to a microneurosurgeon for evaluation of left lingual nerve anesthesia.

The patient also complained of pain radiating into her left tongue when chewing food or brushing her left lower teeth (allodynia) and frequent accidental biting of her tongue. (Allodynia is defined as pain due to a stimulus that does not normally produce pain. Dysesthesia is an unpleasant abnormal sensation, either spontaneous or evoked, and anesthesia dolorosa is pain in an area or a region that is anesthetic.)

PMHX/PDHX/MEDICATIONS/ALLERGIES/SH/FH

Noncontributory.

EXAMINATION

General. The patient is a well-developed and well-nourished woman in no apparent distress.

Maxillofacial. There is no lymphadenopathy, and all extraction sockets are healing well. There are no masses or ulcerations, no fasciculations or atrophic changes of the tongue, and no evidence of recent tongue trauma (scars or lacerations). Inspection of the lingual and buccal aspects of mandible reveals no abnormalities (texture, color, and consistency of mucosa are within normal limits). Palpation and percussion of the lingual surface of the posterior mandible adjacent to the third molar area produced a localized painful sensation that radiated to the left tongue (positive Tinel's sign; a provocative test of regenerating nerve sprouts in which light percussion over the nerve elicits a distal tingling sensation; used as a sign of small fiber recovery but can also be confused with neuroma formation).

Clinical neurosensory. This examination is performed at three levels: A, B, and C (Box 5-3). Cranial nerves II through XII are intact (except left lingual nerve distribution).

In patients with abnormal pain sensations (allodynia, anesthesia dolorosa, dysesthesia), a local anesthetic block is a good predictor of pain relief from microneurosurgical repair of the injured nerve.

IMAGING

Panoramic radiograph (11 weeks postsurgery) reveals no evidence of retained root fragment or foreign bodies. The outline of the socket of the right mandibular third molar is well demarcated and is appropriate for the stage of healing.

LABS

No routine laboratory tests are indicated for routine microneurosurgical evaluation unless dictated by the medical history.

ASSESSMENT

Left lingual nerve neurotmesis or Sunderland fifth-degree injury (Table 5-1) (nerve injury with disruption of all axonal and sheath elements, producing Wallerian degeneration and likely neuroma formation)

Microneurosurgical intervention is indicated for lingual nerve neurorrhaphy (suturing of the two nerve ends together) and possible excision of proximal stump neuroma.

TREATMENT

The two most important factors in successful microneurosurgery are correct patient selection (diagnosis) and prompt evaluation of suspected nerve injuries. Surgical treatment may include nerve exploration with identification of nerve pathology such as a neuroma in continuity, lateral exophytic neuroma, lateral adhesive neuroma, and partial transaction or transaction with a stump neuroma. Specific intraoperative

Table 5-1. **Nerve Injury Classification**

Seddon	Sunderland	Histology	Outcomes
Neurapraxia	First degree	No axonal damage, no demylination or no neuroma	Rapid recovery (days to weeks)
Axonotmesis	Second, third and fourth degree	Some axonal damage, demylination, possible neuroma	Loss of sensation, slow incomplete recovery (weeks to months), microsurgery may help
Neurotmesis	Fifth degree	Severe axonal damage, nerve discontinuity, neuroma formation	Loss of sensation, spontaneous recovery unlikely, microsurgery may help

Box 5-3. **Performance Levels for Clinical Neurosensory**

Level A (Directional and two-point discrimination): Patient unable to feel the direction of the stimulus using a cotton swab and unable to feel a single- versus two-point stimuli applied to the affected side. Control side within normal limits (inability to discriminate two points farther than 6.5 mm apart is considered abnormal).
Level B (Contact detection): Patient does not experience pain to repetitive application of touch/pressure. Control side is within normal limits.
Level C (Pain sensitivity): Exhibits no response to pinprick, noxious pressures, and heat on the left lingual nerve distribution. Control side is within normal limits.

findings will dictate the surgical treatment modality of choice.

Under general nasal endotracheal anesthesia, bupivacaine with epinephrine was injected into the soft tissue of the operative field in addition to an inferior alveolar nerve block for vasoconstriction of the associated proximal vessels. Using 3.5X loop magnification (or an operating microscope) and fiberoptic lighting, incisions were made along the gingival margins of premolar and molar teeth, on both the buccal and lingual aspects of the mandible. The mucoperiosteum was elevated from the region of the bicuspids and posteriorly up the ascending ramus. The periosteum was sharply incised with microscissors, and the lingual nerve was identified and dissected free to reveal a total transection adjacent to the previously removed third molar with a stump neuroma on the proximal segment. There was a defect in the lingual cortex of the mandible. The distal and proximal nerve stumps were freed of surrounding scar tissue, the proximal amputation neuroma was excised, and the distal nerve stump was freshened to ensure viable fascicles (Figure 5-3, *A*). Subsequently, the nerve endings were reanastomosed (neurorrhaphy) in a tension-free manner (tension across the suture line of greater than 25g will significantly compromise regeneration) using 8-0 nylon sutures (Figure 5-3, *B*). The anastomosis

was guarded by a resorbable flexible collagen nerve cuff to avoid fibrous tissue ingrowth (Figure 5-3C). The mucosal incision was closed with chromic sutures, and the patient was extubated.

Postoperatively the patient was closely monitored for adequate wound healing and subsequent neurosensory reeducation exercises. At 1-year follow-up, the patient demonstrated both subjective and objective signs of left lingual nerve sensory function.

COMPLICATIONS

Like other surgical operations, microneurosurgical intervention is not without risks. Careful patient selection is of paramount importance. The indications for microneurosurgical intervention are not always consistent in the literature. However, common indications for surgical exploration and repair of the lingual nerve include the following:

- Abnormal and triggered hyperpathia (a painful syndrome of increased reaction to a stimulus), allodynia, or hyperalgesia (an increased response to a stimulus that is normally painful) that is abolished by an anesthetic block of the suspected nerve
- Constant, deep pain in an anesthetic (anesthesia dolorosa) or a hypoesthetic tongue that is abolished by a local anesthetic block of the suspected nerve
- Intolerable anesthesia or hypoesthesia with no signs of recovery with interval neurosensory testing, persisting beyond 3 months after injury

Patients with tolerable anesthesia/hypoesthesia or with satisfactory neurosensory recovery without intolerable pain or dysfunction may not be candidates for surgical nerve exploration. It is possible for such patients to have a worse outcome, such as the development of anesthesia dolorosa, in a previously anesthetic but nonpainful region. Fortunately, this appears to be a rare event. Most patients with nerve injury whose presurgical symptom is numbness rather than pain do not develop painful sensations after microsurgical nerve repair. More commonly, failure of peripheral trigeminal microneurosurgery is related to the ability to restore the preinjury sensory function. In cases of total nerve severance (neurotmesis or Sunderland fifth-degree), the time lapse from

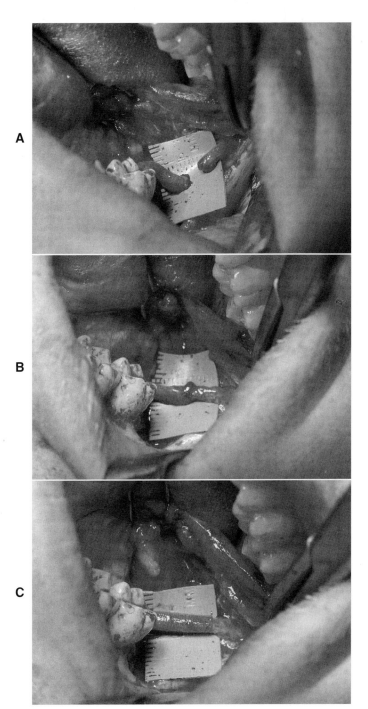

Figure 5-3 **A,** Proximal and distal nerve stumps before reanastomosis. **B,** Neurorrhaphy with 8-0 nylon sutures. **C,** Repair protected by a resorbable flexible collagen nerve cuff.

injury to repair, proper surgical technique (such as tension-free closure), patient age, and health status are among the most important factors for success. Best results are seen when repair is performed within 6 months of the date of injury. In cases of a witnessed nerve severance, immediate primary nerve repair is indicated unless the surgical site is contaminated (e.g., gunshot wound), the patients current medical status is compromised, or the surgeon does not possess the training or instrumentation to complete the repair.

DISCUSSION

The inferior alveolar nerve and the lingual nerve are the sensory nerves most commonly injured during surgical treatment by oral and maxillofacial surgeons. Injury to these nerves is not always avoidable despite knowledge of the anatomy and meticulous surgical technique. The lingual nerve has a more variable and less predictable course. The lingual nerve is positioned above the lingual alveolar crest at the retromolar area in 14% of cases (see the section on third molar odontectomy earlier in this chapter). In other cases, the lingual nerve travels through the submandibular salivary gland. Injuries to the lingual nerve occur less frequently than do injuries to the inferior alveolar nerve. However, the lingual nerve, which is located entirely within soft tissue, is less likely to spontaneously recover from injury compared with the inferior alveolar nerve. This is hypothesized to be due to the position of the inferior alveolar nerve in the bony canal that serves as a conduit for nerve regeneration.

The reported incidence of temporary paresthesia to the lingual nerve from third molar surgery is between 2% and 6%, with approximately less than 25% of these injuries resulting in a permanent deficit. Several factors may be associated with an increased risk of lingual nerve injury, including lingual bone–splitting technique, aggressive curettage of the follicular sac or granulation tissue, excessive lingual bone removal, lingual plate perforation by a drill or an instrument, and deeply placed lingual sutures. Placement of lingual retraction increases the incidence of temporary lingual nerve paresthesia but may decrease the incidence of permanent nerve injury.

Upon injury to a nerve, the distal axonal segment degenerates slowly (Wallerian degeneration). The distal segments are progressively phagocytosed over several months and replaced by scar tissue. Once scar tissue has fully replaced the connective tissue framework, the regenerating proximal axons can no longer recannulate the endoneurial tubules and reinnervate their target tissue. Therefore best results for microneurosurgical repair of nerve severance are achieved when surgery is performed as soon as the diagnosis is confirmed and the patient is willing to proceed with the procedure given the risks and benefits. Within 6 months of the injury, the patient has a reasonable chance of success (80% to 90%) (defined as response to pressure and light touch at normal thresholds, two-point discrimination at a threshold of less than 15 mm, and no hyperesthesia), whereas beyond 12 months, the likelihood of success is very low.

Bibliography

Gregg JM: Surgical Management of lingual nerve injuries, *Oral Maxillofac Clin N Am* 4(2); 417, 1992.

Meyer RA: Application of microneurosurgery to the repair of trigeminal nerve injuries, *Oral Maxillofac Clin N Am* 4(2):405, 1992.

Miloro M: Microneurosurgery. In Miloro M, ed: *Peterson's principles of oral and maxillofacial surgery,* London, 2004, BC Decker.

Robert RC, Bacchetti P, Pogrel MA: Frequency of trigeminal nerve injuries following third molar removal, *J Oral Maxillofac Surg* 63(6):732-735, 2005.

Zuniga JR, Essick GK: A contemporary approach to the clinical evaluation of trigeminal nerve injuries, *Oral Maxillofac Clin N Am* 4(2):353, 1992.

Zuniga JR, Meyer RA, Gregg JM, et al: The accuracy of clinical neurosensory testing for nerve injury diagnosis, *J Oral Maxillofac Surg* 56:2, 1998.

Displaced Root Fragments During Dentoalveolar Surgery

Danielle Cunningham, DDS, and Shahrokh C. Bagheri, DMD, MD

CC

A 41-year-old man is referred to your office for extraction of a nonrestorable left maxillary first molar.

HPI

Four years earlier the patient had a root canal performed due to extensive caries on the left maxillary first molar without any complications (extractions of endodontically treated teeth have a greater probability of root fracture and displacement). He did not pursue restoration of the tooth due to financial reasons and is now referred for extraction of the failed root canal. He presented to his general dentist with a complaint of pain and mild gingival swelling adjacent to the left maxillary first molar.

PMHX/PDHX/MEDICATIONS/ALLERGIES/SH/FH

Noncontributory. The patient does not use tobacco.

Medical comorbidities (such as chronic steroid therapy, smoking cigarettes, diabetes, radiation therapy, or malnutrition) that compromise wound healing may increase the likelihood of persistent oral antral communications requiring repeat surgical closure. However, the regional anatomy of the area, such as the length of the roots, extent of sinus pneumatization, and amount and quality of surrounding bone, is also important.

EXAMINATION

Intraoral. The patient has localized gingival edema and erythema of the left maxillary first molar, with no vestibular fluctuance. There is a 2-mm draining fistula on the buccal gingiva. A large carious lesion is present on the mesial-occlusal surface of the tooth. The left maxillary second and third molars (teeth Nos. 15 and 16) are missing with significant resorption of the posterior maxillary ridge.

IMAGING

The periapical or panoramic radiograph is the minimal imaging modality necessary before the extraction of a tooth. The panoramic radiograph allows better evaluation of the surrounding structures (such as the maxillary sinus). Evaluation of the size and shape of the tooth, degree of sinus pneumatization, and amount of bone is important for assessment of possible risks for oral antral exposure or root fracture.

For this patient, the panoramic radiograph reveals a long palatal root of the left maxillary first molar that appears to partially project into the sinus. There is a loss of continuity of the maxillary sinus in the area of the palatal root (suggestive of a periapical scar secondary to the previous root canal or a pathological process involving the maxillary sinus).

LABS

No laboratory testing is indicated before routine dentoalveolar surgery unless dictated by the medical history.

ASSESSMENT

Nonrestorable carious left maxillary first molar requiring extraction

Preoperative assessment of this patient should alert the surgeon to the increased likelihood of root fracture and/or oral antral communication upon surgical removal of the left maxillary first molar. Well-informed patients are more accepting of necessary secondary procedures (such as oral antral closure, root retrieval form the sinus, or nerve repair).

TREATMENT

After injection of local anesthetic with epinephrine, extraction of the left maxillary first molar was attempted using an elevator and forceps. Removal of the tooth revealed fracture of the palatal root with the root fragment retained within the palatal socket. A root tip pick was used to retrieve the fragment. During elevation, the root tip suddenly disappeared from the surgical field. Evaluation of the socket reveals a dark hole, suggesting that the fragment has dislodged into the maxillary sinus.

Upon diagnosis of a displaced root into the maxillary sinus, several maneuvers may be attempted to retrieve the fragment. It is possible for a fragment to be displaced below the Schneiderian membrane without actual dislodgment into the maxillary antrum. If the membrane appears intact, this diagnosis should be considered. In cases of dislodgment into the sinus, a perforation into the antrum may be visible. Asking the patient to exhale while pinching the nose may demonstrate air or bubbles exiting the socket, confirming the diagnosis of sinus perforation. Immediately upon diagnosis, a small suction tip can be placed at the apex of the extraction socket in an attempt to remove the fragment. The procedure can be repeated with the patient placed in an upright position. If this maneuver fails, the maxillary sinus can be irrigated with normal saline followed by suctioning to allow root retrieval. If the root fragment cannot be visualized, the procedure should be aborted. The following two treatment approaches should be considered:

- The sinus communication is closed and the root fragment is left in place. The patient is subsequently monitored with panoramic radiographs to document the position of the root. In patients who are asymptomatic, with small fragments that are fixed within the antrum, it is possible to simply observe the root with serial radiographs.
- Closure of the sinus perforation followed by immediate or delayed removal of the root fragment via a Caldwell-Luc, transalveolar, or endoscopic sinus surgery.

These treatment options are addressed in more detail below (see Discussion).

COMPLICATIONS

Displacement of a tooth/root fragment into the maxillary sinus in a known complication of maxillary dentoalveolar surgery. Although several preoperative findings can identify patients at risk (see earlier), this complication can occur in any patient. Other possible complications of dentoalveolar surgery are listed in Box 5-4.

Pain and swelling are inevitable consequences of any surgical intervention. However, measures to minimize pain and swelling (preoperative steroids, short operative time, and careful surgical technique) may increase patient comfort and satisfaction.

DISCUSSION

The palatal root of the maxillary first molar is the most likely root to be pushed into the maxillary sinus. There is some controversy regarding the optimal management of displaced root fragments into the maxillary sinus. Many surgeons advocate removal of all root fragments from the sinus regardless of any preexisting sinus or periapical pathology. It is hypothesized that a root tip may act as a foreign body within the sinus leading to polyps or sinusitis. Although there are no randomized trials to evaluate this issue, most authors argue that the decision needs to be made on a case-by-case basis. It is recommended that if the root tip is small (less than 3 mm) and the sinus and the tooth demonstrate no preexisting pathology, only minimal attempts should be made to retrieve the root. The majority of root fragments are fibrosed into the sinus membrane without any long-term sequelae. Case reports of retrieved maxillary implants that had migrated or perforated the sinus mucosa have demonstrated no inflammatory changes in the mucosa (both clinically and radiographically). However, there are other case reports where migration of a cover screw caused acute sinusitis.

A standard procedure used to retrieve foreign bodies from the maxillary sinus is the Caldwell-Luc procedure. A vestibular incision is used to access the canine fossa. A perforation is made in the anterior maxillary wall, allowing

---

Box 5-4.   Complications of Dentoalveolar Surgery

Intraoperative Complications
- Root fracture (increased incidence with age and root canal therapy)
- Injury to adjacent structures (lingual nerve, inferior alveolar nerve, mental nerve, greater palatine artery and vein, and injury to adjacent teeth and restorations)
- Maxillary tuberosity fracture (seen with maxillary second and third molar extractions, with an increasing incidence with age)
- Oral antral communication
- Displacement of the tooth fragments (or entire tooth) outside of the tooth socket. Root fragments can be displaced into the maxillary sinus, inferior alveolar canal, infratemporal fossa (uncommon complication of maxillary third molar extractions), sublingual space (perforation of the lingual cortex above the mylohyoid attachment), or the submandibular space (perforation below the mylohyoid attachment)
- Hemorrhage (bleeding in an otherwise noncoagulopathic patient is almost always easily controlled with local measures)
- Temporomandibular joint pain (secondary to acute temporomandibular joint muscle spasm, especially with preexisting internal derangement)
- Mandibular fracture (this is an uncommon but known complication of mandibular third molar extractions)
- Failure to achieve adequate local anesthesia

Postoperative Complications
- Alveolar osteitis (dry socket)
- Wound infection
- Periodontal complications (loss of gingival attachment levels or development of periodontal pockets)
- Poor wound healing causing delayed recovery
- Alveolar bone abnormalities/irregularities (may require repeat minor alveoplasty)
- Osteoradionecrosis
- Bisphosphonate-induced osteonecrosis of the jaws

---

visualization of the sinus. This can be enlarged to gain access to the sinus as needed. Careful attention to the infraorbital nerve avoids postoperative hypoesthesia.

Access to the maxillary sinus can also be gained via a transalveolar approach, by extending the opening of the extraction socket. Removal of buccal bone beyond the apex of the socket allows exposure of the antral mucosa. If the membrane has not been violated, this tissue plane may be explored; otherwise, an opening can be made through the membrane to allow sinus exploration. The opening is closed primarily using a buccal flap. This technique provides superior exposure to the antral floor (exposing the most likely position of the dislodged tooth). However, if the patient is interested in replacing the edentulous area with an implant, this approach would compromise the alveolar ridge bone, which is important for implant restorations.

Prevention of root displacement is the best treatment. If a root tip is fractured and the clinician suspects the possibility of displacement into the sinus, blind attempts at elevation of the fragment should be avoided. The use of adequate lighting (headlight) and full exposure of the area usually allow successful retrieval of the root from the socket. A variety of methods, including the use of endodontic files to remove root tips, have been described.

It is generally recommended that exposure of the sinus via the oral cavity warrants antibiotic therapy and "sinus precautions," regardless of decision to retain or retrieve a tooth fragment. The sinus flora includes the bacteria *Haemophilus influenzae, Streptococcus pneumoniae,* and *Moraxella catarrhalis.* Nasal decongestants such as oxymetazoline (Afrin) or pseudoephedrine are used to improve sinus drainage. Topical application of oxymetazoline (alpha-agonist) causes arteriolar vasoconstriction, resulting in nasal mucosal shrinkage, which allows for improved drainage. Oxymetazoline should not be used for longer than 3 to 5 days secondary to the development of rhinitis medicamentosa, causing rebound nasal congestion. Pseudoephedrine (sympathomimetic, alpha-adrenergic agonist)-containing decongestants cause vasoconstriction by selectively acting on the peripheral alpha-receptors, without the central nervous system side effects. These medications are frequently available in combination with an antihistamine or antitussive agents.

Extraction of mandibular molars can be complicated by displacement of root tips through a perforated lingual cortex into the submandibular or sublingual space (depending on the attachment of the mylohyoid muscle). The lingual plate at the area of the mandibular third molars can be very thin and, in some instances, fenestrated. Upon identification of a tooth fragment that is likely to be dislodged from the socket, place-ment of a finger along the medial aspect of the lingual cortex can frequently prevent this complication.

If a tooth becomes dislodged into the submandibular/sublingual space, attempts should be made at removal through the extraction socket or the perforation. If this maneuver is unsuccessful, a lingual mucoperiosteal flap can be elevated to allow exploration of the immediate region. Care should be taken not to injure the lingual nerve. In the event of failure to identify the tooth, the procedure should be aborted, and the patient is placed on antibiotics. A time period of 4 to 6 weeks has been recommended to allow the development of fibrosis around the tooth to facilitate removal. A CT scan may be obtained to visualize the exact position of the tooth, allowing careful preoperative planning. For small root fragments (less than 5 mm) that are not associated with any pathology, the surgeon may elect to observe the tooth and only remove the fragment if it becomes symptomatic.

Bibliography

Barclay JK: Root in the maxillary sinus, *Oral Surg Oral Med Oral Pathol* 64:162-164, 1987.

Iida S, Tanaka N, Kogo M, Matsuya T: Migration of dental implant into the maxillary sinus. A case report, *Int J Oral Maxillofac Surg* 29(5):358-359, 2000.

Lee FM: Management of the displaced root in the maxillary sinus, *Int J Oral Maxillofac Surg* 7:374-379, 1978.

Peterson LJ, Ellis E, Hupp JR, Tucker MR: *Contemporary oral and maxillofacial surgery,* St. Louis, 1993, Mosby, pp 279-280.

Speilman AI, Laufer D: Use of a Hedstrom file for removal of fractured root tips, *J Am Dent Assoc* 111(6):970, 1985.

Ueda M, Kaneda T: Maxillary sinusitis caused by a dental implant: report of 2 cases, *J Oral Maxillofac Surg* 50:285-287, 1992.

6 Head and Neck Pathology

Deepak Kademani, DMD, MD, FACS, and Shahrokh C. Bagheri, DMD, MD

This chapter addresses:
- Pleomorphic Adenoma
- Irritation Fibroma
- Acute Herpetic Gingivostomatitis
- Aphthous Ulcers
- Sialolithiasis
- Acute Suppurative Parotitis
- Mucocele
- Presentation of a Neck Mass: Differential Diagnosis
- Oral Leukoplakia
- Osteoradionecrosis of the Mandible

Pathological diseases of the head and neck encompass a wide spectrum of disorders with associated maxillofacial or systemic involvement. Several categories of disorders can be identified, which can frequently assist in formulation of a differential diagnosis:
- Infectious (e.g., bacterial, viral, fungal infections)
- Traumatic etiology (e.g., irritation fibroma)
- Neoplastic: epithelial, connective tissue, glandular, lymphatic, osseous, muscle, and vascular tumors that can be characterized as either benign or malignant tumors; metastatic disease to the head and neck are by definition malignant
- Immunologically mediated disorders (e.g., rheumatoid arthritis)
- Side effects or other medical or surgical therapy (e.g., osteoradionecrosis)
- Cysts of the head and neck (inflammatory and non-inflammatory cysts)
- Pathological processes related to the regional anatomy (e.g., sialolithiasis)
- Congenital malformations (cleft lip and palate)
- Degenerative disorders (osteoarthritis)
- Iatrogenic (e.g., intraoperative damage to a cranial nerve)
- Idiopathic (e.g., aphthous ulcers)
- Vasculitis (e.g., temporal arteritis)

Several of these categories are addressed elsewhere in this book. In this chapter, we have elected 12 teaching cases that represent disorders of infectious, traumatic, neoplastic, anatomic, and idiopathic etiology common in the oral and maxillofacial region. A teaching case discussing the differential diagnosis of a neck mass is provided, and a case of osteoradionecrosis outlines the current controversies and management issues for this complex complication of head and neck radiation.

Pleomorphic Adenoma

Scott D. Van Dam, DDS, MD, and Deepak Kademani, DMD, MD, FACS

CC

A 53-year-old woman (pleomorphic adenoma is most common in the fourth to sixth decades of life, with a slight female predilection) schoolteacher is referred for evaluation of a mass inferior to her left ear.

HPI

Over the past 8 months, she had noticed a progressively enlarging mass anterior and inferior to her left ear (pleomorphic adenoma is the most commonly occurring benign tumor of the major salivary glands. They are typically slow growing, at a rate of less than 5 mm per year). She explains that it has slowly enlarged, prompting her to bring it to her dentist's attention. There is no associated pain, paresthesias, or motor deficits (motor or sensory nerve deficits are not commonly seen with benign salivary neoplasm). She denies any constitutional symptoms including fever, chills, night sweats, appetite changes, and weight loss (systemic symptoms associated with inflammatory or malignant processes).

PMHX/PSHX/MEDICATIONS/ALLERGIES/SH/FH

She sees her dentist yearly for routine maintenance. She drinks alcohol on social occasions, and has never smoked. (There is no known association between tobacco and alcohol as risk factors for the development of pleomorphic adenomas. One potential risk factor is exposure to certain chemicals and dyes, but this association is very weak.)

There is no previous history of head and neck cancer or facial cosmetic surgery (important to be aware of previous surgeries in the area of the pathology). She has completed all her childhood immunizations including the mumps vaccine as part of the MMR vaccine (less likely to have mumps as a cause of parotid swelling).

EXAMINATION

General. The patient is a well-developed and well-nourished 43-year-old woman in no apparent distress.

Vital signs. Her blood pressure is 135/90 mm Hg, heart rate 80, respirations 16, and temperature 36.9°C.

Maxillofacial. Examination of the eyes and ears is unremarkable. The tympanic membranes are clear bilaterally. Cranial nerves II to XII are intact, with no weakness of the muscles of mastication (V). There is no sensory deficit in the V_1-V_3 distributions. Facial mimetic muscles are intact and symmetrical (involvement of the facial or trigeminal nerve would be suggestive of a malignant process).

There is a visible swelling in the left subauricular area that distorts her facial contour. Palpation reveals a well-circumscribed, freely moveable, firm, rubbery 1- to 1.5-cm nontender mass above the angle of the mandible (benign processes are typically slow growing and push rather than infiltrate local structures, as the overlying skin and adjacent structures such as blood vessels and nerves are usually not involved). There is no warmth, erythema, ulceration, or induration of the overlying soft tissue (signs of an inflammatory or a malignant process).

Intraoral. The parotid papillae appear noninflamed bilaterally, with expression of clear saliva from Stenson's duct (purulence drainage from the duct would be indicative of suppurative parotitis). There are no mucosal ulcerations or intraoral extension of the mass (consistent with a benign process).

Neck. No palpable submandibular or cervical lymphadenopathy (palpable lymph nodes would be indicative of a malignant neoplastic process).

IMAGING

Several imaging modalities may be used for the evaluation of a parotid mass, including ultrasound, computed tomography (CT), magnetic resonance imaging (MRI), and sialography. The most commonly used initial studies of choice are CT and MRI.

Histological confirmation is ideally performed preoperatively by means of fine-needle aspiration (FNA). This is best performed by an experienced cytopathologist and can provide diagnostic information guiding definitive treatment. FNA can have a high false-negative rate, and therefore inconclusive results can be repeated using ultrasonographic or CT guidance. Should the FNA continue to be inconclusive, one should proceed with definitive surgical resection of the tumor with facial nerve preservation, if possible. It is not necessary to perform an open biopsy of the parotid gland because 80% of parotid masses are benign and therefore a parotidectomy is appropriate as a diagnostic and treatment modality. Patients should be prepared preoperatively for the potential of facial nerve deficit. If the integrity of the nerve is maintained during the procedure, facial nerve function will return.

Sialography can be used to identify sialoliths and ductal obstruction and to differentiate parenchymal from nodal disease. A CT scan can also help differentiate nodal from parenchymal disease and is particularly useful in assessing

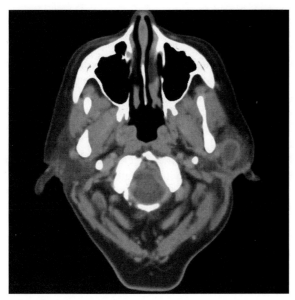

Figure 6-1 Axial CT scan with contrast showing a rim-enhancing mass of the left parotid gland.

larger lesions with atypical ultrasonic features. This is not as reliable as sialography for identification of ductal pathology. MRI offers excellent visualization of the glandular pathology and tumors. It is often the imaging modality of choice. Neither CT nor MRI can reliably outline the surgical anatomy of the mass relative to cranial nerve VII.

A panoramic radiograph can be used as a surveillance imaging tool to exclude the presence of intraductal or glandular calcifications; however, it is not particularly useful in the evaluation of parotid gland lesions.

For this patient, a panoramic radiograph confirmed no observable pathology. A CT scan demonstrated a well-circumscribed mass within the substance of the parotid gland, measuring 1.5 cm in diameter with no homogeneous enhancement following contrast administration (Figure 6-1). There was no evidence of enlarged intraparotid lymph nodes.

LABS

No routine laboratory tests are indicated in the workup of a parotid mass. A complete blood cell count (CBC) may be obtained to evaluate for an elevation of the white blood cell (WBC) count secondary to an infectious process. The minimum preoperative laboratory examination should include the hematocrit and hemoglobin levels. Further laboratory tests would be dictated by the medical and surgical histories.

For this patient, the CBC was within normal limits.

DIFFERENTIAL DIAGNOSIS

The slow circumscribed growth, lack of fixation, and absence of cranial nerve involvement or adenopathy associated with this lesion suggest a benign process. In addition, the absence of any erythema, pain, or warmth, together with a normal WBC count, implies a noninfectious/inflammatory process.

With a swelling in this region, a differential for proliferative processes includes pleomorphic adenoma, Warthin's tumor, monomorphic adenoma, and malignant salivary gland neoplasms (Box 6-1).

ASSESSMENT

FNA demonstrates a combination of ductal cells, chondromyxoid matrix, and dispersed plasmacytoid and lymphocyte-like myoepithelial cells (classic histology for pleomorphic adenoma), confirming the diagnosis of pleomorphic adenoma

Pleomorphic adenomas are characterized by a variety of morphological and histological patterns. It is considered a true "mixed" tumor, referring to the biphasic proliferation of both ductal epithelial and myoepithelial (mesenchymal) cells. The ductal epithelial cells give rise to gland-like epithelial structures, while the myoepithelial cells are responsible for the characteristic pleomorphic extracellular matrix (myxochondroid connective tissue). Within a single tumor, there may be cellular, glandular, myxoid, cartilaginous, and even ossified features. This morphological diversity may only be evident when the lesion is excised and examined in its entirety. Histologically, pleomorphic adenomas may resemble polymorphous low-grade adenocarcinoma, adenoid cystic carcinoma, basal cell adenoma, or epithelial-myoepithelial carcinoma. The connective tissue lining, or "pseudocapsule," is an important feature limiting growth but may be incomplete or infiltrated by tumor cells (tumor pseudopodia).

FNA may show various combinations of three elements: ductal cells, chondromyxoid matrix, and myoepithelial cells.

An aspirate with more than one of these components, especially when coupled with characteristic clinical presentation, makes this a straightforward diagnosis.

TREATMENT

Enucleation of a pleomorphic adenoma of the parotid gland is associated with recurrence rates of up to 40%. The treatment of choice is a superficial parotidectomy, which has resulted in low morbidity with recurrence rates of less than 2% to 3%. An attempt should be made to remove the tumor en bloc while maintaining the integrity of the capsule, with a 5-mm cuff of normal tissue. When the capsule is encountered on the deep aspect, it must be carefully dissected from the facial nerve. Maintaining the capsule is thought to be the key factor in minimizing recurrence. This observation led to the development of extracapsular dissection, in which the tumor and capsule are carefully dissected from the parotid gland. This conservative approach is associated with low rates of morbidity (facial nerve damage and Frey syndrome) with recurrence rates of 2% to 3%. Upon excision, the specimen should be delivered to pathology intact, to allow macroscopic evaluation of the integrity of the capsule. Pleomorphic adenomas of the palate should be excised with a 5-mm margin including the overlying mucosa and underlying periosteum.

For this patient, a superficial parotidectomy with cranial nerve VII preservation was performed through a face-lift incision. The tumor was excised with a 5- to 10-mm margin of uninvolved surrounding tissue, with the exception of the deep margin, where the capsule was carefully dissected off of the facial nerve. The superficial musculoaponeurotic system was carefully repositioned in an attempt to prevent Frey syndrome.

Subsequently, the intact specimen was evaluated using frozen sections by the pathologist, and the diagnosis of pleomorphic adenoma was confirmed. Permanent hematoxylin and eosin–stained sections demonstrated typical histology including gland-like epithelial cells forming nests, chords, and duct-like structures within a heterogeneous stromal background of myxoid, chondroid, and mucoid material along with a distinct fibrous connective tissue lining.

COMPLICATIONS

Early complications can include facial nerve paralysis, hemorrhage, hematoma, infection, skin flap necrosis, trismus, salivary fistula, sialocele, and seroma formation. Long-term complications include Frey syndrome, hypoesthesia of the greater auricular nerve, tumor recurrence, and cosmetic deformity from the soft tissue defect (Box 6-2).

DISCUSSION

Salivary gland tumors are rare, with an overall incidence of 2.5 to 3 per 100,000 per year. The majority of parotid (80%)

Box 6-2.   Complications of Parotidectomy for Pleomorphic Adenoma

Facial nerve injury. Cranial nerve VII can be preserved in most parotidectomies in the setting of benign disease. However, despite correct surgical technique, paresis of this nerve can occur. Careful handling, with minimal skeletonization of the branches, can help reduce anoxia and ischemia intraoperatively. If major trauma to the nerve is avoided, deficits are usually transient (seen in 14% to 40% of cases) and can be expected to resolve.

Recurrence. In a review of 52 studies (804 cases of pleomorphic adenoma), Hickman and coworkers reported a 5-year recurrence free rate of 96.6% and 10-year recurrence-free rate of 93.7%. There is a higher risk of multifocal recurrence (20% to 40% of cases), of which 25% are malignant, when the surrounding tissues are seeded by inappropriate handling of the tumor, such as with open biopsy of major glands, or attempts at enucleation. Such recurrences usually are within the first 10 years after the original surgery. Some recent immunohistochemical studies (Bankamp and Bierhoff, 1999) have claimed that recurrent tumors are characterized by differentiation of the epithelial components, which is related to greater proliferation.

Malignancy and metastasis. The overall rate of malignant transformation for a pleomorphic adenoma has been estimated at about 6%. There are three distinct histological types of mixed tumor with the potential for metastasis:

1. A benign-appearing lesion may become a benign metastasizing pleomorphic adenoma. These lesions tend to recur locally, often multiple times, before metastasizing. This is a rare occurrence.

2. There is a 2% to 3% risk of malignant transformation to carcinoma ex-pleomorphic adenoma. This usually occurs in larger and longstanding benign pleomorphic adenomas (usually about twice the size and present for about twice as long). The average age for presentation of carcinoma ex-pleomorphic adenoma is 60 years, and usually the original pleomorphic adenoma has been present for more than 15 years.

3. Very rarely, malignant change in both ductal and myoepithelial elements gives rise to a true mixed malignant pleomorphic adenoma or carcinosarcoma.

Frey syndrome (auriculotemporal nerve syndrome or gustatory sweating). This is a relatively common long-term complication of parotidectomy. It is characterized by localized sweating and dermal flushing during salivary stimulation. This is thought to be caused by aberrant connections between severed secretomotor parasympathetic fibers as they anastomose with severed postganglionic sympathetic fibers that supply the sweat glands of the face in the auriculotemporal region. Frey syndrome has been reported in as high as 30% to 60% of patients undergoing parotidectomy. However, only 10% of patients have symptoms requiring treatment. Treatment options include surgical disruption of the aberrant neural connections or use of botulinum toxin.

Bankamp DG, Bierhoff E. Proliferative activity in recurrent and nonrecurrent pleomorphic adenoma of the salivary glands. *Laryngorhinootologie* 78(2):77-80, 1999.

and submandibular gland (60%) tumors are benign. Fifty percent of tumors originating form the minor salivary glands, and only 10% of tumors of the sublingual gland are benign. Pleomorphic adenoma compromises about 40% to 70% of all salivary gland tumors. It is the most frequent salivary gland tumor in both children and adults and the most common tumor of both major and minor salivary glands. Approximately 75% of pleomorphic adenomas occur in the parotid gland. Ten percent are found in the submandibular gland, and another 10% are found in the palate. Pleomorphic adenomas make up 60% to 70% of all parotid neoplasms, 40% to 60% of submandibular gland tumors, and 40% to 70% of minor salivary gland tumors.

Pleomorphic adenoma classically presents as a painless, firm swelling. It may be lobulated, irregularly dome shaped, or smooth. The consistency is typically rubbery or semisolid, and there may be isolated areas that are softer. If untreated, it will enlarge slowly over months or years. The connective tissue capsule generally limits growth, but tumors can become very large if neglected.

In the parotid gland, pleomorphic adenoma most commonly presents in the inferior aspect of the superficial lobe. Deep lobe invasion may manifest as a mass of the soft palate or lateral pharyngeal space. CT or MRI scans can help localize tumor or differentiate lymph nodes from tumor.

The most common intraoral sites are the palate and upper lip. When arising from minor glands of the palate, pleomorphic adenomas are most commonly located lateral to the midline at the junction of the hard and soft palate. Minor gland tumors may cause localized pressure resorp-tion of the palate but do not tend to invade the underlying bone.

Bibliography

Allison GR, Rappoport I: Prevention of Frey's syndrome with superficial musculoaponeurotic system interposition, *Am J Surg* 166:407-410, 1993.

Bankamp DG, Bierhoff E. Proliferative activity in recurrent and nonrecurrent pleomorphic adenoma of the salivary glands. *Laryngorhinootologie* 78(2):77-80, 1999

Garcia-Perla A, Munoz-Ramos M, Infante-Cossio P, et al: Pleomorphic adenoma of the parotid in childhood, *J Craniomaxillofac Surg* 30:242-245, 2002.

Howlett DC, Kesse KW, Hughes DV, Sallomi DF: The role of imaging in the evaluation of parotid disease, *Clin Radiol* 57:692-701, 2002.

Stanley MW: Selected problems in fine needle aspiration of head and neck masses, *Mod Pathol* 15(3):342-350, 2002.

Jorge J, Pires FR, Alves FA, Perez DEC, et al: Juvenile intraoral pleomorphic adenoma: report of five cases and review of the literature, *Int J Oral Maxillofac Surg* 31:273-275, 2002.

Kwon MY, Gu M: True malignant mixed tumor (carcinosarcoma) of parotid gland with unusual mesenchymal component: a case report and review of the literature, *Arch Pathol Lab Med* 125:812-815, 2001.

Schreibstein JM, Tronic B, Tarlov E, Hybels RL: Benign metastasizing pleomorphic adenoma, *Otolaryngol Head Neck Surg* 112(4):612-615, 1995.

Speight PM, Barrett AW: Salivary gland tumours, *Oral Dis* 8:229-240, 2002.

Valentini V, Fabiani F, Perugini M, et al: Surgical techniques in the treatment of pleomorphic adenoma of the parotid gland: our experience and review of literature, *J Craniofac Surg* 12(6):565-568, 2001.

Irritation Fibroma

Aric Murphy, DDS, and Deepak Kademani, DMD, MD, FACS

CC

A 30-year-old woman is referred by her local dentist for evaluation of a small mass in her cheek.

HPI

The patient admits to a history of biting her cheek for several months. More recently she has noticed a lesion on her left buccal mucosa. The lesion is not painful, and there is no history of bleeding from the area. She denies any other constitutional symptoms such as fever, weight loss, nausea, and vomiting.

PMHX/PSHX/MEDICATIONS/ALLERGIES/SH/FH

Noncontributory. The patient has no history of tobacco use or alcohol consumption and no significant family history.

EXAMINATION

Maxillofacial. The patient is normocephalic, with no submandibular or cervical lymphadenopathy (lymphadenopathy would be seen in inflammatory or neoplastic conditions).

Intraoral. The tongue, floor of mouth, hard and soft palate, and gingiva are all within normal limits. The uvula is midline, pharyngeal mucosa and tonsils appear normal, and bimanual examination reveals no masses or tenderness. There is an 8-mm pedunculated round, nonulcerated mass along the occlusal plane on the left buccal mucosa. The lesion is slightly pale but has the same consistency as the surrounding mucosa with no erythema (Figure 6-2).

IMAGING

No imaging studies are indicated unless there is suspicion of other pathological processes.

LABS

No routine labs are indicated unless dictated by underlying medical conditions.

DIFFERENTIAL DIAGNOSIS

Despite characteristic clinical findings of a fibroma, the differential diagnosis of a soft tissue mass needs to be considered (Box 6-3).

BIOPSY

For small lesions of less than 1 cm, an excisional biopsy (complete removal with a small rim of grossly normal appearing tissue) is appropriate. For larger lesions (larger than 1 cm), an incisional biopsy (removal of a representative segment of the lesion) can allow for histological confirmation prior to the definitive treatment.

ASSESSMENT

Histologically, the lesion appears as a nodular mass of fibrous connective tissue covered by stratified squamous epithelium; this is consistent with the diagnosis of a traumatic (irritation) fibroma of the buccal mucosa

Occasionally, chronic inflammatory infiltrates can be seen within the connective tissue portion of the lesion.

TREATMENT

Excisional biopsy for histopathological analysis is both diagnostic and the definitive treatment for this patient. With the patient under local anesthesia, a No. 15 surgical blade is used to harvest a 1-mm rim of normal appearing adjacent tissue around the lesion. The entire excision is elliptical in shape to facilitate primary closure. Once the mucosa is incised, a subcutaneous plane under the lesion is developed at the level of the submucosa. The entire specimen is then removed and sent for histological examination. The surgical site is rendered hemostatic and closed in a single-layer fashion.

COMPLICATIONS

There are very few complications that may result from excision of lesions from the buccal mucosa. For all surgical procedures, bleeding and infection are possible, although with good surgical technique and hemostasis, this is rarely a problem. Antibiotics are not routinely required preoperatively or postoperatively for these procedures, as the infection risk is extremely low. It is important for the surgeon to recognize the position of the Stensen's duct and to ensure a minimum of 5-mm distance from the orifice of the duct, to avoid inadvertent injury. In lesions that are particularly close, a lacrimal probe may be placed for identification of the duct, and in some situations, sialoducoplasty for ductal repositioning may be required.

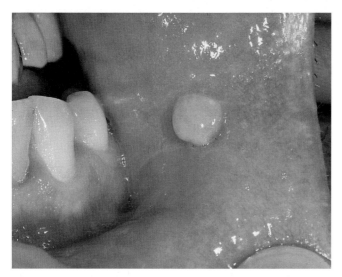

Figure 6-2 Pedunculated round, nonulcerated mass, along the occlusal plane on the left buccal mucosa. *(From Ibsen OAC, Phelan JA: Oral pathology for the dental hygienist, ed 4, Philadelphia, 2004, WB Saunders.)*

DISCUSSION

The oral fibroma (irritational or traumatic) is one of the most common exophytic, soft tissue lesions seen within the oral cavity with an incidence of 12 lesions per 1000 population. It is considered a reactive hyperplasia of fibrous connective tissue in response to local irritation or trauma. These lesions have a limited growth potential, and the lesion may even decrease in size after prolonged removal of irritation or trauma.

Clinically, the fibroma can occur anywhere in the oral cavity, but it is most common in the buccal mucosa along the occlusal plane. Other common sites are the labial mucosa, tongue, and gingiva. Fibromas often appear pink due the absence of vascularity. Most commonly, they appear as a well-circumscribed nodule that is often pedunculated or sessile. Rarely do the lesions exceed 2 cm in the greatest dimension. In some cases, the lesion can appear white due to hyperkeratosis from continual irritation. Occasionally, the fibroma can appear mildly erythematous and even ulcerated, if recently traumatized. Fibromas most commonly occur between ages 30 and 50 years, favoring females to males in a 2:1 ratio in cases submitted for biopsy. Treatment is conservative surgical excision and the prognosis is excellent with

rare recurrence. It is important to submit the lesion for histopathological diagnosis because some benign, and even malignant, tumors can mimic the clinical appearance of the fibroma.

Bibliography

Bouquot JE, Gundlach KK: Oral exophytic lesions in 23,616 white Americans over 35 years of age, *Oral Surg Oral Med Oral Pathol* 62(3):284-291, 1986.
Mandel L, Baurmash H: Irritation fibroma. Report of a case, *NY State Dent J* 36(6):344-347, 1970.
Marx RE, Stern D: *Oral and maxillofacial pathology: A rational for diagnosis and treatment,* Carol Stream, IL, 2003, Quintessence Publishing, p. 395.
Neville BW, Damm DD, Allen CM: *Oral and maxillofacial pathology,* ed 2, Philadelphia, 2002, WB Saunders, pp 438-439.
Regezi JA, Courtney RM, Kerr DA: Fibrous lesions of the skin and mucous membranes which contain stellate and multinucleated cells, *Oral Surg Oral Med Oral Pathol* 39(4):605-614, 1975.
Regezi JA, Sciubba JJ: Connective tissue lesions. In Regezi JA, Sciubba JJ, eds: *Oral pathology,* Philadelphia, 1995, WB Saunders, p 191.

Acute Herpetic Gingivostomatitis

Matthew J. Karban, DMD, and Deepak Kademani, DMD, MD, FACS

CC

A 4-year-old boy presents to the pedodontist because he has had a sore mouth and decreased oral intake for the past 2 days.

Acute herpetic gingivostomatitis is an infection that typically affects children. The most common age of onset is between 6 months to 5 years. A second peak occurs in the early 20s. The majority (90%) of primary infections are asymptomatic. By adulthood, about 60% to 95% of the population is affected by a herpes virus.

HPI

The patient's mother reports that he has been in distress with mouth pain and has not been eating well for the past few days (pain is the most common presenting symptom). The parents noticed multiple vesicles and ulcers in his mouth 2 days earlier. He has had a low-grade temperature over the past 2 days, which they have treated with acetaminophen (in the pediatric population, decreased oral intake is often the first sign of a developing infectious/pathological process).

It is important to distinguish primary and recurrent infection. Primary infection tends to be more severe and can occur anywhere in the oral cavity. Symptoms typically last 1 week and can be associated with malaise, lymphadenopathy, and fever. Recurrent disease occurs sporadically and tends to be limited to the keratinized mucosa.

PMHX/PSHX/MEDICATIONS/ALLERGIES/SH/FH

The patient has never been to the dentist. He does not have any known drug allergies and is not on any medications. The mother admits to having recurrent herpes labialis several weeks ago.

Herpes simplex virus (HSV) is transmitted via direct contact with infected secretions from the saliva and other bodily fluids. The main risk factor is a known exposure to the virus. When HSV-1 comes into contact with the host, the virus migrates to the sensory nerve endings and frequently to the trigeminal ganglia. The virus then enters a latent phase for 7 to 10 days before replication. Recurrent disease with HSV-1 characteristically involves the distribution of the trigeminal nerve.

EXAMINATION

General. The patient is an uncooperative, anxious boy in otherwise good health.

Vital signs. His blood pressure is 105/70 mm Hg, heart rate 100 bpm, respirations 18 per minute, and temperature 38.9° (febrile).

Maxillofacial. He has palpable cervical lymph nodes (this is commonly seen with acute herpetic gingivostomatitis). The face is symmetrical, with no other obvious signs of infection or edema.

Intraoral. Multiple vesicles and ulcerations extend over the buccal and labial alveolar mucosa and dorsal tongue (Figure 6-3) (primary acute herpetic gingivostomatitis can affect both the keratinized and nonkeratinized mucosa, but recurrent infection preferentially involves the keratinized tissue). Ulcerations measure from 1 to 3 mm in diameter and are covered by a pseudomembrane and an erythematous border. The gingiva is erythematous and painful, and there is copious saliva production with drooling.

Extremities: Right thumb displays similar erythematous vesicles and ulcerations (consistent with herpetic whitlow).

IMAGING

No imaging modalities are necessary for the diagnosis and management of acute herpetic ginigivostomatitis.

LABS

The diagnosis of acute herpetic gingivostomatitis is mainly a clinical diagnosis, but several laboratory tests are available for detecting an active herpes viral infection. Some of these tests include viral cultures, direct immunofluorescence, and a Tzanck smear. The Tzanck smear involves unroofing the vesicles and scraping of the tissue bed for cytological examination. Identification of multinucleated epithelial giant cells with eosinophilic viral inclusions is the hallmark feature.

ASSESSMENT

Acute (primary) herpetic gingivostomatitis

TREATMENT

Acute herpetic gingivostomatitis is a self-limiting condition usually resolving within 3 weeks from the onset of symptoms. Treatment predominantly involves observation and palliative care. This may involve topical anesthetics and over-the-counter pain relief such as acetaminophen or ibuprofen. Fluids and electrolyte status should be monitored as needed to avoid dehydration.

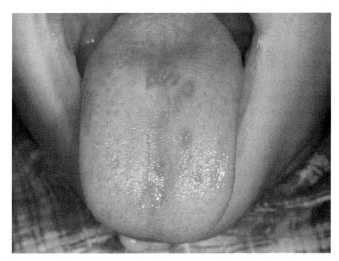

Figure 6-3 Acute herpetic gingivostomatitis of the dorsal tongue. (*From Ibsen OAC, Phelan JA:* Oral pathology for the dental hygienist, *ed 4, Philadelphia, 2004, WB Saunders; courtesy Dr. Edward V. Zegarelli.*)

Pharmacological treatment is often minimal due to the self-limiting course of the herpes virus. In more severe cases, pharmacotherapy can be of use if administered appropriately. Conventional antiviral therapy such as acyclovir, valcyclovir, and pencyclovir have been proved effective and can shorten the healing times by several days.

Primary acute herpetic gingivostomatitis can be managed on an outpatient basis with aggressive oral hydration, analgesia, and topical and systemic antiviral therapy. The main criteria for hospital admission include severe dehydration and pain.

Adult patients are typically managed on an outpatient basis. Severe disease refractory to treatment may indicate an underlying cause of immunosuppression that may require further evaluation for recurrent, persistent or refractory disease.

COMPLICATIONS

The main complications include potential nutritional deficiencies and inadequate fluid intake leading to dehydration, ocular involvement, herpetic whitlow, and central nervous system involvement.

Ocular herpes is relatively rare, affecting 50,000 patients in the United States per year. Stromal keratitis occurs is 25% of patients affected with ocular symptoms, involves inflammation of the deep layers of the cornea, and can lead to globe rupture and blindness. Herpetic whitlow is an intense painful infection of the hand involving one or more fingers that typically affects the terminal phalanx. HSV-1 is the cause in approximately 60% of cases of herpetic whitlow, and HSV-2 is the cause in the remaining 40%. In children, HSV-1 is the most likely causative agent. Infection involving the fingers usually is due to autoinoculation from primary oropharyngeal lesions as a result of finger-sucking or thumb-sucking behavior in patients with herpes labialis or herpetic

gingivostomatitis. In the general adult population, herpetic whitlow is most often due to autoinoculation from genital herpes; therefore, it is most frequently secondary to infection with HSV-2.

Similarly, in health care workers, infection with HSV-1 is more common and usually is secondary to unprotected exposure to infected oropharyngeal secretions of patients. This easily can be prevented by use of gloves and by scrupulous observation of universal fluid precautions.

Although a prodrome of fever and malaise may be observed, most often, the initial symptoms are pain and burning or tingling of the infected digit. This usually is followed by erythema, edema, and the development of 1- to 3-mm grouped vesicles on an erythematous base over the next 7 to 10 days. These vesicles may ulcerate or rupture and usually contain clear fluid, although the fluid may appear cloudy or bloody. Lymphangitis and epitrochlear and axillary lymphadenopathy are not uncommon. After 10 to 14 days, symptoms usually improve significantly and lesions crust over and heal.

After the initial infection, the virus enters cutaneous nerve endings and migrates to the peripheral ganglia and Schwann cells, where it lies dormant. The primary infection usually is the most symptomatic. Recurrences observed in 20% to 50% of cases are usually milder and shorter in duration.

Over 2100 cases of herpetic encephalitis are seen in the United States per year, making it a rare but extremely serious brain disease. HSV-1 is almost always the culprit, except in newborns. In about 70% of infant herpes encephalitis, the disease occurs when a latent HSV-2 virus is activated. Untreated, herpes encephalitis is fatal in over 70% of cases. Fortunately, rapid diagnostic tests and treatment with acyclovir have significantly improved both survival rates (up to about 80%) and complication rates.

DISCUSSION

Acute gingivostomatitis is an oral presentation of HSV-1. The virus typically presents in children between the ages of 6 months to 5 years with a peak incidence at 2 to 3 years of age. Infection is rare before 6 months of age due to the presence of maternal anti-HSV antibodies. Manifestations rarely present into adulthood.

The initial clinical presentation includes fever, nausea, and cervical lymphadenopathy, although it is thought that 90% of all primary infections are subclinical. Patients may proceed to display multiple small yellow- or white-filled vesicles, which develop into 1- to 3-mm ulcers after a few days. These vesicles and ulcers can present on attached and unattached gingiva as well as the tongue. Affected gingiva is erythematous, enlarged, and painful, often leading to constitutional symptoms such as dehydration from lack of adequate oral intake. In adults, acute herpetic gingivostomatitis can also present as pharyngotonsillitis. Diagnosis is primarily based on clinical presentations along with the absence of any previous clinical symptoms and confirmatory laboratory studies.

Bibliography

Ajar AH, Chauvin PJ: Acute herpetic gingivostomatitis in adults: a review of 13 cases, including diagnosis and management, *J Can Dental Assoc* 68(4):247-251, 2002.

Avery DR, McDonald RE: Gingivitis and periodontal disease. In Avery DR, McDonald RE, eds: *Dentistry for the child and adolescent,* ed 7. St Louis, 2000, Mosby, pp 443-446.

Blevins JY: Primary herpetic gingivostomatitis in young children, *Dermatol Nursing* 29(3):199-202, 2003.

Aphthous Ulcers

Ma'Ann C. Sabino, DDS, PhD, Anthony A. Indovina, Jr., DDS, and Deepak Kademani, DMD, MD, FACS

CC

A 25-year-old woman is referred for evaluation of painful ulcerations inside her mouth (aphthous ulcerations affect 20% of the population with a slight female predilection).

HPI

For the past 5 years, the patient reports episodes of ulcers that occur spontaneously and typically last for 3 weeks with intervals of up to 1 to 3 months between episodes. She does not have any history of trauma or known infectious diseases. The ulcers occasionally occur at multiple sites simultaneously. The hallmark feature is that they are slow healing with visible scarring, are extremely painful, and can take as long as 3 weeks to heal.

PMHX/PDHX/MEDS/ALLERGIES/SH/FH

There is no known history of immunosuppression, HIV, malnutrition, cancer, or previous infections of the head and neck region (potential risk factors).

A careful history may identify contributing etiological factors. In some individuals, the ulcers are a secondary or hypersensitivity response to an antigenic stimulus, especially foods, while other ulcers represent a primary autoimmune disorder. Patients with aphthae have a decreased ratio of T-helper (CD4$^+$) cells to T-suppressor/cytotoxic (CD8$^+$) cells in their circulation, and the ulcer bed itself has a high level of CD8$^+$ cytotoxic cells. While this is a likely contributor to the destruction in these ulcers, initiating causes are variable due to multiple contributing factors: familial predisposition, allergy, nutritional imbalances, infectious agents, hormones, trauma, stress, and blood dyscrasias. Individuals with comorbid extraoral diseases such as Behçet disease (ulcerations of the genitalia, ocular and oral mucous membranes), Crohn disease, celiac disease, ulcerative colitis, psoriasis, and ankylosing sponditits are at increased risk of developing aphthous ulcerations. Cyclic neutropenia is responsible for a subgroup of patients with aphthous stomatitis, with the ulcers occurring at points of minor trauma during times when the number of circulating neutrophils is low. Stress may be indirectly responsible for the sores, which were once called "stress ulcers," through its modulation of the immune system. Paradoxically, tobacco smoking, with its own immune modulation, is often protective, probably because of the increased keratinization resulting from local irritation of the oral mucous membranes.

EXAMINATION

General. The patient is a well-developed and well-nourished woman in no apparent distress.

Vital signs. Vital signs are stable and the patient is afebrile (fever is usually not seen with aphthous ulcers).

Maxillofacial. There is no facial swelling or cervical lymphadenopathy.

Intraoral. There are multiple ulcerations at various stages of healing within the oral mucosa measuring between 6 and 12 mm. Two ulcers at the right buccal mucosa appear to coalesce (Figure 6-4). There is also a 7-mm ulcer of the left lateral tongue. The lesions demonstrate a central zone of ulceration covered by a fibrinopurulent membrane that is surrounded by a varying degree of erythema along the margins. There does not appear to be any source of trauma in association with the ulcers (sharp dental restorations or fractured dental cusps).

IMAGING

No imaging studies are indicated for the evaluation of aphthous ulcers.

LABS

Routine laboratory tests are not indicated unless dictated by other underlying medical conditions.

ASSESSMENT

Multiple minor and major aphthous ulcers in an otherwise healthy 25-year-old woman

The diagnosis of aphthous ulcers is usually a clinical diagnosis. In cases of chronic nonhealing ulcers, a biopsy may be indicated to exclude viral and/or neoplastic etiologies. Therefore, all lesions should be followed for observation for adequate healing. Diagnosis is established by clinical history without the need for routine histopathology. Should a biopsy be performed, it would likely show surface mucosal ulceration with an intense inflammatory infiltrate. The ulcer bed would likely have an increased concentration of CD8$^+$ cytotoxic cells.

TREATMENT

There is no definitive cure for aphthous ulcerations. Treatment is directed toward symptomatic relief and is based on

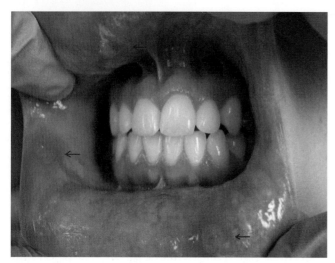

Figure 6-4 Multiple aphthous ulcers of the oral mucosa *(arrows)*.

Minor aphthous ulcer (aka Mikulicz aphthae). Less than 10 mm in size, requiring no treatment and resolving within 7 to 10 days without scarring. Should the ulcer remain after 2 weeks, topical corticosteroid therapy is indicated (see later). Palliative therapy in the form of topical local anesthetic such as 2% viscous lidocaine, diphenhydramine elixir (12.5 mg/ml), or topical benzocaine may be indicated in cases of severe pain associated with minor aphthous ulcers.

Major ulcers (aka periadenitis mucosa necrotica recurrens, Sutton disease). Major aphthous ulcers are by definition greater than 10 mm in diameter with deeper penetration than minor ulcers and therefore heal with scarring. Resolution of major aphthous ulcers may exceed several weeks in length. Treatment of more severe forms of major aphthous ulcers includes the use of topical or systemic corticosteroid therapy (see later). A protocol has been established by Kerr and Ship in the management of aphthous ulcers, especially with reference to those associated with HIV-infected patients.

Herpetiform ulcers. Herpetiform ulcers occur as many (10 to 100) small ulcerations coalescing within a large area of nonkeratinized mucosa that can extend to keratinized mucosa. Its name and clinical characteristic bear resemblance to ulcerations resulting from primary herpes simplex infection. Herpetiform ulcers are distinct from herpetic ulcers in that they lack viral particles and are not preceded by formation of vesicles. Healing occurs within 7 to 10 days.

---

the type of ulcer and response to topical versus systemic therapy. Aphthous ulcers are categorized into three types based on clinical course, size, and shape and are designated as minor, major, and herpetiform (Box 6-4).

Topical corticosteroid therapy. Topical therapy should be discontinued within 2 weeks if no improvement is obs-

erved. Clinicians should be cautious with prolonged use of topical steroids as pseudomembranous candidiasis may develop.

- Fluocinonide 0.05% ointment or gel over ulcer four times daily
- Clobetasol propionate 0.05% ointment over ulcer three times daily
- Dexamethasone elixir 0.5 mg/5 ml swish for 3 minutes and expectorate three times daily

First-line systemic therapy. If topical corticosteroid therapy fails to resolve the pathology, intralesional or systemic corticosteroid therapy is indicated. Intralesional injection of 20 to 40 mg triamcinolone has been shown to be efficacious in reducing pain and resolving recurrent and major aphthous ulcers in HIV-positive patients. Additionally, short-course high-dose ("short-burst") prednisone (40 to 80 mg) therapy for 3 to 7 days without taper has been described with excellent clinical results. Clinicians should be cautioned of the use of systemic corticosteroid therapy during active infections such as tuberculosis, which is prevalent in the HIV-positive population.

Second-line systemic therapy: Thalidomide has been shown to be a potent immunomodulator that is efficacious in treatment of severe forms of recurrent aphthous ulcers. Treatment with thalidomide 200 mg daily for 1 month resulted in a significantly greater number of individuals with complete or partial resolution of ulcers and decreased pain compared with control subjects. However, its use is limited by adverse effects, including constipation, drowsiness, peripheral neuropathy, and excessive fatigue.

COMPLICATIONS

The most common complication of aphthous ulceration is pain leading to difficulty eating. Scar formation can be seen with major aphthous ulcers.

DISCUSSION

Recurrent aphthous ulcerations remain one of the most common oral mucosal disorders. Despite its prevalence, its etiology is largely unknown. The differentiation of aphthous ulcers into minor, major, and herpetiform categories does not have an etiological basis. Mucosal ulcerations may also be manifested in chronic diseases related to immunosuppression, malnutrition, infection, and neoplasm.

Chronic irritation of nonkeratinized oral mucosa by dental appliances (ill-fitting dentures or orthodontic wires), fractured dental cusps, or dental treatment may cause ulcerations to occur; this needs to be differentiated from aphthous ulcerations. Removal of the source of irritation usually allows for resolution of the ulcer.

Deficiencies of iron, vitamin B$_{12}$, and folate have been implicated in the pathogenesis of chronic aphthous ulcers. According to a study by Scully and colleages, 18% to 28% of cases of recurrent aphthous ulcers occurred in patients with these deficiencies compared with 8% in healthy cohorts. In some cases, replacement of the deficiencies results in clinical improvement.

Varicella zoster virus and cytomegalovirus antibody titers have been isolated in patients with recurrent aphthous ulcers, but results are conflicting. The association between the presence of varicella zoster virus or cytomegalovirus and the development of aphthous ulcers has not been demonstrated. The gram-negative *Helicobacter pylori* was previously implicated in the formation of recurrent aphthous ulcers in children and adolescents, but it is no longer considered an important etiological factor. HIV infection has been shown to increase the propensity for developing recurrent aphthous ulcers, especially the major aphthous variant. The relationship between HIV infection and ulcer formation may be related to the decrease in circulating CD4 T-lymphocytes (fewer than 100 cells/mm^3) and resultant immunosuppression related to this disease.

Bibliography

Friedman M, Brenski A, Taylor L: Treatment of aphthous ulcers in AIDS patients, *Laryngoscope* 104(5):566, 1994.

Fritscher AM. Cherubini K, Chies J, Dias AC: The association between *Helicobacter pylori* and recurrent aphthous stomatitis in children and adolescents, *J Oral Pathol Med* 33(3):129, 2004.

Jacobson JM, Greenspan JS, Spritzler J, et al: Thalidomide for treatment of oral aphthous ulcers in patients with human immunodeficiency virus infection. National Institute of Allergy and Infectious Diseases AIDS Clinial Trial Group, *N Engl J Med* 336(21):1487, 1997.

Kerr AR, Ship JA: Management strategies for HIV-associated aphthous stomatitis, *Am J Clin Dermatol* 4(10):669, 2003.

Natah SS, Kontinen YT, Enattah NS, et al: Recurrent apthous ulcers today: a review of the growing knowledge, *Int J Oral Maxillofac Surg* 33:221, 2004.

Scully C, Grosky M, Lozada-Nur F: The diagnosis and management of recurrent aphthous stomatitis: a consensus approach, *J Am Dent Assoc* 134(2):200, 2003.

Sialolithiasis

Derek H. Lamb, DMD, Deepak Kademani, DMD, MD, FACS, and Shahrokh C. Bagheri, DMD, MD

CC

A 48-year-old woman reports to your office complaining of pain and swelling of the right submandibular region (sialoliths, or salivary stones, within the salivary gland ductal system, tend to occur more commonly in the elderly population, with a slight female predominance).

HPI

The patient reports having episodes of mild discomfort of the right submandibular area over the past 7 months (it is not uncommon for symptoms to wax and wane, especially during mealtime, coinciding with gland function). Her pain and swelling increased significantly 2 days earlier, which has prompted her to seek care.

Decreased salivary flow is the most significant risk factor for the development of sialolithiasis (salivary gland stones within a gland or duct) and sialadenitis (inflammation of the salivary gland). Dehydration, poorly controlled diabetes mellitus, certain medications, and radiation therapy are among several factors that can lead to xerostomia (dry mouth) secondary to decreased salivary flow.

PMHX/PSHX/MEDICATIONS/ALLERGIES/SH/FH

Major depression diagnosed 5 years earlier (some of the medications used to treat depression have anticholinergic side effects that include decreased production of saliva).

Type 1 diabetes mellitus was diagnosed 7 years ago. The patient's most recent Hb_{A1c} was 9% and her blood glucose levels range between 200 and 300 mg/dl (both indicative of poorly controlled diabetes, which is associated with an increased risk of sialolithiasis secondary to osmotic diuresis causing dehydration. The decreased immune function seen with diabetes is also a risk factor for the development of sialadenitis).

She has no known history of autoimmune disorders such as Sjögren syndrome or a history of radiation therapy (both are risk factors for xerostomia).

Medications include amitriptyline (tricyclic antidepressant with anticholinergic side effects, including xerostomia) and regular and NPH insulin as adjusted by her endocrinologist. The patient admits to drinking alcohol socially (chronic excessive alcohol consumption may predispose to the development of sialoliths secondary to frequent episodes of dehydration. Alcohol suppresses the antidiuretic hormone [ADH], causing polyuria).

EXAMINATION

General. The patient is a well-developed and well-nourished alert woman in mild discomfort (secondary to pain).

Vital signs. Her blood pressure is 143/89 mm Hg (elevated secondary to anxiety), heart rate 110 (tachycardia secondary to anxiety), respirations 15 per minute, and temperature 37.1°C (sialadenitis can present with fever secondary to inflammation of the gland).

Neck. There is mild to moderate tender right submandibular swelling (Figure 6-5). The area is firm and warm to touch on the overlying skin (dolor, tumor, calor, and rubor secondary to localized inflammation). Several palpable cervical lymph nodes are detected on the ipsilateral neck (enlarged lymph nodes are not uncommon secondary to localized inflammation of the submandibular gland. Lymphadenopathy due to a neoplastic process is also possible, but these are usually nontender due to the noninflammatory etiology).

Intraoral. Bimanual palpation reveals a 2- to 3-cm palpable tender mass of the right posterior floor of the mouth consistent with the location of the submandibular gland. Decreased salivary flow is observed relative to the contralateral gland at the opening of Wharton's duct (strong evidence of dysfunction or obstruction of the right submandibular gland).

IMAGING

The majority of sialoliths are radiopaque and are visible on plain radiographs (panoramic or occlusal radiograph) or CT scans. Some calculi may be radiolucent (not visible radiographically) secondary to the lack of mineralization or smaller size. If there is a high index of suspicion for a sialolith despite negative imaging, a sialogram may be considered. This was frequently used in the past, but it has been largely replaced by CT and ultrasound imaging. Sialography is contraindicated in the setting of acute infection. Ultrasonography and magnetic resonance sialography are other imaging modalities that have been more recently applied for identification of sialoliths.

In the absence of documented caliculi, kinks and strictures should be considered as possible causes of salivary obstruction. Sialography and sialendoscopy can be useful in diagnosing such anatomical impediments to salivary flow.

For this patient, a panoramic radiograph revealed a 1-cm radiopaque lesion of the right submandibular area consistent with a sialolith (Figure 6-6). (It is not uncommon, however, for the sialolith to be undetectable on a panoramic radiograph

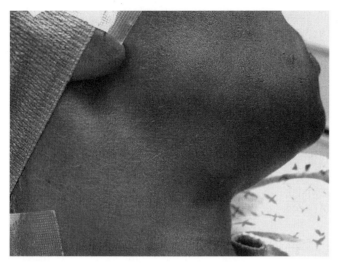

Figure 6-5 A view of the right neck demonstrating swelling of the right submandibular region.

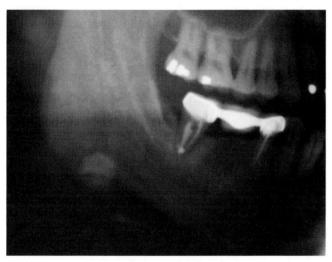

Figure 6-6 Panoramic radiograph demonstrating a well-demarcated radiopaque lesion in the area of the right mandibular angle.

due to overlap with the body of the mandible or due to the radiolucent nature of a sialolith). A CT scan with intravenous contrast was also obtained to outline the anatomy of the submandibular gland in preparation for surgical excision. The CT scan also revealed a 10-mm stone within the body of the submandibular gland (Figure 6-7).

LABS

No laboratory studies are indicated in the evaluation and treatment of sialolithiasis unless dictated by the medical history. In the management of sialadenitis, a WBC count may be beneficial for monitoring the progression of an infectious process. In cases of suspected sepsis, adjunctive laboratory studies such as blood cultures and complete metabolic panels can be obtained to guide medical and supportive therapy.

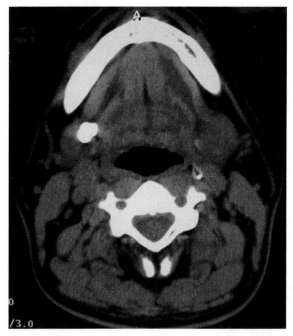

Figure 6-7 Contrast-enhanced CT scan demonstrating an 10-mm radiopaque lesion within the body of the submandibular gland consistent with a sialolith.

ASSESSMENT

Sialolithiasis within the right Wharton's duct with associated localized chronic sialadenitis (inflammation of the submandibular gland)

TREATMENT

There is a considerable body of literature with regard to the treatment of sialolithiasis. These have included transductal surgical removal, ductal dilation, lithotripsy, laser ablation, endoscopic retrieval, sialadenectomy (submandibular gland excision), or a combination of these approaches. The size and location of the stone, history of prior treatments, existing medical conditions, availability of resources, and surgeon preference are among the factors to be considered for optimal treatment planning. Transductal surgical removal is probably the most common technique; up to 70% of sialoliths can be removed by this method. Surgical access to the posterior portion of the duct and the risk for injury to the lingual nerve are among factors limiting the use of this technique.

In select cases, small stones along the anterior portion of Wharton's duct can be managed conservatively with antiinflammatory agents and antibiotics. Moist heat, sialogogues (cholinergic agonists), and certain foods such as hard tart candies or sour lemon drops can be used adjunctively to ameliorate symptoms. Palpable sialoliths can often be "massaged" out, relieving symptoms and alleviating the need for further treatment (although recurrence is not uncommon). Anticholinergics (which decrease salivary gland production) should be avoided when possible. If these measures are unsuccessful, ductal dilation followed by manual expression of the stone may be used to facilitate stone removal. Larger stones in the posterior third of the duct or within the glandular parenchyma that foresee problematic transoral surgical access may be best served by removal of the submandibular gland and ligation of Wharton's duct.

The choice of treatment is based on individual clinical and radiographic findings as well as surgical judgment. The most important factor in the treatment of sialolithiasis is the presence or absence of clinical symptoms. In the absence of symptoms, treatment may not be necessary. In the presence of signs and symptoms (pain, swelling, purulent drainage) of ductal or glandular obstruction treatment is typically medical with hydration, systemic antibiotics, and sialogogues to stimulate salivary flow for cleansing of the ductal system.

In this case, given the diagnosis of chronic sialadenitis and the presence of a large sialolith, it was elected to excise the submandibular gland transcutaneously (intraoral removal of the submandibular gland has been reported, but the transcutaneous approach is the most commonly used procedure), along with removal of the existing sialolith. With the patient under general endotracheal anesthesia, an incision was made 1.5 to 2 cm below the inferior border of the mandible (to avoid the marginal mandibular branch of the facial nerve) and dissection was carried through the platysma muscle. The investing layer of deep cervical fascia was incised at the inferior most extent of the dissection. The facial artery and vein were ligated, and the gland was removed along with the capsule (which is an extension of the fascia that surrounds the gland). The submandibular duct was identified and the duct was ligated. The lingual nerve was identified, as it makes its course from lateral to medial (passing inferior to Wharton's duct). The crossing of these two structures takes place in the area of the first and second molars, lateral to the hypoglossal nerve. The surgical specimen (submandibular gland) was sent to pathology for histological examination (Figure 6-8). A drain was placed to prevent hematoma formation (the decision to place a drain is not uniform among surgeons and depends on intraoperative and patient-related factors). This was removed the next day. The pathology report confirmed the presence of submandibular calculi within the gland parenchyma that showed extensive fibrosis and destruction of glandular architecture.

COMPLICATIONS

Depending on the severity of the presenting symptoms and the chronology of the disease process, sialolithiasis may be treated with a variety of methods. A common complication in all modalities that spare the submandibular gland is recurrent, new-onset, or nonresolving sialadenitis. The initial pathological insult may irreversibly damage the gland (fibrosis of glandular architecture), rendering it incapable of function and thereby prone to sialadenitis. Therefore in cases of multiple recurrences with nonsurgical therapy or in patients with significant comorbid medical conditions such as diabetes that increase the risk of infection, consideration should be given to excision of the gland. In select cases, excision of the gland may be the treatment of choice at the initial presentation. In either scenario, most surgeons elect not to remove the gland during acute episodes of infection, because the existing inflammation can complicate surgical dissection and increase the chances of nerve injury, postoperative infection, and fistula formation. If there is clinical or radiographic evidence of purulence around the gland, an incision and drainage may be performed initially to gain control of the acute process.

A significant complication associated with surgical excision of major salivary glands is nerve injury. Removal of the submandibular gland may be associated with damage to the lingual and hypoglossal nerves or the marginal mandibular branch of the facial nerve. Facial nerve injury is also a complication of parotidectomy (although sialolithiasis of this gland is far less common).

The submandibular glands produce up to 70% of the saliva, so decreased salivary output may be one consequence of sialadenectomy. Patients sometimes complain of subjective xerostomia following submandibular gland excision. This is rarely of any clinical consequence, especially in cases where the contralateral gland is functioning well.

Postoperative pain and swelling should be managed as with other maxillofacial procedures using a combination of opioids, over-the-counter analgesics (such as nonsteroidal antiinflammatory drugs), and steroids as deemed necessary by the treating surgeon. The use of postoperative antibiotics should be based on the status of host factors, preexisting infections, clinical findings, and experience of the surgeon. Postoperative infection should be managed with antibiotics using culture and sensitivity studies when available and incision and drainage as needed.

DISCUSSION

Sialolithiasis is the most common nonneoplastic disease of the salivary glands and the most common cause of salivary gland obstruction. Patients frequently complain of recurrent pain and swelling of the gland, particularly around meal-

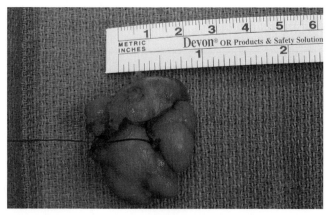

Figure 6-8 Gross specimen of the excised submandibular gland, demonstrating the enlarged and firm gland structure consistent with sialadenitis.

times. Salivary gland calculi are estimated to occur in 1% to 2% of the population. However, the prevalence of symptomatic sialolithiasis is 0.45%. They are most common within the body of the submandibular gland or Wharton's duct (80% to 90%). From 5% to 10% of sialoliths occur in the parotid gland/duct, and the remaining 0% to 5% are located within the sublingual or minor salivary glands.

The higher incidence of submandibular sialoliths is likely secondary to the thicker, mucoid secretions of the gland as well as the long, convoluted, and superiorly directed path of the duct along the anterior floor of the mouth. Wharton's duct has two noteworthy bends (areas more likely to develop sialolithiasis): the genu (knee area), which is located at the posterior border of the mylohyoid muscle, and around the punctum, where the duct makes an acute turn before emptying into the oral cavity. The diameter of the duct ranges from 2 to 4 mm and is narrowest at the punctum.

The etiology of sialolithiasis is not clear. A popular theory is that mineralization occurs around a nidus of organic matter and may be the initial etiological factor. Bacteria, foreign bodies, ductal epithelial cells, and collections of mucus are thought to be probable sources of this organic matrix. Their retention in the gland and ductal system is likely due to morphoanatomical abnormalities such as ductal stenosis (obstruction), strictures (constriction), or diverticula (outpouching). Irregular salivary composition is thought to contribute to mineralization around these structures. High concentrations of substances such as calcium combined with low levels of crystallization inhibitors in the saliva are thought to play a role in the continued growth of the calculi, which ultimately may result in obstruction.

Bibliography

Berini-Aytes L, Gay-Escoda C: Morbidity associated with removal of submandibular gland, *J Craniomaxillofac Surg* 20:216-219, 1992.

Escudier MP, McGurk M: Symptomatic sialoadenitis and sialolithiasis in the English population, an estimate of the cost of hospital treatment, *Br Dent J* 186:463-469, 1999.

Grases F, Santiago C, Simonet BM, Costa-Bauza A: Sialolithiasis: mechanism of calculi formation and etiologic factors, *Clin Chim Acta* 334(1-2):131-136, 2003.

Jacob RF, Weber RS, King GE: Whole salivary flow rates following submandibular gland resection, *Head Neck* 18:242, 1996.

Marchal F, Dulguerov P: Sialolithiasis management: the state of the art, *Arch Otolaryngol Head Neck Surg* 129:951, 2003.

Marchal F, Kurt AM, Dulguerov P, et al: Histopathology of submandibular glands removed for sialolithiasis, *Ann Otol Rhinol Laryngol* 110:494-499, 2001.

McGurk M, Escudier MP, et al. Modern management of salivary calculi, *Br J Surg* 92(1):107-112, 2005.

Nahlieli O, Shacham R, et al: Diagnosis and treatment of strictures and kinks in salivary gland ducts, *J Oral Maxillofac Surg* 59(5):484-490; discussion, 490-492, 2001.

Acute Suppurative Parotitis

David G. Molen, DDS, MD, Deepak Kademani, DMD, MD, FACS, and Shahrokh C. Bagheri, DMD, MD

CC

A 25-year-old man presents to the emergency department complaining of right facial swelling. You are consulted for management of a presumed odontogenic infection.

HPI

He reports awakening with painful right facial swelling 48 hours earlier. He has noticed a foul taste in his mouth (secondary to oral mucosal dehydration and purulent drainage from Stenson's duct), and has had no appetite. He admits to limited oral intake over the past 24 hours. Over the past 12 hours, he has begun to feel weak and light-headed and has developed chills. He has not been to a dentist in over 10 years and acknowledges having several "bad teeth."

PMHX/PDHX/MEDICATIONS/ALLERGIES/SH/FH

The patient is a known alcoholic (risk factor for acute suppurative parotitis) who is presently living in a homeless shelter. He is unaware of any major medical problems or allergies and is not currently taking any medications.

EXAMINATION

General. The patient is a thin (dehydration and malnutrition) man who appears older than his stated age; he is trembling (chills) and appears to be in pain.

Vital signs. His blood pressure is 128/85 mm Hg, heart rate 110 (mild tachycardia secondary to elevated temperature), respirations 16 per minute, and temperature 39.5°C (febrile).

Maxillofacial. He has obvious facial asymmetry, with swelling of the soft tissues over the right preauricular area and angle of the mandible (Figure 6-9). The tissue is indurated, erythematous, and exquisitely tender to palpation (signs of inflammation). He has palpable, mobile, tender lymph nodes in the right precervical chain. His maximum interincisal opening is 25 mm (trismus).

Intraoral. He is partially edentulous with most of his remaining teeth grossly carious, including the right mandibular second and third molars. The oral mucous membranes are dry (consistent with dehydration). There is no visible or palpable fluctuance, suppuration, or swelling around any teeth or in the buccal vestibules or floor of mouth. The uvula is midline, with no fullness of the lateral pharyngeal spaces.

Palpation of his involved tissues extraorally produces purulence from Stensen's duct on the right. The contralateral duct produces clear saliva, as do both submandibular ducts.

Skin. There is decreased skin turgor with tenting (sign of dehydration, a predisposing factor for acute suppurative parotitis).

IMAGING

A panoramic radiograph is the initial screening study of choice to rule out possible odontogenic sources of infection. CT with intravenous contrast is indicated when the source and extent of infection is unclear. Contrast-enhanced CT will assist in determining the proper management strategies.

In this patient, the panoramic radiograph reveals multiple grossly carious teeth, consistent with the clinical examination. There are no frank periapical lesions, and no other pathology is noted. Contrast-enhanced CT (which can be rapidly performed and will delineate the suspected infectious process when performed with intravenous contrast) shows diffuse enlargement of the right parotid parenchyma with stranding. There are no discreet lesions or loculations within the gland and no involvement of the adjoining potential fascial spaces (Figure 6-10). A sialogram is contraindicated in this setting. (increased risk of ductal or glandular rupture and typically is extremely painful in the patient with acute parotitis).

LABS

A CBC with differential is indicated to evaluate the presenting WBC count. A basic metabolic panel is indicated to rule out metabolic and electrolyte derangements associated with chronic alcohol abuse, dehydration, and malnutrition. Liver function tests may be indicated in chronic alcohol abusers. Blood cultures may be indicated in patients presenting with signs of sepsis. Gram stain and culture and sensitivity of the purulent exudates (if present) ensure that proper antibiotic coverage is maintained.

In this patient, the WBC count was elevated at $17 \times 10^9/L$. Serum electrolytes include Na^+ at 153 mEq/L (hypernatremia), K^+ 3.6 mEq/L, Cl^- 112 mEq/L, HCO_3 20 mEq/L, blood urea nitrogen 28 mg/dl, creatine 1.4 mg/dl, and Mg^{2+} 1.3 mg/dl.

Liver function tests. Results were aspartate amino transferase of 180 U/L, alanine aminotransferase 90 U/L, gamma-glutamyl transpeptidase 90 U/L, and alkaline phosphatase 98 U/L.

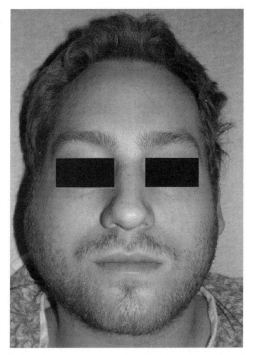

Figure 6-9 Frontal view showing facial asymmetry, with swelling of the soft tissues over the right preauricular area and angle of the mandible.

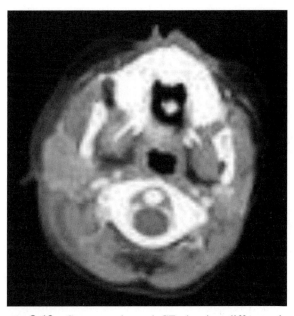

Figure 6-10 Contrast-enhanced CT showing diffuse enlargement of the right parotid parenchyma with stranding.

Microbiology

- **Gram stain.** Reveals gram-positive cocci in clusters and gram-negative bacilli
- **KOH.** Few hyphae noted (normal finding)
- **Cultures of purulence from Stenson's duct.**
  Staphylococcus aureus identified after 48 hours

The patient's electrolyte values are consistent with dehydration (elevated Na^+, blood urea, and creatine), which is common in alcoholics (alcohol suppresses ADH, causing water loss

from the kidneys). Low magnesium and elevated liver enzymes, with the aspartate amino transferase/alanine aminotransferase ratio 2:1 or greater, are also common with chronic alcohol abuse.

ASSESSMENT

Acute suppurative parotitis with associated dehydration in an alcoholic patient

TREATMENT

The management of patients with acute suppurative parotitis is primarily medical, consisting of rehydration with intravenous fluids, initiation of empiric antibiotic therapy, nutritional support, and stimulation of salivary flow. Surgical intervention may be necessary when demonstrated areas of loculation are present within the gland. Over 80% of cases are caused by *Staphylococcus aureus;* therefore, empiric first-line antibiotic treatment includes the β-lactamase–resistant penicillins, first-generation cephalosporins, or clindamycin. A review by Brook found strict anaerobes to be the causative agent in 43% of cases of acute suppurative parotitis; cultures and sensitivities should be followed closely and antibiotic therapy adjusted accordingly, for a total course of 10 to 14 days. Most patients should respond to aggressive medical management within 3 to 5 days. Extraoral incision and drainage of the capsule of the parotid may be indicated for failure to respond to medical therapy. Follow-up after resolution with sialography and/or repeat CT scan to determine possible underlying treatable explanations for the episode (stones, duct strictures, or tumor) may be indicated.

COMPLICATIONS

There are rare reports of patients with acute suppurative parotitis developing cervical necrotizing fasciitis. Possible infectious complications also include facial nerve dysfunction, septicemia, mastoiditis/osteomyelitis, and spread into adjacent fascial spaces with possible airway compromise. The reported mortality rate of acute suppurative parotitis approaches 25%. Acute suppurative parotitis is also seen as a complication of chronic recurrent parotitis, which may ultimately necessitate superficial or total parotidectomy (see Discussion). In the setting of acute suppurative parotitis, the criterion for parotidectomy is recurrence after two episodes of medical management; elective parotidectomy should be performed only after a period of 4 to 6 weeks of quiescence to allow for identification and preservation of the facial nerve in a noninflamed surgical field.

DISCUSSION

The term "parotitis" is a generic designation for parotid swelling with an inflammatory component. The aim of diagnosis should be to categorize the patient with parotitis into one of three possible subcategories to guide management (Box 6-5):

Box 6-5.   Categorization of the Patient With Parotitis Into One of Three Possible Subcategories to Guide Management

Acute (bacterial) suppurative parotitis. This is caused by colonization of the gland by oral bacteria which have migrated in a retrograde fashion through Stensen's duct. Patients almost invariably have a comorbid state, causing decreased salivary flow and/or immunosuppression. Common contributors to this relatively uncommon condition are diabetes, alcoholism, autoimmune disorders (e.g., Sjogren), medications (e.g., tricyclic antidepressants, anticholinergics, or diuretics), dehydration, malnutrition, neoplasm, or ductal obstruction. It is most common in debilitated elderly patients (nursing home or hospitalized patients) but has been described in all populations. The hallmark of ASP is frank suppuration along with the cardinal signs of inflammation; tumor (swelling), rubor (redness), calor (heat), dolor (pain), and *functio laseo* (loss of function). Sialography can be beneficial at follow-up in diagnosing ductal disorders or obstructions, it should be avoided in the acute stage. The increased pressure can be exquisitely painful, and can potentially rupture an already dilated duct.

Nonsuppurative parotitis (NSP) (parotid sialadenitis). The list of other causes of parotid inflammation and swelling that will not cause frank suppuration is lengthy and includes viruses, granulomatous inflammation, and autoimmune disorders. Although frank suppuration is not present, the gland can still be milked for discharge, which can be sent for viral or microbial studies. The most common viral cause of parotitis is paramyxovirus (mumps), although others must be considered (Epstein-Barr virus, coxsackievirus, herpes simplex, cytomegalovirus). HIV can cause bilateral parotid enlargement secondary to intraglandular lymphadenopathy. The most common cause of granulomatous parotid inflammation is *Mycobacterium tuberculosis.* Other mycobacterium, *Actinomycosis* species, and cat-scratch disease *(Bartonella henselae)* may need to be considered. Autoimmune states head the list of "other" causes and usually lead to bilateral parotid swelling. Common culprits are Sjogren disease, systemic lupus erythematosus, diabetes, cystic fibrosis, and collagen vascular disease. Nonsuppurative infectious states should be treated accordingly, while noninfectious inflammation is usually addressed by treating the underlying disease state and avoiding low-flow salivary states and antisialogogue medications whenever possible.

Chronic recurrent parotitis (CRP). This entity has been described as a nonspecific parotid sialadenitis with episodes of swelling and remission or persistent swelling with recurrent infection, either unilaterally or bilaterally. The overlap with the two previously discussed disease states is the cause of much confusion, and often times the diagnosis of CRP is delayed until further investigations and resolution of the presenting complaint, especially with recurrent episodes. A state of CRP can also be initiated by many of the same diseases that contribute to ASP and NSP. Diagnosis is made upon discovery of characteristic changes within the ductal and parenchymal architecture of the gland. These changes can be noted on sialography, CT, MRI, scintigraphy, or combinations thereof. Early findings include ectasia and dilatation of peripheral ducts, progressing to "sausaging" of the primary duct, and continuing to destruction of parenchyma with extravasation of contrast material in late stages. Treatment is usually supportive when patients are symptomatic, and includes antibiotics when appropriate, sialogogues, short-term oral steroids (dexamethasone) and dilatation of Stensen's duct with lacrimal probes to encourage drainage. Lavage with normal saline or penicillin solutions has been advocated to facilitate resolution of symptoms due to stasis of salivary flow or presence of sialoliths. The treatment of last resort for troublesome recurrent or refractory cases is parotidectomy, either superficial or total, and should not be entertained until conservative treatment options have been exhausted. Both operations have risks of facial nerve dysfunction, with a slightly greater risk with total parotidectomy.

- Acute (bacterial) suppurative parotitis
- Nonsuppurative parotitis (parotid sialadenitis)
- Chronic recurrent parotitis

Bibliography

Antoniades D, Harrison J, Epivatianos A, Papanayotou P: Treatment of chronic sialadenitis by intraductal penicillin or saline, *J Oral Maxillofac Surg* (62)4:431-434, 2004.

Baurmash H: Chronic recurrent parotitis: A closer look at its origin, diagnosis, and management, *J Oral Maxillofac Surg* (62)8:1010-1018, 2004.

Brook I: Acute bacterial suppurative parotitis: microbiology and management, *J Craniofac Surg* 14(1):37-40, 2003.

Fattahi T, Lyu P, Van Sickels J: Management of acute suppurative parotitis, *J Oral Maxillofac Surg* 60(4):446-448, 2002.

Marioni G, Bottin R, Tregnaghi A, et al: Craniocervical necrotizing fasciitis secondary to parotid gland abscess, *Acta Otolaryngol* 123(6):737-740, 2003.

Motamed M, Laugharne D, Bradley PJ: Management of chronic parotitis: a review, *J Laryngol Otol* 117(7):521-526, 2003.

Nahlieli O, Bar T, Shacham R, et al: Management of chronic recurrent parotitis: Current therapy, *J Oral Maxillofac Surg* (62)9:1150-1155, 2004.

O'Brien CJ, Murrant NJ: Surgical management of chronic parotitis, *Head Neck* 15(5):445-449, 1993.

Pou AM, Johnson JT, Weissman J: Management decisions in parotitis, *Comprehensive Therapy* 21(2):85-92, 1995.

Mucocele

David M. Weber, DDS, MD, and Deepak Kademani, DMD, MD, FACS, and Shahrokh C. Bagheri, DMD, MD

CC

A 20-year-old patient presents to office complaining of a painless mass of her lower lip. (Mucoceles are more common in young adults, but can be seen in all ages, including infants. There is no gender predilection.)

HPI

The patient was recently evaluated by her general dentist and was subsequently referred for evaluation and treatment of a persistent mass of her lower lip. The lesion was noticed 1 month earlier and has gradually increased to its current size (some patients give a history of recurrent swelling that periodically ruptures). The mass developed after trauma to the lower lip during function and has proved to be a site of continued trauma due to its persistence.

Although trauma (such as lip biting) had been associated with mucoceles, a positive history of trauma is frequently lacking.

PMHX/PDHX/MEDICATIONS/ALLERGIES/SH/FH

Noncontributory. There is no association with preexisting medical conditions and the incidence of mucoceles.

EXAMINATION

Maxillofacial. There is asymmetrical prominence of the patient's lower lip (most common site). There are no other areas of swelling or lymphadenopathy.

Intraoral. Examination reveals no pathology of the hard or soft palate, tongue, floor of the mouth, or buccal mucosa. A soft, 1-cm painless mass is appreciated just inferior and medial to the right labial commissure (Figure 6-11). The mass is fluctuant, soft, and nontender with a bluish mucosal discoloration. There is some evidence of trauma to the mass from the adjacent dentition. The tissue overlying the mass has become fibrotic as a result of repetitive trauma.

IMAGING

No imaging studies are indicated unless there is suspicion of other pathological processes.

LABS

No routines labs are indicated unless dictated by underlying medical conditions.

DIFFERENTIAL DIAGNOSIS

Despite characteristic clinical findings, in addition to the mucocele, the differential diagnosis of a soft tissue mass needs to be considered.

The differential diagnosis would include an irritation fibroma. This lesion is commonly pink and nonfluctuant and does not have history of intermittent swelling and rupturing (as opposed to a mucocele). Otherwise, it has a differential that is similar to a fibroma (see the section on irritation fibroma earlier in this chapter).

BIOPSY

Although the clinical examination can be highly suspicious of a mucocele, histopathological analysis is the only confirmatory test. An excisional biopsy (removal of entire lesion) is both diagnostic and the definitive treatment.

ASSESSMENT

An excisional biopsy was performed under local anesthesia confirming the diagnosis of a mucocele

Histopathological examination of a mucocele would demonstrate spillage of mucin surrounded by dense granulation tissue, which may be seen in association with minor salivary glands. An inflammatory response (neutrophils) may be observed.

TREATMENT

The above patient was seen in the clinic for excisional biopsy under local anesthesia. Care was taken to evert the lower lip with finger pressure against the skin. This provides increased exposure of the mass on the mucosal surface. A straight-line incision is made perpendicular to the vermillion border over the length of the mass on the mucosal surface. This is followed with careful, blunt, and sharp dissection around the mucocele and the offending gland. The surgical specimen was labeled and sent to pathology, and a diagnosis of a mucocele was confirmed.

Alternative surgical approach to treatment of mucocele includes excision or marsupialization with a carbon dioxide laser. Cryotherapy has also been used for the treatment of mucoceles. Direct application of liquid nitrogen is made with a cotton-tip applicator. A major advantage with this technique is compliance with pediatric patients.

COMPLICATIONS

The most common complication associated with treatment of mucocele is its recurrence. This can be minimized by the

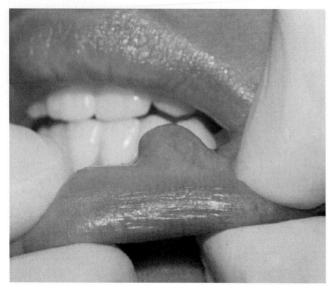

Figure 6-11   A 1-cm painless mass seen just inferior and medial to the right labial commissure.

removal of any adjacent minor salivary glands. With patients who experience problematic recurrence, a carbon dioxide laser can be used to ablate the surgical field, which is left to heal by secondary epithelialization. Excision or dissection of larger mucoceles of the lower lip can pose a risk to the labial branch of the mental nerve, resulting in postoperative neurosensory dysfunction.

DISCUSSION

Mucoceles, also called mucus retention cysts, or mucus extravasation phenomenon, by definition, are cavities filled with mucus produced by trauma to minor salivary glands. With functional trauma to the soft tissue and underlying glands, mucus leaks into the adjacent tissues, creating a mucocele. It is the most common lesion affecting the oral mucosa. It can grow to a few millimeters in size and rarely is larger than 1.5 cm. The lower lip is the most common site of a mucocele due to its susceptibility to trauma. Seldom are they seen in the upper lip even though it has an equivalent number of minor salivary glands. In a recent study of distribution of mucoceles in 263 patients, 78% occurred in the lower lip and 3% occurred in the upper lip. These findings are consistent with previous studies. Mucoceles do not have an epithelial lining (in contrast to salivary duct cysts). The extravasation of mucus produces a wall of inflamed fibrous tissue.

Bibliography

Baurmash H: Mucoceles and ranulas, *J Oral Maxillofac Surg* 61:369-378, 2003.

Harrison JD: Salivary mucoceles, *Oral Surg Oral Med Oral Pathol* 39:268-278, 1975.

Ishimaru M: A simple cryosurgical method for treatment of oral mucous cysts, *Int J Oral Maxillofac Surg* 22:353-355, 1993.

Jinbu Y: Mucocele of the glands of Blandin-Nuhn: clinical and histopathologic analysis of 26 cases, *Oral Surg Oral Med Oral Pathol Oral Radiol Endod* 95:467-470, 2003.

Kopp WK, St-Hilaire H: Mucosal preservation in the treatment of mucocele with CO2 laser, *J Oral Maxillofac Surg* 62:1559-1561, 2004.

Sela J, Ulmansky M: Mucous retention cyst of salivary glands, *J Oral Surg* 27(8):619-623, 1969.

Presentation of a Neck Mass: Differential Diagnosis

Kevin L. Rieck, DDS, MS, MD, and Shahrokh C. Bagheri, DMD, MD

CC

A 63-year-old man is referred for evaluation of a mass in his neck.

HPI

The patient reports a several-month history of a midline submandibular neck swelling that he associated with an abscessed tooth. A mandibular tooth was subsequently removed by his dentist, but the patient indicates no improvement. He reports that the area is slightly tender (swellings of neoplastic origin are unlikely to be painful or tender). He explains that the swelling under his jaw had been present for many months (chronic process) but became bothersome over the past several weeks. There are no associated symptoms of hoarseness or dysphagia (would be seen with impingement of a mass on the vocal cords or posterior oropharynx). There is no history of recent weight loss (cachexia could be a sign of a malignant process). He does not have any complaints of airway obstruction or difficulty breathing (expanding mass could progressively impinge on the airway).

PMHX/PDHX/ MEDICATIONS/ALLERGIES/SH/FH

He has no significant past medical or surgical history. There is no family history of similar presentations. He does not have any risk factors for neoplastic causes of his neck mass (smoking, alcohol). His abscessed tooth could cause submandibular swelling, but this would be unlikely due to persistence of symptoms after removal of the infectious source.

Patients should be questioned regarding a history of malignancies that may present with a metastatic lesion in the neck.

EXAMINATION

General. The patient is a well-developed and well-nourished patient in no apparent distress.

Vital signs. Vital signs are stable and he is afebrile (fever and the associated elevation in baseline heart rate can be secondary to an infectious etiology). Tumors can also cause fever either secondary to associated inflammation/infection or due to the release of inflammatory mediators such as tumor necrosis factor.

Maxillofacial. There is a soft, doughy midline swelling of the submandibular area measuring 6 cm in diameter. The mass appears freely movable with no clear attachment to the overlying skin. No fluctuance or frank fluid component is appreciated within the mass upon bimanual examination. It is not warm to palpation (seen with inflammation). The overlying skin appears normal (Figure 6-12). No palpable cervical adenopathy is noted.

Intraoral. Partial edentulism is noted with no gross areas of decay in the remaining dentition. There are no soft tissue lesions within the oral cavity. Salivary flow appears normal and without evidence of obstruction or erythema at the orifices of the submandibular and parotid ducts (important finding that makes sialadenitis unlikely). The muscles of mastication and temporomandibular joints are unremarkable. Bimanual intraoral examination also reveals the palpable mass in the midline floor of mouth that appears to be contiguous with the anterior neck mass. The mass does not elevate with tongue protrusion or swallowing (elevation of the mass would be consistent with a thyroglossal duct cyst).

IMAGING

Panoramic, lateral cephalometric or lateral neck films are rarely used in evaluating a neck mass. The panoramic radiograph should be used as a screening tool for evaluation of the dentition if there is suspicion of an odontogenic source of infection.

For this patient the panoramic radiograph demonstrated no source of odontogenic or osseous pathology. The contrast-enhanced CT scan showed a 5-cm cystic appearing mass in the anterior midline neck between the mandible and the hyoid bone (Figure 6-13). Several spherical densities were noted within the lesion. There was no evidence of adenopathy. The mass appeared discreet and not attached to the overlying skin.

LABS

No specific laboratory tests are indicated in the absence of pertinent medical history.

DIFFERENTIAL DIAGNOSIS

The differential diagnosis of a neck mass can be quite extensive and can include any or all of the intricate structures within the neck. There are several considerations in distinguishing between inflammatory and/or infectious causes, anatomical variants, congenital lesions, and benign or malignant processes. One of the most important aspects in assessing a neck mass is a thorough patient history. The age of the patient is an important initial consideration. An adult patient over the age of 40 has an 80% chance that a nonthyroid neck

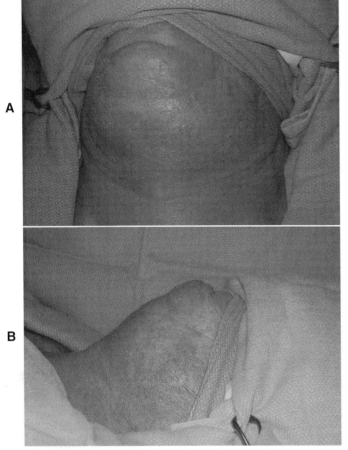

Figure 6-12 Frontal view (**A**) and profile (**B**) swelling of the submandibular area measuring 6 cm in diameter. The overlying skin appears normal.

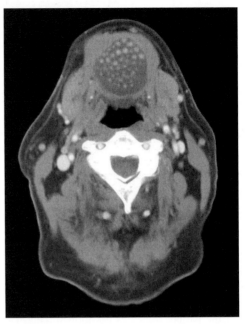

Figure 6-13 Contrast-enhanced CT scan showing a 5-cm cystic appearing mass in the anterior midline neck between the mandible and the hyoid bone.

mass will be neoplastic, of which 80% of cases are metastatic squamous cell carcinoma from the aerodigestive tract. Figure 6-14 is a flow chart for the diagnosis of a neck mass that uses age and location as distinguishing factors.

In general it is useful to consider four broad categories: anatomical, inflammatory and/or infectious, congenital, and neoplastic (Box 6-6).

One must maintain a high index of suspicion for metastatic disease processes. These commonly include squamous cell cancers of the head and neck, lung, thyroid, and salivary glands malignancies. Melanoma may also present in this area. Primary neck tumors presenting as a neck mass typically result from salivary gland lesions, lymphoma, or thyroid masses. Benign masses result from several of the tissues in the neck. These can include lipomas, neural tumors, vascular lesions, sebaceous cysts, and fibromas.

ASSESSMENT

A well-circumscribed soft tissue mass of the anterior midline neck

An FNA was performed that revealed scant cellular material. Diagnosis would require surgical exploration with an excisional biopsy.

TREATMENT

This 63-year-old man underwent a cervical exploration under general anesthesia in the hospital setting. Prior to any incision, the lesion was aspirated and returned several milliliters of a viscous yellowish fluid. A transverse incision was made in the anterior neck well below the mass. Subcutaneous skin flaps were raised and the platysma muscle was identified. Blunt dissection was performed around the mass. The mylohyoid muscle was identified and divided in the midline. No communication with the oral cavity was encountered. The mass was removed and submitted for permanent histopathological examination (Figure 6-15). A drain was placed in the neck defect and the wound was closed in standard layered fashion.

The pathological diagnosis revealed the lesion to be a dermoid cyst. These cysts can have tremendous histological variability. There is a connective tissue wall that may have a thin lining of epithelial cells. This can exhibit keratinization, and the lumen may be filled with keratin as well as sebaceous fluid. Glandular components from apocrine or sebaceous tissue may also be present.

COMPLICATIONS

Several complications can occur in performing neck surgery. Hematomas; seromas; wound infections; injury to branches of the facial, trigeminal or hypoglossal nerves; and atypical scar formation are all possible sequelae. Surgeons must have a thorough understanding of anatomy in order to effectively recognize and manage lesions and complications in this complex area.

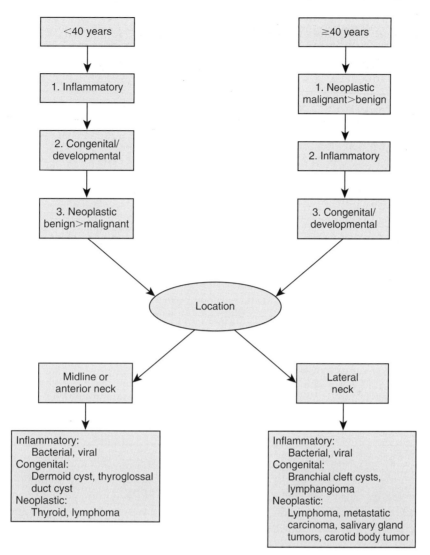

Figure 6-14 Evaluation of a neck mass using age and location as distinguishing factors.

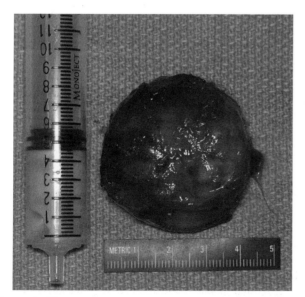

Figure 6-15 Surgical specimen later diagnosed as a dermoid cyst.

DISCUSSION

The diagnostic challenge in assessing the neck mass can be overwhelming. It is important to have a consistent system in both history taking and examination aspects of the approach to this complex anatomic region. Onset, duration, size fluctuations, or progression and any associated symptoms must be elucidated from the patient when possible. Similarly, the association of squamous cell carcinoma with alcohol and tobacco abuse has been well documented, and the patient's present and past use of these products should be noted. Any recent exposure to infectious diseases, trauma, animals (cats), dental work, or surgical intervention should be determined.

The adult patient presenting with a neck mass should have a thorough history taken to assist the diagnosis. Supplemental evaluation with ultrasound, CT scan, MRI, or positron emission tomography scans, in addition to a fine needle aspirates of the mass can be extremely useful

Box 6-6.	The Four Major Categories for the differential diagnosis of a Neck Mass

- **Anatomical.** Several anatomical structures are palpable in certain patients. These include the transverse process of C1, the hyoid bone, thyroid and cricoid cartilages, and prominent or atherosclerotic carotid bulbs.
- **Inflammatory and/or infectious.** This category encompasses several causes for a neck mass, which is generally a reactive process. Cervical adenitis can arise from bacterial, viral, parasitic, and fungal sources. *Staphylococcus aureus,* cutaneous skin infections, Epstein-Barr virus, and herpes simplex viruses are frequent culprits. Other inflammatory causes include infectious and/or obstructive lesions of the salivary glands. Sialadenitis and associated sialolithiasis of the major salivary glands can cause significant swelling within the neck.
- **Congenital lesions or masses.** These are frequently recognized at an early age but may also present later in life with the onset of new symptoms. Several common disorders are encountered: thyroglossal duct cyst, branchial cleft cyst or fistula, cystic hygroma, dermoid cyst, lymphangioma, and ranula. Other rare conditions such as thymic mass, laryngoceles, and teratomas can occur.
  - ○ **Thyroglossal duct cysts** are midline or anterior neck masses. These frequently appear post upper respiratory tract infection. The mass itself moves with swallowing or tongue protrusion. The cyst, thyroglossal tract, and midportion of the hyoid bone are removed in the Sistrunk procedure to treat this condition.
  - ○ **Dermoid cysts** are midline masses that lie deep to the cervical fascia and tend to be slow growing. They are above the hyoid bone and do not move with protrusion of the tongue.
  - ○ **Branchial cleft cysts** are remnants of the branchial arch apparatus present during embryogenesis.
  - ○ **First branchial cleft cysts** (two types are possible).
    - **Type I cysts** tend to occur in the preauricular or postauricular region and connect the skin to the external auditory canal.
    - **Type II cysts** are near the mandibular angle and closely associated with the parotid gland.
  - ○ **Second branchial cleft cysts** are the most common of the branchial cleft cysts. The cyst or opening to the cyst is usually found at the anterior edge of the sternocleidomastoid muscle.
  - ○ **Third branchial cleft cysts** are very rare. These are also found along the anterior border of the sternocleidomastoid muscle but ultimately empty into the piriform sinus.
  - ○ **Fourth branchial cleft cysts** can occur and have an extensive course through the neck looping around the hypoglossal nerve and aortic arch.
- **Neoplastic.** Neoplastic lesions in the neck are common and have certain characteristics that set them apart from other conditions. Masses fixed to the underlying structures and matted nodes are ominous findings for malignancy.

in further defining the lesion. Suspected inflammatory or infectious conditions should respond to broad-spectrum antibiotics. Suspected neoplastic masses should be evaluated with contrast-enhanced CT scans and an FNA of the mass.

This patient tolerated the surgical procedure well and had an uneventful postoperative course. Histopathological evaluation confirmed the diagnosis of a dermoid cyst. This is thought to result from entrapment of midline epithelial tissue during the closure of the mandibular and hyoid branchial arches. In this location, they are rarely present at birth and typically present in young adulthood. As in this case, these cysts typically feel dough-like, but this can vary with the actual contents of the cyst. They can be either above or below the mylohyoid muscle. Surgical extirpation is the recommended treatment and recurrence is rare.

Bibliography

Armstrong WB, Giglio MF: Is this lump in the neck anything to worry about? *Postgrad Med* 104(3):63-78, 1998.

Cummings CW, et al: *Otolaryngology—head and neck surgery,* Vol 2, ed 2, St. Louis, 1993, Mosby, pp 1543-1565.

Gujar S, et al: Pediatric head and neck masses, *Top Magn Reson Imaging* 15(2):95-101, 2004.

Prakash PK, Hanna FW: Differential diagnosis of neck lumps, *Practitioner* 246(1633):252-254, 259, 2002.

Prisco MK: Evaluating neck masses, *Nurse Pract* 25(4):50-51, 2002.

Schwetschenau E, Kelley DJ: The adult neck mass, *Am Fam Phys* 66(5):831-838, 2002.

Shafer WG, et al: *Oral pathology,* ed 4. Philadelphia, 1983, WB Saunders, pp 75-79.

Thawley SE, Panje WR, et al: *Comprehensive management of head and neck tumors,* Vol 2, Philadelphia, 1987, WB Saunders, pp 1230-1240.

Oral Leukoplakia

Derek Lamb, DMD, Deepak Kademani, DMD, MD, and Shahrokh C. Bagheri, DMD, MD

CC

A 53-year-old man is referred to your office by his general dentist for evaluation of an intraoral lesion that was found during a routine dental examination. The prevalence of oral leukoplakia increases with age and has a strong male predilection.

HPI

The patient presents with a painless, asymptomatic white lesion (leukoplakia) of the right buccal mucosa (lip vermilion, buccal mucosa, and gingiva are the most common sites). He was not aware of the lesion until his general dentist detected it during a routine oral exam. The lesion has been present for an unknown duration. He denies any history of trauma, cheek biting (morsicatio buccarum), or parafunctional habits (chewing tobacco, snuff, sunflower seeds, or other foreign objects that may cause frictional keratosis). He denies any history of fevers, weight loss, dysphagia, or other constitutional symptoms.

PMHX/PSHX/MEDICATIONS/ALLERGIES/SH/FH

The patient's history is significant for a 44 pack per year history of smoking (higher incidence in patients using tobacco on a routine basis).

EXAMINATION

General. The patient is a white man who appears his stated age. He is well nourished with no signs of cachexia (seen with advanced malignant disease or malnutrition).

Maxillofacial. There is a 1.3×0.8-cm well-circumscribed, slightly elevated white plaque of the right mid buccal mucosa just inferior to the occlusal plane (presents as linea alba on the buccal mucosa). The lesion is soft, nonindurated, nonulcerated, and nonadherent to underlying tissues (firm, indurated, ulcerated, and/or fixed lesions can be a sign of invasive carcinoma). The lesion does not rub off with gauze (white lesions that can be scraped off have a separate differential diagnosis) and does not form a bulla with firm pressure (negative Nikolsky sign). No Wickham striae are present (seen in lichen planus). The lesion does not diminish or disappear when stretched (seen in leukoedema). No other lesions or masses are noted. He is partially edentulous with poor oral hygiene and no grossly carious teeth.

Neck. No cervical or submandibular lymphadenopathy was noted.

IMAGING

Imaging for soft tissue lesions is based on the clinical presentation and differential diagnosis. This lesion is a superficial mucosal lesion that does not appear to invade underlying structures; therefore, no imaging studies are required.

LABS

No routine laboratory studies are indicated for a planned biopsy or workup of a white lesion in an otherwise healthy patient.

DIFFERENTIAL DIAGNOSIS

The working differential diagnosis of a white lesion of the buccal mucosa that cannot be scraped off should include hyperkeratosis with or without dysplasia (histological diagnosis), lichen planus, morsicatio buccarum (chronic cheek biting), frictional keratosis, nicotine stomatitis, leukoedema, and white sponge nevus. The diagnosis of leukoplakia is one of exclusion, presenting as a white plaque that cannot be removed, and requires a biopsy for histological confirmation. Because leukoplakia is considered a premalignant lesion with risk of malignant transformation, squamous cell carcinoma is included in the differential diagnosis.

BIOPSY

Definitive diagnosis requires an incisional or excisional biopsy depending on the size and character of the lesion. Typically, lesions less than 1 cm can be easily excised and closed primarily, whereas an incisional biopsy is indicated in larger lesions or when a malignancy is suspected.

In this patient, an excisional biopsy was performed under local anesthesia (direct infiltration into the lesion should be avoided to prevent distortion of the specimen), which showed full-thickness (from basal layer to surface mucosa) epithelial dysplasia with cellular atypia, loss of rete peg formation with mucosal atrophy, and superficial parakeratosis. The integrity of the basement membrane was maintained, indicating carcinoma in situ (if the dysplastic cells invaded through the basement membrane into the underlying submucosa, invasive squamous cell carcinoma would be the correct diagnosis).

ASSESSMENT

Oral leukoplakia with biopsy-proved diagnosis of carcinoma in situ ($T_{is}N_0M_0$, stage 0 squamous cell carcinoma) of the right buccal mucosa

133

TREATMENT

Traditionally, the first line of treatment of white oral lesions has been identification and elimination of possible etiological factors. This is then followed by a 2-week period of observation. Persistent lesions with no identifiable cause undergo biopsy to establish a diagnosis. The resulting diagnosis should dictate the subsequent management. Toluidine blue may be used to identify potential biopsy sites that are more likely to exhibit dysplastic changes. Exfoliative cytology can be used for the evaluation of mucosal lesions (advantage of being less invasive and not requiring local anesthesia). However, a biopsy is required for a definitive diagnosis.

Current treatment is aimed at prevention of malignant transformation and resolution of the lesion. Biopsy-proved hyperkeratosis (gives the lesion the white textured appearance) without dysplasia can be closely observed for changes, while hyperkeratosis with mild to moderate dysplasia can be treated with carbon dioxide laser ablation. Severe dysplasia or carcinoma in situ requires wide local excision. Laser excision, ablation, or a combination of the two can also be performed depending on the location of the leukoplakia. Chemopreventive measures (β-carotene, vitamin A, or retinoids) have been shown to cause regression of existing lesions and prevention of other lesions in the aerodigestive tract (therapy must be maintained indefinitely and therefore patient compliance is low). Photodynamic therapy, although not available in the United States, is showing some promise in the treatment of precancerous and malignant lesions.

This patient underwent an excisional biopsy of the lesion under local anesthesia. An elliptical incision was made around the entire lesion and into the submucosa (the junction of the basement membrane and submucosa is important in the evaluation for possible invasive carcinoma). Normal appearing tissue surrounding the area is also included in the biopsy specimen to ensure clear margins. Electrocautery is used to provide hemostasis of the surgical bed. The wound is close primarily. The surgical specimen is oriented with sutures of different length placed at the anterior and superior margins.

The histopathological report confirmed carcinoma in situ, which requires a wide local excision of the entire lesion for histological documentation.

COMPLICATIONS

The main concern with oral leukoplakia is the risk of malignant transformation. Leukoplakia is a premalignant lesion implying that it is "a morphologically altered tissue in which cancer is more likely to occur than in its normal counterpart." The rate of malignant transformation of oral leukoplakia (homogeneous type) is between 3% and 6%. Erythroplakia, which is much less common than leukoplakia, has a much higher transformation rate (20% to 90%), and always requires surgical excision. Consequently, it is very important for these patients to be followed closely for any mucosal changes allowing prompt treatment to reduce the morbidity and mortality from malignant transformation.

DISCUSSION

The World Health Organization defines leukoplakia as "a white patch or plaque that cannot be characterized clinically or pathologically as any other disease." It is, therefore, a diagnosis of exclusion. Leukoplakia is a condition that is frequently encountered in the oral cavity and is most commonly found on the lip vermillion, buccal mucosa, and gingiva. However, lesions of the floor of the mouth, tongue, and lower lip are most likely to exhibit dysplasia and are associated with a higher rate of malignant transformation. The prevalence in the general population is estimated to vary from less than 1% to more than 5%. Its presence has been associated with tobacco smoking (although the rate of malignant transformation with smokeless tobacco has not definitively been shown to be higher), sanguinaria, ultraviolet radiation, and microorganisms such as *Treponema pallidum* (mucous patch of stage 2 syphilis), *Candida albicans*, and human papilloma virus.

Lesions may present as a white patch (leukoplakia), a white patch with red dots (speckled leukoplakia), or a mixed red and white lesion (erythroleukoplakia). Those lesions with areas of mixed erythema frequently contain advanced dysplasia or invasive squamous cell carcinoma (biopsy of mixed lesions should include the red component). Leukoplakic lesions are classified histopathologically according to the degree of dysplasia or histology of the cellular and other epithelial elements. Mild dysplasia is cellular atypia that is limited to the basilar and parabasilar epithelial layers. Moderate dysplasia involves the basal layer up to the midportion of the spinous layer. Severe dysplasia is atypia that extends more than halfway through the epithelium but does not involve the full thickness. Carcinoma in situ is defined as dysplasia of the entire epithelial layer without invasion of the basement membrane into the underlying tissue.

Most leukoplakias do not transform into carcinomas, and recent studies have attempted to identify molecular markers for malignant transformation. Potential areas that have been explored are DNA ploidy status, loss of heterozygosity utilizing microsatellite markers, *p53* mutations and aberrant expression, inappropriate expression of other oncogenes such as cyclin D1, and differentiation markers such as keratins and cell surface carbohydrates including blood group antigens.

Another aggressive form of this disease is proliferative verrucous leukoplakia. Interestingly, proliferative verrucous leukoplakia is not associated with tobacco use, and it has a strong female predilection. It has a high recurrence rate and a tendency to slowly spread to involve multiple oral sites. Proliferative verrucous leukoplakia has a high rate of malignant transformation (to verrucous or squamous cell carcinoma).

Figure 6-16 demonstrates a case of severe leukoplakia under the denture-bearing tissue. There was evidence of moderate dysplasia upon biopsy of the midpalatal area.

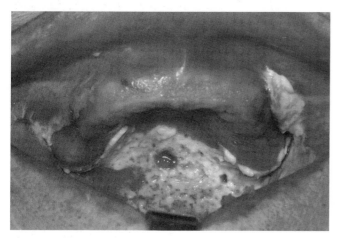

Figure 6-16 Extensive leukoplakia of the palate in a different patient that showed evidence of moderate dysplasia upon biopsy.

Bibliography

Saito T, Suguira C, Hirai A, et al: Development of squamous cell carcinoma from preexisting oral leucoplakia with respect to treatment modality, *Int J Oral Maxillofac Surg* 30:49-53, 2001.

Silverman S Jr: Leukoplakia, dysplasia, and malignant transformation [Editorial], *Oral Surg Oral Med Oral Pathol* 82:117-125, 1996.

Slaughter DP, Southwick HW, Smejkal W: Field cancerization in oral stratified squamous epithelium: clinical implications of multicentric origin, *Cancer* 963-968, 1953.

Vigliante CE, Quinn PD, Alwai F: Proliferative verrcucous leukoplakia: a case report with characteristic long term progression, *J Oral Maxillofac Surg* 61:626-631, 2003.

Osteoradionecrosis of the Mandible

Abtin Shahriari, DMD, MPH, and Shahrokh C. Bagheri, DMD, MD

CC

A 67-year-old man is referred to your office for evaluation of exposed bone of the left posterior mandible subsequent to full-mouth extraction (osteoradionecrosis is more commonly seen in the elderly and in the posterior mandible).

HPI

The patient has a history of squamous cell carcinoma of the left tonsillar fossa treated with a total dose of 7300 centiGray (cGy) of external radiation 1 year earlier (cGy is the unit for radiation that has replaced the equivalent unit of rad). Full-mouth extraction was performed 9 months after completion of radiation therapy. During the past 3 months, he has developed a nonhealing painful wound of the left mandible. He has been on several different antibiotics and oral chlorohexidine with no apparent resolution. His current pain level has been difficult to manage with opioid analgesics. In addition, he reports to have lost over 10 pounds in the past 2 months (due to decreased oral intake). One month ago, he heard a cracking noise on his left mandible with associated pain (suggestive of a pathological fracture). More recently, the skin overlying his mandible has developed an orocutaneous fistula.

The most important factor for the development of osteoradionecrosis is the radiation dose. High-dose radiotherapy (above 7200 cGy) is likely to reach the clinical threshold for the development of osteoradionecrosis, compared to a moderate dose (5000 cGy to 6400 cGy). Patients are generally at a progressively increasing risk with doses above 5000 cGy.

The risk of developing osteoradionecrosis is also related to other factors, including location of the primary tumor, size of the tumor, proximity of the tumor to bone, condition of the dentition, and type of treatment (external beam radiotherapy, brachytherapy, surgery, or chemotherapy). Other medical comorbidities that influence wound healing such as the nutritional status and extrinsic factors such as tobacco or alcohol abuse are likely to play a role. However, the radiation dose and time elapsed since radiation therapy are the most significant risk factors.

PMHX/PDHX/MEDICATIONS/ALLERGIES/SH/FH

The patient has a 40-year history of tobacco and alcohol use (risk factors for oral squamous cell carcinoma).

He has no history of oral or intravenous bisphosphonate use or adjuvant chemotherapy.

Osteonecrosis of the jaws secondary to bisphosphonate use can have a similar clinical presentation as osteoradionecrosis despite a different pathophysiology (see Chapter 2, section on bisphosphonate related osteonecrosis of the jaws). Metastatic disease to the mandible (prostate, kidney) is rare but can present as a nonhealing wound. Primary malignant tumors of bone, osteomyelitis, and fibro-osseous lesions can present as exposed bone, but most of these conditions are easily distinguished from osteoradionecrosis by an accurate history and clinical and radiographic examination.

EXAMINATION

General. The patient is a cachectic, thin man in mild distress (generalized muscle wasting is an indication of the poor nutritional status but is also related to the wasting associated with advanced malignant processes).

Vital signs. Vital signs are stable and he is afebrile (lack of fever is not uncommon with osteoradionecrosis).

Maxillofacial. There is minimal left facial edema, with hyperemic skin (secondary to the effects of radiation) overlying the mandible posteriorly. The left mandible is painful to palpation. The maximal jay opening is less than 25 mm (due to radiation fibrosis and pain). There is no cervical or submandibular lymphadenopathy (positive nodes may be seen with acute infections or recurrence of the primary tumor). There is a draining orocutaneous fistula of the left neck, with surrounding erythema.

Intraoral. His oral hygiene is poor. The extraction sockets of the posterior left mandible have not healed, and there is approximately 1.5 cm of exposed bone. The oral mucous membranes are dry (radiation-induced xerostomia secondary to the effects of radiation on salivary glands). The mandible shows intersegmental mobility across the area of exposed bone (indicative of mandible fracture).

Pulmonary. He has a barrel-shaped chest with distant breath sounds and mild bilateral scattered rhonchi (physical findings consistent with emphysema secondary to prolonged tobacco use).

Although this patient is edentulous, radiation caries is commonly seen on teeth remaining in the path of radiation and is probably related to pulpal necrosis combined with the effects of xerostomia from radiation.

IMAGING

The panoramic radiograph is the initial imaging study of choice for evaluation of the mandible, and may be the only

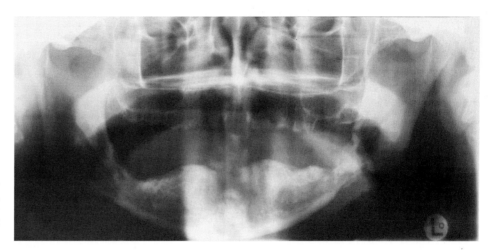

Figure 6-17 A panoramic radiograph demonstrates an undefined poorly demarcated sclerotic radiolucent lesion with a fracture at the left angle.

study necessary for suspected osteoradionecrosis. A CT scan of the mandible may also be used to more accurately delineate the areas of bony involvement.

For this patient, the panoramic radiograph demonstrates an undefined poorly demarcated sclerotic radiolucent lesion with a fracture at the left angle (Figure 6-17).

LABS

Laboratory tests for the preoperative workup of osteoradionecrosis should include a CBC to assess for leukocytosis secondary to any acute infection and baseline hematocrit and hemoglobin levels. Other tests are ordered based on the medical history and extent of anticipated surgery. An albumin and prealbumin level may be obtained if there is a suspicion of malnutrition (as seen with chronic alcohol use). Nutritional status should be supplemented as needed.

This patient had a WBC count of 11,000 cells/mm^3. The prealbumin level was 8 mg/dl, which is consistent with malnutrition (normal range, 16 to 30 mg/dl). The basic metabolic panel was within normal limits.

ASSESSMENT

Stage III osteoradionecrosis of the left posterior mandible, with a pathological fracture and an orocutaneous fistula compounded by generalized malnutrition

TREATMENT

There is some controversy regarding the optimal treatment of osteoradionecrosis. The description of the pathophysiology of osteoradionecrosis by Marx in 1983 (hypoxia, hypocellular, hypovascular) is generally well accepted. As radiation energy passes through normal tissue, it immediately kills a small number of cells, which incur internal damage to their DNA, RNA, enzyme systems, and cell membranes. These cells may not be replaced when they die (due to impaired cell division). Consequently the tissue become less cellular (hypocellular), less vascular (hypovascular), and less oxygenated (hypoxic). Marx has further popularized the use of hyperbaric oxygen

therapy for treatment of early and advanced osteoradionecrosis using a hyperbaric oxygen protocol (described later). Hyperbaric oxygen therapy is administered in a pressurized chamber most commonly at 2.4 atmospheres (ATA), which is equal to the pressure under 45 feet of water. The patient breathes 100% oxygen for a predetermined amount of time (90 minutes at 2.4 ATA is considered one dive). The increase in partial pressure (Pao$_2$) of the inspired air increases the amount of oxygen dissolved in blood and subsequently increases the oxygen delivered to tissue. The increased oxygen gradient at the cellular level stimulates angiogenesis, and therefore vascularity. Hyperbaric oxygen may also have a oxygen-dependent bactericidal function affecting the function of leukocytes (oxygen tension less than 30 mm Hg significantly impairs the ability of the leukocytes to kill the phagocytosed organism). Absolute contraindications of hyperbaric oxygen include untreated pneumothorax, optic neuritis, fulminant viral infections, and congenital spherocytosis.

With the advent of microvascular surgery and the recent advances in this field, many surgeons recommend resection of the necrotic mandibular (or maxillary) segment and immediate reconstruction using microvascular free flaps without the use of hyperbaric oxygen. Until further studies regarding the outcome, morbidity, cost, and effectiveness of these two dramatically different treatment philosophies are available, the optimal treatment of osteoradionecrosis remains partially unclear. The two methodologies are briefly described next:

Hyperbaric oxygen protocol. This protocol developed by Marx is based on categorizing osteoradionecrosis into three stages. Patients presenting with exposed bone are designated as having stage I osteoradionecrosis. These patients would receive 30 dives of hyperbaric oxygen. If the bone softens and granulation tissue develops, the patient is designated as a stage I responder and is treated by minimal local debridement followed by 10 more dives. However, if the patient does not respond, he is designated as having stage II, which is treated by surgical debridement followed by 10 additional dives. If there is persistence of dehiscence and exposed bone, he is designated as having stage III osteoradionecrosis. This requires a continuity resection, jaw stabilization, and soft tissue flap as needed. Patients presenting with a pathological fracture, orocutaneous fistula, or osteolysis of the inferior border of the mandible are also designated as having stage III osteoradionecrosis.

Microvascular techniques. A vast body of literature supports the treatment of early and late osteoradionecrosis using free vascular tissue transfer into the irradiated field with success rates of over 95%. Microvascular surgery (free flaps) allows the surgeon to bring in hard and soft tissues with independent blood supply anastomosed outside of the radiated field. Commonly used donor sites include the free fibular osteocutaneous flap (see Chapter 11, section on fibular free flap for mandibular reconstruction), radial forearm fasciculocutaneous flap (see Chapter 11, section on radial forearm free flap), the deep circumflex iliac artery osteomyocutaneous flap using the iliac crest, and the anterolateral thigh (soft tissue transfer). The arterial and venous blood supply of the transferred tissue (flap) is anastomosed into the available vessels within the head and neck (most commonly, the carotid or associated branches and the jugular venous system).

An advantage of microvascular flaps with respect to osteoradionecrosis is the ability to bring in new blood supply independent of the compromised host bed. This eliminates the need for multiple costly hyperbaric oxygen treatments.

This patient was taken to the operating room for resection of the fracture segment and associated necrotic tissue and fistula (Figure 6-18, A). A free fibula flap was harvested (Figure 6-18, B) and inserted into the defect along with anastomosis of the vessels to the facial artery and internal jugular vein. The postoperative panoramic radiograph and clinical photograph demonstrate the position of the fibular graft and soft tissue closure 4 weeks postsurgery (Figure 6-18, C and D).

COMPLICATIONS

Radiotherapy can be highly effective in the treatment of head and neck cancer. However, the effects of direct and scattered radiation on adjacent normal tissue are associated with significant side effects that further affect the already compromised quality of life of a cancer patient. Radiation-induced damage should be anticipated and prevented whenever possible. Early management can ameliorate the long-term effects. Radiation-induced damage is the result of the deleterious effects of radiation, not only on the oral mucosa but also on the adjacent salivary glands, bone, dentition, and masticatory musculature. Radiation mucositis is an acute complication representing the inflammatory response to acute radiation injury. This is a self-limiting condition that may develop in the last 3 weeks of radiotherapy and may extend for about 1 month thereafter. During this period, topical viscous 2% lidocaine gel as well as systemic analgesic may be needed for pain control, along with the use of chlorhexidine gluconate antiseptic rinses. Radiation caries is seen as hard and black erosions of the teeth structure mostly at the gingival margin, cusp tips, and incisal surfaces, presenting only in the direct path of radiation. Even the best oral hygiene, dental care, and fluoride treatment will not totally prevent this condition.

The chronic complications of radiotherapy include mucosal fibrosis and atrophy, salivary gland dysfunction, soft tissue necrosis, osteoradionecrosis, dysgeusia (distortion or decrease in sense of taste), ageusia (loss of taste function), muscular fibrosis (causing trismus), xerostomia, and fungal and bacterial infections. Radiation-induced xerostomia is caused by the direct damaging effects of radiation on both major and minor salivary gland structures located within the path of radiation. Dysphagia (difficulty swallowing) is one of the most troubling and least treatable chronic complications of radiation. Last, there can be significant effects of radiation on jaw growth and development of teeth in the younger population.

Complications directly related to osteoradionecrosis include chronic pain, drug dependency, trismus, nutritional deficiencies, pathological fractures, orocutaneous fistulas, disfigurement due to loss of soft tissue and bone, loss of time from work and family, and the psychological stigma of having a nonhealing wound.

DISCUSSION

Osteoradionecrosis is defined as a radiation-induced necrosis of bone and associated soft tissue.

This is a well-known complication of radiation therapy that predominantly involves the mandible, although it can be seen in the maxilla. This condition has frustrated maxillofacial surgeons and radiation oncologists since the 1950s with the popularization of radiation therapy for head and neck cancer. Osteoradionecrosis was initially thought to have an infectious etiology, but subsequent studies have shown infection to be a secondary process related to the hypovascular, hypoxic, and hypocellular nature of radiated tissue and the subsequent inability to resist infection. The incidence and prevalence of osteoradionecrosis of the jaws after radiation therapy for the treatment of oral and oropharyngeal cancer is uncertain and has been reported between 1% and 30% in the literature. The incidence increases as more time is elapsed from surgery. Recent studies, along with the development of improved radiation technology such as intensity-modulated radiation therapy (IMRT) and other methods that expose the normal tissue to lower doses of radiation for head and neck cancer, suggest a lower incidence than previously reported. Intensity-modulated radiation therapy is an exciting new modality in radiation technology that is applied in the head and neck. It uses dose-volume relationships with computer imaging to substantially localize the delivered radiation and reduce the dose received by the mandible, with the goal of reduction of osteoradionecrosis.

The advantages of intensity-modulated radiation therapy include the following:
- Delivery of high doses to the target volume
- Relatively sparing of normal structures in the head and neck because of the sharp dose gradient
- Accurate delivery of radiation

The main disadvantages are the greater preparation needed compared to conventional plans from the perspective of physician contouring and physics design and requirement of a

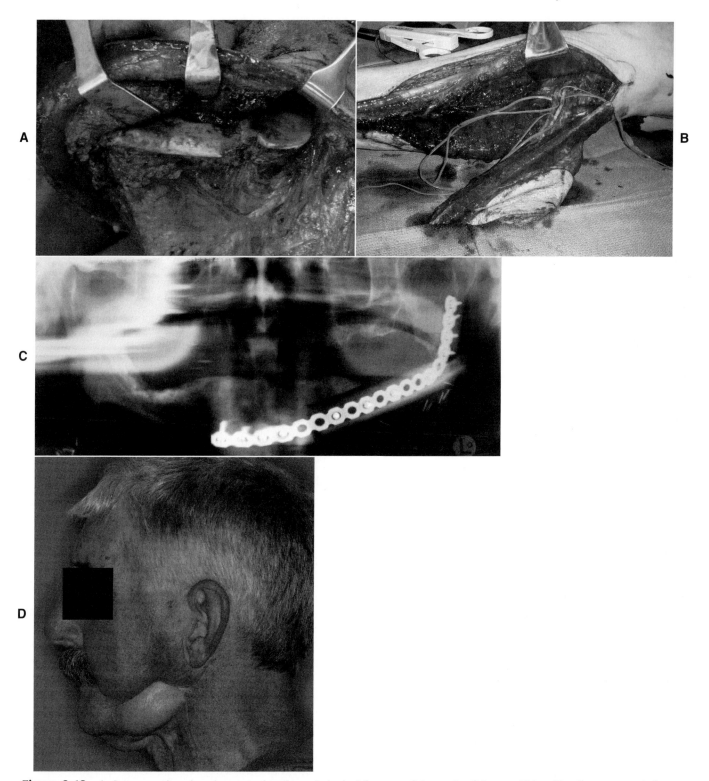

Figure 6-18 **A,** Intraoperative view demonstrating the pathological fracture of the angle of the mandible with adjacent necrotic bone. **B,** Harvest of a free fibula osteomyocutaneous flap. **C,** Postoperative panoramic radiograph showing inset of the free fibula for mandibular reconstruction. **D,** Profile view of the patient showing the inset of the soft tissue flap and closure of the orocutaneous fistula. *(Courtesy Dr. R. Bryan Bell, DDS, MD.)*

thorough understanding of target selection and delineation on the part of the treating physician. The use of intensity-modulated radiation therapy is expected to translate into a further reduction of the risk of osteoradionecrosis.

Osteoradionecrosis can be categorized into three different types based on etiology and chronology:

1. Early trauma-induced osteoradionecrosis, which develops either soon after radiation or months afterward (attributed to the combined effects of radiation injury with surgical trauma and physiological demands of wound healing)
2. Spontaneous osteoradionecrosis (unassociated with any surgical or traumatic event, occurring secondary to high-dose radiation)
3. Late trauma-induced osteoradionecrosis, usually associated with surgical procedures over 2 years since radiotherapy

The highest incidence of osteoradionecrosis has been seen with oral cancer of the tongue, retromolar region, and floor of the mouth. This is probably due to the proximity of the mandibular bone within the radiated field.

Prevention of osteoradionecrosis is currently the best modality of treatment. Upon diagnosis of head and neck cancer, radiation therapy is usually initiated as soon as possible. General dental evaluations should be conducted promptly to treat and control for caries and initiate fluoride tray treatments. It is generally recommended that grossly carious and periodontally diseased mandibular teeth that are in the direct path of radiation 5000 cGy or greater should be removed at least 14 to 21 days before the initiation of radiation therapy. Restorable maxillary teeth that do not have severe periodontal disease do not require preradiation extraction. A retrospective study by Curi reviewed 104 patients who were treated for osteoradionecrosis of the jaws. All patients had a history of osteoradionecrosis of at least 3 months' duration with a minimum follow-up of 1 year. In this group, osteoradionecrosis was seen predominantly in the mandible compared with the maxilla (20:1). This is attributed to the greater blood supply and thinner bone of the maxilla. In cases where a severe toothache or a dental abscess occurs during radiation therapy, treatment should not be interrupted. The decayed tooth should be restored with noninvasive methods such as pulpotomies, pulpectomies, endodontic treatment, and analgesics. In cases of an acute odontogenic abscess, an incision and drainage in addition to endodontic therapy and antibiotics is recommended. There generally is a 4-month period after radiation, the "golden window" that allows for definitive care, including extractions. The effects of radiation damage to the tissue are time dependent and take several months to affect wound healing.

There are three basic types of radiotherapy protocols. External beam radiotherapy is the most common (includes intensity-modulated radiation therapy), followed by interstitial (or implant-seeded) radiotherapy. The third type is the neutron beam radiotherapy, which is the most damaging to the normal tissue as well as tumor cells. The latter is rarely used due to its complications. Radiation entails high linear energy transferred to tissue with the intent to kill cancer cells.

The external beam radiotherapy is usually achieved with cobalt-60 radiation-emitting beta-particles that collide with water molecules, splitting them into free radicals such as superoxide $O^{\cdot}$, and hydroxyl OH^{-}, which react with DNA, RNA, enzyme systems, and cell membranes. Most cells survive but incur internal damage to the cell structures, resulting in impairment of cell division. Consequently, the tissue becomes progressively less cellular, less vascular, and hypoxic.

There has been some controversy over the prophylactic use of hyperbaric oxygen therapy before extraction of teeth in a previously irradiated field. Hyperbaric oxygen therapy dates back to 1930s, when the United States Navy studied the use of oxygen to treat divers who had decompression sickness and arterial gas embolism.

In clinical practice, it has been used both for treatment and prophylactically for management and prevention of compromised wound healing. The benefit of prophylactic hyperbaric oxygen therapy before the extraction of teeth in previously irradiated tissue has been questioned, given the lower incidence of osteoradionecrosis reported in recent years. Despite the growing body of scientific evidence supporting hyperbaric oxygen therapy in wound healing, its precise application remains a controversial issue. This controversy has resulted in a continuing skepticism among some practitioners.

Further scientific studies are necessary to address the optimal application of hyperbaric oxygen therapy in prevention and treatment of osteoradionecrosis.

Bibliography

Ang E, Black C, Irish J, et al: Reconstructive options in the treatment of osteoradionecrosis of the craniomaxillofacial skeleton, *Br J Plast Surg* 56:92, 2003.

Annane D, Depondt J, Aubert P, et al: Hyperbaric oxygen therapy for radionecrosis of the jaw: a randomized, placebo-controlled, double-blind trial from the ORN96 Study Group, *J Clin Oncol* Dec 15;22(24):4893-900, 2004; Epub Nov 1, 2004.

Buchbinder D, St Hilaire H: The use of free tissue transfer in advanced osteoradionecrosis of the mandible, *J Oral Maxillofac Surg* 64:961, 2006.

Cordeiro PG, et al: Reconstruction of the mandible with osseous free flaps: a 10 year experience with 150 consecutive patients, *Plast Reconstr Surg* 104:1314, 1999.

Curi MM, Dib LL: Osteoradionecrosis of the jaws: a retrospective study of the background factors and treatment in 104 cases, *J Oral Maxillofac Surg* 55:540, 1997.

Hidalgo DA: A review of 716 consecutive free flaps for oncologic surgical defects: refinement in donor site selection and technique, *Plast Reconstr Surg* 102:722, 1998.

Marx RE: A new concept in the treatment of osteoradionecrosis, *J Oral Maxillofac Surg* 41:351, 1983.

Peleg M, Lopez EA: The treatment of osteoradionecrosis of the mandible: the case of hyperbaric oxygen and bone graft reconstruction, *J Oral Maxillofac Surg* 64:956, 2006.

Puri DR, Chou W, Lee N: Intensity-modulated radiation therapy in head and neck cancers: dosimetric advantages and update of clinical results, *Am J Clin Oncol* 28:415, 2005.

Reuther T, Schuster T, Mende U, Kubler A: Osteoradionecrosis of the jaws as a side effect of radiotherapy of head and neck tumour patients: a report of a thirty year retrospective review, *Int J Oral Maxillofac Surg* 32:289, 2006.

Sciubba PJ, Goldenberg D: Oral complications of radiotherapy, *Lancet Oncol* 7:17, 2006.

Studer G, Studer SP, Zwahlen RA, Huguenin P: Osteoradionecrosis of the mandible: minimized risk profile following intensity-modulated radiation therapy (IMRT), *Strahlenther Onkol* 182:283, 2006.

Sulaiman F, Huryn MJ, Zlotolow MI: Dental extractions in the irradiated head and neck patient: a retrospective analysis of Memorial Sloan-Kettering Cancer Center protocols, criteria, and end results, *J Oral Maxillofac Surg* 61:10, 2003.

Wahl MJ: Osteoradionecrosis prevention myths, *Int J Radiat Oncol Biol Phys* 64:661, 2006.

Martin B. Steed, DDS, and Shahrokh C. Bagheri, DMD, MD

"What the mind does not know the eye cannot see."

The modern management of maxillofacial trauma has evolved with the advent of new biomaterials, improved diagnostic imaging, and refined instrumentation with associated techniques. The approach to maxillofacial trauma is in part related to the surgeon's training and available facilities, but the basis of evaluation of the trauma patient who has sustained maxillofacial injuries remains unchanged. The importance of adherence to Advanced Trauma Life Support (ATLS) protocols and comprehensive physical examination cannot be overemphasized. The use of bone grafts and placement of dental implants allows oral and maxillofacial surgeons to be in a unique position to offer complete rehabilitation beyond the immediate surgical repair of the fractured segments. An understanding of occlusion and related musculoskeletal apparatus is essential for correct management of facial fractures that involve the dentate segments. The goal of maxillofacial trauma surgery is restoration of the preinjury level of function and optimal cosmetic outcome. In addition, practitioner emphasis of prevention and public health measures such as strict seatbelt laws, airbags, protective sporting gear, helmets, and restriction of alcoholic beverages while operating motor vehicles will reduce the incidence of traumatic injuries.

In this chapter we present a series of cases representing the spectrum of maxillofacial injuries as they are encountered in the most classic way. Although most of the cases presented (except for the panfacial trauma case) represent isolated injury patterns, it is important to recognize that injuries can present in any combination.

It is not our intent to provide an exclusive approach to the evaluation and management of these injuries but rather to emphasize common patterns of presentations, treatment options, complications, and discussion of other pertinent factors. In clinical practice, three interdependent factors are related to a successful outcome—the patient, the injury, and the surgeon. These are different every time.

The Facial Injury Severity Scale (FISS) is a tool used to designate the severity of facial injuries (Box 7-1). This is a numerical value of the sum of all facial fractures and fracture patterns. The FISS is a predictor of severity of facial injury as measured by the operating room charges required for treatment and the length of hospital stay.

The Glasgow Coma Scale (GCS) score is a universally used system for evaluation of neurological status (Box 7-2).

Box 7-1.   Facial Injury Severity Scale (FISS)

Mandible

Dentoalveolar	1 point
Each fracture of the body/ramus/symphysis	2 points
Each fracture of condyle/coronoid	1 point

Mid face

Each midfacial fracture is designated 1 point, unless part of a complex fracture pattern

Dentoalveolar	1 point
Le Fort I	2 points
Le Fort II	4 points
Le Fort III	6 points
(Unilateral Le Fort fractures are assigned half the numeric value)	
Naso-orbital-ethmoid	3 points
Zygomaticomaxillary complex	1 point
Nasal	1 point
Orbital floor/rim fracture	1 point

Upper face

Orbital roof/rim	1 point
Displaced frontal sinus/bone fracture	5 points
Nondispalaced frontal sinus/bone fractures	1 point
Facial laceration >10 cm long	1 point

Bagheri SC, Dierks EJ, Kademani D, et al: Application of a Facial Injury Severity Scale in craniomaxillofacial trauma, *J Oral Maxillofac Surg* 64:404-414, 2006.
The FISS is the summation of the above points in an individual patient.

Box 7-2.   Glasgow Coma Scale (GCS)

Eye Opening (E)

4 = Spontaneous
3 = To voice
2 = To pain
1 = None

Verbal Response (V)

5 = Normal conversation
4 = Disoriented conversation
3 = Words, but not coherent
2 = No words . . . only sounds
1 = None

Motor Response (M)

6 = Normal (follows command)
5 = Localizes to pain
4 = Withdraws to pain
3 = Decorticate posture
2 = Decerebrate
1 = None

Total = E + V + M

Subcondyle Mandibular Fracture

Timothy M. Osborn, DDS, and Brett A. Ueeck, DMD, MD

CC

You are asked to evaluate a 21-year-old man who reportedly fell and hit his chin. He presents to the local emergency department explaining that, "I fell and cut my chin."

Direct trauma to the chin is the most common etiology of condyle fractures associated with isolated blunt trauma. The impact at the symphysis area is transmitted to the condylar head against the glenoid fossa and subsequently causes a fracture at the weaker subcondylar area.

HPI

During routine daily exercise, the patient reports jumping over a fence, when he tripped and landed on his chin and right hand earlier this morning. He was seen at a local emergency department for the deep cut on his chin. He also complains of inability to open wide and pain in front of his right ear. He denies losing consciousness (would be indicative of intracranial injury) or neck pain (the association between mandible fractures and cervical spine injuries, although infrequent, is well established, and any neck pain warrants further evaluation). In addition, he describes a sore right wrist.

Although subcondylar fractures associated with blunt trauma can occur in isolation, more than half of fractures are associated with a contralateral parasymphysis or angle fracture. Characteristically, the mandible fractures at the point on impact (symphysis or angle) and at the subcondylar area.

PMHX/PDHX/MEDICATIONS/ALLERGIES/SH/FH

Noncontributory.

EXAMINATION

General. The patient is a well-developed and well-nourished man in no apparent distress.

Maxillofacial. There is a 3-cm hemostatic laceration at the submental region (point of impact). Upon opening the mandible deviates to the right (due to the unopposed contralateral lateral pterygoid muscle). The maximal interincisal opening is limited to 20 mm, with associated pain. Palpation of the right preauricular region also elicits pain (pain at the preauricular area with a history of trauma to the symphysis is highly suggestive of a subcondylar fracture).

Intraoral. Left lateral excursive movement is limited to 2 mm (excursive movement of the mandible to the left requires the function of the right lateral pterygoid against an intact condylar neck). There are no associated intraoral lacerations or dental trauma (fractures of the teeth are not uncommon with forceful closure of the mandible at the time of trauma). Occlusal examination shows premature contacts on the right side, with a posterior left open bite (secondary to collapse of the vertical height of the mandible on the right).

Extremities. There is pain to passive range of motion (ROM) of the right wrist.

IMAGING

Depending on the facility, initial imaging for evaluation of the mandible may include a computed tomography (CT) scan, panoramic radiograph, or plain-view mandibular series that includes lateral and posteroanterior cephalometric films, a reverse Towne's view, and oblique views of the mandible. Many rural hospitals still use a plain-view series of the mandible. Most hospitals use a CT scan, which has become the gold standard imaging modality. A CT scan allows the entire face to be evaluated in one study. The mandible can also be evaluated in several different anatomical planes. The axial and coronal planes are the two most commonly used views. The coronal plane can be very helpful for condylar process fractures, while the axial planes are useful for the body. Direct coronal imaging requires hyperextension of the neck and should not be obtained in patients with a suspicion of cervical spine injury. Three-dimensional reconstructions are extremely valuable and allow preoperative planning in a more sophisticated manner for complex cases such as gunshot wounds or severely comminuted fractures. A panoramic film is the single best plain film for evaluating the entire mandible at once. In combination with a reverse Townes view, the sensitivity for detecting a condylar process fracture increases. However, all modalities have limitations and surgeons should use imaging studies based on individual cases and available resources.

For this patient, a CT scan was obtained as the initial study, demonstrating a right subcondylar fracture on coronal and axial views (Figure 7-1). A plain wrist film was also obtained, which revealed a right-sided fracture of the distal radius (Colles fracture).

LABS

No routine laboratory testing is indicated unless dictated by the medical history.

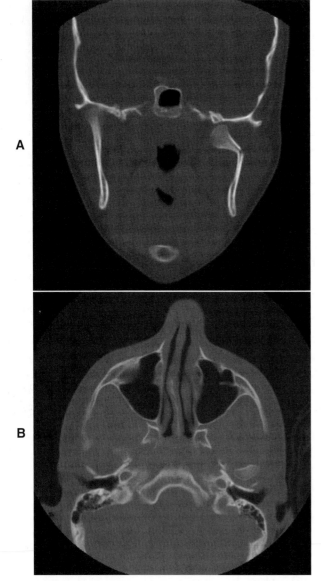

Figure 7-1 **A,** Coronal view of the ramus and condyle showing an anteromedial displaced subcondylar fracture on the right side. **B,** Axial view at the level of the glenoid fossae. Notice the absence of the condyle from the fossa on the right.

ASSESSMENT

Right subcondylar fracture of the mandible, and associated chin laceration; Colles fracture of the right wrist; FISS score of 1

TREATMENT

The treatment of fractures of the mandibular condyle is one of the most widely debated topics in the maxillofacial literature. Several variables should be considered when determining treatment and predicting the prognosis, including the level of fracture, degree and direction of displacement, age of patient, medical status, concomitant injuries, and status of the dentition. Assael has developed a comprehensive list of considerations affecting treatment selection and outcome, all of

which should be considered in evaluation of patients prior to institution of therapy. While the comprehensive discussion of these considerations is beyond the scope of this chapter, the variables can be divided into patient, surgeon, and third party categories. The age, gender, medical status, compliance, associated injuries, and fracture type are a few of the patient-specific variables. The surgeon's ability and resources, as well as resources to cover the expense of treatment, are also pertinent to successful treatment.

The primary goal in the treatment of any fracture is adequate stabilization allowing for fracture healing and primary osseous union. In treatment of mandibular condyle fractures, the goals of treatment are:

- Pain-free mouth opening with return to an acceptable interincisal opening
- Pain-free functional movement
- Restoration of occlusion
- Facial and jaw symmetry, and establishment of facial height
- Minimal visible scarring

Preinjury alignment of the mandibular condyle within the glenoid fossa is not essential for adequate rehabilitation after mandibular condyle fractures. The pull of the lateral pterygoid muscle characteristically displaces the condyle anteriorly and medially, and therefore closed reduction (more correctly termed "closed treatment") typically does not reduce the condyle into its original position.

The treatment options are categorized into surgical and nonsurgical modalities. The surgical treatment includes open reduction with or without internal fixation; however, most advocate that if an open approach is taken, fixation should be applied. Endoscopic reduction and fixation of condyle fractures has gained popularity during the past decade. The use of this technique requires the familiarity with the endoscope and the ability to convert the procedure to an open method if endoscopic reduction fails to successfully complete the procedure. The options of nonsurgical treatment include closed reduction (closed treatment) with maxillomandibular fixation (CR-MMF) or diet modification with ROM exercises. In the treatment of facial fractures, patients older than 10 years are treated in a similar manner as adults; however, it is rarely advocated that children and teenagers undergo open reduction of condyle fractures; soft diet with mobilization is the treatment of choice in patients 15 years old or younger. If the occlusion is unstable and not reproducible, a short period of intermaxillary fixation (2 weeks) can be advocated.

For this patient, the occlusion was reestablished easily with minimal manipulation, and after extensive discussion of procedures, alternatives, risks, and benefits, the patient was placed in MMF for 4 weeks, without any complications.

COMPLICATIONS

The complications of treating fractures of the mandibular condyle are well described in the literature and are often used as the basis of comparison for surgical versus nonsurgical treatment. One of the most severe late complications can be temporomandibular joint (TMJ) ankylosis (fusion between the mandibular condyle and the glenoid fossa). Patients with TMJ ankylosis often have a history of facial trauma. Prevention of ankylosis was discussed by Zide and Kent in 1983. They advocated appropriate physiotherapy early in the phase of nonsurgical treatment. Other types of late mandibular dysfunction have been cited as complications of closed reduction, including chronic pain, malocclusion, internal derangement, asymmetry, limited mobility, and gross radiographic abnormalities (however, radiographic abnormalities in the absence of pain or functional impairment have no clinical significance). Long-term complications of open reduction and internal fixation (ORIF) are scar perception, facial nerve palsy/ paralysis, loss or failure of fixation, Frey syndrome, avascular necrosis, TMJ dysfunction, and facial asymmetry. The early complications are few and can include early failure of fixation, malocclusion, pain, and infection.

DISCUSSION

As is common with most traumatic injuries, fractures of the mandibular condyle occur in men (78%) between the ages of 20 and 39 (60%). The majority of the fractures are unilateral

(84%); fewer are bilateral (16%); 14% of fractures are intracapsular, 24% are in the condylar neck, and 62% are subcondylar fractures. For children 10 years or younger, 41% of fractures are intracapsular, which dramatically influences the profile of treatment and potential complications in children. Another important difference between children and adults is anatomical. Adults have a relatively narrow condylar neck and thick articular surface, while the pediatric patient has a relatively broad condylar neck and thin articular surface in an active osteogenic phase.

Many studies have compared various outcomes of surgical versus nonsurgical therapy, with most of the debate being centered on ORIF and CR-MMF (closed treatment). The outcomes studied included perception of pain, occlusal function, asymmetry, maximal interincisal opening/ROM, muscle activity, malocclusion, midline deviation, radiographic changes, and nerve dysfunction. Brandt and Haug in 2003 conducted a review of the literature (Table 7-1) regarding open versus closed treatment and suggested indications for closed and open reduction. If a patient has an acceptable ROM, good occlusion, and minimal pain, observation or CR-MMF is preferred regardless of the level of the fracture. They

Table 7-1.	**Review of the Literature for Open Versus Closed Treatment of Mandibular Subcondylar Fractures**		
Author	**Total No. of Patients**	**Follow-up**	**Results**
Hidding et al	20 ORIF/54 CR-MMF	5 yr	Deviation 64% CR-MMF versus 10% ORIF
			Anatomical reconstruction 93% ORIF versus 7% CR-MMF
			No differences in headaches mastication or MIIO
Konstantinovic and Dimitrijevic	26 ORIF/54 CR-MMF	2.5 yr	100% of ORIF were 81% to 100% of ideal
			77.7% of CR-MMF were 81% to 100% of ideal
			No difference in deviation or MIIO
Oezman et al	20 ORIF/10 CR-MMF	2 yr	MRI revealed 30% disc displacement in CR-MMF and 10% in ORIF
			MRI revealed 80% of CR-MMF with maligned or deformed condyles
Worsae and Thorn	61 CR-MMF/40 ORIF	2 yr	39% Complication rate in CR-MMF—asymmetry, malocclusion, reduced MIIO, headaches, pain 4%
			Complication rate in ORIF—malocclusion, impaired mastication, pain
Haug and Assael	10 CR-MMF/10 ORIF	6 yr	No statistically significant differences found for ROM, occlusion, contour, or motor or sensory function
			ORIF associated with perceptible scars
			CR-MMF associated with chronic pain
Throckmorton et al	14 CR-MMF/62 ORIF	3 yr	No perceivable differences noted between CR-MMF versus ORIF for mandibular motion or muscle activity
Palmieri et al	74 CR-MMF/62 ORIF	3 yr	ORIF patients had greater mobility
Ellis et al	65 CR-MMF	6 wk	Position of condylar process is not static
Ellis et al	61 ORIF	6 mo	Anatomical reduction possible, but changes in the condylar process position may result from a loss of fixation
Ellis et al	77 ORIF/65 CR-MMF	3 yr	CR-MMF had significantly greater percentage age of malocclusion
Ellis and Throckmorton	81 CR-MMF/65 ORIF	3 yr	CR-MMF had shorter posterior facial and ramus heights on the side of injury
Ellis et al	93 ORIF/85 CR-MMF	3 yr	ORIF—17.2% facial nerve weakness at 6 weeks with 0% at 6 mo and 7.5% scarring judged as hypertrophic
Ellis and Throckmorton	91 CR-MMF/64 ORIF	3 yr	No difference noted between ORIF versus CR-MMF for maximum bite forces

Modified from Brandt M, Haug RH: Open vs closed reduction of adult mandibular condyle fractures: a review of the literature regarding the evolution of current thoughts on management, *J Oral Maxillofac Surg* 61:1324-1332, 2003.

also suggest that condylar displacement and ramus height instability are the only orthopedic indications for ORIF of condylar fractures. Based on their review, they concluded that under similar indications and conditions, ORIF is the preferred approach.

Haug and Assael described the indications and contraindications for open treatment of condylar fractures in 2001. Their absolute indications for ORIF are patient preference (when no absolute or relative contraindications coexist), when manipulation and closed reduction cannot reestablish pretraumatic occlusion and/or excursions, when rigid internal fixation is being used to address other fractures affecting the occlusion, the rare instance of intracranial impaction of the proximal condylar segment, and when stability of the occlusion is limited. Among the absolute contraindications are condylar head fractures (including single fragment, comminuted, and medial pole) and when medical illness or systemic injury adds undo risk to an extended general anesthesia. Condylar neck fractures were among the relative contraindications.

When the decision is made to use nonsurgical techniques, there is no consensus on the use of immobilization and for the duration of immobilization. One can find literature supporting anywhere from 0 to 6 weeks of closed treatment. A period of MMF is typically instituted for one of three reasons:

1. Patient comfort
2. To promote osseous union
3. To help reduce the fractured segment

A method for treating fractures with no occlusal disturbances, acceptable ROM, and minimal pain is to place the patient in early full function along with functional physiotherapy. If the patient demonstrates occlusal discrepancy, Erich arch bars can be placed for MMF or guiding elastics. For pediatric patients in a mixed dentition stage who demonstrate an occlusal discrepancy, there may be a need for circum-mandibular wires and/or circum-zygomatic or piriform wires to obtain adequate stabilization.

Regardless of the type of treatment, patients should undergo postoperative physical therapy. Functional therapy is needed to improve ROM, asymmetrical movements, scarring within the joint, or other TMJ dysfunctions. If there is limitation in mouth opening, tongue blades or other sequentially enlarging devices to gradually improve range of mandibular opening can be used. For patients with asymmetrical mouth opening, it is recommended that they function on the contralateral side. Patients can be encouraged to observe their opening and closing in the mirror and to use their hand to help correct any asymmetrical movement. The overall goal is to achieve early full function.

When the decision is made to use ORIF, many advocate a retromandibular approach. This approach affords excellent exposure to the ramus-condyle unit for reduction and fixation. The approach was first described by Hinds and Girotti in 1967 and later adapted for use in the treatment of mandibular condyle fractures. An incision of 3 cm is made parallel to the posterior border of the mandible starting 1 cm below the ear lobe. Dissection proceeds through skin, subcutaneous tissue, and platysma down to the parotid capsule. The tail of the parotid is released and elevated with blunt dissection if necessary to avoid violation of the parotid capsule. The posterior mandible and pterygomasseteric sling are identified. The periosteum at the posterior border of the mandible is incised and dissected in a subperiosteal plane. Both sides of the fracture are exposed to facilitate reduction and fixation. One can also use a similar approach when utilizing endoscopy. This approach allows excellent exposure to the ramus condyle unit, minimal visible scarring, and low incidence of facial nerve damage. Other surgical approaches to the mandibular condyle include a preauricular (or endaural) incision, intraoral incision, or Risdon-type incision, depending on the fracture pattern and location.

Multiple modalities have been used to rigidly fix mandibular condyle fractures. Studies have evaluated the biomechanical behavior of dynamic compression plates, locking plates, mini–dynamic compression plates, adaptation plates, and single and double miniplates. Both mini–dynamic compression plates and double miniplates have been shown to be stable for fixation. It has also been shown that resorbable plates are effective and provide reliable stability in ORIF of condylar fractures. Many surgeons recommend that fixation be applied with the use of one or two 2.0-mm plates with two or three bicortical screws on both sides of the fracture. Lag screw fixation can be used in appropriate situations.

Treatment of fractures of the mandibular condyle requires consideration of many factors. Many techniques are available to surgeons and patients. One must always use the simplest approach with the lowest risk of morbidity to accomplish the goals of treatment.

Bibliography

Assael LA: Open versus closed reduction of adult mandibular condyle fractures: an alternative interpretation of the evidence, *J Oral Maxillofac Surg* 61:1333-1339, 2003.

Beekler DM, Walker RV: Condylar fractures, *J Oral Surg* 27:563, 1969.

Behnia H, Motamedi MHK, Tehranchi A: Use of activator appliances in pediatric patients treated with costochondral grafts for temporomandibular joint ankylosis: an analysis of 13 cases, *J Oral Maxillofac Surg* 55:1408, 1997.

Brandt MT, Haug RH: Open versus closed reduction of adult mandibular condyle fractures: a review of the literature regarding the evolution of current thoughts on management, *J Oral Maxillofac Surg* 61:1324-1332, 2003.

Choi BH, Yi CK, Yoo JH, et al: Clinical evaluation of 3 types of plate osteosynthesis for fixation of condylar neck fractures, *J Oral Maxillofac Surg* 59:734-737, 2001.

Chossegros C, Cheynet F, Blanc JL, Bourezak Z: Short retromandibular approach of subcondylar fractures: clinical and radiologic long-term evaluation, *Oral Surg Oral Med Oral Pathol Oral Radiol Endod* 82:248-252, 1996.

Ellis E, McFadden D, Simon P, et al: Surgical complications with open treatment of mandibular condylar process fractures, *J Oral Maxillofac Surg* 58:950, 2000.

Ellis EE, Dean J: Rigid fixation of mandibular condyle fractures, *Oral Surg Oral Med Oral Pathol Oral Radiol Endod* 76:6-15, 1993.

Ellis EE, Throckmorton GS: Treatment of mandibular condylar process fractures: biologic considerations, *J Oral Maxillofac Surg* 63:115-134, 2005.

El-Sheikh MM, Medra AM, Warda MH: Bird face deformity secondary to bilateral temporomandibular joint ankylosis, *J Craniomaxillofac Surg* 24:96, 1996.

Eppley BL: Use of resorbable plates and screws in pediatric facial fractures, *J Oral Maxillofac Surg* 63(3):385-391, 2005.

Haug RH, Assael LA: Outcomes of open versus closed treatment of mandibular subcondylar fractures, *J Oral Maxillofac Surg* 59:370-375, 2001.

Haug RH, Gilman PP, Goltz M: A biomechanical evaluation of mandibular condyle fracture plating techniques, *J Oral Maxillofac Surg* 60:73-80, 2002.

Hinds EC, Girotti WJ: Vertical subcondylar osteotomy: a reappraisal, *Oral Surg Oral Med Oral Pathol Oral Radiol Endod* 80:394-397, 1967.

Ikemura K: Treatment of condylar fractures associated with other mandibular fractures, *J Oral Maxillofac Surg* 43:810, 1985.

Ivy RH, Curtis L: *Fractures of the jaws,* Philadelphia, 1931, Lea and Febiger, p 78.

Manisali M, Amin M, Aghabeigi B, Newman L: Retromandibular approach to the mandibular condyle: a clinical and cadaveric study, *Int J Oral Maxillofac Surg* 32:253-256, 2003.

Posnick JF, Wells M, Pron GE: Pediatric facial fractures: evolving patterns of treatment, *J Oral Maxillofac Surg* 51:836, 1993.

Schüle H: Injuries of the temporomandibular joint. In: Krüger E, Schilli W, editors: *Oral and maxillofacial traumatology,* Vol 2, Chicago, 1986, Quintessence, pp 45-70.

Suzuki T, Kawamura H, Kasahara T, Nagasaka H: Resorbable poly-L-lactide plates and screws for the treatment of mandibular condyle process fractures: a clinical and radiologic follow-up study, *J Oral Maxillofac Surg* 62:919-924, 2004.

Thoren H, Hallikainen D, Iizuka T, Lindquist C: Condylar process fractures in children: a follow-up study of fractures with total dislocation of the condyle from the glenoid fossa, *J Oral Maxillofac Surg* 59:768-773, 2001.

Villareal PM, Monje F, Junquera LM, et al: Mandibular condyle fractures: determinants of outcome, *J Oral Maxillofac Surg* 62:155-163, 2004.

Zide MF. Kent JN: Indications for open reduction of mandibular condyle fractures, *J Oral Maxillofac Surg* 41(2):89-98, 1983.

Combined Mandibular Parasymphysis and Angle Fractures

Michael S. Wilkinson, DMD, Shahrokh C. Bagheri, DMD, MD, and Brett A. Ueeck, DMD, MD

CC

You are asked by the trauma physician at your local emergency department to evaluate a 23-year-old male patient for facial fractures (mandible fractures are more common in males in the third decade of life). His chief complaint is that, "My jaw hurts, and my teeth do not come together like before."

HPI

The patient was riding his motor cross bike earlier today when he crashed and landed on his face. He was not wearing a helmet, but he denies any loss of consciousness. He was able to get up from the scene and ride his bike to the emergency department. He explains that his lower face and jaw are painful, his teeth do not occlude correctly, and his left lower lip is anesthetic.

Assault, motor vehicle accidents, and sporting injuries are the most common etiologies of mandible fractures. Malocclusion is the single most important historic information suggestive of a mandible or dentoalveolar fracture. Paresthesia of the distribution of the third division of the trigeminal nerve (V_3) is common and can be due to neuropraxia, axontemesis, or neurotemesis of the mental or inferior alveolar nerve at the fracture site.

PMHX/PDHX/MEDICATIONS/ALLERGIES/SH/FH

He smokes one pack of cigarettes a day and drinks alcohol on the weekends. He denies all other habits (both alcohol and tobacco use have been associated with an increased risk of infectious complications with mandible fractures).

EXAMINATION

Primary Survey

Airway and cervical spine control. Speaking without difficulty (in cases of multiple fragmented mandible fractures, the upper airway can become acutely compromised due to posterior collapse of the tongue with loss of a stable genioglossus insertion at the genial tubercle). The cervical spine examination is within normal limits (Haug and associates report an association between cervical spine injuries and mandible fractures. The stability of the cervical spine is crucial throughout the care of the patient).

Breathing and oxygenation. The patient's breathing is unlabored, with an oxygen saturation of 97% on room air.

Circulation. There is no active bleeding.

General. He is semisupine on an emergency department bed with oxygen.

Vital signs. His blood pressure is 116/78 mm Hg, heart rate 70 bpm, respirations 12 per minute, and temperature 37°C.

Secondary Survey

Neurological. The patient is alert and oriented times 3, and his GCS score is 15.

Maxillofacial. The facial structures are grossly symmetrical. Examination of the eyes (pupils, visual acuity, visual fields, and extraocular movements) are within normal limits. External ears are without deformity. The tympanic membranes are clear (external auditory canal lacerations, tympanic plate rupture, and fracture of the posterior wall of the joint should be ruled out). The remainder of the facial bones are stable except the mandible, which demonstrates mobility in the parasymphysis region on the right and in the left angle regions. Facial edema is present bilaterally with tenderness to palpation at the fracture sites. This motion causes pain. Cranial nerves II through XII are intact with the exception of anesthesia of V_3 on the left side. His neck is nontender and demonstrates full range of active motion with no neck pain (important to rule out cervical spine injury).

Intraoral. His dentition is in moderate repair and he has obvious steps in his occlusal plane between the right mandibular central incisor and the right mandibular lateral incisor and distal to the left mandibular second molar. There are multiple lacerations involving the gingiva in the associated areas. He has an obvious malocclusion, and there is hematoma formation in the anterior floor of the mouth.

IMAGING

Most practitioners consider CT scanning to be the gold standard imaging modality for evaluation of mandible fractures. A CT scan allows the entire face to be evaluated in one study. Facial bones including the mandible can be evaluated in several different anatomical planes. The axial and coronal planes are the two most commonly used views. The coronal plane can be very helpful for condylar process fractures, whereas the axial views are useful for the corpus. Patients with suspicion of cervical spine injury should not have the neck hyperextended for direct coronal imaging; instead, digitally reconstructed coronal images can be used.

Despite the popularity of CT imaging, in many facilities the initial imaging studies may consist of a panoramic radiograph or a plain-view series of the mandible (posteroanterior, reverse Towne's, and bilateral lateral oblique radiographs). Many rural hospitals still use a plain-view series of the mandible. Therefore familiarity with plain radiographs is important.

A panoramic radiograph is the imaging modality of choice for patients presenting at the surgeon's office. This radiograph is inexpensive and is the single best plain film for evaluation of the entire mandible. Nondisplaced or minimally displaced fractures of the condyle or the symphyseal area may be difficult to detect on a panoramic radiograph. When combining a reverse Townes view and/or an anteroposterior radiograph of the mandible, there are similar sensitivity and specificity as a CT scan. The decision to order different imaging modalities should be based on available resources, physical examination findings, and the cost and knowledge of limitations related to particular studies.

For this patient, a panoramic radiograph demonstrates fractures at the left angle and right parasymphysis area (Figure

7-2, *A*). A posteroanterior view of the mandible shows severe displacement at the left angle (explaining the anesthesia of the left V₃) and fracture at the right parasymphysis (Figure 7-2, *B*). Notice that the degree of lateral displacement is not evident on the panoramic radiograph.

LABS

Routine laboratory testing is not mandatory before surgical correction of mandible fractures unless dictated by underlying medical conditions. In cases of infected mandible fractures, a white blood cell (WBC) count may be obtained.

ASSESSMENT

Open mandibular fractures at the right parasymphysis (nondisplaced), and left angle (severely displaced); FISS of 4; also an associated injury to his left inferior alveolar nerve

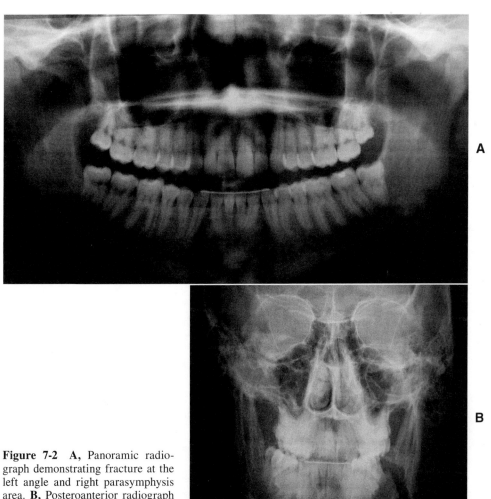

Figure 7-2 A, Panoramic radiograph demonstrating fracture at the left angle and right parasymphysis area. **B,** Posteroanterior radiograph of the skull showing severe lateral displacement of the mandible angle on the left. The fracture at the right parasymphysis is also evident.

most consistent with neurotmesis or Sunderland's class 5 injury

TREATMENT

The treatment of mandible fractures has a long and complicated history dating back to 1600 BC. The mandible is unique in that it is singled out as the bone in the face requiring special attention to various aspects of treatment (occlusion, aesthetics, function), to achieve a good result. The important points in treating mandible fractures are immobilization of the fractures, the appropriate use of antibiotics, and restoration of form and function.

Mandible fractures at the angle and parasymphysis involving the teeth-bearing segments are considered open fractures. Treatment should be rendered in a timely fashion, as soon as the patient is stable and operating room facilities are available. Preoperative antibiotics have been shown to decrease the incidence of postoperative infectious complications and should be initiated regardless of the time interval before definitive surgery can be completed. The use of postoperative antibiotics remains largely practitioner dependent, and no good evidence exists guiding its necessity and potential benefits for the duration of treatment.

More important in the prevention of infection is the proper application of fixation. Movement at the fracture site increases not only the chance of infection but also the development of fibrous union, malunion, or nonunion. Rigid fixation is the key to good outcome. However, the use of semirigid fixation techniques, when correctly applied, can also provide a successful outcome. Lag screws are also a strong form of fixation and provide the very good rigidity, but the technique is not applicable to all fractures. Locking versus nonlocking fixation plates provides continued rigidity, if the contact area at the screw/plate–bone interface is reduced due to bony remodeling. In addition, locking plates do not require precise adaptation to the bony anatomy, because the screw is "locked" into special threads within the plate. Closed reduction of mandible fractures continues to be an acceptable form of treatment and, in certain patients, provide the best option. Closed reduction does not offer the benefit of early function, and the patient must tolerate a prolonged period of intermaxillary fixation.

When treating cases where the mandible has more than one fracture, consideration should be given to the sequence of fixation. It is generally advocated to fixate the fracture segments involving dentate segments to ensure correct occlusal relationship before fixation of nondentate segments. In this case, the parasymphysis fracture was repaired first, to correctly establish arch form and occlusion.

This patient was treated with ORIF under general anesthesia in an ambulatory care facility (Figure 7-3). Arch bars were applied, and subsequently the occlusion and arch form were reestablished. Fixation at the parasymphysis fracture was completed by placing a plate at the superior border (zone of tension) and a plate at the inferior border (zone of compression). The fracture at the angle was reduced and fixated using rigid fixation plates at the superior and inferior border. No postoperative MMF was used. He was allowed to function and maintain a soft-chew diet. The use of antibiotics consisted of perioperative intravenous penicillin. The patient was sent home with a prescription for Peridex (chlorhexidine) and oral analgesics. The postoperative course was otherwise uncomplicated.

Similarly, the fracture could be treated using a single lag screw placed according to the Niederdellman method, as shown in Figure 7-4.

COMPLICATIONS

Mandibular angle fractures are generally more prone to the development of complications compared with the body, symphyseal, or parasymphyseal areas. Multiple complications may arise but most commonly include loose hardware necessitating removal, infection, malocclusion, delayed union, and fibrous union. Damage to the inferior alveolar and lingual nerves can be a complication of the initial injury or a

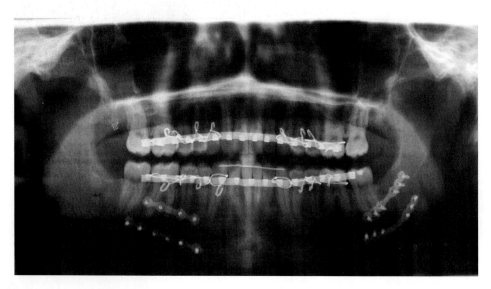

Figure 7-3 Postoperative panoramic radiograph demonstrating rigid fixation of the fracture segments.

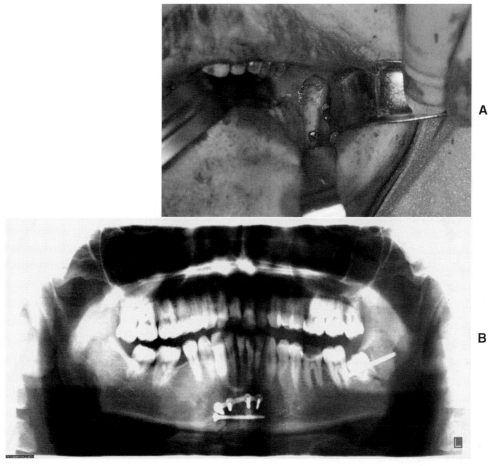

Figure 7-4   A, Intraoperative view of a different patient with an angle fracture treated with a single lag screw. **B,** Postoperative panoramic radiograph of the patient in A showing fixation at the angle using a lag screw, and also at the parasymphysis using a lag screw and a superior border plate.

consequence of treatment. Infection rates for angle fractures reportedly range from 2% to over 19%.

DISCUSSION

There are a variety of treatment options for the treatment of mandible fractures that primarily differ in the method of fixation (number, size, and location of fixation plates and screws). Traditionally, mandible fractures have been successfully treated with closed reduction using intermaxillary fixation. This method results in relatively few complications. However, this modality is associated with a delay to functional rehabilitation relative to the more modern techniques of ORIF.

ORIF failed to attain widespread use before the 1960s mainly due to early reports of metal corrosion of steel plates and screws, metal fatigue, and screw loosening. The advent of biocompatible materials such as vitallium and titanium, along with orthopedic biomechanical studies ascribing the benefits of compression osteosynthesis, increased interest in open treatment of mandible fractures. Many practitioners prefer open versus closed reduction of parasymphysis/angle fractures of the mandible. The treatment of subcondylar fractures has caused a series of controversies that are addressed

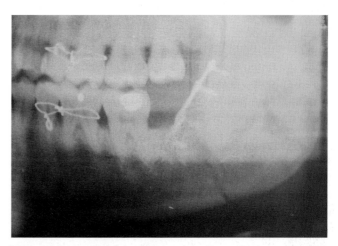

Figure 7-5   Postoperative panoramic radiograph of a patient with a left angle mandible fracture. The left angle is treated by the Champy technique with semirigid fixation using a four-hole plate.

in a separate section (see the section on subcondyle mandible fracture earlier in this chapter).

Considerable variation arises when comparing methods of fixation. For example, dynamic compression plating (Schmoker and Spiessl), monocortical noncompression miniplate (Michelet), superior border mandibular angle plate (Champy) (Figure 7-5), lag screw (Niederdellmann and associates), and rigid locking reconstruction plate techniques have all been described. Consensus for optimal treatment of mandibular parasymphysis/angle fractures remains elusive, with each method exhibiting pros and cons and a paucity of prospective randomized trials for direct comparison.

Angle fractures produce the highest frequency of complications among mandibular fractures. Infection, malunion, nonunion, and damage to adjacent structures (nerve, tooth) all plague reduction of this anatomical site. Thus many practitioners espouse the concept of absolute rigidity of the bony segments for rapid, uncomplicated healing. Early on, AO/ASIF (Arbeits-gemeinschaft für Osteosynthesefragen/Association for the Study of Internal Fixation) established principles recommended superior and inferior border dynamic compression plates. On the other end of the spectrum, Champy recommended a single noncompression miniplate at the superior border for angle fractures based on his studies demonstrating the tendency of the superior border to separate from unfavorable muscle pull (tension zone) and the inferior mandibular border to compress (compression zone) with an interposed neutral zone or "line of zero force." Contrary to the principles of interfragment rigidity for optimal healing, some studies describe decreased complications with less rigid techniques, such as the Champy technique.

Niederdellmann in the 1970s described the use of lag screws for treatment of mandibular angle fractures with placement of the screw through the impacted third molar, if present, and subsequent removal of the tooth and screw after healing. Due to technique sensitivity and difficulty, the Niederdellmann lag screw technique remains less popular.

Several studies attribute an associated increased risk of angle fractures with the presence of impacted third molars. Management of teeth in the line of fracture has previously sparked some controversy. Extraction is undoubtedly indicated in cases where the tooth in the line of fracture is deeply carious, harbors periodontal or pericoronal infection, prevents bony reduction of the fracture, demonstrates severe root exposure, or is fractured. However, in the absence of the above conditions, extraction of the tooth has shown a statistically significant benefit. Ellis in 2002 reported a relatively increased, but statistically not significant, risk of postoperative complications (namely, infection) with teeth left present in the line of fracture, resulting in need for infection management and/or removal of hardware. Other studies recommend that tooth buds in the line of fracture should be preserved unless infection occurs, requiring subsequent removal.

Overall, mandibular angle fractures are common and relatively easily treated with a variety of conventional techniques. The surgeon should keep in mind the potential complications and adhere strictly to the sound principles regardless of the technique selected.

Bibliography

Alpert B: Complications in the treatment of facial trauma, *Oral Maxillofac Clin North Am* 11(2):255, 1999.

Ellis E: Lag screw fixation of mandibular fractures, *J Craniomaxillofac Trauma* 3:16, 1997.

Ellis E: Outcomes of patients with teeth in the line of mandibular angle fractures treated with stable internal fixation, *J Oral Maxillofac Surg* 60:863, 2002.

Ellis E: Treatment methods for fractures of the mandibular angle, *J Craniomaxillofac Trauma* 2:28, 1996.

Ellis E, Walker L: Treatment of mandibular angle fractures using two noncompression miniplates, *J Oral Maxillofac Surg* 52:1032, 1994.

Gear A, et al: Treatment modalities for mandibular angle fractures, *J Oral Maxillofac Surg* 63:655, 2005.

Halmos D, Ellis E, Dodson TB: Mandibular third molars and angle fractures, *J Oral Maxillofac Surg* 62:1076, 2004.

Haug RH, et al: Cervical spine fractures and maxillofacial trauma, *J Oral Maxillofac Surg* 49:725, 1991.

Lamphier J, et al: Complications of mandibular fractures in an urban teaching center, *J Oral Maxillofac Surg* 61:745, 2003.

Leonard MS: History of the treatment of maxillofacial trauma, *Oral Maxillofac Clin North Am* 2(1):1, 1990.

Murthy A, Lehman J: Symptomatic plate removal in maxillofacial trauma: a review of 76 cases, *Ann Plast Surg* 55:603, 2005.

Niederdellmann H, Akuamoa-Boateng E, Uhlig G: Lag-screw osteosynthesis: a new procedure for treating fractures of the mandibular angle, *J Oral Surg* 39:938, 1981.

Potter J, Ellis E: Treatment of mandibular angle fractures with a malleable noncompression miniplate, *J Oral Maxillofac Surg* 57:288, 1999.

Prein J, editor: *Manual of internal fixation in the cranio-facial skeleton,* Berlin/Heidelberg, 1998, Springer.

Tate GS, Ellis E, Throckmorton G: Bite forces in patients treated for mandibular angle fractures: implications for fixation recommendations, *J Oral Maxillofac Surg* 52:734, 1994.

Zygomaticomaxillary Complex Fracture

Shahrokh C. Bagheri, DMD, MD, and Chris Jo, DMD

CC

A 28-year-old (peak incidence second or third decades) man (male:female ratio is 4:1) is admitted to the local emergency department 4 hours after he was hit on his left side of his face with a fist (left zygoma most commonly affected). He complains of left-sided facial pain, blurry vision, and inability to open his mouth fully (trismus present in about one-third of patients).

HPI

The patient claims that he was minding his own business when he was suddenly "jumped" and beaten in the face with a fist by an unknown individual. He does not report losing consciousness. He was subsequently brought to the emergency department by the emergency medical services (EMS) personnel.

PMHX/PDHX/MEDICATIONS/ALLERGIES/SH/FH

He has a positive history of alcohol abuse (more common in the trauma population) and an 8 pack-year history of tobacco use.

EXAMINATION

The patient's ATLS primary survey is negative, and his GCS score is 15.

General. He is alert and oriented times 3. The patient is a well-developed and well-nourished man in mild distress.

Vital signs. His blood pressure is 130/84 mm Hg, heart rate 120 bpm (tachycardia), respirations 16 per minute, and temperature 37.6°C.

Maxillofacial. There is tenderness over the left zygoma and subconjunctival ecchymoses and edema around the left eye (present in 50% to 70% of cases). There is a palpable step along the zygomaticofrontal (ZF) suture and infraorbital rim, with flattening over the zygomatic arch, as well as visible depression over the malar eminence and hypoesthesia of the left maxillary branch (V_2) of the trigeminal nerve (50% to 90% of cases).

Eyes. The pupils are equal, round, and reactive to light and accommodation (PERRLA) (cranial nerves II and III), with no ptosis (cranial nerve III). There is no proptosis (tense proptosis may be indicative of a retrobulbar hematoma, a surgical emergency). Careful examination of the pupils reveals a downward displacement of the left pupil suggestive of loss of osseous support along the orbital floor and/or increase in orbital volume. The lateral palpebral fissure appears grossly displaced inferolaterally (producing an anti-mongoloid slant). Examination of the extraocular muscles demonstrates a decrease in range of motion in the extremes of upward and downward gaze (mostly due to edema). Visual fields are intact by confrontation (cranial nerve II). Examination of left eye confirms binocular diplopia (10% to 40% of cases). Visual acuity is 20/25 bilaterally (cranial nerve II), there is no hyphema (blood in the anterior chamber of the eye), and the fundoscopic examination is within normal limits.

Intraoral. There is ecchymosis of the maxillary buccal sulcus on the left.

IMAGING

The CT scan (bony windows) is the gold standard for evaluation of zygomatic fractures, using axial and coronal sections. Reconstructed parasagittal views through the orbit can be valuable to assess the orbital floor in the antero-posterior dimension. Direct coronal imaging may not be feasible given the status of the cervical spine in the acute setting.

In this case, axial sections (Figure 7-6, *A*) reveal a significantly displaced left zygoma with fractures at the anterior maxillary wall and zygomaticotemporal (ZT) and zygomaticosphenoid (ZS) sutures. Coronal CT (Figure 7-6, *B*) reveals fractures at the right ZF suture and zygomaticomaxillary (ZM) buttress and disruption of the left orbital floor with displacement of orbital contents into the maxillary sinus. A three-dimensional computer reconstruction, although not necessary, can also be helpful in treatment planning (Figure 7-6, *C*).

LABS

No routine laboratory testing is necessary for the management of isolated zygomaticomaxillary complex (ZMC) fractures, unless dictated by the medical history. A blood alcohol level and urine drug screen should be obtained in cases of suspected alcohol or drug intoxication.

This patient had a blood alcohol level of 150 mg/dl (alcohol is commonly implicated in the trauma population) and a negative urine drug screen.

ASSESSMENT

Isolated fracture of the left ZMC; FISS score of 1

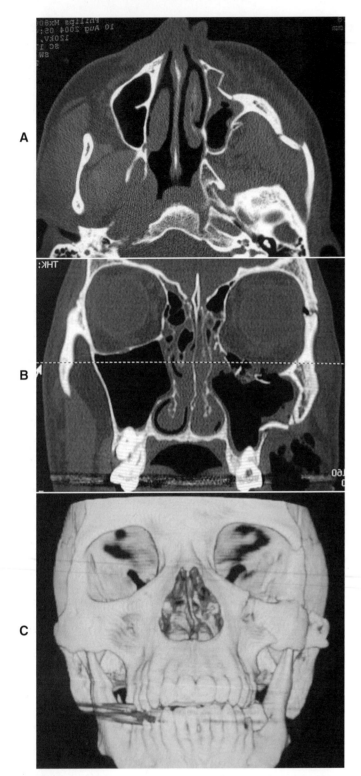

Figure 7-6 A, Axial bony window CT scan demonstrating a depressed left ZMC fracture. **B,** Reformatted coronal CT scan demonstrating a left ZMC fracture with mild herniation of orbital contents through the displaced orbital floor fracture. **C,** Three-dimensional reconstruction CT scan demonstrating the degree of displacement of the left ZMC.

TREATMENT

The goal of treatment is reduction of the fracture to its anatomical position to achieve both optimal functional and aesthetic rehabilitation. The ZS is not commonly fixated, but adequate reduction at this suture is a good indicator of overall three-dimensional position of the zygoma. The degree of displacement and comminution, the age of the patient, preexisting skin creases or lacerations, in addition to the status of the globe should be taken into account for surgical treatment planning. As with any surgery, the best treatment is that which achieves the best outcome with the least intervention. Extensive dissection and plating at multiple sutures may provide a very stable zygoma, yet the anatomical demands on the zygoma may be equally met with more conservative approaches in select cases. In a study by Zachariades and colleagues, 1270 patients with ZMC fracture were reviewed, and they concluded that the best results are achieved with semirigid fixation with miniplates at one or more sites.

This patient was taken to the operating room for ORIF. Fixation was used at the ZF suture via an upper blepharoplasty (supratarsal fold) incision and at the maxillary buttress via the maxillary buccal vestibular approach. The zygomatic arch was also reduced via the same incision using a Goldman elevator. Subsequently, the orbital floor and rim were explored and reconstructed via the transconjunctival approach using a titanium mesh and plate. A bilateral forced duction test was performed at beginning and the completion of the procedure.

COMPLICATIONS

Complications of ORIF of ZMC fractures can be divided into functional and aesthetic categories, which can be related to the surgical approach. The most feared, but fortunately rare, complication is blindness secondary to retrobulbar hemorrhage (0.3%). Retrobulbar hematoma may present as tense proptosis, eye pain, elevated intraocular pressures, and visual disturbances (decreased red-green color perception, followed by decreased visual acuity) that may require surgical decompression via a lateral canthotomy and inferior cantholysis. It is also possible that the initial trauma irreversibly affects the vision. Orbital complications such as ectropion and enophthalmos can be most concerning to the patient and the surgeon. The incidence of ectropion following a subcilliary incision varies considerably in the literature. However, most series have reported a greater incidence of ectropion with this incision compared with the transconjunctival approaches. A great majority of cases of ectropion are transient and resolve with nonsurgical interventions.

Enophthalmos can be a difficult aesthetic problem to correct and predict. Our ability to predict the incidence of enophthalmos (based on clinical and radiographic parameters) is a key measure in determining the need for orbital floor exploration. This is weighed against the aesthetic and functional risks to the eye and periorbital tissue from orbital floor exploration/reconstruction. It is unclear what amount of orbital floor disruption would predictably cause enophthalmos. However, it is generally accepted that disruption of over 50% of the floor along with loss of support at the equator of the globe will cause future enophthalmos if untreated. Therefore, careful consideration must be given to orbital floor exploration upon treatment planning.

Dysfunction of the infraorbital nerve is common and intuitively related to the severity of the initial trauma, the status of the nerve, and the complexity of dissection/stretching of the soft tissue. Persistent diplopia is uncommon because most cases of binocular diplopia resolve after the resolution of edema; however, persistent diplopia beyond 7 days will require further investigation to rule out inferior rectus entrapment.

It is important to distinguish between monocular diplopia (double vision with the unaffected eye closed) and binocular diplopia (double vision with both eyes open). Monocular diplopia may be caused by trauma to the globe such as lens dislocation or retinal detachments. This would require emergent ophthalmologic consultation, whereas binocular diplopia (which is far more common) is generally caused by extraocular muscle dysfunction secondary to edema or entrapment or globe malposition.

Aesthetic complications such as hypertrophic scars and inadequate bony reduction can be addressed surgically at the appropriate time.

DISCUSSION

Understanding the anatomy of the zygoma is essential in the treatment of ZMC fractures. By definition, the four articulating sutures (ZF, ZT, ZM, and ZS) are disrupted in this fracture. Therefore the commonly applied term "tripod fracture" is a misnomer and does not correctly describe this fracture.

Much controversy exists regarding the optimal treatment of ZMC fractures. Not unlike any other condition, treatment needs to be individually tailored to both the patient and the surgeon's experience. In the preoperative evaluation of the patient with a ZMC fracture, the ophthalmologic examination is of paramount importance. Ophthalmology consult should be obtained on select cases as dictated by the physical examination findings.

Another area of controversy is the amount of fixation necessary for adequate reduction (ranging from none to four-point fixation). The ZF and the ZM sutures are the most commonly fixated areas. All ZMC fractures involve the orbital floor (composed of the orbital segment of the maxilla, zygomatic bone, and orbital process of the palatine bone). However, as mentioned, not all ZMC fractures warrant orbital floor exploration/reconstruction. Entrapment of the extraocular muscles warrants orbital floor exploration. On examination of the eye, though, one should be careful to distinguish impaired extraocular movement secondary to generalized edema, which is very common and frequently impairs all directions of gaze, from inferior rectus entrapment, which is rare and usually demonstrates strict impairment of upward gaze.

Bibliography

Adekeye DO: Fractures of the zygomatic complex in Nigerian patients, *J Oral Surg* 38:596, 1980.

Ellis E, El-Attar A, Moos KF: An analysis of 2,067 cases of zygomatico-orbital fractures, *J Oral Maxillofac Surg* 43:428, 1985.

Fisher-Brandeis E, Dielert E: Treatment of isolated lateral midface fractures, *J Maxillofac Surg* 12:103, 1984.

Foo GC: Fractures of the zygomatic malar complex: a retrospective analysis of 76 cases, *Singapore Dent J* 9:1, 1984.

Larsen OD, Thompsen M: Zygomatic fractures II. A follow-up study of 137 patients, *Scand J Plast Reconstruct Surg* 12:59, 1978.

Lundin K, Ridell A, Sandberg N: One thousand maxillofacial and related fractures at the ENT-Clinic in Gothenburg: a two year prospective study, *Acta Otolaryngol* 75:359, 1973.

Nysingh JG: Zygomatico-maxillary fractures with a report of 200 consecuetive cases, *Arch Chir Neerl* 12:157, 1960.

Ord RA: Post-operative retrobulbar hemorrhage and blindness compicating trauma surgery, *Br J Oral Surg* 19:202, 1981.

Rake PA, Rake SA, Swift JQ, Schubert W: A single reformatted oblique sagittal view as an adjunct to coronal computed tomography for the evaluation of orbital floor fractures, *J Oral Maxillofac Surg* 62(4):456-459, 2004.

Wisenbaugh JM: Diagnostic evaluation of zygomatic complex fractures, *J Oral Surg* 28:204, 1970.

Zachariades N, Mezitis M, Anagnostopoulos D: Changing trends in the treatment of zygomaticomaxillary complex fractures: a 12-year evaluation of methods used. *J Oral Maxillofac Surg* 56:1152-1156; discussion 1156-1157, 1998.

Zygomatic Arch Fracture

Jaspal Girn, DMD, and Martin Steed, DDS

CC

A 33-year-old man presents to the emergency department complaining of left facial swelling, pain, and difficulty opening his mouth.

The epidemiology of isolated midfacial fracture varies greatly and is dependent on the geographic region, population density, socioeconomic status, and type of facility in which the research was conducted. Trends that transcend these factors include an increased incidence in men aged 21 to 30 years and a preponderance of the left over right-sided injuries when the etiology involves personal altercation, because most assailants are right-handed and use this hand to strike the opponent on the left side.

HPI

The patient reports that he was assaulted on the way home several hours earlier by an unknown assailant and was hit on the left side of his face with a hard object one time (isolated zygomatic arch fractures are most frequently due to assault). He denies any loss of consciousness, nausea, or vomiting and experienced no changes in his vision (it is important to question the patients about any signs of transient neurological impairment for suspicion of possible intracranial injury). He explains that he has difficulty opening his mouth, and any attempt to stretch open his mouth causes severe pain.

PMHX/PDHX/MEDICATIONS/ALLERGIES/SH/FH

The patient denies any significant past medical history and takes no medications. He admits to drinking several glasses of beer that night (a history of alcohol abuse is frequently elicited in the trauma population. The clinician should also keep an index of suspicion for other drugs of abuse).

EXAMINATION

The evaluation of the patient as dictated by the ATLS protocol revealed no findings except for the maxillofacial injuries outlined below (despite obvious isolated maxillofacial injuries, the evaluation of the patient should be comprehensive).

General. The patient is a well-developed and well-nourished man in no apparent distress.

Vital signs. Vital signs are stable and he is afebrile (abnormal vital signs in an otherwise healthy patient may be due to anxiety or autonomic stimulation secondary to substance abuse).

Neurological. The patient is alert and oriented with a GCS score of 15.

Maxillofacial. There are no scalp lacerations or contusions. Examination of the eyes reveals no abnormalities (visual acuity, visual fields, papillary response, and extraocular movements). There are no palpable step deformities of the orbital rims, nasal bones, maxilla, or mandible. There is no evidence of posterior or anterior epistaxis (bleeding from the nose [epistaxis] and subconjunctival ecchymosis can be seen with zygomatic arch fractures). There is mild left facial edema and tenderness anterior to the tragal cartilage of the ear (an indentation and loss of normal convex curvature would be evident in the left malar area after the acute edema subsides). The TMJs are not painful to palpation or function. The cranial nerve examination including the sensory branches of the trigeminal nerve (V_1, V_2, and V_3) are intact bilaterally (gross sensory deficits can be evaluated by asking the patient to identify soft and sharp sensation at different regions of the face).

Intraoral. Maximal intraincisal opening is measured at 15 mm (trismus commonly associated with zygomatic arch fractures is seen in 45% of cases). The maxilla and mandible are stable, and the occlusion is reproducible. There is tenderness upon palpation of the posterior aspect of the left maxillary vestibule. Mandibular lateral excursive movements demonstrate limitation of the right side (less than 5 mm); with normal lateral excursion toward the left (11 mm) (limitation of movement of the left mandibular condyle secondary to the fractured zygomatic arch impairs excursive movement of the mandible to the contralateral side).

IMAGING

Many radiological studies are available for evaluation of the zygomatic arch; the gold standard is the facial CT scan. Axial images of the zygomatic arch are ideal for assessment of fractures of the arch. Reformatted or direct coronal views can also allow visualization of the segments. Three-dimensional reconstructed views are not essential but permit visualization of the displaced fractures in all planes. If facial CT is not available, standard plain-film facial series should be obtained including the submentovertex (Figure 7-7) view, which, when correctly obtained, allows for excellent visualization of the zygomatic arch. The submentovertex view is directed from the submandibular region to the vertex (top) of the skull. The film is placed behind the patient's head in the supine position and the cone is directed from underneath the genial region so that the beam will bisect the mandibular angles, capturing the

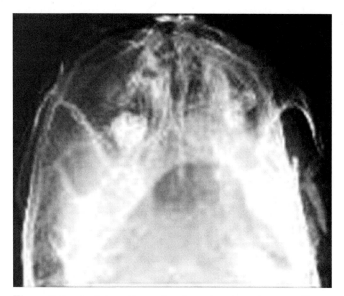

Figure 7-7 A plain radiograph submentovertex view revealing a left zygomatic arch fracture.

entire skull. This film should not be obtained in the trauma patient with suspicion of cervical spine injury because it would require hyperextension of the neck.

In this patient, a bony window facial CT scan (Figure 7-8, *A*) revealed an isolated medially displaced fracture of the left zygomatic arch that is clearly demonstrated on the three-dimensional reconstructed view (Figure 7-8, *B*) (this is the most common pattern of zygomatic arch injury and includes fractures at three points).

LABS

No routine laboratory tests are indicated for the evaluation and treatment of isolated zygomatic arch injuries unless dictated by other systemic injuries or medical conditions. Blood alcohol level and a urine drug screen should be considered in cases of suspected substance abuse.

ASSESSMENT

Isolated medially displaced fracture of the left zygomatic arch; FISS score of 1

TREATMENT

Various intraoral and transcutaneous approaches have been advocated for reduction of zygomatic arch fractures.

Transcutaneous approaches include the Gillies (temporal) approach, described first in 1927, which has been a popular technique for reduction of the zygomatic arch (described later). Alternatively, incisions in the area of the ZF suture (lateral brow or supratarsal fold incisions) can be used to gain access for placement of an instrument medial to the arch. Several methods for reduction of the arch through a percutaneous approach have been described, including:

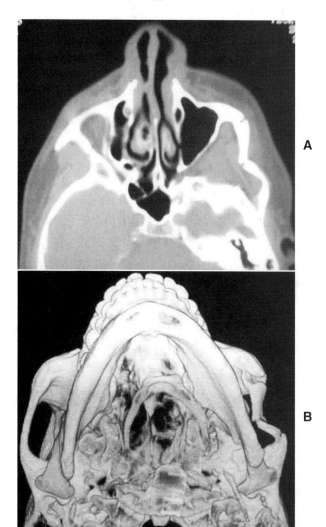

A

B

Figure 7-8 **A,** An axial CT scan bony window cut of a depressed left zygomatic arch fracture. **B,** A reconstructed facial CT scan bony window cut revealing a depressed left zygomatic arch fracture.

- The use of a J-shaped bone hook elevator through a preauricular stab incision
- Towel clip reduction using two stab incisions superior and inferior to the fractured arch
- Passing a wire or heavy suture medial to the arch to allow lateral force for reduction

ORIF can be done via a hemicoronal approach, but this should be reserved for severely displaced/comminuted fractures that are not amendable to more conservative approaches.

Transoral approaches include the Keen or buccal sulcus approach, in which a small incision is made in the mucobuccal fold beneath the zygomatic buttress of the maxilla. A periosteal elevator is inserted into the incision and, using a side-to-side sweeping motion, contact is made with the infratemporal surface of maxilla, zygoma, and zygomatic arch in a supraperiosteal manner. Subsequently, a heavier instrument can be inserted into the incision site and, using lateral and anterior controlled force, the fracture is reduced. Another intraoral technique is the lateral coronoid or Quinn approach. In this approach, a 3- to 4-cm incision is made intraorally along the anterior border of the ramus. The incision is deepened superiorly, following the lateral aspect of temporalis muscle with blunt dissection. A flat-bladed heavy instrument is inserted to elevate the arch. Care must be taken to ensure the instrument is lateral to the coronoid process. Regardless of the method used, following reduction of the zygomatic arch, the area requires protection to prevent displacement. Commonly used materials include metal eye patches or aluminum finger splints, which are secured in place with sutures. If reduction of the arch is questioned, a submentovertex radiographic view can be obtained while the patient is still in the operating room to assess the adequacy of reduction.

This patient was taken to the operating room for surgical reduction of the right zygomatic arch fracture using the Gillies (temporal) approach. A temporal incision (2 cm in length) was made adjacent to the bifurcation of the superficial temporal artery, 2.5 cm superior and 2.5 cm anterior to the helix. The incision was made through skin and subcutaneous tissue, angled from the anterosuperior to posteroinferior direction, down to the glistening white deep temporal fascia. The temporal fascia was incised horizontally to expose the temporalis muscle. Next, the broad end of a No. 9 periosteal elevator was inserted between the temporalis muscle and the temporalis fascia and swept back and forth until the medial aspect of the zygomatic arch was felt. At this point, the periosteal elevator was removed and a Rowe zygomatic elevator was inserted and pulled laterally and superiorly for reduction of the zygomatic arch (another commonly used instrument in the urethral sound). Reduction is confirmed by palpation with the nonoperating hand. The Rowe elevator is then swept back and forth to ensure reduction of the arch. The incision is closed in two layers.

Attempts to reduce isolated arch fractures more than 10 days from the initial injury date may be difficult secondary to progressive healing. Severely comminuted and displaced zygomatic arch fractures and displaced fractures that present late may require ORIF through either a hemicoronal approach or an extended preauricular incision.

COMPLICATIONS

Early complications of zygomatic arch injuries include damage to the temporal branch of the facial nerve, as it runs in a superior/anterior tangential direction at the level of the zygomatic arch. Intraoperative bleeding may be encountered if the superficial temporal artery is injured.

Long-term complications can be differentiated into functional and cosmetic. Cosmetic deformities due to asymmetry of the malar region may result if a depressed zygomatic arch fracture is not diagnosed or if it is inadequately elevated. A rare functional complication is ankylosis between the coronoid process and the zygomatic arch, causing limitation of mouth opening.

DISCUSSION

The zygomatic arch is formed by the temporal process of the zygoma and the zygomatic process of the temporal bone that are joined at the ZT suture. The glenoid fossa and articular eminence are located at the posterior aspect of the zygomatic process of the temporal bone. The point of least resistance to fracture is not at the ZT suture but is approximately 1.5 cm more posteriorly in the zygomatic process of the temporal bone.

The most common symptoms associated with zygomatic arch fractures are indentation or flattening over the zygomatic arch and limitation of mouth opening. This limitation is most likely due to spasm of the temporalis muscle from impinging displaced fragments and not from the direct impingement of the translating coronoid process by zygomatic arch fragments. Most often, fractures of the zygomatic arch are incomplete, or greenstick fractures, and may require no surgical intervention if minimally displaced. Depending on the severity of the fracture, medical comorbidities, associated injuries, and the experience of the surgeon, arch fractures can be treated either under general anesthesia in the hospital or using intravenous sedation techniques in the office setting.

Bibliography

Carter T, Bagheri S, Dierks EJ: Towel clip reduction of the depressed zygomatic arch fracture, *J Oral Maxillofac Surg* 63:1244, 2005.

Dingman RO, Natvig P: *Surgery of facial fractures.* Philadelphia, 1964, WB Saunders, pp 211-245.

Ellis E, El-Attar A, Moos KF: An analysis of 2,067 cases of zygomatico-orbital fractures, *J Oral Maxillofac Surg* 43:417, 1985.

Gilles HD, et al: Fractures of the malar-zygoma compound, with a description of a new x-ray position, *Br J Surg* 14:651, 1927.

Keen WW: *Surgery: Its principles and practice,* Philadelphia, 1909, WB Saunders.

McLoughlin P, Gilhooly M, Wood G: The management of zygomatic complex fractures—results of a survey, *Br J Oral Maxillofac Surg* 32:284, 1994.

Ogden GR: The Gillies method for fractured zygomas: an analysis of 105 cases, *J Oral Maxillofac Surg* 49:23, 1991.

Quinn JH: Lateral coronoid approach for intra-oral reduction of fractures of the zygomatic arch, *J Oral Surg* 35:321, 1977.

Zingg M, Laedrach K, Chen J, et al: Classification and treatment of zygomatic fractures: a review of 1025 cases, *J Oral Maxillofac Surg* 50:778, 1992.

Nasal Fracture

Eric P. Holmgren, MS, DMD, MD, and Samuel L. Bobek, DMD

CC

A 22-year-old man presents to the emergency department complaining that, "I think I broke my nose, and I can't breathe out of it."

Nasal bone fracture is the most common facial fracture, due to the relatively little force required to fracture this bone and its prominent position in the face. The most common cause of nasal fractures is blunt trauma to the face from interpersonal violence and sporting injuries.

HPI

The patient was involved in an altercation at a bar several hours before presentation. He received a single blow from a right fist to the left side of his nose. He does not report falling to the ground or losing consciousness. Immediately postinjury, he experienced approximately 30 minutes of brisk epistaxis (highly suggestive of nasal bone or septal fractures and lacerations of the nasal mucosa), which progressively slowed down. His pain is localized to his nasal complex. He complains of difficulty breathing through both nostrils but otherwise denies any diplopia, visual changes, or paresthesias. He states that his nose now appears crooked and was perfectly straight before this injury (preinjury appearance can be determined by a detailed history or ideally by evaluation of preinjury photographs). He also denies neck or back pain, headache, nausea, vomiting, or dizziness (review of system questions should inquiry about symptoms suggestive of possible intracranial or ocular injury).

PMHX/PDHX/MEDICATIONS/ALLERGIES/SH/FH

The patient has an unremarkable medical history. A thorough nasal history is important when evaluating nasal or nasalseptal fractures. There is no previous history of facial fractures, nasal surgeries, or preexisting nasal deformities (preexisting nasal form and function are paramount for surgical treatment planning). He denies a prior history of chronic nasal obstruction (would be suggestive of prior septal deviation). He denies any history of cocaine use (cocaine compromises nasal mucosal blood flow and predisposes to septal perforation).

EXAMINATION

His ATLS primary survey is negative, and his GCS score is 15.

General. The patient is a well-developed and well-nourished man in mild distress from pain and nasal obstruction.

Eyes. The pupils are equal, round, reactive to light and accommodation (PERRLA), and the extraocular muscles are intact. Visual acuity is 20/20 in both eyes (OS [ocular sinister, or left eye], OD [ocular dexter, or right eye]). Visual fields are intact by confrontation, without monocular or binocular diplopia. There is no evidence of hyphema (blood in the anterior chamber of the eye), no chemosis (subconjunctival edema), or subconjunctival hemorrhage. The patient exhibits bilateral infraorbital edema that is more severe on the left. There is no epiphora (large "crocodile" tears suggestive of lacrimal apparatus injury). The intercanthal distance is normal, measuring 31 mm (range, 30 to 33 mm) (increased intercanthal distance would be suggestive of nasoorbito-ethmoid [NOE] fracture).

Maxillofacial. There is minimal edema of the nose with an obvious deviation of the dorsum to the right (Figure 7-9) (with moderate to severe edema, treatment may be best delayed to allow for resolution of the edema). The bony nasal dorsum is tender to palpation with bony crepitus over the radix and upper dorsum. The alar base appears normal and coincident with the remainder of the face. Nasal tip projection is adequate with no signs of lateral or columellar collapse. The upper, middle, and lower thirds of the nose do not collapse with digital pressure (Brown-Guss provocation). There is no evidence of cerebrospinal fluid rhinorrhea (cerebrospinal fluid leakage would be indicative of fracture of the cribiform plate).

Intranasal. Using a fine suction, several blood clots were evacuated from the nares. Nasal speculum examination using a headlight and prior application of topical vasoconstrictor (oxymetazoline [Afrin] spray or 4% cocaine) reveals a 2-cm left nostril mucosal laceration over the cartilaginous septum with obvious lateral displacement. There is no septal hematoma (blood collection between the perichondrium and quadrangular cartilage, which can disrupt the blood supply to the cartilage resulting in septal necrosis, septal abscess formation, and a subsequent saddle nose deformity). The turbinates are intact and the inferior meatus is identified. (When available, an endoscopic intranasal examination provides the most information when evaluating the nasal septum.)

IMAGING

Although imaging studies may not be necessary to diagnose nasal fractures, studies are recommended to evaluate the degree of displacement and comminution (especially of the nasal septum) and to rule out other facial fractures. The CT

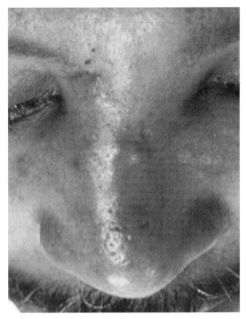

Figure 7-9 A preoperative photo (bird's eye view) showing displacement of the nasal complex to the right.

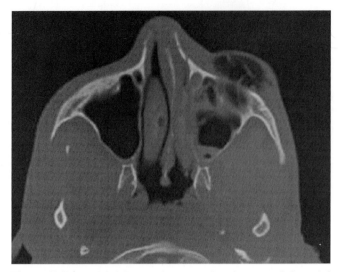

Figure 7-10 Axial CT scan demonstrating fracture of the nasal bones and septal deviation to the left.

scan is the gold standard imaging modality for the evaluation of nasal bones and associated structures. Clinical examination of acute nasal fractures in the setting of edema is often difficult, and accurate diagnosis using CT imaging becomes important. Routine plain films are rarely used in diagnosis and characterization of nasal fractures unless CT imaging is unavailable. Plain films have a low specificity (false-positive rates as high as 66%) and are limited in their inherent ability to distinguish old versus new fractures (only 15% of nasal bone fractures heal by ossification). Additionally, plain films cannot detect cartilaginous injuries, which occur more often in the pediatric population.

In this patient, a facial CT scan demonstrates bilateral nasal bone fracture with deviation to the right and bowing of the septum (Figure 7-10). Preinjury photographs can be extremely helpful to delineate injury displacement and serve as a guide in surgical correction.

LABS

No routine laboratory tests are necessary for the diagnosis and management of nasal fractures unless dictated by the medical history. In patients with suspicion of drug or alcohol abuse, a toxicology screen (including cocaine metabolites) and a blood alcohol level should be obtained. In patients with unusual bleeding that cannot be controlled with nasal packs, coagulation studies (PTT, PT, INR, platelet count) should be obtained to evaluate for underlying blood dyscrasias (von Willebrand disease is the most common bleeding disorder that can be previously undiagnosed).

ASSESSMENT

Bilateral nasal bone and nasal septal fracture; FISS score of 1

TREATMENT

Treatment for nasal bone fractures begins with a detailed nasal history and control of hemorrhage. Information regarding previous nasal trauma, surgery, deviation, and obstruction should be obtained. The mechanism, injuring agent, direction of blows, timing of injury, and postinjury epistaxis should be obtained. A preinjury photograph can be very helpful. A detailed history will allow the surgeon to better evaluate the extent of the nasal deformity, including septal deviation. Preexisting nasal deformities can complicate the reduction of the bony nasal pyramid, which may potentially drift back toward the preinjury state. This is especially true in cases of preinjury deviated nasal septum (see Discussion). The anticipated difficulty of reduction is an important factor in choice of anesthesia (local versus general).

Control of epistaxis can be achieved with one of the many choices of nasal packings with or without the aid of vasoconstrictors or electrocautery. The placement of anterior and posterior nasal packing should be precise, and the surgeon must be aware of potential complications such as infection, dehydration, and altered ventilation from obstructive and physiological derangements in pulmonary mechanics. Ribbon gauze or Merocel sponges can be used to pack anterior bleeds. Posterior bleeds usually require an anteroposterior pack, which frequently includes a balloon as a means for tamponade. Nasal packs are usually left in place for a maximum of 24 to 48 hours. The patient is admitted to the hospital for observation and antibiotics are initiated. If the epistaxis is persistent, FloSeal (Baxter) or other local hemostatic agents can be considered. Adequate control of blood pressure and the patient's pain can assist in the management of epistaxis. Silver nitrate or electrocautery is usually not helpful in traumatic bleeds where the hemorrhage is not from a punctuate source.

A thorough external and internal nasal examination will preclude the need for any adjunctive radiographic studies. Undetected and untreated septal injuries have been attributed to cause postreduction nasal deformities, and a thorough endonasal examination with a rigid endoscope or a speculum examination is recommended. This should be done after adequate anesthesia and decongestion of the nasal mucosa is achieved with 2% lidocaine with oxymetazoline or 4% cocaine.

Treatment options include open versus closed reduction. Timing of repair can be immediate or delayed. Immediate repair should be done if there is no significant edema that would compromise the assessment of surgical intervention. In the presence of significant edema, surgery should be postponed for the edema to resolve. In cases of delayed repair, it is generally recommended that nasal bone fractures be treated within 10 days of injury for optimal results (earlier in the pediatric population).

The surgeon should have an algorithm to follow in the case of a difficult or unstable closed reduction. An uncomplicated displaced nasal bone fracture with no preexisting nasal or septal deformity will be most amenable to closed reduction. This can be attempted with any number of instruments (Boies elevator, Walsham's forceps, Asch forceps, etc.). If the nasal pyramid snaps into position and is stable, an external nasal splint is applied (either an Aquaplast thermal splint or a Denver metal splint). If there is continued memory or drift of the nasal pyramid, further intervention is indicated until a stable reduction is achieved. First, a septoplasty procedure should be considered, especially in patients with a prior history nasal obstruction. Nasal osteotomies are performed if there is continued drift. The upper lateral cartilages can be released from the nasal septum if there continues to be drift of the nasal structures. (The upper lateral cartilages will splint bones toward initial preexisting deformity. Therefore release of upper lateral cartilage from septum allows nasal bones to remain midline.) This can be followed by fracturing the bony septum (the anterior extension of the perpendicular plate of the ethmoid and vomer) opposite to the deviation by pushing the bony pyramid toward the contralateral lateral canthus. The final attempt at correcting any residual deformity can be accomplished with a cartilage camouflage graft in the depressed area. External nasal splint for 1 to 2 weeks and endonasal packing (Bacitracin-impregnanted $^1/_2$-inch NuGauze [Johnson & Johnson]) for 2 to 3 days will assist in further stabilizing the fractures.

In this patient, the nasal bones were treated with closed reduction using a Boies elevator. The nasal bony pyramid reduced into correct anatomical position with a distinct "snapping" sound and remained in stable position. The nasal septal fracture was treated with closed reduction back to a stable midline position. There was no immediate memory or drift noted after reduction (preinjury nasal and nasal septal deformities predispose the nasal complex to drift). An external nasal split was applied for 1 week (Figure 7-11).

COMPLICATIONS

The most common and problematic postinury or postoperative complication is a postreduction nasal deformity. Most authors believe that an undiagnosed or untreated nasal septal

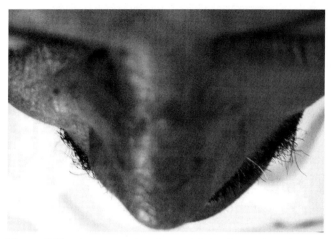

Figure 7-11 A postoperative photograph (bird's eye view) 6 weeks after the procedure.

fracture/deviation has a significant role in causing this complication. The incidence of posttraumatic nasal deformity has been reported at around 14% to 50%. The algorithm presented here is aimed at reducing the incidence of postreduction deformities with special attention to the nasal septum. Nasal obstruction due to collapse of the nasal valve and formation of synecchiae can cause significant breathing and chronic sinus problems.

The presence of a septal hematoma is an urgent complication in the setting of nasal trauma. The mucosa overlying the nasal septum is highly vascular. Kiesselbach's plexus (Little's area) is a vascular area in the anterior septum where terminal branches of the internal and external carotid arteries meet. The anterior ethmoidal, septal branch of the superior labial, sphenopalatine, and greater palatine arteries compose this plexus. Injury to this area can cause a septal hematoma in the subperichondrial plane, disrupting the vascular supply to the septum. A septal hematoma requires immediate evacuation with dependent drainage and intranasal packing to prevent reaccumulation. Undetected or untreated septal hematomas can lead to abscess formation, septal necrosis, and resultant fibrosis and deformity (saddle-nose deformity).

Other complications include unremitting epistaxis, synecchiae formation, scar contracture, nasal airway obstruction, cerebrospinal fluid rhinorrhea, and toxic shock syndrome (the latter is very rare).

DISCUSSION

The nasal bone is reported to be the most common facial fracture. The nose can be divided into three vaults. The upper vault is comprised of the paired nasal bones, frontal processes of the maxilla, and the perpendicular plate of the ethmoid bone. This structure is also referred to as the bony pyramid. The middle vault includes the upper lateral cartilages and the midportion of the nasal septum (quadrangular cartilage). The lower vault includes the nasal tip, lower lateral (alar) cartilages, and the inferior portion of the nasal septum. These vaults can be tested individually for stability by applying digital pressure, which will cause the vault to collapse if it is unstable. This is called the Brown-Gruss provocation.

It is important to remember that the nasal septum is attached to both the bony nasal pyramid and the upper and lower lateral cartilages. Any septal deformity has the potential to transmit forces to the bony and cartilaginous portions of the nose and cause a postreduction deformity. The nasal septum is composed of the perpendicular plate of the ethmoid bone, vomer, nasal crests of the maxilla, palatine bones, and the quadrangular cartilage. Treatment of nasal fractures in the pediatric patient should follow the same protocol because normal growth will resume after septal repair/surgery.

The indications for primary open reduction of nasal fractures include the following:

- Inability for the septum to remain in the reduced position
- Considerable displacement of cartilaginous structures
- Bilateral fractures with dislocation of nasal dorsum and septal pathology
- Fractures of cartilaginous pyramid with or without dislocation of the upper lateral cartilages
- Anticipation of cartilage or bone grafting

Nasal fractures should be diagnosed and treated with close consideration to function and esthetics. The simplicity of closed reduction techniques should not replace more invasive surgical interventions. Untreated septal injuries can significantly complicate airway flow and the aesthetic outcome.

Bibliography

Chegar B, Tatum S: Nasal fractures. In: *Cummings otolaryngology: Head and neck surgery,* ed 4, Philadelphia, 2005, Elsevier, pp 962-979.

Deeb G, Dierks E: *Use of CT in diagnosing nasal fractures.* Presented at the 82nd Annual Meeting of the American Association of Oral and Maxillofacial Surgeons, San Francisco, CA, October 2000.

de Vries N, van der Baan S: Toxic shock syndrome after nasal surgery: is prevention possible? A case report and review of the literature, *Rhinology* 27(2):125-128, 1989.

Indreasano AT, Beckley ML: Nasal fractures. In: Fonseca RJ, editor: *Oral and maxillofacial trauma,* ed 3, Philadelphia, 2004, WB Saunders, pp 737-750.

Mondin V, Rinaldo A, Ferlito A: Management of nasal bone fractures, *Am J Otolaryngol* 26(3):181-185, 2005.

Logan M, O'Driscoll K, Masterson J: The utility of nasal bone radiographs in nasal trauma, *Clin Radiol* 49(3):192-194, 1994.

Oluwasanmi AF, Pinto AL: Management of nasal trauma—widespread misuse of radiographs, *Clin Perform Qual Health Care* 8(2):83-85, 2000.

Rhee SC, Kim YK, Cha JH, et al: Septal fracture in simple nasal bone fracture, *Plast Reconstr Surg* 113(1):45-52, 2004.

Ridder GJ, Boedeker CC, Fradis M, Schipper J: Technique and timing for closed reduction of isolated nasal fractures: a retrospective study, *Ear Nose Throat J* 81(1):49-54, 2002.

Rohrich RJ, Adams WP Jr: Nasal fracture management: minimizing secondary nasal deformities, *Plast Reconstr Surg* 106(2):266-273, 2000.

Weber R, Keerl R, Hochapfel F, et al: Packing in endonasal surgery, *Am J Otolaryngol* (5):306-320, 2001.

Frontal Sinus Fracture

Martin B. Steed, DDS, and Shahrokh C. Bagheri, DMD, MD

CC

You are called by the trauma team to evaluate a 25-year-old man status post high-speed motor vehicle collision and to manage his facial trauma.

HPI

The patient was the unrestrained driver in a high-speed, head-on collision with another vehicle. No air bag was deployed, with subsequent significant steering wheel and windshield damage. The patient was found to be unconscious and was not arousable. He was intubated at the scene due to a GCS score of 7 (high index of suspicion for a severe intracranial injury) and was life-flighted to your Level I trauma center for evaluation and treatment.

PMHX/PDHX/MEDICATIONS/ALLERGIES/SH/FH

All histories are unknown (when possible, history should be obtained from available family members).

EXAMINATION

Primary Survey

The primary survey is accomplished via ATLS protocol. The patient is sedated and intubated and has spontaneous respirations. He wears a transport cervical collar, and his pupils are equal and reactive. His GCS score is 10T on arrival. He is otherwise hemodynamically stable.

Secondary Survey

Vital signs. His blood pressure is 115/64 mm Hg, heart rate 115 bpm (tachycardia), respirations 12 per minute, and temperature 37.6°C.

Maxillofacial. There is a stellate laceration through the frontalis muscle measuring over 10 cm in combined length at the left forehead and supraorbital regions. Bony crepitance is noted upon palpation of the supraorbital rims, nasal bones, and frontal bone (indicative of comminuted fractures). There is a flow of blood tinged fluid from the left nare (possible cerebrospinal fluid rhinorrhea). The maxilla is stable. The dental occlusion is difficult to assess secondary to oral endotracheal intubation. A cervical-spine collar is in place (correctly sized and applied).

Eyes. Pupils are equal and reactive to light consensually (5 mm → 2 mm). There is evidence of bilateral subconjunctival hemorrhage, no evidence of hyphema (blood in the anterior chamber of the eye, which may be difficult to detect in the supine patient), and normal fundi with no evidence of papilledema (edema of the optic nerve seen with increased intracranial pressure or intracranial pressure). The intraocular pressures were normal at 16 mm Hg OU as measured with an orbital tonometer.

IMAGING

CT scan is the diagnostic modality of choice for the evaluation of frontal sinus injury, but it is not a reliable predictor of nasofrontal duct injury.

A head and facial helical CT scan without contrast was obtained after the primary and secondary surveys were completed. The head CT scan reveals a 4 × 1-cm left subarachnoid hemorrhage with no midline shift and two regions of increased enhancement of the frontal lobe. The fine-cut axial face CT scan reveals a comminuted frontal bone fracture involving both the anterior and posterior tables of the frontal sinus (Figure 7-12, *A*), nasal bone fracture, bilateral supraorbital rim, and left infraorbital rim fractures. Three-dimensional reconstruction demonstrates the overall fracture patterns (Figure 7-12, *B*). The cervical-spine CT reveals no obvious fractures with good alignment of the cervical vertebrae. (The incidence of facial fractures accompanied by spinal injuries, while low, is of significant concern to the craniomaxillofacial surgeon.)

LABS

Standard laboratory tests for the evaluation of multisystem trauma patients include: complete blood cell count (CBC), complete metabolic panel, arterial blood gas analysis, urine analysis, and coagulation studies (PT, PTT, and INR). A urine drug screen and blood alcohol level are indicated in patients with decreased mental status.

Laboratory values are within normal limits except for mildly low hemoglobin/hematocrit (secondary to blood loss from the scalp laceration and fluid resuscitation). One milliliter of the blood-tinged transudate from the patient's left nare was collected and sent for laboratory analysis. The sample tested positive for beta-2 transferrin (diagnostic for cerebrospinal fluid).

ASSESSMENT

Subarachnoid hemorrhage with intracerebral contusion; comminuted frontal sinus fracture with significant displacement of the anterior and posterior tables (greater than one

165

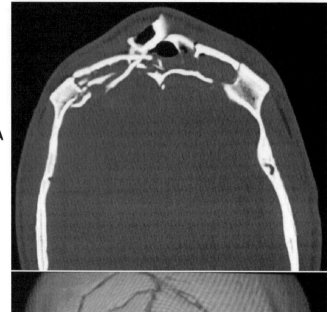

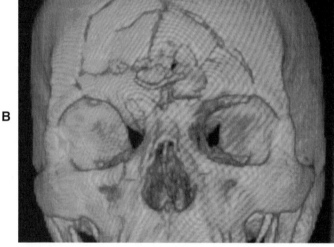

Figure 7-12 A, Preoperative axial CT scan demonstrating comminuted displaced anterior and posterior sinus wall fractures. **B,** Three-dimensional reconstruction of preoperative CT scan demonstrating a comminuted frontal bone fracture with a step deformity at the supra-orbital rims bilaterally. There is also evidence of fractures at the inferior orbital rims bilaterally.

table thickness), nasal bone and bilateral supraorbital rim fractures, with associated left frontal stellate skin laceration, evidence of cerebrospinal fluid rhinorrhea, and possible nasofrontal duct injury or obstruction; FISS score of 10 (displaced frontal sinus fracture [5], bilateral supraorbital rim fractures [2], left infra orbital rim fracture [1], nasal bone fracture [1], and forehead laceration over 10 cm [1]

TREATMENT

The primary indications for repair of a fractured sinus are:
- Displaced anterior sinus wall fractures with resultant aesthetic deformity
- Displaced posterior table fractures (greater than one table thickness displacement)
- Nasofrontal duct injury

However, these indications are not absolute and each case needs treatment planned on an individual basis.

A variety of treatment modalities have evolved to treat frontal sinus fractures; options include observation, trephination, frontoethmoidectomy (Lynch or Knapp procedure), frontal sinus collapse (Reidel) procedure, osteoplastic flap, sinus obliteration, ORIF with preservation of the sinus and its drainage, or cranialization (removal of the posterior table, allowing the brain parenchyma to occupy the frontal sinus).

The ability of the surgeon to evaluate or predict the function of the nasofrontal ducts is critical. If the decision is made to observe a fracture and/or the nasofrontal ducts are not obliterated, then it is imperative to follow the patient with interval CT imaging to assess the adequate drainage of the sinus. Some surgeons examine the status of the nasofrontal ducts intraoperatively by injecting dye into the duct and observing its presence in the nasal cavity. However, the accuracy of this test is questionable.

In this case, the presence of a displaced posterior table fracture, dural tear, and cerebrospinal fluid leak lends itself well to a cranialization procedure through a bicoronal flap in coordination with the neurosurgical team. The supraorbital rims and nasal bone were reconstructed and rigidly fixated with titanium plates (Figure 7-13, *A*). The posterior table was removed, the dural tears were repaired, and the sinus mucosa was obliterated and meticulously removed with the aid of a pear-shaped bur (to remove all remnants of the peripheral sinus mucosa). The mucosa at the nasofrontal ducts was inverted, and the ducts were plugged with a small piece of free temporalis fascia. An anteriorly based pericranial flap (based on the deep branches of the supratrochlear and supraorbital vessels) was used to facilitate separation of the brain from the nasal environment (Figure 7-13, *B*). The craniotomy defect was reconstructed with rigid fixation plates (Figure 7-13, *C*).

The patient did well postoperatively. A postoperative CT demonstrated excellent restoration of frontal region contour (Figure 7-14). His neurological examination improved, and he was discharged home 11 days after surgery.

COMPLICATIONS

Complications of frontal sinus fracture repair can be characterized as early if it occurs within the first few weeks of surgical intervention or late if it occurs beyond this period. Early complications after frontal sinus fracture repair include cerebrospinal fluid leak, meningitis, transient frontal region paresthesia, diplopia, and pain in the frontal region. Inadequate reduction of the anterior wall of the sinus will result in aesthetic contour defects (a common complication). By far the most feared early complication is meningitis. The incidence of meningitis can be as high as 6% postoperatively. These patients are uniquely susceptible to the consequences of meningitis as they are neurologically compromised, and early diagnosis of the condition may elude the clinician. To minimize the morbidity and potential mortality from meningitis, this condition needs to be diagnosed without delay. Change

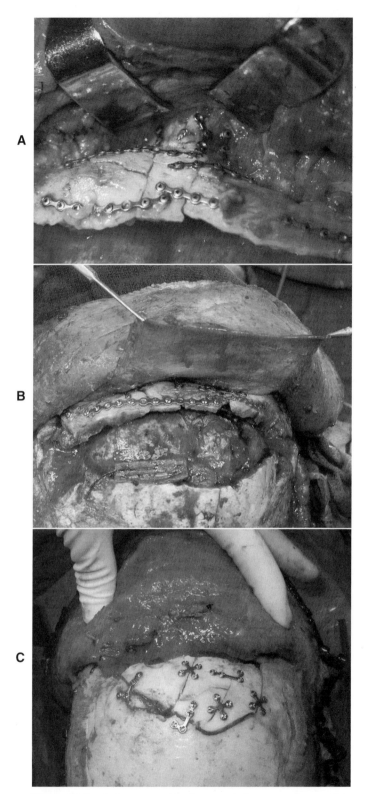

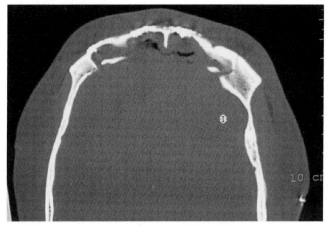

Figure 7-14 Postoperative axial CT scan demonstrating the removal of the posterior sinus wall and cranialization of the frontal lobe into the previous sinus space, with good reduction of the anterior sinus wall and restoration of proper contour.

Figure 7-13 **A,** Intraoperative photograph demonstrating cranialization (posterior table has been removed and the supraorbital bar reconstructed. **B,** Anterior based pericranial flap—an anteriorly pedicled pericranial flap (based on the supratrochlear and supraorbital vessels) before insetting. **C,** Intraoperative photograph demonstrating anterior based pericranial flap inset and restoration of superior frontal region contour.

in mental status, fever, and/or neck rigidity should prompt an immediate lumbar puncture after a brain CT. The patient should be stabilized medically and administered broad-spectrum antibiotics that possess good cerebrospinal fluid penetrance (such as nafcillin). The antibiotics should be altered based on the cerebrospinal fluid cultures.

Late frontal sinus fracture complications can occur more than 10 years after the initial incident. Mucopyoceles causing meningitis are the most feared late sequelae of frontal sinus trauma. Retained mucosa left in the fracture line can result in the formation of a mucocele, which upon bacterial contamination can develop into a mucopyocele. Mucopyoceles can potentially spread infection to the orbit and brain. Reoperation with complete removal of the mucocele and reconstruction to isolate the splachnocranium (that part of the skull that is derived from the branchial [or pharyngeal] arches and comprises the bones of the face) from the orbit and nasal cavity is the method of choice for management of mucoceles. Endoscopic marsupialization of mucoceles has been attempted after infectious complications of frontal sinusitis with limited success rates. Under normal circumstances, both the nasofrontal duct and frontal recess are widely patent. Following traumatic disruption of the area, even partial obstruction of the duct often results in stasis of secretions, increasing the risk of delayed frontal sinus infectious complications.

In a study of 727 patients with facial fractures receiving formal ophthalmologic consultation, Holt found that 89% of those with frontal sinus fractures had associated eye injuries.

DISCUSSION

The frontal sinus develops as an outgrowth from the nasal chamber in utero and exists only as a small cephalic evagination of the middle meatus until after birth. Between ages 1 and 2 years, this evagination begins to invade the frontal bone. The adult frontal sinus averages 28 mm in height, 27 mm in width, and 17 mm in depth, but asymmetry is common and the size is variable. The sinus commonly has a vertical septum at its center, although several septa may be present. The drainage of the frontal sinus is also variable but begins in the posteromedial floor on either side of the septum. A true identifiable duct may be absent in up to 85% of patients, and when present, it opens at different sites within the nose. Van Alyea found that in 55% of patients, the frontal sinus drained directly into the frontal recess, and in 30%, it opened above the ethmoidal infundibulum. In 15%, the frontal sinus was continuous with the ethmoidal infundibulum, and in 1%, it drained above the ethmoid bulla.

The chief blood supply to the frontal sinus is a diploic branch from the supraorbital artery and branches of the anterior ethmoidal artery. It drains through the angular and anterior facial veins externally and through the posterior sinus wall via the foramen of Breschet posteriorly.

Frontal sinus fractures most often result from blunt trauma, although penetrating injuries also occur. Schultz and colleagues found that 70% of frontal sinus fractures resulted from automobile accidents, while 20% resulted from assault. The force necessary to fracture the anterior wall of the frontal sinus (800 to 1600 N) is two to three times greater than that required to fracture the zygoma, mandible, or maxilla.

Significant intracranial injury occurs more often with frontal sinus injuries than with injury to the maxilla or mandible secondary to the proximity to the brain and the force necessary to fracture the frontal bone.

Nasal secretions with a glucose level greater than 30 mg/dl may be indicative of cerebrospinal fluid. Other indicators used to identify nasal secretions as originating from cerebrospinal fluid include low protein and potassium concentrations (however, glucose, protein, and potassium levels are not a reliable means of identifying cerebrospinal fluid secondary to variability). The "halo" test can also be performed by placing a drop of the fluid onto a clean bedsheet or onto filter paper and observing whether a clear halo forms around the central stain. Beta-2 transferrin is the laboratory test of choice for distinguishing cerebrospinal fluid because detection of a beta-2 transferrin band by immunofixation electrophoresis is diagnostic for cerebrospinal fluid. This test should be considered when there is suspicion of cerebrospinal fluid otorrhea or rhinorrhea. Beta-2 transferrin is not detected in normal serum, tears, saliva, sputum, or nasal secretions.

Bibliography

Bagheri SC, Dierks EJ, Kademani D, et al: Application of a Facial Injury Severity Scale (FISS) in cranio-maxillofacial trauma, *J Oral Maxillofac Surg* 64:408-414, 2006.

Bell RB, Dierks EJ, Homer L, Potter BE: Management of cerebrospinal fluid leak associated with craniomaxillofacial trauma, *J Oral Maxillofac Surg* 62(6):676-684, 2004.

Gerbino G, Roccia F, Benech A, et al: Analysis of 158 frontal sinus fractures: current surgical management and complications, *J Craniomaxillofac Surg* 28:133, 2000.

Helmy ES, Koh ML, Bays RA: Management of frontal sinus fractures, *Oral Surg Oral Med Oral Pathol* 69:137-148, 1990.

Holt GR: Ethmoid and frontal sinus fractures, *Ear Nose Throat J* 62:33-42, 1983.

Lee D, Brody R, Har-El G: Frontal sinus outflow anatomy, *Am J Rhinol* 11:283, 1997.

Manolidis S: Frontal sinus injuries: associated injuries and surgical management of 93 patients, *J Oral Maxillofac Surg* 62:882-891, 2004.

Nahum AM: The biomechanics of maxillofacial trauma, *Clin Plast Surg* 2:59-64, 1975.

Rice DH: Management of frontal sinus fractures, *Curr Opin Otolaryngol Head Neck Surg* 12:46-48, 2004.

Schultz RC: Frontal sinus and supraorbital fractures from vehicle accidents, *Clin Plast Surg* 2:93-106, 1975.

Van Alyea OE: Frontal sinus drainage, *Ann Otol Rhinol Laryngol* 55:267-277, 1946.

Naso-Orbital-Ethmoid Fracture

Martin B. Steed, DDS, and Shahrokh C. Bagheri, DMD, MD

CC

A 21-year-old man arrives via EMS responders to the emergency department status post high-speed motor vehicle collision.

HPI

The EMS personnel report that the patient was an unrestrained driver traveling at 60 mph through a red light at an intersection when he hit an oncoming vehicle. The driver side airbag did not deploy, resulting in the direct collision of the upper midface with the steering wheel and causing a positive "steering wheel deformity." (The incidence of NOE fractures has decreased with the advent of airbags. However, the impact of the midface with the steering wheel continues to be a common cause of NOE fractures.) The patient had a transient loss of consciousness but has remained coherent, alert, and oriented during transport to the emergency department (need to rule out intracranial injury/hemorrhage). He complains of a severe headache, poor vision, and pain in the midface. The trauma team has requested a consultation for management of the patient's midfacial soft tissue lacerations and evaluation for facial fractures.

PMHX/PDHX/MEDICATIONS/ALLERGIES/SH/FH

The patient has a prior history of substance abuse (cocaine) according to telephone contact with family member.

A history of cocaine abuse is important to the reconstructive maxillofacial surgeon because it may imply previous nasal septal perforation or compromised local vasculature of the nasal structures due to repeated episodes of vasoconstriction from nasal cocaine abuse. In addition, chronic or recent history of cocaine abuse has cardiovascular implications, rendering the patient at increased risk for coronary vasospasm and cardiac arrhythmias. Illicit drugs are commonly implicated in motor vehicle accidents.

EXAMINATION

The initial evaluation of a trauma patient should be completed by following the ATLS protocol.

Primary Survey

The patient's primary survey is intact, with a GCS score of 15. The patient has been able to easily maintain his airway (severe posterior nasal hemorrhage can compromise the airway and be a significant source of blood loss).

Secondary Survey

General. The patient is a well-developed and well-nourished man in moderate distress, requesting pain medications and supporting a partially soaked 4 × 4 dressing held over the bridge of his nose and right eye.

Vital signs. His blood pressure is 150/84 mm Hg (hypertensive), heart rate 125 bpm (tachycardia), respirations 16 per minute, and temperature 37.6°C.

Maxillofacial. There is significant bilateral midface and periorbital edema with a 10-cm horseshoe (U)-shaped laceration to the frontal region down to bone. A second 8-cm horizontal laceration extends through the right upper eyelid, across the nasal bridge (nasion) and through the left upper eyelid (Figure 7-15). There are several small arterial bleeders within each laceration. Facial abrasions extend over the left malar (zygoma) region. The patient exhibits a positive bowstring test on the left (movement of bone fragment at insertion of medial canthal tendon upon lateral pull on the upper eyelid). The intercanthal distance is 42 mm (distance between the left and right medial canthus—this may be acutely influenced by edema), with an interpupillary distance of 62 mm (normal intercanthal distance is usually half the interpupillary distance).

Nose. There is bright red blood in the bilateral nares (epistaxis), with obvious crepitus of the nasal complex upon palpation. The nasal bones are comminuted, displaced, and unstable, with a widened nasal bridge. Nasal speculum examination reveals the nasal septum to be deviated to the right with no evidence of a septal hematoma (examination may be difficult in the awake patient). There is clear fluid obtained from the right nare that was sent for laboratory evaluation of cerebrospinal fluid (beta-2 transferrin).

Maxilla. The examination reveals bilateral hypoesthesia of the infraorbital nerve distributions (cranial nerve V_2). The maxilla is nonmobile, and the patient's occlusion is intact. The patient has a full complement of teeth, with no grossly carious lesions and no mobile dentoalveolar segments.

Eyes. There is severe bilateral chemosis and subconjunctival hemorrhage. The patient is unable to open either eye, and examination requires careful lid elevation. There is blunting of the bilateral medial palpebral fissures. There is no obvious epiphora (excessive tearing from the eye), but no attempts are made at primary probing of any of the canaliculi.

OD examination reveals a reactive pupil with hyphema (blood in the anterior chamber of the eye). The OD pupil appears round and the visual acuity is limited to light perception. OS visual acuity is 20/200.

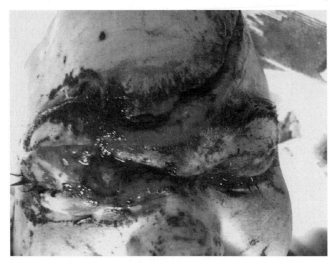

Figure 7-15 Preoperative photograph demonstrating frontal and orbital/nasal bridge lacerations, increased intercanthal distance, severe depression of nasal bridge unit, bilateral midfacial edema, and periorbital ecchymosis.

Physical examination of suspected NOE fractures should be detailed toward assessing the degree of telecanthus and early identification of concurrent ocular and neurological injuries. Soft tissue intercanthal distances greater than 35 mm are suggestive of a displaced NOE fracture, and distances greater than 40 mm are diagnostic. Crepitus or movement upon palpation of the medial orbital rim indicates instability and the presence of a fracture; clinical "bowstring" examinations can demonstrate whether the canthal bearing bone fragment is displaced and mobile.

IMAGING

The imaging modality of choice in the diagnosis and evaluation of midface fractures is a noncontrast helical CT scan with thin cuts (1.5 to 2.0 mm) of the face. Due to overlapping bony architecture, plain films fail to demonstrate the degree and location of bony disruption. Thin cuts are usually required to determine the extent of the NOE injury. Of surgical importance is the determination of the position and status of the frontal process of the maxilla, as this region bears the insertion of the medial canthal tendon.

A facial helical CT scan without contrast was obtained. Axial bony windows show bilateral fractures at the NOE region with avulsion of several bony segments and bilateral medial orbital wall fractures (Figure 7-16, *A*). The orbital floors appear intact bilaterally. There is evidence of a 1-cm punctuate subarachnoid hemorrhage, with no midline deviation. A three-dimensional reconstruction view permits visualization of the lines of fracture (Figure 7-16, *B*).

LABS

A complete trauma panel was obtained, and the results were remarkable for an elevated WBC count of 15,100 cells per microliter (likely secondary to demargination of leukocytes

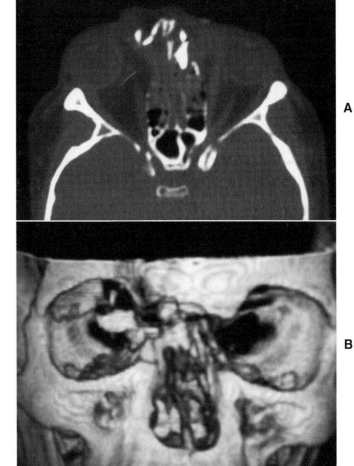

A

B

Figure 7-16 **A,** Preoperative axial bony CT window demonstrating fracture of the nasal bones with severe displacement of the bilateral nasal bones and comminution of the frontal process of the maxilla. The view also demonstrates fracture of the lamina papyracea and bilateral medial orbital walls. **B,** Preoperative anterior three-dimensional CT reconstruction demonstrating severe displacement and comminution of a bilateral NOE fracture.

in the setting of acute trauma), and a urine toxicology screen was positive for cocaine metabolites.

The beta-2 transferrin test performed on the nasal fluid was negative (decreasing the likelihood of cerebrospinal fluid rhinorrhea).

ASSESSMENT

- *Type I NOE fracture of the right side (right medial canthal tendon attached to one large segment of bone)*
- *Type III NOE fracture of the left side (significant comminution and complete avulsion of left medial canthal tendon).*
- *11-cm U-shaped frontal region laceration through frontalis muscle to frontal bone with no evidence of frontal sinus fracture*
- *10-cm linear horizontal laceration through both upper eyelids and probable left nasolacrimal tract injury*

- *OD grade I traumatic hyphema (less than one-third of the anterior chamber of the right eye filled with blood)*
- *Punctate subarachnoid hemorrhage*
- *FISS of 5 (NOE = 3, facial laceration over 10 cm = 1 + 1)*

TREATMENT

The goals of surgical correction of NOE fractures are to restore the patient to the preinjury level of function and cosmesis. This becomes extremely challenging in the treatment of complex and comminuted NOE fractures with concomitant injuries.

Adequate exposure is essential for the precise reduction and fixation required for correction of NOE fractures. Most commonly, a combination of a coronal flap with or without lower eyelid incisions is adequate. Placement of incisions in areas over the radix or lateral aspect of the nasal bridge should be avoided due to unfavorable scarring. Most often, the fractured segments can be fixated to a curved titanium plate that extends from the nasofrontal junction along the frontal process of the maxilla onto the medial portion of the inferior orbital rim. The canthal tendon is rarely avulsed from bone and is usually attached to a sizable bony fragment that can be reduced to a correctly adapted plate. In cases where the medial canthal tendon is in fact avulsed, a canthopexy must be accomplished primarily through transnasal wiring or by securing a permanent suture to a transnasal wire, as described by Herford.

The treatment of this patient demonstrates many of the principles of the management of NOE fractures. Upon completion of the primary and secondary surveys and diagnostic imaging, the patient was evaluated by the neurosurgical team and the ophthalmology service. The patient required no surgical intervention for the small subarachnoid hemorrhage and no intracranial pressure monitoring in light of consistently normal serial neurological examinations. The ophthalmologic team concurred with the presence of a grade I traumatic hyphema and the high likelihood of a nasolacrimal apparatus injury, which may require subsequent treatment. He was found to have no evidence of a ruptured globe or traumatic optic neuropathy.

The patient was taken to the operating room and orally intubated. A coronal flap was not used secondary to the excellent exposure through the existing lacerations (Figure 7-17, *A*). It must be stressed that this is usually not the case. Access is paramount in the proper reduction and fixation of NOE fractures, and a large number of comminuted NOE fractures benefit from immediate bone grafting. Each of these requirements is met through the use of a coronal incision, which provides large amounts of access and allows the concurrent harvest of cranial bone grafts for immediate grafting of the nasal dorsum or medial orbital walls.

Careful intraoperative examination revealed a 1 × 1-cm fiberglass foreign body within the right upper eyelid. A Jones type I (fluorescein dye into eye) or Jones type II (dye into puncta/canaliculi) test can be performed intraoperatively to assess the lacrimal function. The nasolacrimal apparatus may be injured in 20% of patients with NOE fractures. It is

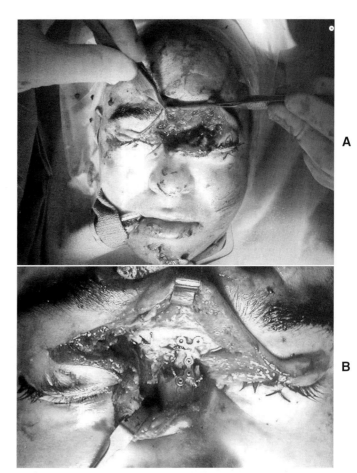

Figure 7-17 A, Intraoperative photograph demonstrating access through facial lacerations. **B,** Intraoperative photograph after ORIF of the NOE complex.

especially susceptible when telecanthus is present secondary to a loss of the protective influence provided by the anterior limb of the medial canthal ligament. Open reduction and anatomical fixation of the fracture segments usually result in reestablishment of the lacrimal drainage. Intraoperative repair may be completed through the use of a stent such as a Crawford tube, which acts to bridge the two severed ends of the canaliculi, and careful closure of the pericanalicular tissues. Delayed assessment may be done with fluorescein dye, instrument probing, or dacrocystography. Refractory or uncorrected epiphora often necessitate correction through a dacrocystorhinostomy at a later date. In this procedure, the tear drainage pathways are reconnected to the inside of the nose. A small incision is usually placed approximately midway between the corner of the eye and the bridge of the nose. The lacrimal sac is located, incised, and then connected to the nasal mucosa, creating a new tear drainage pathway. A stent is then placed in the newly created tear drainage pathway for a few months to prevent scarring of the tear drainage ducts, which might otherwise result in failure of the surgery. The tubes can usually be removed in the office with little, if any discomfort, or need for anesthesia.

The lacerations were meticulously washed out with pulse irrigation. The NOE fractures were confirmed to be a type I on the right side with the medial canthus attached to a large segment of bone and a type III on the left side with complete avulsion of the medial canthal ligament attachment. A 2.0 X-shaped plate was applied to secure the nasal bones to the frontal bone (Figure 7-17, *B*). The medial orbital rims were also reconstructed using rigid mini fixation plates. Twenty-six–gauge wires were used to directly secure the left and right medial canthal tendons to stable bone posterior and slightly superior to the insertion of the preinjured tendon. This is done to overcome the forces of migration, relapse, and telecanthus. Intranasal splints (i.e., Doyle) were placed and sutured in place anteriorly through the membranous septum. The lacerations were closed in layers with special attention to the upper eyelid regions, where the levator muscle and its insertion were evaluated and maintained. The patient underwent consistent neurological checks postoperatively and underwent a second CT head scan on postoperative day one, which showed no change in his punctuate subarachnoid hemorrhage. He was discharged on the third postoperative day.

COMPLICATIONS

Intraoperative

Intraoperative complications are often best avoided by a thorough preoperative evaluation and examination. Concomitant ocular injuries must be identified and evaluated before general anesthetic induction and surgical manipulation of the globe and adnexal structures. Neurosurgical consultation must be obtained in case of neurological changes and/or radiographic evidence of intracranial injury. In the case of severe bleeding from midfacial injuries, the use of bilateral posterior nasal packs can be lifesaving.

Early

Nasolacrimal obstruction present as epiphora secondary to inadequate tear drainage. This may require secondary correction with a dacrocystorhinostomy procedure.

Late

The majority of complications resulting from NOE fractures are cosmetic in nature and are the result of nontreated or inadequately treated NOE fractures. Perhaps the most common is a residual "saddle defect" or shortened and retruded nose. This is secondary to the loss of dorsal nasal support in the upper bony and lower cartilaginous dorsum. The importance of immediate primary dorsal bone grafting has been emphasized in the literature. It is important when placing the graft as a strut to position it inferiorly underneath the lower lateral cartilage to provide support for the inferior portion of the nose and prevent palpation of the graft after healing is complete. The graft is secured superiorly with screws or plate fixation. Attention should be given to fixation of the graft superiorly to avoid overprojection at the nasofrontal region or at the nasal tip.

Telecanthus is best managed through correct reduction of the bone fragments that carry the medial canthal tendon insertions or, in the case of type III fractures, meticulous reduction of the insertions themselves with overcorrection. Septal deviation may require immediate correction or a septoplasty at a later date. Enophthalmos most often results from an increase in the orbital volume due to untreated medial orbital wall or orbital floor fractures. These injures should be addressed concurrently or secondarily with NOE reconstruction.

DISCUSSION

Fractures of the NOE region are among the most complex maxillofacial injuries in both diagnosis and treatment. The superior limits of this region are defined medially by the cribiform plate and laterally by the roof of the ethmoid sinuses. The anterior cranial fossa and contents lie above. The lateral limits comprise the medial orbital walls and are made up primarily of the lacrimal bone and the orbital plate of the ethmoid. The anterior limits consist of the frontal bone and, more laterally, the frontal process of the maxilla. Posteriorly lies the sphenoid bone and its sinus, while inferior is the lower border of the ethmoid sinuses. An NOE fracture involves the central midface—the nasal bones, frontal process of the maxilla, and ethmoid bones. In 1973 Epker coined the term "naso-orbito-ethmoid" to describe this midfacial injury. Prior to 1960, most textbooks offered little guidance in the treatment of these injuries, and early investigations focused on closed treatment using external nasal dressings following nasal manipulation. ORIF has proved to be an important advancement in the management of these fractures and, combined with proper reduction of the medial canthal tendon and primary nasal dorsum bone grafting, has improved the cosmetic result of even severe injuries.

A detailed classification scheme by Markowitz defined the injury pattern with respect to the medial canthal tendon and the fragment of bone upon which it inserts. Three distinct patterns are identified. A type I injury is the simplest form of NOE fracture and involves only one portion of the medial orbital rim with its attached medial canthal tendon. Type II fractures have a comminuted central fragment with the fracture lines remaining external to the medial canthal tendon insertion. Type III fractures have comminution involving the central fragment of bone where the medial canthal tendon inserts. Variants of type I, II, and III fractures may occur in bilateral fractures.

In a 1985 study by Holt, 67% of 727 patients with facial fractures sustained some degree of ocular injury, while most series report the incidence to be in the range of 20% to 25%. A high degree of suspicion should be present in patients with significant NOE fractures, and full fundoscopic examination should be accomplished. Slit-lamp examinations, when possible, allow evaluation of adnexal structures. The nasolacrimal apparatus may also be injured in about 20% of patients with NOE fractures.

NOE fractures are an uncommon but aesthetically challenging maxillofacial injury. The importance of precise reduction and primary bone grafting in the setting of inadequate dorsal nasal support and comminution cannot be overemphasized.

Bibliography

Ellis E III: Sequencing treatment for naso-orbito-ethmoid fractures, *J Oral Maxillofac Surg* 51:543-558, 1993.

Fedok FG: Comprehensive management of nasoethmoid-orbital injuries, *J Craniomaxillofac Trauma* 1:36-48, 1995.

Gruss JS: Naso-ethmoid-orbital fractures: classification and role of primary bone grafting, *Plast Reconstr Surg* 75:303-317, 1985.

Herford AS, Ying T, Brown B: Outcomes of severely comminuted (type III) nasoorbitoethmoid fractures, *J Oral Maxillofac Surg* 63:1266-1277, 2005.

Holt GR, Holt JE: Nasoethmoid complex injuries, *Otolaryngol Clin North Am* 18:87-98, 1985.

Leipziger LS, Manson PN: Nasoethmoid orbital fractures. Current concepts and management principles, *Clin Plast Surg* 19:167-193, 1992.

Markowitz BI, Manson PN, Sargent L, et al: Management of the medial canthal tendon in nasoethmoid orbital fractures: the importance of the central fragment in classification and treatment, *Plast Reconstr Surg* 87:843-853, 1991.

Sargent LA, Rogers GF: Nasoethmoid orbital fractures: diagnosis and management, *J Craniofac Trauma* 5:19-27, 1999.

Le Fort I Fracture

Martin B. Steed, DDS, and Shahrokh C. Bagheri, DMD, MD

CC

A 26-year-old man presents to the emergency department with the chief complaint of, "they hit my face with a brick and got my wallet. My face hurts . . . I was bleeding from my nose, but it has stopped."

HPI

You are called by the emergency department team to evaluate the patient. He reports being struck in the face at the level of his upper lip and teeth just below the nose by an unknown man who was walking the opposite way on the sidewalk (the vast majority of Le Fort I injuries are from blunt, as opposed to penetrating, trauma). He explains that he was hit one time in the face with a brick and subsequently fell to his knees, without any loss of consciousness (lower likelihood for intracranial injury in the absence of loss of consciousness).

PMHX/PDHX/MEDICATIONS/ALLERGIES/SH/FH

The patient smokes one pack of cigarettes daily and drinks alcohol regularly (both contribute to an increased relative risk of postoperative infections. A history of alcohol abuse is more frequently encountered in the trauma population). The remainder of his medical history is noncontributory.

EXAMINATION

The initial evaluation of a trauma patient should be completed by following the ATLS protocol.

Primary Survey

His primary survey is intact (control of the airway and hemorrhage are both part of the primary survey. Compromised airway and life-threatening hemorrhage are unlikely with isolated Le Fort I injuries; however, they can be seen with more complex facial fractures [higher FISS]).

Secondary Survey

General. The patient is a well-developed and well-nourished man in no apparent distress and holding a blood-soaked cloth under his nose.

Vitals. His blood pressure is 115/64 mm Hg, heart rate 115 bpm, respirations 12 per minute, and temperature 37.6°C (mild tachycardia can be due to a compensatory response to volume loss from prolonged oropharyngeal bleeding, and/or from the sympathetic response associated with pain and anxiety).

Eyes. Pupillary response, visual acuity, visual fields, and extraocular movements are all within normal limits (a complete eye examination is mandatory in all midface fractures). There is no evidence of subconjunctival hemorrhage or hyphema (blood in the anterior chamber of the eye).

Maxillofacial. The examination reveals moderate bilateral midface edema with left facial abrasions extending over the lip region. There is mild hypoesthesia of the bilateral infraorbital nerve distributions (cranial nerve V_2). The maxilla is mobile with no simultaneous movement of the nasal bones upon palpation (would be seen in Le Fort II or III injuries). Examination of the teeth reveals premature posterior occlusal contacts and a 5-mm anterior open bite (Figure 7-18). There is no evidence of mobile dentoalveolar segments. The remaining facial skeleton, including the nasal bones, is intact and stable upon palpation. Nasal speculum examination reveals a deviated nasal septum to the right, with no evidence of a septal hematoma (a hematoma needs to be drained to prevent subsequent necrosis of the septal cartilage and possible saddle-nose deformity).

IMAGING

The imaging modality of choice for the diagnosis and evaluation of suspected maxillary Le Fort I–level fractures is a noncontrast maxillofacial CT scan with thin cuts (axial views with coronal reconstructions). Direct coronal imaging or coronal reconstructions are helpful (patients with suspected cervical-spine injuries should not hyperextend the neck for direct coronal imaging).

For this patient, a facial helical CT scan without contrast was obtained after the primary and secondary surveys were completed. Axial bony window cuts show bilateral pterygoid plate, anterior and lateral maxillary wall, and posterior nasal septal fractures, with opacification of the maxillary antrum (Figure 7-19, *A*). A moderate amount of soft tissue edema and subcutaneous emphysema is noted. Coronal reconstruction views demonstrate bilateral fractures through the lateral walls of the maxillary sinuses (Figure 7-19, *B*). A three-dimensional reconstruction view allows clear visualization of the lines of fracture at the Le Fort I level (Figure 7-19, *C*).

LABS

A complete trauma panel was obtained and the results were remarkable for an elevated WBC count of 16,900 cells per microliter (increased WBCs or leukocytosis in the acute

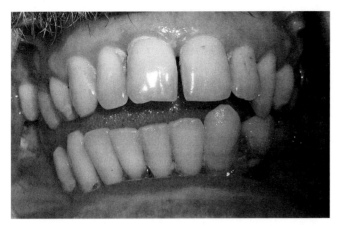

Figure 7-18 Posttraumatic anterior open bite and malocclusion.

setting is most likely secondary to physiological stress, due to catecholamine-induced demargination of WBCs).

ASSESSMENT

Isolated Le Fort I maxillary fracture; FISS of 2

TREATMENT

The goal of treatment of Le Fort I injuries is to reduce the displaced maxillary bone with its dentition to allow for uneventful healing, reestablishment of the patient's preexisting occlusal function, and aesthetics. Treatment of a particular fracture needs to be individualized and includes several options, mainly either ORIF or CR-MMF. The use of surgical splints should be considered, especially with segmental maxillary fractures. The degree of comminution at the anterior and lateral maxillary walls needs to be assessed for possible reconstructive measures.

To this date, most surgeons consider ORIF the gold standard. As a general principle, early reduction and fixation is preferable. After a 7- to 10-day period, some difficulty may be encountered in mobilizing the maxilla in order to achieve appropriate reduction, especially if the fracture is associated with significant impaction. Consideration should also be given to osteotomizing the maxilla if the fracture is incomplete or significant time has elapsed since the original insult. Attempting to mobilize the incompletely fractured maxilla can result in unfavorable fractures, often distant from the site of injury. After MMF is established, it is critical to establish passive reduction of the maxilla (maxillomandibular complex) with the condyles seated in a correct position; otherwise, an anterior open bite will develop after rigid fixation has been applied and the intermaxillary fixation is released. If adequate bone contact is available, plating system applied bilaterally at the piriform rims and zygomatic buttress areas is usually sufficient for stabilization. However, if more comminution is present and less bone contact is available, immediate bone grafting or secondary bone grafting reconstructive procedures should be considered.

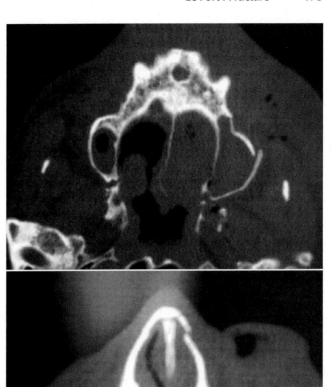

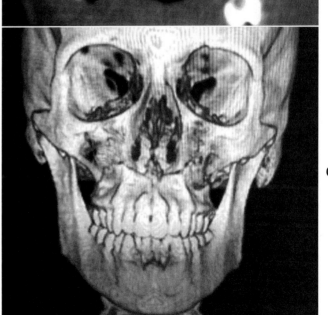

Figure 7-19 A, Preoperative axial bony CT window demonstrating fractures of the pterygoid plates, anterior maxillary walls, subcutaneous emphysema, and opacification of the maxillary sinuses. **B,** Preoperative coronal bony CT window through the anterior maxilla and nasal vault demonstrating fracture at the Le Fort I level. **C,** Preoperative anterior three-dimensional reconstruction demonstrating a horizontal fracture of the maxilla at the Le Fort I level.

In this patient, maxillomandibular arch bars were placed. An intraoral circumvestibular maxillary incision was made to gain access to the fractured segments. After appropriate mobilization of the maxilla, the patient was placed into MMF. The maxillomandibular complex was guided passively using the arc of rotation of the condyle into proper anatomical reduction, while the patient was paralyzed to ensure that the condyles are appropriately positioned (failure to seat the condyles may result in postoperative anterior open bite). The deviated septum was reduced onto the nasal crest of the maxilla and sutured to a hole drilled through the anterior nasal spine. Subsequently, the maxilla was stabilized with fixation at the piriform rim and ZM buttress regions bilaterally (four plates). MMF was then released, and the occlusion was found to be as planned and reproducible.

COMPLICATIONS

Complications of Le Fort I injuries are related to the severity of the initial injury, as well as host-related factors, but can be categorized into intraoperative, early, and late complications.

Intraoperative

- Bleeding can occur as a result of damage to any number of the vessels that are located in the vicinity, especially when significant disimpaction or an osteotomy is required for reduction of the segment. Potential sources of bleeding include the anterior and posterior superior alveolar, nasopalatine, and descending palatine arteries and, uncommonly, the internal maxillary artery. Packing, cauterization, and ligation are usually sufficient in controlling most situations. In cases where hemorrhage cannot be controlled, external carotid artery ligation can be performed. Arterial angiography with embolization should also be considered.

- Maxillary hypoperfusion is uncommon but can occur especially when the maxilla is fractured in multiple pieces and/or when surgical splints are used. Early reduction and stabilization with rigid internal fixation may help improve outcome. In addition, consideration should be given to positioning the maxilla back into the preoperative position (in trauma situations). Postoperative use of hyperbaric oxygen has been suggested, but its benefits remain unclear. If prefabricated occlusal splints are used, they should be checked to avoid impingement on the soft tissues (and possibly the blood supply) of the palate.

- Malpositioning of the maxilla can occur when the bony interferences are not appropriately evaluated and the maxillomandibular complex is not seated passively with the condyles in the correct position. This will result in a postoperative anterior open bite.

Early

- Control of nasal bleeding can be obtained in the immediate postoperative period by using a variety of techniques for nasal packing. A speculum and a good light source are essential in order to determine an anterior versus posterior origin. If adequate control is not achieved, exploration in the operating room or interventional radiology for angiographic evaluation may be necessary.

- Malocclusion can result from improper intraoperative maxillary positioning, early hardware failure, or undiagnosed mandibular or maxillary segmental fractures. Careful examination and appropriate imaging modalities help in discerning the etiology of malocclusion for surgical repositioning and refixation.

- Infraorbital nerve paresthesia can be the result of nerve injury at the initial trauma, especially when fracture patterns extend through the infraorbital foramen, or from intraoperative traction or manipulation for adequate reduction. Nasal septal deviation can result from improper repositioning of the nasal septum onto the nasal crest of the maxilla, undiagnosed nasal septal injuries, or preoperative septal deformities. This can result in increased airway resistance, nasolacrimal obstruction, and aesthetic complaints by the patient.

- Loss of vision can result from an unfavorable fracture pattern of the maxilla or from the initial trauma, compounded by surgical manipulation of the segment during repositioning. The orbital process of the palatine bone makes up a portion of the bony orbit and has been hypothesized as possible cause (this is very rare for Le Fort I fractures but more common with Le Fort III injuries).

- Early postoperative infection can result from foreign bodies, necrotic teeth, or bony segments but is also related to host factors (malnutrition, immunocompromised state, chronic alcohol use). Management should be directed at appropriate antibiotic selection, incision and drainage, and removal of any possible source.

Late

- Malocclusion, if not addressed early, will typically present with an anterior open bite, posterior premature contacts, and an overall Class III skeletal appearance. Once union has developed, small discrepancies can be treated with orthodontics, while larger ones will need to be addressed by orthognathic surgery.

- Late postoperative bleeding (especially with an intermittent pattern) should be taken seriously. Pseudoaneurysm formation should be high on the differential diagnosis and can be evaluated by angiography.

- Epiphora (excessive tearing) can result from damage or obstruction of the nasolacrimal duct (the nasolacrimal duct drains beneath the inferior turbinate 11 to 17 mm above the nasal floor and 11 to 14 mm posterior to the piriform aperture). Epiphora can be managed by a dacrocystorhinostomy procedure.

- Nonunion or fibrous union will cause the maxilla to demonstrate mobility, which can often be subtle. Management should be directed at refixating the maxilla with rigid internal fixation, skeletal fixation, extraskeletal fixation, and/or MMF.

DISCUSSION

Maxillary fractures most frequently occur as a result of blunt trauma from assault, sporting injuries, and motor vehicle accidents. They are frequently seen in conjunction with other facial and systemic injuries. The Le Fort classification is frequently used to describe midface fracture patterns. In 1901, Rene Le Fort published the results of his experiments based on 35 cadavers whose heads were subjected to different forms of force. Based on these findings, he concluded that the midface commonly fractures in three predictable patterns. A Le Fort level I fracture involves the anterior and lateral walls of the maxillary sinus, lateral nasal walls, the pterygoid plates, and the nasal septum (see Figure 7-25). It should be noted that isolated Le Fort fractures are relatively uncommon and that fractures occur in a variety of combinations of Le Fort I, II, or III with unilateral (hemi–Le Fort) and bilateral fractures. The "pure" Le Fort I fracture is typically bilateral and is composed of the maxilla with associated alveolar bone and part of the palatine bone posteriorly. Unilateral fractures are seen with an additional fracture between the midpalatal suture.

The blood supply to the maxilla is from the descending palatine artery, which contributes to the greater and lesser palatine arteries, the terminal branch of the nasopalatine artery, and from the anterior, middle, and posterior superior alveolar arteries. Extensive research has been done with regard to the blood supply of the fractured maxilla, mostly in association with orthognathic maxillary procedures. In experiments done by Bell and later by Bays and Dodson, it has been shown that the maxilla (along with its associated dentition and periodontium) maintains an adequate blood supply even after complete downfracture and ligation of the descending palatine artery. The maxilla remains pedicled to the palate receiving contributions from the ascending pharyngeal artery (a branch of the external carotid artery) and the ascending palatine artery (a branch of the facial artery), which in turn then anastomose with greater and lesser palatine arteries.

Patients with suspicion of maxillary fractures should be approached using the ATLS protocol. Because other bodily injuries may be present, the initial evaluation and stabilization of the patient are best performed by a trauma team experienced in the management of the multisystem trauma. Proper diagnosis should begin with careful history and physical examination. The mechanism of injury should be considered. Symptoms associated with a Le Fort I fracture may include facial pain, infraorbital hypoesthesia, malocclusion, or epistaxis. Clinical signs suggestive of a Le Fort I fracture include facial edema, ecchymosis, abrasions, lacerations, active epistaxis, palpable crepitus, mobile maxilla, and step deformities. Intraoral examination could identify fractured teeth, vestibular ecchymosis, mucosal lacerations, palatal edema and/or ecchymosis (especially with fractures associated with midpalatal suture), and malocclusion (typically, an anterior open bite with posterior occlusal premature contacts secondary to the vector of impact and the pull of lateral and medial pterygoid muscles).

Bibliography

Bagheri SC, Dierks EJ, Kademani D, et al: Comparison of the severity of bilateral Le Fort injuries in isolated midface trauma, *J Oral Maxillofac Surg* 63:1123-1129, 2005.

Bagheri SC, Dierks EJ, Kademani D, et al: Application of a Facial Injury Severity Scale in craniomaxillofacial trauma, *J Oral Maxillofac Surg* 64:404-414, 2006.

Bays RA: Complications of orthognathic surgery. In: Kaban LB, Pogrel MA, Perrott DH, et al, eds: *Complications in oral and maxillofacial surgery,* Philadelphia, 1997, WB Saunders, pp 193-221.

Bays RA, Reinkingh MR, Maron G: Descending palatine artery ligation in LeFort osteotomies, *J Oral Maxillofac Surg* 51(suppl): 142, 1993.

Bell WH: Revascularization and bone healing after anterior maxillary osteotomy, *J Oral Surg* 27:249, 1969.

Bell WH, Fonseca RJ, Kennedy JW, et al: Bone healing and revascularization after total maxillary osteotomy, *J Oral Surg* 33:253, 1975.

Bell WH, Levy BM: Revascularization and bone healing after posterior maxillary osteotomy, *J Oral Surg* 29:313, 1971.

Cunningham LL Jr, Haug RH: Management of maxillary fractures. In: Miloro M, Ghali GE, Larsen PE, et al, eds: *Peterson's principles of oral and maxillofacial surgery,* ed 2, Hamilton, Ontario, 2004, BC Decker, pp 435-443.

Dodson TB, Bays RA, Biederman GA: In-vivo measurement of gingival blood flow following LeFort I osteotomy, *J Dent Res* 71:603, 1992.

Dodson TB, Bays RA, Neuenshwander MC: Maxillary perfusion during LeFort I osteotomy after ligation of the descending palatine artery, *J Oral Maxillofac Surg* 55:51-55, 1997.

Dodson TB, Neuenschwander MC, Bays RA: Intraoperative assessment of maxillary perfusion during LeFort I osteotomy, *J Oral Maxillofac Surg* 54:827, 1994.

Dodson TB, Neuenschwander MC, Bays RA: Intraoperative measurement of maxillary gingival blood flow during LeFort I osteotomy, *J Oral Maxillofacial Surg* 51(suppl 3):138, 1993.

Ellis E III: Passive repositioning of maxillary fractures, *J Oral Maxillofac Surg* 62:1477-1485, 2004.

Gruss JS, Mackinson SE: Complex maxillary fractures: role of buttress reconstruction and immediate bone grafts, *Plast Reconstr Surg* 78:9, 1986.

Gruss JS, Philips JH: Complex facial trauma: the evolving role of rigid fixation and immediate bone graft reconstruction, *Clin Plast Surg* 16:93-104, 1989.

Haug RH, Adams JM, Jordan RB: Comparison of the morbidity with maxillary fractures treated by maxillomandibular and rigid internal fixation, *Oral Surg* 80:629, 1995.

Iida S, Kogo M, Sugiura T, et al: Retrospective analysis of 1502 patients with facial fractures, *Int J Oral Maxillofac Surg* 30:286-90, 2001.

Lew D, Sinn DP: Diagnosis and treatment of midface fractures. In: Fonseca RJ, Walker RV, Betts NJ, et al, eds: *Oral and maxillofacial trauma,* ed 2, Philadelphia, 1997, WB Saunders, pp 661-667.

Perciaccante VJ, Bays RA: Maxillary orthognathic surgery. In: Miloro M, Ghali GE, Larsen PE, et al, eds: *Peterson's principles of oral and maxillofacial surgery,* ed 2, Hamilton, Ontario, 2004, BC Decker, pp 1179-1204.

Plaiser BR, Punjabi AP, Super DM, Haug RH: The relationship between facial fractures and death from neurologic injury, *J Oral Maxillofac Surg* 58:708-712, 2000.

Top H, Aygit C, Sarikay A, et al: Evaluation of maxillary sinus after treatment of midfacial fractures, *J Oral Maxillofac Surg* 62:1229-1236, 2004.

Vaughan ED, Obeid G, Banks P: The irreducible middle third fracture: a problem in management, *Br J Oral Surg* 21:124, 1983.

You ZH, Bell WH, Finn RA: Location of the nasolacrimal canal in relation to the high Le Fort I osteotomy, *J Oral Maxillofac Surg* 50:1075-1080, 1992.

Le Fort II Fracture

Martin B. Steed, DDS, and Chris Jo, DMD

CC

A 43-year-old man arrives via EMS responders at the emergency department status post high-speed motor vehicle collision and has complaints of headache and pain in the mid and lower face (blunt trauma [motor vehicle collision, assault] is the most common etiology of Le Fort II injuries).

HPI

The patient was the unrestrained passenger seat occupant in a head-on collision with a telephone pole, without loss of consciousness (negative loss of consciousness reduces the likelihood of a closed head injury) or prolonged extrication. The patient had a GCS score of 15 at the field. He was transported to the state Level I trauma hospital via ambulance for complete assessment and evaluation. You are consulted to evaluate the patient for his facial injuries.

PMHX/PDHX/MEDICATIONS/ALLERGIES/SH/FH

His past medical history is significant for hypertension, which is controlled with metoprolol (β_1-selective blocker [cardioselective]).

EXAMINATION

The initial evaluation of a trauma patient should be completed by following the ATLS protocol.

Primary Survey

There were no significant findings (control of the airway and hemorrhage are both part of the primary survey. Compromised airway and life-threatening hemorrhage are unlikely with isolated Le Fort I or II injuries; however, they can be seen with more complex facial fractures [higher FISS]). In a series of 22 patients with isolated Le Fort II injuries, Bagheri and associates reported that two patients (9%) required a tracheostomy, one (4.5%) required neurosurgical intervention, and one (4.5%) patient died as a consequence of the facial trauma.

Secondary Survey

General. The patient is a well-developed and well-nourished male in no apparent distress, with a transport cervical-collar in place (Figure 7-20). He has a GCS score of 15. He is alert and oriented to time, place, and person.

Maxillofacial. There is moderate bilateral midface and periorbital edema with left facial abrasions extending over the left lip. There is significant periorbital ecchymoses (left greater than right). Bony crepitus is detected upon palpation at the nasofrontal junction and nasal bones (indicative of nasal bone fractures). The maxilla is grossly mobile (indicative of a Le Fort fracture). There is mobility and increased bony crepitance at the nasofrontal junction upon mobilizing the maxilla with bimanual manipulation (indicative of a Le Fort II or III fracture pattern). There are step deformities and pain upon palpation at the inferior orbital rims bilaterally (consistent with a Le Fort II fracture). There are no step deformities, bony crepitus, or pain upon palpation at the lateral orbital rims or zygomatic arches bilaterally (reduces the likelihood of ZMC or Le Fort III fractures). There is hypoesthesia along the infraorbital nerve distribution bilaterally (commonly seen after fractures of the anterior maxillary wall, inferior orbital rim, and orbital floor).

Intraoral and occlusion. The dentition is in good repair. There is a 4-mm anterior open bite and bilateral posterior prematurities (indicative of maxillary or mandibular fractures). The dentoalveolar segments are stable (rules out dentoalveolar fracture). The mandible is stable, without any signs of fracture (pain, ecchymoses, step deformity, bony crepitance, mobility, or deviation).

Eyes. Extraocular movements are intact, and pupils are equal round and reactive to light and accommodation (PERRLA). Visual acuity is 20/20 in both eyes (OS and OD). There is no subconjunctival hemorrhage or hyphema (blood in the anterior chamber of the eye), and there is no proptosis or enophthalmos. Fundoscopic examination reveals no abnormalities.

Intranasal. There is bright red blood in the bilateral nasal cavities. The nasal septum is deviated to the right with no evidence of a septal hematoma.

IMAGING

Mandatory trauma plain-film radiographic series in the acute setting include cross-table cervical-spine, portable anteroposterior chest radiography, and an anteroposterior pelvis radiograph. Other studies are added as needed, including cervical-spine series (in suspected cervical-spine injury), thoracic and lumbar spine series (indicated in motor vehicle collisions with ejection, in rollover accidents, or in symptomatic patients), and extremity radiographs (when fracture or dislocation is suspected).

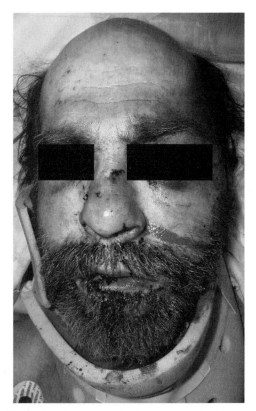

Figure 7-20   A patient immediately upon arrival to the emergency department. Note is made of the bilateral periorbital ecchymoses and midfacial edema.

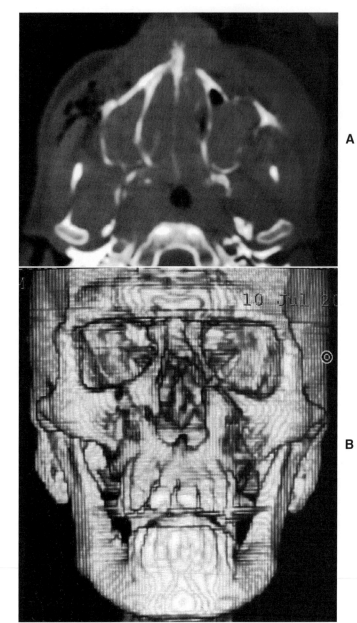

Figure 7-21   A, Preoperative coronal bony CT window demonstrating fractures of the pterygoid plates, comminuted fracture of the bilateral maxillary anterior walls, subcutaneous emphysema, and fluid levels within the bilateral maxillary sinuses. **B,** Preoperative anterior three-dimensional reconstruction demonstrating a pyramidal fracture (Le Fort II level) with fractures of the maxilla extending superiorly to the bilateral orbital rims and through the medial lower third of the orbits onto the nasal frontal junction.

Axial-cut bony window CT scans (with or without coronal reconstructions) are the gold standard radiographic examination for midfacial fractures. Direct coronals are useful but should be avoided in patients with suspected cervical-spine injury (patient's head needs to be hyperextended for direct coronal CT). Three-dimensional reconstructions are helpful adjuncts as they provide the most graphic representation of the fractures, degree of displacement, and orientation of fragments.

A facial helical CT scan without contrast was obtained after the primary and secondary surveys were completed. Axial bony windows showed bilateral fractures extending through the pterygoid plates, the anterior and lateral maxillary walls, and an air-fluid level in the bilateral maxillary sinuses (consistent with blood in the sinuses). A moderate amount of soft tissue edema and emphysema is noted (Figure 7-21, *A*). Coronal views revealed bilateral infraorbital rim fractures continuing posteriorly through the medial orbital walls and separation of the nasofrontal suture. Sagittal views demonstrated a left orbital floor defect. Three-dimensional reconstruction views allow clear visualization of the lines of fracture (Figure 7-21, *B*).

arterial blood gas, urine analysis, and coagulation studies (PT/PTT/INR). A urine drug screen and blood alcohol level can be of value. In this patient, all laboratory values were within normal limits.

LABS

Standard laboratory tests for the evaluation of multisystem trauma patients included CBC, complete metabolic panel,

ASSESSMENT

Isolated midface fracture consistent with the Le Fort II pattern, with concomitant left orbital floor defect and dis-

placed nasal septal fracture; FISS score of 5 (Le Fort II fracture = 4, orbital floor fracture = 1)

TREATMENT

A variety of treatment modalities have been advocated for the treatment of Le Fort II–level fractures, but they are generally categorized into open versus closed reduction techniques, or a combination of the two. The majority of Le Fort–type fractures commonly occur in conjunction with other facial, neurological, or orthopedic injuries. Among many factors, each case is treated based on the individual fracture patterns, medical comorbidities, associated systemic trauma, status of the airway, hemorrhage, and available resources. Several factors that are important in the management of Le Fort II injuries are outlined here. (Readers are advised to also refer to the Le Fort I and III and panfacial fracture cases discussed in this chapter.)

- Le Fort fractures that are complicated by a palatal fracture may benefit from the use of surgical splints, to achieve an optimal postoperative occlusion.
- The degree of comminution at the anterior and lateral maxillary walls may complicate reduction at the ZM buttress. This may require immediate or secondary bone grafting techniques.
- The absence of mandible fractures and an intact dentition significantly facilitates the treatment of this (and most midface injuries involving the dentate segments). Placement of the patient in intermaxillary fixation will allow accurate alignment of the midface structures. In the presence of mandible fracture(s), treatment needs to be dictated by anatomical alignment at stable segments.
- All fracture sites do not need to be visualized or fixated for proper alignment of the segments. Adequate fixation at the bilateral ZM and/or orbital rim areas may alleviate the need for fixation at the nasofrontal suture (thereby avoiding a coronal or other unsightly incisions). If the segment is unstable despite fixation at these areas, exposure of the nasofrontal area may be necessary using a variety of approaches (coronal, upper blepharoplasty, lynch, direct, or existing lacerations).
- A maxillary vestibular incision provides access to the ZM buttresses and can frequently provide sufficient access to the inferior orbital rims for alignment and fixation. Various periorbital incisions (transconjunctival with or without lateral canthotomy and subciliary incisions are the most commonly used) can provide access to the inferior orbital rim and orbital floor.
- Commonly, midface fractures are comminuted Le Fort patterns that require additional fixation of the fragmented segments in a "stable to unstable" fashion. Infrequently, immediate bone grafting to reconstruct severely comminuted or avulsed bony segments is required.
- The airway should be secured for safe anesthetic administration, optimal surgical care, ease of intubation, and decreased morbidity. In cases of severe midface fractures, early tracheostomy may be necessary. Unstable midface structures and posterior nasopharyngeal hemorrhage can make intubation challenging. Management of the intraoperative airway must be anticipated as patients with Le Fort II fractures often necessitate both MMF and nasal septal correction, making the choice between oral and nasal tubes difficult. Submental intubation techniques can be considered via a transcutaneous incision penetrating the anterior floor of the mouth.

This patient underwent an awake fiberoptic intubation with a nasoendotracheal tube. There was no severe bleeding into the oropharynx. The tube was changed to an oral tube during the case to allow correction of the nasal septum after the bone fractures were reduced and fixated. Care must be taken in placing nasoendotracheal tubes in patients with midface fractures that may have basilar skull components, as there have been isolated reports of intracranial placement of the endotracheal tube.

ORIF of the maxilla was accomplished in concert with closed treatment of the nasal bone fracture. An intraoral circumvestibular maxillary incision was made to gain access to the fractured maxillary segments. Bilateral transconjunctival incisions with lateral canthotomy and cantholysis were also used to gain access to the bilateral infraorbital rim region and allow for proper reduction and stabilization of the infraorbital rims (Figure 7-22, *A*). The left orbital floor was explored and a 1.5 × 2-cm floor defect was reconstructed using a titanium mesh. No direct visualization of the nasofrontal junction was necessary in this case, and the nasal bones were reduced in a closed manner. Upon appropriate maxillary mobilization, proper reduction was achieved after the establishment of MMF. The maxillomandibular complex was manipulated passively into proper reduction, while ensuring that the condylar heads were appropriately positioned. The nasal tube was then changed to an oral endotracheal tube to allow easier manipulation of the nasal complex. The deviated septum was not reduced easily (may be indicative of preexisting nasal septal deformity), necessitating a Killian incision and subperichondrium dissection with judicious septal cartilage resection. This allowed for ideal reduction of the septum. Subsequently, the maxilla was stabilized with four-point fixation (at the right piriform rim, bilateral infraorbital rims, and bilateral ZM buttress regions. Secondary to good bone contact, L-shaped and curved plates were used from a 2.0-mm plating set (Figure 7-22, *B*). MMF was then released and occlusion was found to be stable and reproducible. The incisions were meticulously closed. The nose was stabilized with a Denver splint (thermoplastic splints can also be used). A postoperative posteroanterior radiograph demonstrates the position of the rigid fixation plates (Figure 7-23).

COMPLICATIONS

Complications of Le Fort II injuries are related to the severity of the initial injury and host-related factors but can be categorized into intraoperative, early, and late complications.

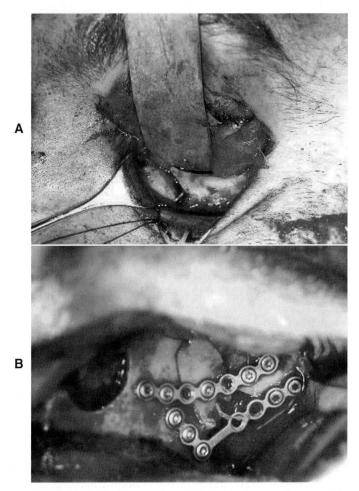

Figure 7-22 **A,** Transconjunctival approach to expose the right infraorbital rim fracture for alignment and fixation. **B,** Plating of the left maxillary buttress through a maxillary vestibular incision.

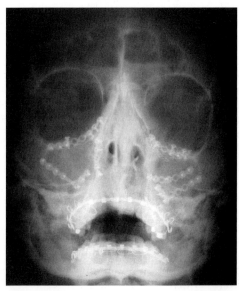

Figure 7-23 Postoperative posterior-anterior radiograph demonstrating reduction and fixation of the Le Fort II fracture.

Intraoperative

- Bleeding can occur as a result of damage to any number of the vessels that are located in the vicinity, especially when significant disimpaction or an osteotomy is required for reduction of the segment. Potential sources of bleeding include the anterior and posterior superior alveolar, nasopalatine, and descending palatine arteries and, uncommonly, the internal maxillary artery. Packing, cauterization, and ligation are usually sufficient in controlling most situations. In cases where hemorrhage cannot be controlled, external carotid artery ligation can be performed. However, arterial angiography with embolization should be strongly considered.

- Maxillary hypoperfusion is uncommon but can occur, especially when the maxilla is fractured in multiple pieces, and/or when surgical splints that impinge on the palatal mucosa compromise the blood flow are utilized. Early reduction and stabilization with rigid internal fixation may help improve the outcome. Postoperative use of hyperbaric oxygen has been suggested, but its benefits remain unclear. If prefabricated occlusal splints are used, they should be checked to avoid impingement on the soft tissues of the palate.

- Malpositioning of the maxilla can occur when the bony interferences are not appropriately evaluated and the maxillomandibular complex is not seated passively with the condyles in correct position. This results in a postoperative anterior open bite. Infrequently, osteotomies are required to completely disimpact and reduce the midface.

Early

- In the immediate postoperative period, control of nasal bleeding can be obtained using a variety of nasal packs. A nasal speculum and a good light source are essential in order to determine the anterior or posterior origin. If adequate control is not achieved, exploration in the operating room or interventional radiology for angiographic evaluation may be necessary.

- Malocclusion can result from improper intraoperative maxillary positioning, early hardware failure, or undiagnosed mandibular or maxillary segmental fractures. Thorough examination and appropriate imaging modalities help in discerning the etiology of malocclusion for surgical repositioning and refixation.

- Nasal septal deviation can result from improper repositioning of the nasal septum onto the septal crest of the maxilla, undiagnosed nasal septal injuries, or preoperative septal deformities. The septum is by definition fractured in Le Fort II injuries, and special care must be taken to identify and reduce deviations.

- Loss of vision can result from an unfavorable fracture pattern of the maxilla or from the initial trauma, compounded by surgical manipulation of the segment during repositioning. The orbital process of the palatine bone makes up a portion of the bony orbit and has been hypothesized as a possible cause.

- Early postoperative infection can result from foreign bodies, necrotic teeth, or bony segments but is also related to host factors. Management should be directed at appropriate antibiotic selection, incision and drainage, and, when possible, removal of the source.

Late

- Malocclusion, if not addressed early, will typically present with an anterior open bite, posterior premature contacts, and an overall Class III skeletal appearance. Once union has developed, small discrepancies can be treated with orthodontics, while larger ones need to be addressed by orthognathic surgery.
- Late postoperative bleeding (especially with an intermittent pattern) should be taken seriously. Pseudoaneurysm formation should be high on the differential diagnosis and can be evaluated by angiography.
- Epiphora (excessive tearing) can result from damage or obstruction of the nasolacrimal duct (the nasolacrimal duct drains beneath the inferior turbinate 11 to 17 mm above the nasal floor and 11 to 14 mm posterior to the piriform aperture). Epiphora can be managed by a dacrocystorhinostomy procedure.
- Nonunion or fibrous union will cause the maxilla to demonstrate mobility, which can be subtle. Management should be directed at rigidly refixating the maxilla with rigid internal fixation, skeletal fixation, and/or MMF.

DISCUSSION

Patients with a suspected maxillary fracture should be approached in a manner consistent with ATLS protocol. The initial evaluation and stabilization of the patient are best performed by a trauma team experienced in the management of the multisystem trauma patient. Airway management in patients sustaining a Le Fort II injury is paramount as patients with higher-level Le Fort injuries have less readily accessible sources or bleeding, often mandating a surgical airway. Clinicians treating midface trauma should be prepared to establish a surgical airway both acutely and in more controlled settings.

The proper diagnosis should begin with careful history and physical examination. The mechanism of injury should be carefully assessed and obtained from the patient in detail. In a review of isolated midface fractures by Bagheri and colleagues, a statistically significant difference in the Injury Severity Score was detected between patients with Le Fort I versus II or III injuries. In their series of 67 patients, 3 patients (4.5%) died—1 patient with a Le Fort II (Injury Severity Score of 24) and two with Le Fort III fractures (both with an Injury Severity Score of 35). In addition, patients with Le Fort II or III fractures had a significantly higher probability of intensive care unit admission or immediate operative intervention (86.4% and 82.1%, respectively) than did patients with Le Fort I injuries (50%). This may be reflective of more severe airway compromise, uncontrollable hemorrhage, or neurosurgical complications.

Symptoms associated with a Le Fort II fracture include facial pain, infraorbital hypoesthesia (which usually results secondary to direct trauma to the infraorbital nerve or from the surrounding edema), malocclusion, and epistaxis. Clinical signs suggestive of a Le Fort II fracture include facial edema, ecchymosis, abrasions, lacerations, active epistaxis, palpable crepitus, and step deformities at the bilateral infraorbital rims. Intraoral examination should identify fractured teeth, vestibular ecchymosis, mucosal lacerations, palatal edema and/or ecchymosis (especially with fractures associated with mid-palatal suture), and malocclusion (typically, an anterior open bite with posterior occlusal premature contacts secondary to the vector of impact and the pull of lateral and medial pterygoid muscles).

Maxillary fractures at the Le Fort II level are pyramidal in shape. They involve the nasal bones, maxilla (including pterygoid plates), orbital rim, palatine bones, and the lower two-thirds of the nasal septum zygoma. The base of the pyramid is the pterygoid plates, and the fracture lines extend superiorly through the ZM suture and the medial inferior third of the nasal bones and cross the midline at the nasofrontal suture.

Treatment is analogous to that of other Le Fort injuries, but special attention must be given to early control of the airway and hemorrhage and correct surgical management of the orbital component, nasal complex, and nasal septum.

Bibliography

Bagheri SC, Dierks EJ, Kademani D, et al: Comparison of the severity of bilateral Le Fort injuries in isolated midface trauma, *J Oral Maxillofac Surg* 63:1123-1129, 2005.

Baker SP, O'Neill B, Haddon W Jr, et al: The Injury Severity Score: a method for describing patients with multiple injuries and evaluating emergency care, *J Trauma* 14:187, 1974.

Haug RH, Adams JM, Conforti PJ, et al: Cranial fractures associated with facial fractures: a review of mechanism, type and severity of injury, *J Oral Maxillofac Surg* 52:729, 1994.

Haug RH, Prather J, Indresano AT: An epidemiologic survey of facial fractures and concomitant injuries, *J Oral Maxillofac Surg* 48:926, 1990.

Haug RH, Savage JD, Likavek MJ, et al: A review of 100 closed head injuries associated with facial fractures, *J Oral Maxillofac Surg* 50:218, 1992.

Haug RH, Wible RT, Likavek MJ, et al: Cervical spine fractures and maxillofacial trauma, *J Oral Maxillofac Surg* 49:725, 1991.

Lee FK, Wagner LK, Lee YE, et al: The impact-absorbing effects of facial fractures in closed-head injuries, *J Neurosurg* 66:542, 1987.

Le Fort R: Etude experimentale sur les fractures de la machoire superieure, *Rev Chir Paris* 23:208, 1901.

Ng M, Saadat D, Sinha UK: Managing the emergency airway in Le Fort fractures, *J Craniomaxillofac Trauma* 4:38, 1998.

Plasier BR, Punjabi AP, Super DM, et al: The relationship between facial fractures and death from neurologic injury, *J Oral Maxillofac Surg* 58:708, 2000.

Smoot EC 3rd, Jernigan JR, Kinsley E, et al: A survey of operative airway management practices for midface fractures, *J Craniofac Surg* 8:201, 1997.

Tessier P: The classic reprint. Experimental study of fractures of the upper jaw. Rene Le Fort M.D., *Plast Reconstr Surg* 50:497, 1972.

Turvey TA: Midfacial fractures: a retrospective analysis of 593 cases, *J Oral Surg* 35:887-891, 1977.

Le Fort III Fracture

Chris Jo, DMD, Shahrokh C. Bagheri, DMD, MD, and Martin B. Steed, DDS

CC

A 37-year-old man is transported to the emergency department by EMS personnel status post motor vehicle accident (most common etiology of Le Fort III injures). You are called down to the trauma bay for evaluation of facial injuries.

HPI

The patient was an unrestrained driver (higher risk for more severe facial injuries) involved in a high-speed, head-on collision with another vehicle. There was no roll-over or ejection (lower risk of cervical, thoracic and lumbar spine injury), but significant damage was done to the front side of the car with 6-inch intrusion and steering wheel deformity (evidence of significant energy transfer to the head and neck). Upon arrival of the EMS personnel, the patient was hunched over the steering wheel and had a GCS score of 13. Fifteen minutes later (rapid transport time has reduced prehospital morbidity) at the emergency department, his primary survey was intact, vital signs were consistent with mild volume loss (tachycardia and hypotension), and a repeat GCS score was 11 (moderate head injury). He recalls striking the steering wheel with his upper face and admits to loss of consciousness for an unknown period of time (indicative of a closed head injury). Otherwise, he does not recall the events surrounding the accident. Secondary to decreasing mental status and uncontrolled nasopharyngeal hemorrhage, the patient was orally intubated with in-line cervical spine stabilization in the emergency department (approximately 40% of patients with Le Fort III injuries require advanced airway interventions).

PMHX/PDHX/MEDICATIONS/ALLERGIES/SH/FH

The patient's histories are unknown (when possible, information may be obtained from family members).

EXAMINATION

ATLS Primary Survey

Airway and cervical spine control. The patient was orally intubated with a transport cervical-collar in place. (In a review of 563 patients with maxillofacial injuries, Haug and colleagues found that concomitant cervical-spine fractures occurred in 2% of patients. Of those with cervical-spine fractures, 91% had mandibular fractures. Bagheri and associates found a 1.5% incidence of cervical-spine fractures in a series of 67 patients with isolated midface fractures.)

Breathing and oxygenation. He was intubated and on mechanical ventilation with clear and equal breath sounds bilaterally and with oxygen saturation of 99% on an FIO_2 of 100%.

Circulation and hemorrhage control. His blood pressure is 105/71 mm Hg and heart rate of 115 bpm (mild hypotension and tachycardia are indicative of mild volume depletion; Class II hypovolemic shock is indicative of 15% to 30% blood volume loss, which is characterized by a normal mean arterial blood pressure, decreased pulse pressure, decreased urine output [20 to 30 ml/hr], and anxiety). Moderate hemorrhage was observed in the nasopharynx and oral cavity (blood pooling in the nasopharynx can arise from the posterior, commonly from Woodruff's plexus, or anteriorly from Kiesselbach's plexus. Nasal bleeds can be a source of significant blood loss if not controlled). The oral and nasal cavities were rapidly packed to control the acute hemorrhage (hemorrhage control and fluid resuscitation are initiated). Control of hemorrhage and adequacy of resuscitation must be frequently reassessed. This patient responded well to a 2-L bolus of lactated Ringer's, and the anteroposterior nasal packs controlled the bleeding.

Disability and dysfunction. On the AVPU scale (A, awake; V, responds to voice; P, responds to pain; U, unresponsive) assessment, the patient is responsive to pain. His GCS score was E3, M5, V1T = 9T. The right pupil is 4 mm and reactive, and the left pupil is flaccid with irregular and nonreactive (indicative of globe rupture). Sedation should be discontinued for an accurate assessment of mental status as needed.

Exposure and environmental control. The patient's clothing is removed, and a warm blanket or other warming devices are used to prevent hypothermia.

ATLS Secondary Survey

Allergy—*m*edications—*p*ast medical history—*l*ast meal—*e*vents leading to presentation (A-M-P-L-E) history is taken from available sources.

General. The patient is a well-developed man who is intubated and sedated, with a cervical-collar in place.

Neurological. There is no evidence of cerebrospinal fluid rhinorrhea or otorrhea; the GCS score is 9T. Sequential neurological examination of the intubated patient is more challenging than that in the conscious patient. All sedation should be withheld before the neurological evaluation. For this reason, propofol is the sedative drug of choice, allowing for rapid emergence and hourly AVPU assessment and GCS scoring. Pupils are checked for size and responsiveness (large, unresponsive pupils are indicative of increased intracranial pressure). Motor strength and responsiveness are assessed on all four extremities (motor weakness can be indicative of intracranial or spinal derangement). In the intubated patient, a high index of suspicion for intracranial hemorrhage and edema should be maintained. Any acute deterioration in neurological status warrants a STAT head CT or an intracranial monitoring device. An initially low-yield neurological examination (unconscious and unresponsive), the need for deep sedation, paralysis, or severe head injury with evidence of elevated intracranial pressure warrants an intracranial pressure–monitoring device.

Eyes. There is significant periorbital edema, with OS greater than OD. OD examination shows a pupil that is round, reactive, and sluggish (4 mm → 2 mm). OS examination shows a pupil that is large, irregular, and nonreactive, and the globe is flaccid (ruptured globe). Visual acuity cannot be assessed. There is severe bilateral periorbital ecchymosis (raccoon eyes, indicative of anterior basilar skull fracture).

Maxillofacial. The examination shows significant facial edema and ecchymosis, with step deformity at the lateral orbital rims bilaterally and at the nasofrontal junction with notable crepitus. Infraorbital rims are intact without step deformities. The maxilla is grossly mobile with associated mobility and crepitus palpated at the nasofrontal junction and lateral orbital rims bilaterally (indicative of maxillary/midface disjunction at the Le Fort III level). Intercanthal distance is 32 mm with a negative bowstring test (normal intercanthal distance is 30 to 34 mm and varies between races [increased for African and Asian descent] and gender [females less than males] depending on the study). There is no dystopia (disturbance in globe position relative to the normal globe position in the vertical and horizontal planes) or enophthalmos (loss of anteroposterior projection in globe position) (however, enophthalmos and dystopia are hard to assess in the presence of significant edema). Tympanic membranes are clear and intact, and there is no Battle's sign (ecchymosis in the mastoid region indicative of posterior basilar skull fracture). There is a laceration of the lower face that involves the full thickness of the lip (8 cm) and multiple other abrasions.

Intraoral. Occlusion is difficult to assess secondary to orotracheal intubation. Ecchymosis at the posterior soft palate bilaterally (Guerin's sign, indicative of pterygoid plate disjunction/fracture). The mandible is stable, without step deformities. The dentition is in good repair.

IMAGING

Mandatory trauma plain-film radiographic series in the acute setting include cross-table cervical-spine, portable anteroposterior chest radiography, and an anteroposterior pelvis radiograph. Other studies are added as needed, including cervical-spine series (in suspected cervical-spine injury), thoracic and lumbar spine series (indicated in motor vehicle accident with ejection or roll-over or in symptomatic patients),

and extremity radiographs (when fracture or dislocation is suspected).

Axial-cut bony window CT scanning (with coronal reconstructions) is the gold standard radiographic examination for midfacial fractures. Direct coronal views are useful but should be avoided in patients with suspected cervical-spine injury (patients head needs to be hyperextended for direct coronal CT). Three-dimensional reconstructions are helpful adjuncts as they provide the most graphic representation of the fractures, degree of displacement, and orientation of fragments.

In this patient, CT studies reveal fracture lines extending from the nasofrontal suture through the medial wall of the orbit and the superior orbital fissure, along the lateral orbital wall in the area of the ZF suture, extending along the ZS suture, and ending at a separation of the pterygomaxillary junction (pterygoid plates). There is also a fracture of the zygomatic arches bilaterally (near the ZT sutures). This is a classic description of a pure Le Fort III fracture pattern.

An initial head CT for baseline evaluation and follow-up repeat scan are warranted for patients at risk for intracranial hemorrhage. In this patient, this is indicated due to the loss of consciousness and decreased mental status (as measured by GCS). His scan demonstrated bifrontal lobe contusions with no epidural or subdural hematomas. There was no evidence of increased intracranial pressure by CT scan. An interval head CT showed no evolution of the intracranial injury (Intracranial injury is the most common concomitant injury, seen in up to 50% of cases with midfacial fractures). An initial head CT that is negative may require a repeat head CT at 12 to 24 hours (closed head injuries may not have early CT findings and may likely present after 24 hours).

LABS

Standard laboratory tests for the evaluation of multisystem trauma patients included CBC, complete metabolic panel, arterial blood gas, urine analysis, and coagulation studies (PT/PTT/INR). A urine drug screen and blood alcohol level are indicated in patients with decreased mental status.

This patient demonstrated decreased hemoglobin (11.2 g/dl) and hematocrit (32.6%) (indicative of blood loss and fluid resuscitation). Arterial blood gas analysis showed a mild base deficit −3.5 (base deficit is one of the parameters monitored for adequacy of resuscitation in hypovolemic shock and is a better indicator of acute blood loss than hemoglobin/hematocrit). There was also a mild elevation in his blood urea nitrogen and creatinine (indicative of prerenal azotemia secondary to blood loss) and a positive blood alcohol level (common in the trauma patients). The remainder of his laboratory tests were within normal limits.

ASSESSMENT

Isolated midface fracture consistent with the Le Fort III pattern complicated by significant nasopharyngeal hemorrhage, closed head injury, a ruptured left globe, and laceration of the lower face and lip; FISS score of 6

TREATMENT

Treatment of the patient begins with the ATLS protocol. Establishment of a secure airway, cervical-spine stabilization, and control of hemorrhage from the maxillofacial region is paramount. An emergency surgical airway may be necessary (discussed later) if oral endotracheal intubation fails. Intubation can be difficult due to the altered anatomy, edema, and hemorrhage from the nasopharynx. For posterior nasal hemorrhage, posterior nasal packing can be used to tamponade the bleeding; a variety of methods and equipment can be used. A Foley catheter or cuffed endotracheal tube can be carefully inserted into the nares and passed beyond the nasopharynx; the balloons are then inflated, and the catheter/tube is advanced out until the balloons are snug against the posterior nasal aperture. Anterior nasal packing can also be achieved by various methods, including ribbons, sponges, or plain gauze. Special anteroposterior nasal packs are available (e.g., Rhino Rocket; Shippert Medical) but are more expensive and not readily available in all emergency departments or operating rooms. Figure 7-24 shows a patient with bilateral Le Fort III fracture with cervical-collar and a tracheostomy in place, a ruptured left globe, and multiple nasal and oral packings.

A single-piece Le Fort III fracture is a relatively simple (but less common) fracture to reduce and rigidly fixate than a comminuted fracture. Reduction should be achieved at the lateral orbital rim (ZF suture area), nasofrontal region, and zygomatic arch (ZT suture area). Not all reduced areas need to be rigidly fixated. The locations, amount, and size of fixation vary among surgeons and also depend on the severity of the displacement. With the advent of miniplate rigid fixation,

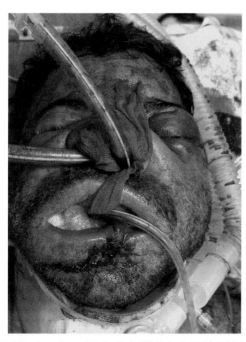

Figure 7-24 A patient with Le Fort III fracture with multiple nasal and oral packing used to control posterior nasal and pharyngeal hemorrhage. The airway has been secured with a tracheostomy.

the need for wire fixation has become obsolete. A key and often challenging step in the surgical correction of Le Fort fractures is disimpaction of the maxillofacial unit to allow passive positioning of the segment. This can be achieved by different techniques. The Rowe disimpaction forceps is a popular instrument used for mobilizing and reducing the maxillary unit.

After the maxillary segment is mobilized, the patient is placed into MMF, and the intact mandibular arch of rotation is used to determine the anatomical reduction of the facial and cranial units. Intraoperative MMF may not be possible in the setting of orally placed endotracheal tube. Oral intubation can be done if there is an edentulous space, where the endotracheal tube can pass with the patient in MMF, or via a submental intubation technique, where the endotracheal tube is passed through the floor of the mouth and exits the skin in the submental space. Nasotracheal intubation or tracheotomy are alternative options. If prolonged postoperative intubation is expected, a tracheotomy would be favored. If the patient is expected to be extubated at the completion of the procedure, consideration should be given to nasotracheal intubation. There are isolated reports of gastric or nasoendotracheal tubes being passed intracranially in patients with severe facial fractures that include the base of skull. However, there is insufficient evidence to exclude this technique in the hands of skilled personnel. It is believed that a trained anesthesiologist in the operating room can safely nasally intubate a patient without the risk of intracranial injury. Emergency cricothyroidotomy may be required in cases of acute airway obstruction. In a review of 64 patients with Le Fort fractures, Ng and associates found that hemorrhage into the upper airway was the most common reason for airway embarrassment. A third of these patients required an emergency surgical airway. Bagheri and colleagues found an overall incidence of tracheostomy in 22.4% of patients with midfacial fractures. Sixty-six percent of their patients with Le Fort III fractures required a tracheostomy.

Incision designs should allow adequate access for evaluation and possible fixation of the nasofrontal region, lateral orbital rim, and zygomatic arches. Existing lacerations can be used for access and may substitute for the need for the coronal incision. This incision is ideal and provides sufficient access to the frontal area (nasofrontal junction and lateral orbital rims) and zygomatic arches; it will also allow for complete visualization, reduction, and fixation. However, not all Le Fort III fractures need to be treated with a coronal incision. An adequately reduced Le Fort III fracture may not require fixation at every involved suture (such as the nasofrontal), and therefore the coronal incision is not always mandatory. The lateral orbital rims can also be approached via a lateral brow or upper blepharoplasty (supratarsal fold) incision. This will not give direct access to the zygomatic arches, and reduction in this area cannot be visually confirmed. In absence of direct visualization of the fracture segments, the occlusion and the mandibular arch of rotation need to be reliable sources for adequate reduction, and consideration of a larger plate (2.0) at the lateral orbital rim would be prudent. Comminution at any areas of this fracture will make optimal visualization essential, thus favoring a coronal incision. Not uncommonly, an intracranial pressure–monitoring device will be in place, either a Camino bolt or an external ventriculostomy drain. These devices may be avoided by a releasing incision in the coronal flap.

Most commonly, Le Fort III fractures are comminuted and not bilaterally symmetrical and must be described by the individual components. Le Fort III facial fractures can present in all possible combinations (comminuted, unilateral, displaced, or nondisplaced including Le Fort I, II, or III, ZMC, orbital floor/rim, nasal, and NOE fractures. All these fractures are discussed in isolation or in conjunction with other fractures elsewhere in this book).

COMPLICATIONS

Major complications secondary to surgical correction of Le Fort III fractures are rare. Ill effects secondary to the initial trauma are usually the most devastating component (i.e., loss of airway, loss of vision, intracranial, cranial nerve, or vascular injuries). Bagheri and associates found that of their 67 patients with midfacial fractures, 4.5% required ophthalmologic surgical intervention. Two required repair/exoneration of a ruptured globe, and a third required intervention for a lens dislocation with scleral laceration repair. All three of these patients had Le Fort III fractures. Ten patients (14.9%) required neurosurgical intervention, of whom 70% had Le Fort III injuries.

Cerebrospinal fluid leak secondary to a tear in the dura mater can be an initial or a late presenting sign. This can present as cerebrospinal fluid rhinorrhea or otorrhea. Le Fort III fractures can involve a fracture of the cribiform plate and dural tear, resulting in a cerebrospinal fluid leak. In a study, Bell and associates reported an overall cerebrospinal fluid leak incidence of 4.6% in patients with severe facial trauma and/or basilar skull fractures. In their study, cerebrospinal fluid otorrhea was almost three times more common than cerebrospinal fluid rhinorrhea; however, in Le Fort III fractures, cerebrospinal fluid rhinorrhea was more likely. The vast majority (84.6%) of cerebrospinal fluid leaks resolved without surgical intervention in 2 to 10 days. Cerebrospinal fluid rhinorrhea is often described as a "tram line" running from the nose. Leaks are usually self-limiting, and reducing the fracture may assist in slowing down the flow, to allow closure of the dura. A bedside cursory evaluation of nasal secretions can be performed to suggest whether the mixture of fluid contains cerebrospinal fluid. If cerebrospinal fluid is placed on a linen sheet, it forms concentric circles (halos); this test is neither sensitive nor specific. Beta-transferrin is the most sensitive laboratory test to identify cerebrospinal fluid. Neurosurgery should be consulted for all cerebrospinal fluid leaks, which can be initially observed for resolution. Persistent cerebrospinal fluid leaks, defined as leaks lasting longer than 7 days, can be managed by cerebrospinal fluid diversion techniques, in which a ventriculostomy drain or a lumbar drain is placed to reroute the leak allowing the dural tear to heal. Significant

leaks that are refractory to initial treatment may require a bifrontal craniotomy and direct dural repair. Bell and associates reported an overall incidence of persistent cerebrospinal fluid leaks of 0.8% (six patients, of whom four required surgical intervention). The use of prophylactic antibiotics is controversial in the case of cerebrospinal fluid leaks or pneumocephalus. Current data suggest that prophylactic antibiotics may not be indicated in either situation.

Other complications of a Le Fort III fractures include nonunion, malunion, cosmetic deformity, unsightly scars and hair loss (secondary to coronal incision), malocclusion, infection (local wound abscess, meningitis, cerebral abscess, and epidural empyema have been reported), facial nerve palsy (weakness to temporal branch of facial nerve [cranial nerve VII] secondary to a coronal incision), and trigeminal nerve injury (V_1 hypoesthesia, dysesthesia, or anesthesia secondary to coronal incisions).

DISCUSSION

Le Fort is credited for identifying and classifying the classic facial fracture patterns (Le Fort I, II, and III) (Figure 7-25) through the study of human cadaver heads. Despite this classification system, even Le Fort made the observation that fracture patterns are commonly unilateral, in combination with other level fractures, and/or comminuted. This is also true in clinical practice. Knowledge of the fracture lines and patterns has significantly helped surgeons develop reconstructive strategies in trauma, craniofacial, and orthognathic surgery. A pure Le Fort III fracture results from blunt trauma at the level of the nasofrontal junction and upper lateral orbital rims. It is less common for a Le Fort III fracture to present without comminution or combination with other Le Fort level or maxillofacial fractures. The literature on Le Fort III fractures is sparse, primarily due to the low incidence of a "pure" Le Fort III fracture as originally described by Le Fort. However, the right amount of force in the right location can propagate a craniofacial disjunction.

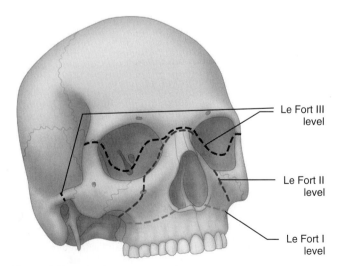

Figure 7-25   The fracture levels for Le Fort I, II, and III.

Le Fort III fractures are also referred to as complete craniofacial disjunctions or separation, in which the facial skeleton is disarticulated from the cranial base. This type of fracture involves the nasal bones, zygomas, maxilla, palatine bone, and pterygoid plates of the sphenoid bone. The fracture lines travel along the areas of least resistance, but not necessarily coincident with, the suture lines (as described in the radiographic findings).

Paul Tessier, the "father of craniofacial surgery," and other craniofacial surgeons have popularized the principles of wide exposure and direct viewing of the fracture segments. Vertical and horizontal buttresses of the face and their articulations were used for alignment and fixation. The introduction of rigid miniplate fixation devices has obviated the need for elaborate external fixation devices used in combination with interfragment wiring. Immediate bone grafting is another principle introduced by Tessier to reconstruct comminuted or missing bony structures.

Bibliography

Bagheri SC, Dierks EJ, Kademani D, et al: Comparison of the severity of bilateral Le Fort injuries in isolated midface trauma, *J Oral Maxillofac Surg* 63:1123-1129, 2005.

Bagheri SC, Dierks EJ, Kademani D, et al: Application of a Facial Injury Severity Scale (FISS) in cranio-maxillofacial trauma, *J Oral Maxillofac Surg* 64:408-414, 2006.

Bähr W, Stoll P: Nasal intubation in the presence of frontobasal fractures: a retrospective study, *J Oral Maxillofac Surg* 50:445-447, 1992.

Bell RB, Dierks EJ, Homer L, Potter BE: Management of cerebrospinal fluid leak associated with craniomaxillofacial trauma, *J Oral Maxillofac Surg* 62(6):676-684, 2004.

Haug RH, Wible RT, Likavek MJ, et al: Cervical spine fractures and maxillofacial trauma, *J Oral Maxillofac Surg* 49:725, 1991.

Horellou MF, Mathe D, Feisse P: A hazard of naso-tracheal intubation, *Anaesthesia* 33:73-74, 1978.

Kreiner B, Stevens MR, Bankston S, Piecuch JF: Management of panfacial fractures, *Oral Maxillofac Surg Knowledge Update* 3:63-81, 2001.

Le Fort R: Experimental study of fractures of the upper jaw. Pars I, II and II. *Rev Chir De Paris* 23:208-227, 360-379, 479-507, 1901; translated by Tessier P: *Plast Reconstr Surg* 50:600-607, 497-506, 1972.

Manson PN, Clark N, Robertson B, Crawley WA: Comprehensive management of pan-facial fractures, *J Craniomaxillofac Trauma* 1(1):43-56, 1995.

Manson PN, Hoopes JE, Su CT: Structural pillars of the facial skeleton: an approach to the management of Le Fort fractures, *Plast Reconstr Surg* 66:53-61, 1980.

Marlow TJ, Goltra DD, Schabel SI: Intracranial placement of a nasotracheal tube after facial fracture: a rare complication, *J Emerg Med* 15:187-191, 1997.

Ng M, Saadat D, Sinha UK: Managing the emergency airway in Le Fort fractures, *J Craniomaxillofac Trauma* 4:38, 1998.

Orbital Trauma: Fracture of the Orbital Floor

Martin B. Steed, DDS, and Shahrokh C. Bagheri, DMD, MD

CC

A 36-year-old man is seen at the emergency department status post assault. He explains that he was "jumped, robbed, beaten and punched in the left eye." You are asked to evaluate the patient for maxillofacial injuries.

HPI

The patient was returning from work when he was assaulted. He received a right hand blow with a fist to the left upper face (common pattern of injury). He reports no loss of consciousness but has difficulty seeing out of his left eye, and his cheek is numb (hypoesthesia of the V_2 cutaneous distribution is suggestive of an orbital floor, ZMC, or and anterior maxillary wall fracture).

PMHX/PDHX/MEDICATIONS/ALLERGIES/SH/FH

Noncontributory. The patient has no previous history of maxillofacial trauma.

Patients with a previous history of orbital floor reconstruction are at a higher risk of globe rupture with subsequent trauma to the globe because the reconstructed orbital floor is less likely to fracture. The energy delivered to the eye is absorbed by the globe (as opposed to being dispersed by fracture of the floor), causing more devastating injuries (blindness).

EXAMINATION

The initial evaluation of a trauma patient should be completed using the ATLS protocol.

Primary Survey

The patient's airway is intact, with a GCS score of 15.

Secondary Survey

General. The patient is a well-developed and well-nourished man in no acute distress.

Vital signs. His blood pressure is 135/84 mm Hg, heart rate 108 bpm (tachycardia), respirations 16 per minute, and temperature 37.6°C.

Maxillofacial. There is moderate left midface edema with left V_2 hypoesthesia. There is no loss of malar projection (seen with displaced ZMC fractures). The intercanthal distance is 32 mm with a negative bowstring test (seen with NOE fractures).

Eyes. Examination of the left eye (OS) reveals subconjunctival hemorrhage and chemosis (inflammation and edema of the conjunctiva) and mild periorbital edema (Figure 7-26). His visual acuity is OD 20/20 and OS 20/40 (commonly attributed to conjunctival edema) determined using a 14-inch near card. Pupils are equal round and reactive to light (5 mm → 3 mm) with accommodation (PERRLA). Assessment of direct and consensual visual reflexes reveals no abnormalities. Evaluation of the extraocular muscles of the left eye reveals restriction of upward gaze (suggestive of inferior rectus entrapment). There is no evidence of monocular diplopia within 30 degrees of primary gaze (monocular diplopia should be investigated for retinal detachment or lens dislocation). He does report binocular diplopia within 20 degrees of primary gaze. This is commonly seen secondary to edema or extraocular muscle entrapment. Slit-lamp examination was accomplished after administration of a topical mydriatic agent and fluorescein dye to the eye with a cobalt blue light in an anterior-to-posterior sequence. This revealed no abnormalities of the bilateral adnexa (eyelids and lacrimal system) and no corneal abrasions, opacities, or foreign bodies. There was no evidence of blood within the anterior chamber (hyphema) and no evidence of injury to the iris (traumatic iridialysis) or lens (dislocation or subluxation). (Use of mydriatic agents [to dilate the pupil of the eye] is relatively contraindicated in patients who have sustained head injuries due to the need for multiple-interval neurological examinations.)

A tonometer pen revealed a globe tension pressure of 12 mm Hg. (Tonometry measures the intraocular pressure, which, when high, is indicative of a retrobulbar hemorrhage. A low value is suggestive of scleral [globe] rupture. Normal intraocular pressure ranges from 11 to 20 mm Hg.)

Fundoscopic examination of the posterior segment (vitreous, retina, and optic nerve) revealed no vitreous or retinal hemorrhage. There were no apparent tears or foreign bodies. A forced duction test was accomplished after administration of a topical anesthetic and revealed true incarceration of infraorbital contents. This test involves the use of one or two fine forceps to carefully move the eye in the directions of gaze and feel for mechanical restriction. Further measurements of globe position include those based upon reference to the surrounding bone (Hertel exophthalmeter using the ZF region or the Naugel exophthalmeter using the frontal bone). If these bony landmarks are displaced or significant soft tissue edema is present, then reliable readings are difficult to obtain.

The remainder of the maxillofacial examination reveals hypoesthesia of the left V_2 distribution. No palpable bony step deformities of the left orbital rim were noted.

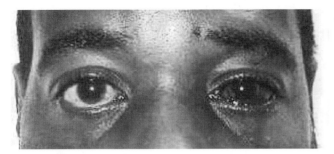

Figure 7-26 Preoperative photo demonstrating left subconjunctival hemorrhage and incidental finding of arcus senilis (a cloudy opaque arc or circle around the edge of the eye, often seen in the eye of the elderly).

IMAGING

The imaging modality of choice for the evaluation of orbital fractures is a noncontrast helical CT scan.

For this patient, a facial helical CT (1-mm cuts) without contrast was obtained after the primary and secondary surveys were completed. Coronal views demonstrate fracture of the left orbital floor with complete opacification of the maxillary sinus (Figure 7-27, *A*). Sagittal views demonstrate the location of the fracture in an anterior posterior dimension (Figure 7-27, *B*). Three-dimensional reconstruction views add little information for the preoperative planning of orbital floor fractures, except for teaching purposes.

LABS

For the management of isolated orbital floor injuries, no routine laboratory testing is indicated unless dictated by the medical history. When evaluated as part of the multisystem trauma patient, routine laboratory tests include CBC, complete metabolic panel, liver function tests, and coagulation studies.

ASSESSMENT

Isolated fracture of the left orbital floor, with entrapment of the inferior rectus muscle; FISS score of 1

TREATMENT

The indications for surgical repair of orbital floor and/or wall fractures are dependent on several factors:
- Correction or prevention of a cosmetic deformity (enophthalmos or inferior dystopia); disruption of greater than 50% of the orbital floor is likely to cause cosmetically apparent enophthalmos
- Correction of unresolved diplopia (7 to 11 days) in the setting of soft tissue prolapse with a positive forced duction test
- Immediate correction of diplopia in the setting of muscle (inferior rectus) incarceration and a positive forced duction test

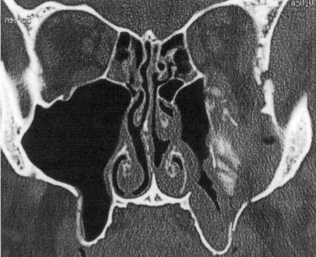

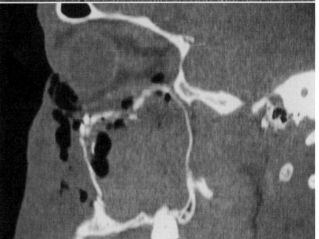

Figure 7-27 A, Preoperative CT scan coronal cut/bone window revealing a left orbital floor fracture. **B,** Preoperative CT scan sagittal cut demonstrating a left orbital floor fracture with evidence of an intact orbital rim.

- Immediate correction in the symptomatic pediatric patient with an orbital floor "trapdoor" fracture that has elicited the oculocardiac reflex (the oculocardiac reflex can be seen with true entrapment)

For this patient, he demonstrates binocular diplopia within 20 degrees of primary gaze, a positive forced duction test with concurrent evidence of greater than 50% orbital floor disruption, and a high likelihood of cosmetically significant postinjury enophthalmos. He was taken to the operating room 4 days after the assault, to allow for partial resolution of soft tissue edema. A preseptal (between the septum and the overlying orbicularis oculi muscle) transconjunctival incision was used without the need for a lateral canthotomy (Figure 7-28, *A*). Once the bony defect was isolated (Figure 7-28, *B*), a titanium mesh was fitted and properly contoured and fixated (Figure 7-28, *C* and *D*). A forced duction test, which was confirmed with the contralateral side, showed full mobility of the eye in all directions. The incision was closed with 5-0 fast-absorbing gut suture. A frost suture was placed. A postoperative CT scan was obtained (Figure 7-29), which revealed

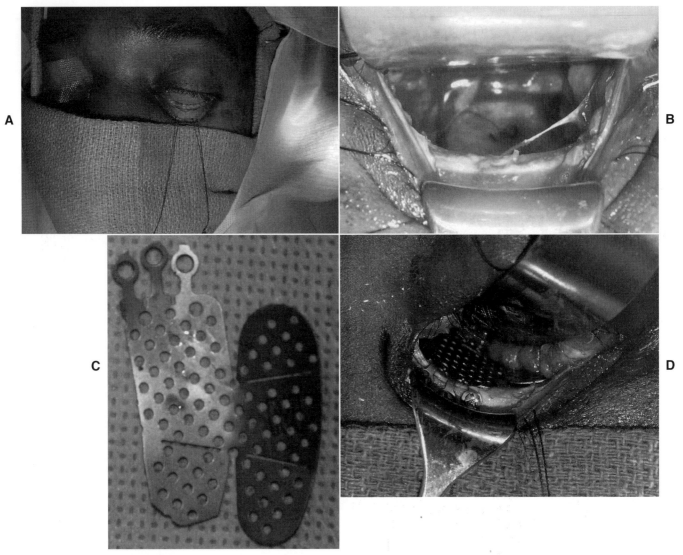

Figure 7-28   A, Intraoperative photograph of a transconjunctival incision. Note the retraction suture placement through tarsal plate to minimize lower lid injury and scleral shield to prevent inadvertent corneal abrasion. **B,** Orbital floor defect seen through the transconjunctival incision. **C,** Titanium mesh plate for reconstruction. **D,** Mesh implant in place restoring the orbital floor contour.

proper positioning and contour of the reconstruction plate. The patient did well postoperatively with no apparent enophthalmos or diplopia upon follow-up at 6 weeks.

COMPLICATIONS

Orbital floor fractures are seen in isolation or in association with other facial injuries. Complications can be related to the impact or the initial injury, concomitant injuries, the surgical repair, or a combination and can be categorized into early and late complications:

Early

- **Corneal abrasion.** Clinical suspicion should be raised upon complaint of ocular pain, photophobia, and a foreign body sensation. Corneal abrasions are diagnosed upon clinical examination with fluorescent dye viewed under cobalt blue light. Treatment includes patching the

eye (24 hours) and administration of a topical cycloplegic (e.g., homoatropine 5%) for ciliary body spasm.
- **Hyphema.** This is defined as blood within the anterior chamber from damage to blood vessels within the ciliary body or rupture of blood vessels within the iris. Hyphema is graded upon the extent to which it vertically fills the anterior chamber. Grade I is designated as less than one-third, grade II is between one-third and one-half, grade III is one-half to near total, and grade IV is total (eightball) fill of the anterior chamber. Treatment is directed toward the control of bleeding, and prevention of rebleeds. This is especially important in patients with sickle cell anemia, or sickle cell trait, where sickling (distorted red blood cells causing obstruction of blood flow in the microvasculature) leads to increased intraocular pressures and optic nerve damage.
- **Superior orbital fissure syndrome.** Compression of the contents of the superior orbital fissure accounts for the

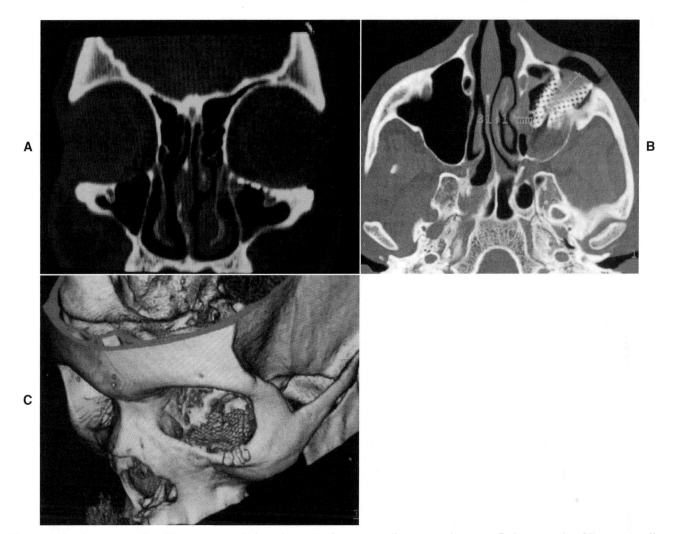

Figure 7-29 **A,** Postoperative CT scan (coronal view) demonstrating proper alignment and contour. **B,** Postoperative CT scan revealing length of plate from infraorbital rim. **C,** Postoperative CT scan (three-dimensional reconstruction) demonstrating contour of titanium mesh.

manifestations of this syndrome. Clinical findings include loss of forehead sensation, loss of corneal reflex, ophthalmoplegia, upper lid ptosis, edema (secondary to venous obstruction), and proptosis. This syndrome must be differentiated from orbital apex syndrome (which also involves the optic nerve causing loss of vision).

- **Lens dislocation.** Subluxation of the lens may occur due to disruption of the lens zonule fibers. The lens margin is often visible, but visual acuity may be compromised, and monocular diplopia can be present. Zonular disruption can cause dislocation of the lens either posteriorly or anteriorly. Patients who are symptomatic with posterior dislocation can be treated with an aphetic contact lens or with an intraocular lens implantation. An anteriorly dislocated lens is an ophthalmic emergency, due to possible blockage of the aqueous flow, resulting in acute glaucoma. Attempts at repositioning the lens can be done by a skilled ophthalmologist by maximally dilating the pupils, placing the patient in a supine position, and indenting the cornea with a gonioprism.

- **Retrobulbar hemorrhage.** Retrobulbar hemorrhage is an ocular emergency, and prompt diagnosis and treatment are essential to prevent loss of vision. This emergent clinical entity can occur after a traumatic injury to the orbit or postoperatively after orbital or eyelid surgery. The orbit is a relatively closed compartment and orbital pressure can rise rapidly with hemorrhage. Untreated, orbital compartment syndrome may develop causing ischemia of the optic nerve. Patients with increased orbital pressure present with pain, decreased vision, diplopia, ophthalmoplegia (restricted extra ocular movements), proptosis, ecchymosis around the eye, chemosis, resistance to retropulsion, and an afferent pupillary defect. An emergent lateral canthotomy with inferior cantholysis is indicated, allowing the orbital contents to expand anteriorly.

- **Traumatic optic neuropathy.** Traumatic optic neuropathy presents as a sudden loss of vision secondary to either blunt or penetrating trauma to the orbit that cannot be explained by other ocular pathological changes. The damage to the nerve is either direct (hemorrhage or compression), shearing (acceleration of the nerve at the optic canal where it is tethered to the dural sheath), or through transmission of a shock wave through the orbit along the course of the optic nerve. Many treatment modalities have been advocated, including high-dose intravenous steroids, optic canal decompression, and optic nerve sheath fenestration. The largest study looking at traumatic optic neuropathy, The International Optic Nerve Trauma Study, was conducted by Levin and colleagues in 1999. They concluded that the use of corticosteroids in patients with traumatic optic neuropathy did not change the outcome (loss of visual acuity), compared with the control group that did not receive any steroid therapy.

- **Ruptured globe.** Globe rupture occurs when the integrity of its outer membranes is disrupted by blunt or penetrating trauma. A peaked, teardrop-shaped, or otherwise irregular pupil may indicate a ruptured globe. A full-thickness laceration to the cornea or sclera constitutes a globe perforation, requiring repair in the operating room setting. Prolapse of the iris through a full-thickness corneal laceration may be seen as a dark discoloration at the site of injury. Scleral buckling is indicative of rupture with extrusion of ocular contents. Intraocular pressure will likely be low, but direct measurement is contraindicated to avoid pressure on the globe. Globe rupture represents a major ophthalmologic emergency that requires surgical intervention.

- **Blindness.** This is a known but uncommon complication of facial trauma, with a reported incidence of only 2% to 5%. In a review of the University of Maryland shock trauma experience of facial trauma over 11 years, the researchers discovered that 2,987 of the 29,474 admitted patients (10.1%) sustained facial fractures and that 1,338 of these fractures (44.8%) involved one or both of the orbits. One thousand two hundred forty of these patients underwent operative repair of their facial fractures. Three patients (0.24%) experienced postoperative complications that resulted in blindness. In their data, blindness was attributable to intraorbital hemorrhage in 13 of 27 cases (48%). Five other patients experienced visual loss with unspecified mechanisms related to increased intraorbital pressure. Within the restricted confines of the optic canal, even small changes in pressure may potentially cause ischemic optic neuropathy.

Late

Late complications of orbital floor fractures and repair can be the result of injuries sustained at the time of the traumatic event, or complications associated with the repair itself.

- **Lacrimal system injury.** Epiphora (excessive tearing due to impaired drainage) can occur. Eyelid lacerations, particularly those extending medially, should be thoroughly evaluated for lacrimal drainage system injury,

canthal tendon disruption, or injury to the tarsal plate and levator aponeurosis. Fractures through the lacrimal apparatus (NOE) can also cause epiphora.

- **Unresolved diplopia.** Diplopia that has a neuromuscular origin (such as cranial nerve III palsy) should be observed for spontaneous recovery over 6 months. Elective strabismus surgery can be considered if the diplopia is unresolved. Acute entrapment of the extraocular muscles causing diplopia needs to be addressed soon after the injury.

- **Enophthalmos.** Enophthalmos results from an increase in orbital volume and will persist if the orbital volume is not restored adequately. This occurs in large unrepaired fractures, particularly when multiple walls are involved. It is most commonly seen with significant involvement (disruption) of the medial orbital wall.

- **Ectropion.** Ectropion is the outward eversion of the lid margin away from the globe. This can results in corneal irritation, exposure, and abnormalities of lacrimal outflow. The prevention of ectropion begins with minimizing vertical tension when closing lid lacerations and/or periorbital skin incisions. The use of the transconjunctival incision with resuspension of the suborbicularis oculi fat and meticulous repair of lid lacerations reduces the incidence of this complication. Cicatricial ectropion occurs from scarring of the anterior lamella while involutional ectropion results from horizontal lid laxity, usually due to age-related weakness of the canthal ligaments and pretarsal orbicularis.

- **Entropion.** Entropion is the malposition of the lid resulting in inversion of the lid margin. Cicatricial entropion occurs as a result of scarring of the palpebral conjunctiva, with consequent inward rotation of the eyelid margin.

- **Unaesthetic Scar.** Cutaneous placement of periorbital incisions such as the infraorbital incision carries the risk of an unaesthetic scar.

DISCUSSION

The management of orbital floor fractures remains controversial. The indications and timing for surgical intervention have proved difficult to study and evaluate. Isolated orbital wall fractures account for 4% to 16% of all facial fractures. If fractures that extend outside the orbit (ZMC, NOE) are included, this would compromise 30% to 50% of all facial fractures.

The optimal management of orbital fractures necessitates an intimate knowledge of the complex anatomy of the region. The orbit is a quadrilateral pyramid, with an average volume of 30 cm³ and height and width at the rim averaging 40 mm and 35 mm, respectively. The average length of the medial wall is 40 to 45 mm (rim to optic canal). Seven bones make up the orbits: the sphenoid, maxillary, lacrimal, ethmoid, frontal, zygomatic, and palatine bones. The orbital process of the frontal bone and the lesser wing of sphenoid make up its roof. The floor is made up of the orbital plates of the maxilla, zygoma, and the palatine bone. The zygoma and the greater and lesser wings of sphenoid form the lateral wall. The medial wall is formed by the frontal process of maxilla, lacrimal, sphenoid, and ethmoid (lamina papyracea) bones.

The distances to known orbital landmarks are crucial to avoiding postoperative complications and aid in intraoperative dissection. These measurements are averages and may be altered by posttraumatic changes of the orbital rim. The average distance from the orbital rim to the orbital apex is 40 to 45 mm. The subperiosteal dissection along the orbital walls can safely be extended up to 25 mm posteriorly along the inferior and lateral rims.

Two theories have been advocated with regard to the physiological mechanism of orbital floor fractures. The hydraulic theory, advocated by Smith and Regan in 1957, proposed that a generalized increased orbital content pressure resulted in direct compression of the orbital floor, thereby fracturing the thin orbital bone. Fujino later disputed this theory and proposed that a direct compression force or buckling force transmitted via the orbital rim was the causative factor for orbital floor fractures. This theory of bone conduction mechanism of injury was first proposed by Le Fort and Lagrange at the turn of the twentieth century. In a series of dried human cadaver experiments during the mid-1970s, Fujino convincingly demonstrated the occurrence of orbital floor fractures with direct blows to the orbital rim without fracturing the orbital rim itself. Recent studies, such as that by Waterhouse and associates, have revealed that orbital fractures may occur by way of the "buckling" or "hydraulic" mechanism, with a combination of the two mechanisms being the most likely etiology dependent upon the direction of the striking force.

A recent study by Fan and colleagues demonstrated a high correlation between the increment of orbital volume and the degree of enophthalmos. An increase of 1 cm^3 of the orbital volume elicited 0.89 mm of enophthalmos. The authors concluded that the measurement of orbital volume in patients with orbital blowout fractures could be used to predict the degree of late enophthalmos and that this may be accomplished through the use of computer assisted volumetric measurements.

The approaches to the orbit include the transconjunctival (with or without a lateral canthotomy and cantholysis), the subcilliary, lower lid crease, and the transcaruncular. The transconjunctival approach has been shown to result in fewer cases of postoperative ectropion and may be used in conjunction with the transcaruncular approach to gain further access to the medial orbit. Attention to the medial orbital wall is paramount in completely treating orbital fractures and preventing enophthalmos. Endoscopic approaches are also being studied to gain access to the orbital floor for assessment and reconstruction.

The literature provides support for notable clinical differences in orbital floor fracture patterns between pediatric patients and adults. Jordan and associates coined the term "white-eyed blowout fracture" in patients 16 years or younger with minimal soft tissue injury, severe diplopia, extraocular muscle limitation, and extremely small extrusion of tissue around the orbit seen on CT imaging. Diplopia, extraocular muscle limitation, and trapdoor fractures were more frequent in children than in adult patients and can be accompanied by nausea and vomiting.

The choices of reconstruction materials for repair of orbital bony contour are numerous and remain controversial. Many autogenous (split calvarial bone, iliac crest, septal cartilage or rib), alloplastic (titanium mesh, porous polyethylene [MEDPOR], PGA/PLLA, Gelfilm), and allogeneic (lyophilized cartilage or dura, banked bone) materials have been used and advocated. The use of autogenous materials is thought to decrease the risk of infection and/or extrusion, while alloplastic materials offer superior ease in intraoperative handling and contouring.

It is highly recommended to institute a multidisciplinary approach to complex orbital trauma, and consultation with ophthalmology and/or oculoplastic services should be considered. Many posterior segment injuries may be subtle and need to be identified before exploration and reconstruction of the bony orbital architecture.

Bibliography

Appling WD, Patrinely JR, Salzer TA: Transconjunctival approach vs subciliary skin-muscle flap approach for orbital fracture repair, *Arch Otolaryngol Head Neck Surg* 119:1000-1007, 1993.

Burnstine MA: Clinical recommendations for repair of orbital facial fractures, *Curr Opin Ophthalmol* 14:236-240, 2003.

Erling BF, Iliff N, Robertson B, Manson PN: Footprints of the globe: a practical look at the mechanism of orbital blowout fractures, with a revisit to the work of Raymond Pfeiffer, *Plast Reconstr Surg* 103:1313-1316, 1999.

Fan X, Li J, Zhu J, et al: Computer-assisted orbital volume measurement in the surgical correction of late enophthalmos caused by blowout fractures, *Ophthal Plast Reconstr Surg* 9:207-211, 2003.

Friedrich RE, Heiland M, Bartel-Friedrich S: Potentials of ultrasound in the diagnosis of midfacial fractures, *Clin Oral Invest* 7:226-229, 2003.

Fujino T: Experimental "blow-out" fracture of the orbit, *Plast Reconstr Surg* 54:81-82, 1974.

Girotto JA, Gamble W, Robertson B, et al: Blindness after reduction of facial fractures. *Plast Reconstr Surg* 102(6):1821-1834, 1998.

Goldenberg-Cohen N, Miller NR, Repka MX: Traumatic optic neuropathy in children and adolescents, *J AAPOS* 8:20-27, 2004.

Holt JE, Holt GR, Blodgett JM: Ocular injuries sustained during blunt facial trauma, *Ophthalmology* 90:14-18, 1983.

Holtmann B, Wray RC, Little AG: A randomized comparison of four incisions for orbital fractures, *Plast Reconstr Surg* 67:731-737, 1981.

Jordan DR, Allen LH, White J, et al: Intervention within days for some orbital floor fractures: the white-eyed blowout, *Ophthal Plast Reconstr Surg* 14:379-390, 1998.

Le Fort R: Experimental study of fractures of the upper jaw. Pars I, II and II. *Rev Chir De Paris* 23:208-227, 360-379, 479-507, 1901; translated by Tessier P: *Plast Reconstr Surg* 50:600-607, 497-506, 1972.

Levin LA, Beck RW, Joseph MP, et al: The treatment of traumatic optic neuropathy: the International Optic Nerve Trauma Study, *Ophthalmology* 106:1268-1277, 1999.

Lorenz P, Longaker M, Kawamoto H: Primary and secondary orbit surgery: the transconjunctival approach, *Plast Reconstr Surg* 103:1124-1128, 1999.

Rhee JS, Kilde J, Yoganadan N, Pintar F: Orbital blowout fractures: experimental evidence for the pure hydraulic theory, *Arch Fac Plast Surg* 4:98-101, 2002.

Shere JL, Boole JR, Holtel MR, et al: An analysis of 3,599 midfacial and 1,141 orbital blowout fractures among 4,426 United States Army soldiers, 1980-2000, *Otolaryngol Head Neck Surg* 130:164-170, 2004.

Shorr N, Baylis HI, Goldberg RA, Perry JD: Transcaruncular approach to the medial orbit and orbital apex, *Ophthalmology* 107:1459-1463, 2000.

Smith B, Regan WF Jr: Blow-out fracture of the orbit; mechanism and correction of internal orbital fracture, *Am J Ophthalmol* 44(6):733-739, 1957.

Waterhouse N, Lyne J, Urdang M, Garey L: An investigation into the mechanism of orbital blowout fractures, *Br J Plast Surg* 52(8):607-612, 1999.

Westfall CT, Shore JW, Nunery WR, et al: Operative complications of the transconjunctival inferior fornix approach, *Ophthalmology* 98(10):1525-1528, 1991.

Wray RC, Holtmann B, Ribaudo JM, et al: A comparison of conjunctival and subciliary incisions for orbital fractures, *Br J Plast Surg* 30:142-145, 1977.

Panfacial Fracture

Chris Jo, DMD, Martin B. Steed, DDS, and Shahrokh C. Bagheri, DMD, MD

CC

A 49-year-old man is transported to the emergency department by EMS personnel status post pedestrian-versus-automobile accident. You are called by the trauma team for the evaluation and management of his facial injuries.

HPI

The patient arrives to the emergency department intubated. The driver of the automobile and another eyewitness report that the patient was walking alongside a busy intersection and suddenly jumped into the path of the vehicle traveling at approximately 35 mph. The front end of the car struck his thighs and then his face hit the hood and windshield, causing significant damage to the automobile. He was launched several feet into the air and landed in a prone position on the pavement. He had a GCS score of 3 on the scene and was orally intubated by the EMS personnel for airway protection (airway intubation is warranted for a GCS score of 8 or less, which is indicative of a severe head injury). Upon your arrival to the emergency department, the patient was being actively resuscitated by the trauma team according to the ATLS protocol, and the orthopedic team was evaluating multiple extremity fractures.

PMHX/PDHX/MEDICATIONS/ALLERGIES/SH/FH

The patient's histories are unknown (when present, information may be obtained from family members).

EXAMINATION

The initial evaluation of a trauma patient should be dictated by the ATLS protocol.

Primary Survey

Airway and cervical spine control. He was orally intubated with a transport cervical-collar in place. (In a review of 563 patients with maxillofacial injuries, Haug and associates found that concomitant cervical-spine fractures occurred in 2% of patients. Of those with cervical-spine fractures, 91% had mandibular fractures. Bagheri and colleagues found a 1.5% incidence of cervical-spine fractures in a series of 67 patients with isolated midface fractures.)

Breathing and oxygenation. Oral endotracheal tube in good position (confirmed by portable chest radiograph) on mechanical ventilation. The right hemithorax showed no chest rise or breath sounds and was hypertympanic to percussion (indicative of a pneumothorax, also confirmed by portable chest radiograph). A chest tube was placed to reexpand the right lung. Oxygen saturation was 90% on 100% inspired oxygen (suggestive of a ventilation-perfusion mismatch).

Circulation and hemorrhage control. His blood pressure is 90/70 mm Hg, and his heart rate is 125 bpm (moderate hypotension and tachycardia consistent with Class III shock) (Class III hypovolemic shock is indicative of a 30% to 40% loss of blood volume, which is characterized by a heart rate over 120 bpm; decreased systolic blood pressure, mean arterial blood pressure, pulse pressure, and urine output [5 to 15 ml/hr]; and altered mental status). A small amount of bleeding was observed from the nasopharynx, which was easily controlled with bilateral nasal packs. The magnitude of bleeding did not clinically correlate with the estimated blood loss and volume depletion (need to be suspicious of other sources of bleeding). The abdomen was soft and nondistended and the focused abdominal sonography for trauma (FAST) was negative (FAST examination is used in the hypotensive blunt trauma patient and evaluates the perihepatic, pericardiac, perisplenic, and pelvic windows for presence of free intraperitoneal fluid or cardiac tamponade), ruling out intraabdominal hemorrhage (hypovolemic) and cardiac tamponade (obstructive) as the source of shock. Bilateral femur deformities (each femur fracture can be a source of 1.5 to 2 L of blood loss) and other open extremity fractures can be a source of significant blood loss and hypovolemic shock. Fractures should be reduced and stabilized to reduce the amount of hemorrhage in the initial resuscitation phases. Fluid resuscitation should begin with crystalloid intravenous fluid boluses to maintain organ perfusion. Transfusion of packed red blood cells should be considered in Class III hemorrhagic shock.

Disability and dysfunction. On the AVPU scale, the patient is unresponsive, off sedation, with a GCS score of E1, M1, V1T = 3T. Pupils were equal, 7 mm with a sluggish reaction to light (large pupils with a sluggish reaction to light reflex may indicate a closed head injury and elevated intracranial pressures). Sedation should be discontinued for an accurate assessment of mental status as needed. Initial head CT revealed moderate contusions in the frontal and occipital lobes (coup, countercoup injury indicative of rapid acceleration-deceleration injury). A Camino bolt was placed to monitor the intracranial pressure, which revealed a mildly elevated opening pressure at 22 mm Hg (normal intracranial pressure is 15 mm Hg or below).

Exposure and environmental control. The patient's clothing was removed, and a warm blanket and other warming devices were used to prevent hypothermia.

Secondary Survey

(A-M-P-L-E history is taken from available sources.)

General. He is a well-developed male who is intubated and sedated, with a cervical-collar in place.

Neurological. His GCS score is 3T (off sedation). Pupils are 7 mm, equal, and sluggish (this was covered during the primary survey, but should be repetitively monitored for changes). The intracranial pressure–monitoring device (such as an intra-intraparenchymal Camino bolt or an external ventriculostomy drain) gives a precise moment-by-moment assessment of intracranial pressures. A sustained intracranial pressure of over 25 mm Hg warrants intervention to reduce the pressure (intravenous mannitol, hyperosmolar therapy with 3% NaCl, elevation of head of bed, hyperventilation to reduce the $Paco_2$ to the low range of normal). Therapy is aimed at not only reducing intracranial pressure (below 20 mm Hg) but also maintaining cerebral perfusion pressures (cerebral perfusion pressure = mean arterial pressure – intracranial pressure), which should be maintained greater than 70 mm Hg (35% reduction in mortality) to prevent secondary brain injury. Invasive hemodynamic monitoring is indicated when hyperosmolar therapy is initiated to maintain an acceptable blood pressure and cerebral perfusion pressure (mortality increase 20% for each 10–mm Hg loss of cerebral perfusion pressure).

Maxillofacial. There is significant upper and lower facial edema. Two-centimeter full-thickness laceration extends over the bridge of the nose (indicating blunt trauma to the upper midface), and there is 5-cm full-thickness stellate laceration over the lower lip and chin.

Eyes. There is significant periorbital edema. Visual acuity cannot be assessed. The patient has bilateral periorbital ecchymosis (raccoon eyes, indicative of anterior basilar skull fracture) and bilateral subconjunctival hemorrhage and chemosis. Intercanthal distance is 36 mm without blunting of the medial canthus (increased intercanthal distance is indicative of an NOE fracture or avulsion of the medial canthal tendon. Normal intercanthal distance is 30 to 34 mm and varies among races and genders). The bowstring test is negative (clinical test for evaluation of the medial canthal attachment). Bilateral step deformities are present at the lateral and inferior orbital rims (step deformity and bony crepitus indicate the presence of fractures).

Nose. Nasal bridge demonstrates crepitus with gross mobility. Endonasal examination reveals edematous nasal mucosa with mild bleeding. The anterior nasal septum is midline with no septal hematoma (septal hematoma requires immediate incision and drainage to prevent necrosis of the septal cartilage and potential perforation and saddle nose deformity). No cerebrospinal fluid rhinorrhea or otorrhea is noted. The maxilla is grossly mobile with bony crepitus at the anterior maxillary walls and the ZM buttresses. No step deformity or crepitus was appreciable at the zygomatic arches bilaterally (does not exclude possibility of fractures).

Intraoral. There is bilateral maxillary vestibular ecchymosis (indicative of fractures of ZM buttresses). There are multiple missing maxillary teeth and a step deformity with an associated gingival laceration between the left mandibular lateral and central incisors (teeth Nos. 23 and 24), with gross mobility of the mandibular segments. The patient has an anterior open bite with no distinct mandibular posterior stop and bilateral posterior prematurities (indicative of bilateral condylar fractures and/or Le Fort level fracture), with the oral endotracheal tube exiting between the edentulous spaces. Ecchymosis at the posterior soft palate bilaterally (Guerin's sign, indicative of pterygoid plate disjunction/fracture).

IMAGING

Mandatory trauma plain-film radiograph series in the acute setting include cross-table cervical-spine, portable anteroposterior chest radiography, and an anteroposterior pelvis radiograph. Other studies are added as needed, including cervical-spine series (in suspected cervical-spine injury), thoracic and lumbar spine series, and extremity radiographs (depending on the mechanism of injury).

Axial-cut, bony window CT scans (with coronal reconstructions) are the gold standard radiographic examination for midfacial fractures. Direct coronal views are useful but should be avoided in patients with suspected cervical-spine injury (patient's head needs to be hyperextended for direct coronal CT). Three-dimensional reconstructions are helpful adjuncts as they provide the most graphic representation of the fractures, degree of displacement, and orientation of fragments. A panoramic radiograph is always helpful, but in the unstable patient with C-T-L spine precautions, it may not be possible.

In this patient, head and facial helical CT scans without contrast were obtained after the primary and secondary surveys were completed. The head CT scan reveals moderate frontal lobe and occipital lobe contusions without evidence of intracerebral hemorrhage or midline shift (should be repeated in 12 to 24 hours to monitor for any changes). The fine-cut axial face CT scan reveals bilateral nasal bone, lateral orbital rims and walls, and bilateral zygomatic arch fractures (Figure 7-30, A and B). There are fractures at the pterygoid plates and along the anterior and posterior maxillary sinus and lateral nasal walls (Figure 7-30, C). Coronal reconstruction views anteriorly demonstrate fractures at the nasofrontal junction, a Le Fort I level fracture, and a midpalatal split (Figure 7-30, D). Coronal views of the midface demonstrate severe comminution of the midface including at the NOE, orbital floors, and ZF junction (Figure 7-30, E). Scans of the mandible demonstrate bilateral condylar neck fractures (Figure 7-30, F and see Figure 7-30, C) and a midline mandibular symphysis fracture. Figure 7-30, G shows the three-dimensional reconstructed view, which also demonstrates fracture of the anterior table of the frontal sinus, confirmed on the axial views.

The CT scan of the cervical spine was negative. The anteroposterior chest radiograph shows evolving bilateral

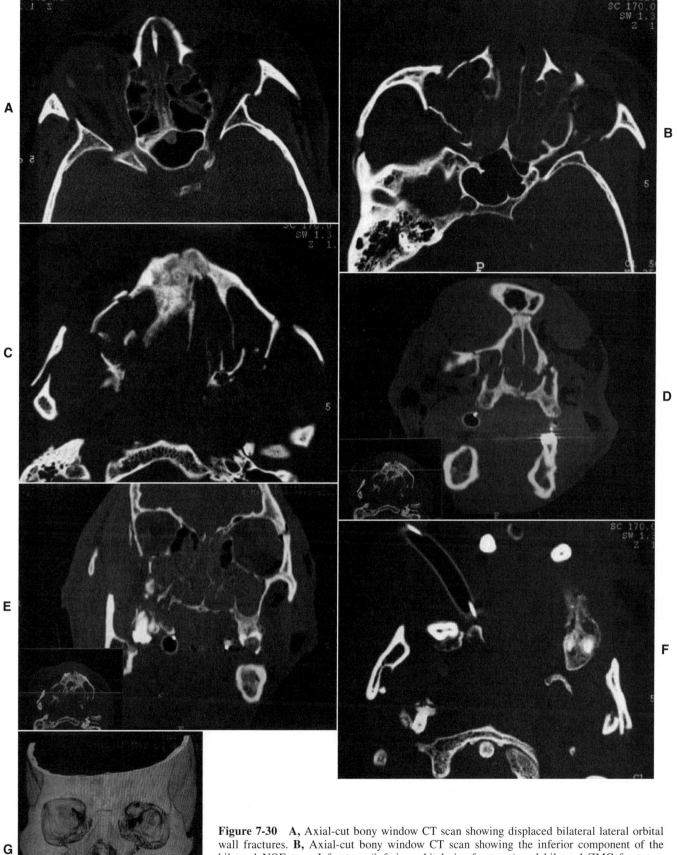

Figure 7-30 **A,** Axial-cut bony window CT scan showing displaced bilateral lateral orbital wall fractures. **B,** Axial-cut bony window CT scan showing the inferior component of the bilateral NOE type I fracture (inferior orbital rim fractures) and bilateral ZMC fractures. **C,** Axial-cut bony window CT scan showing a right subcondylar fracture, a palatal split of the maxilla, pterygoid plate fractures/disjunction, and maxillary sinus wall comminution. **D,** Coronal reconstruction CT scan showing Le Fort I fracture with a palatal split and bilateral NOE type I fracture. **E,** Coronal reconstruction CT scan showing bilateral lateral orbital rim fractures, a comminuted Le Fort I fracture, nasal septal comminution and nondisplaced orbital floor fractures. **F,** Axial-cut bony window CT scan showing a left subcondylar fracture. **G,** Three-dimensional CT reconstruction demonstrating the spatial relationship of the fractures. The symphysis and anterior frontal sinus fractures are seen clearly in this view.

pulmonary contusions and a chest tube in good position without any residual pneumothorax.

LABS

Standard laboratory tests for the evaluation of multisystem trauma patients included: CBC, complete metabolic panel, arterial blood gas, urine analysis, and coagulation studies (PT/PTT/INR). A urine drug screen and blood alcohol level are indicated in patients with decreased mental status.

This patient demonstrated decreased hemoglobin (9.2 g/dl) and hematocrit (26.6%) (suggestive of blood loss; however, acutely, hemoglobin/hematocrit may not be an accurate measure due to a delay in volume redistribution). Arterial blood gas analysis showed a moderate base deficit of −5.5 mEq (base deficit is one of the parameters monitored for adequacy of resuscitation in hypovolemic shock and is a better indicator of acute blood loss than hemoglobin/hematocrit). The complete metabolic panel demonstrated a mild elevation in his blood urea nitrogen (30 mg/dl) and creatinine (1.9 mg/dl) levels (indicative of prerenal azotemia secondary to blood loss) and a negative blood alcohol level and urine drug screen (alcohol and drug intoxication must be considered and ruled out as the source for altered mental status). The remainder of his laboratory tests were within normal limits.

ASSESSMENT

Panfacial fracture involving the frontal bone, midface, and mandible, FISS of 17, complicated by a Class III hemorrhagic shock, closed head injury, multiple extremity fractures, and right pneumothorax with bilateral pulmonary contusions

The maxillofacial injures are classified as follows (FISS designation given in parentheses):

Upper face	Fracture of the anterior wall of the frontal sinus and frontal bar (5)
Midface	Bilateral ZMC fractures (2 × 1)
	Bilateral NOE fractures (type I) (3)
	Le Fort I fracture (2), with a midpalatal split (1).
Mandible	Bilateral subcondylar (2 × 1) and symphysis (2) fractures.

TREATMENT

Treatment begins with initiation of the ATLS protocol and stabilization of the patient. Maxillofacial injuries compromising the airway should be promptly evaluated. Tracheotomy should be readily considered for panfacial fractures. Submental intubation is also a viable alternative. A cricothyrotomy is usually reserved for an acute airway emergency. The control of hemorrhage from the maxillofacial region is part of the ATLS protocol. Nasal packing and pressure dressings should be applied as needed.

Treatment of panfacial fractures can be challenging and should begin after completion of the ATLS protocol with a thorough maxillofacial and radiographic examination. Once the diagnosis is made, a treatment plan must be developed to expose the necessary fractures for alignment and fixation. Selective exposure of necessary fractures is employed for stabilization using rigid fixation (before the advent of rigid fixation, it was common for all fracture sites to be exposed). The surgeon must develop a preoperative plan to expose, examine, align, fixate, and reconstruct the facial skeleton in an orderly fashion. This may include immediate bony reconstruction with bone grafting techniques. If necessary, the entire facial skeleton can be visualized by combining multiple approaches.

Once the fracture sites have been exposed, the principle of using the buttresses of the facial skeleton to help align the fractures from "stable-to-unstable" segments is used. Different concepts and strategies regarding the order of stabilization have been advocated in the past; these include top-to-bottom, bottom-to-top, inside-to-out, and outside-to-in. With the advent of miniplates and rigid internal fixation, a broader range of reconstructive possibilities permit new definitions of optimal sequencing in facial reconstruction. Goals for linking together fragmented bones together came into existence. Starting with stable bone, fractured and displaced segments are fixated to adjacent stable, nondisplaced bone in a piecemeal fashion.

The following treatment sequence was used for this patient:

- **Management of the airway.** Due to the severity of this patient's head injury and anticipation of prolonged mechanical ventilation, an open tracheotomy was initially performed.
- **Exposure of fractures.** Maxillary and mandibular arch bars were applied but not tightened (leaving the arch bars slightly loose on the least dentate segment of the fracture will allow for adjustment at a later time when the proper occlusion and horizontal facial width have been established). Subsequently, all fractures necessary for alignment and fixation are exposed in a systematic fashion.
  - A transoral exposure of the maxillary and mandibular fractures was accomplished with a maxillary circumvestibular incision (from first molar to first molar) and a genioplasty type incision (the midpalatal fracture can also be accessed via a parasagittal palatal incision if it needs to be rigidly fixated). The midface was degloved to expose the body of the zygomas, bilateral ZM buttress, the pyriform rim (nasomaxillary buttress), the inferior portion of the NOE fracture, and the inferior orbital rims (inferior orbital rims can be plated from this access), while skeletonizing and protecting the infraorbital neurovascular bundles. The mandibular symphysis fracture was exposed by degloving the anterior mandible to the inferior border anterior to the mental foramina. Both mental nerves (and associated three branches) were identified and

protected (some surgeons prefer an extraoral approach via a submental incision, which decreases mental nerve injury and gives better visualization of the lingual cortex reduction to prevent splaying). If a fracture exists in the posterior mandible (body, angle, or ramus), submandibular (Risdon), retromandibular (or Hinds), or intraoral incisions can be used.

- Second, a coronal incision (also referred to as the bicoronal incision in the literature) was made to access the frontal bone and sinuses, superior and lateral orbital rims (supraorbital bar), the NOE complex, and the zygomatic arches. It will also provide access for a cranial bone graft (the parietal area offers the thickest bicortical width reducing the risk of entry into the cranium) harvest if needed. This incision was extended into bilateral preauricular (some surgeons prefer an endoaural approach) incisions for access to the mandibular condyle and better access to the zygomatic arch and body.
- Next, the inferior orbital rims and inferior component of the NOE fractures were exposed via transconjunctival approach. Various periorbital incisions can be used for access to the inferior orbital rims, orbital floor and medial orbital walls, inferior components of the NOE, and lateral orbital rims. The lower eyelid incisions can be transcutaneous or transconjunctival. The trancutaneous approaches include the subciliary, subtarsal, and inferior orbital rim (unfavorable scarring) incisions. The subciliary incision can be a skin-only flap, skin-muscle flap, or stepped flap. The stepped flap is recommended when using this approach because it has a lower incidence of postoperative lower eyelid malposition (ectropion, entropion, and scleral show). The transconjunctival incision can be done with or without a lateral canthotomy and inferior cantholysis depending on the amount of access needed. This incision can be extended medially via a transcaruncular incision for greater exposure of the medial orbital wall. The transconjunctival incision is preferred by most surgeons because it has the lowest incidence of transient and permanent postoperative lower eyelid malposition. If a coronal incision is not used, the lateral orbital rim can be exposed via an upper blepharoplasty incision or a lateral brow incision. Paranasal lynch incisions can be used to access NOE fractures; however, it is associated with poor cosmesis.
- **Alignment and fixation of fractures.** After exposure of all necessary fractures, attention is turned to the dentoalveolar segments and occlusion. Due to the fracture of the dentate segment (parasymphysis/symphysis) of the mandible along with the maxillary palatal split, it can be difficult to restore the proper lower facial width and occlusion. In this case, the surgeons chose to rely on proper reduction of the symphysis fracture (guided by direct visualization of the lingual cortex reduction and correct position of the condylar

heads in the glenoid fossa) to define the lower facial third width and occlusion. Proper horizontal width of the maxilla is obtained by placing the dentoalveolar segments into intermaxillary fixation with a properly reduced mandible. Typically, fractures through dentate segments are addressed first. However, when dealing with a symphysis (parasymphysis) and bilateral (or unilateral) subcondylar fractures, it may be wise to reduce and rigidly fixate the subcondylar fractures prior to addressing the symphysis fracture. This will allow the surgeon to visualize and keep the condylar heads in the glenoid fossa as the symphysis fracture is reduced and fixated (assisted by gentle digital pressure at the mandibular angles). When subcondylar fractures are addressed after fixation of the symphysis, there may be undetected splaying of the lingual cortex at the symphysis causing the subsequent condylar displacement and fixation lateral to the fossa. With the occlusion set and the mandibular symphysis and condylar neck fractures reduced and fixated, the mandible's arc of rotation is used to guide the proper reduction of the midface fractures (the vertical dimension of the maxilla cannot be established by the mandible).

- Using the "stable-to-unstable" principle, the most cephalad fractures are addressed next, using the anterior cranial vault as the stable point of fixation. The frontal bar and anterior table of the frontal sinus should be reconstructed first, starting at the lateral orbital rims (frontozygomatic suture area) and working medially toward the radix (the frontal sinus should also be addressed according to the type of injury and should be done after reconstructing the frontal bar, see the section on frontal sinus fracture in this chapter). Then, the zygomatic arches are fixated bilaterally (accurate reduction of the zygomatic arches is important for restoring proper anteroposterior projection of the midface). The superior portion of the NOE fracture (near the nasofrontal junction) is then reduced and fixated to the stable frontal bar, and the inferior portion is addressed later via the periorbital and/or maxillary vestibular access (some surgeons prefer to use a long C-shaped plate to vertically span the entire NOE fracture and simultaneously fixate it to the inferior orbital rims and frontal bar). Otherwise, comminuted NOE fractures are typically addressed last after reduction and stabilization of the surrounding bony structures.
- The orbital rim fractures are reduced and fixated via the transconjunctival incisions. The orbital floor can be explored and reconstructed (cranial bone graft or alloplastic orbital floor plate/mesh) if indicated. In this case, the inferior component of the NOE fracture is coincident with the inferior orbital rim fracture, which is part of the ZMC fractures.
- Once the upper and midface has been reduced and stabilized, the fractured maxilla at the Le Fort I level is then reduced and fixated to the now reduced and

stable midface, using the buttresses (ZM and nasomaxillary) as a guide for reduction and with the patient in MMF. Miniplates are placed at the ZM buttresses and pyriform rims bilaterally. Further stabilization may be required for palatal split situations, such as this case. Palatal vault fixation, intermaxillary fixation, or a palatal strap splint can be used to prevent horizontal collapse of the maxilla.

- **Primary bone grafting.** Finally, primary bony reconstruction with immediate cranial bone grafts can be done at this time. Areas that are highly comminuted or missing bony segments require one-piece bone grafts to replace the defects in bone volume and to support the overlying soft tissue. This need may arise to reconstruct the nasal dorsum, orbital rims, orbital floors, maxillary sinus walls, ZM buttress area (usually comminuted in high impact injuries), and any other area of avulsed or severely comminuted bone.
- **Soft tissue repair and resuspension.** Soft tissue injuries should be addressed last. Layered closure of incisions/lacerations and resuspension of stripped periosteum and suspensory ligaments of the face are important to provide a natural soft tissue drape.

COMPLICATIONS

Major complications secondary to the surgical correction of panfacial fractures can be difficult to assess and are dependent on the severity of the initial traumatic insult. Damage secondary to the initial trauma itself is usually the most devastating (i.e., death, loss of vision, intracranial injury, cranial nerve deficits, cervical-spine injury, etc.). The most troubling complication to the maxillofacial trauma surgeon is a poor cosmetic and/or functional outcome. Wide exposure for proper alignment of facial substructures, rigid fixation, and immediate bone grafting reconstructive techniques have significantly reduced the incidence of postoperative facial deformities. However, despite accurate reduction of facial fractures, the soft tissue envelope can exert undesirable forces in the form of scar formation and wound contracture. This can lead to a progressive migration of the bony infrastructure of the face and to late postoperative deformities. It is important for patients to realize that full functional and cosmetic outcome may require multiple operations and revisions.

Complications of panfacial repair also include: cerebrospinal fluid leaks, nonunion, malunion, cosmetic deformity (telecanthus, orbital dystopia, loss of malar projection, increased mid or lower facial width, nasal deformity), malocclusion, infection (local wound abscess, meningitis, cerebral abscess, epidural empyema), facial nerve palsy, anosmia, and trigeminal nerve injury (hypoesthesia, dysesthesia, anesthesia).

DISCUSSION

The term "panfacial fracture" is frequently used incorrectly. By definition, panfacial fractures involve the upper, middle, and lower thirds of the face. Traditionally, the facial skeleton is divided into thirds or upper and lower halves. More recently, Manson and others have described four anatomical areas of the face: the frontal area (including the frontal bar), the upper midfacial area (including the ZMC and NOE), the lower midfacial area and occlusion (including the maxilla at the Le Fort I level and the maxillary and mandibular dentoalveolar segments), and the basal mandibular area (including the condyle, ramus, body, and symphysis). Nonetheless, when there is a fracture in each of these four anatomical areas, it is considered a true panfacial fracture. Comminution is a common feature for all midfacial fractures especially at the anterior maxillary sinus wall and in the ZM buttress area.

It is of paramount importance to maintain the three dimensions of the facial skeleton: the height (from vertex to menton), the width (bizygomatic width), and the anteroposterior projection. Reconstruction of the anatomy using alignment and fixation of the facial vertical and horizontal buttresses is key. The horizontal buttresses as described by Manson and associates include the frontal bar, infraorbital rim, zygomatic arch, maxillary alveolar bone, and mandibular buttresses. The vertical buttresses include the orbital, frontonasomaxillary, frontozygomaticomaxillary, pterygomaxillary, and mandibular buttresses.

In the past, it has been advocated to wait until the edema resolves before fixation of facial fractures. Surgeons have found that waiting can make the surgical efforts more difficult and now advocate immediate repair once the patient is stabilized. Panfacial fractures frequently occur concomitantly with closed head injuries, mandating neurosurgical evaluation and possible treatment prior to any maxillofacial intervention. A team approach in conjunction with the neurosurgeons is important in the cases requiring cranialization of the frontal sinus. It is important to reconstruct the frontal bar and superior aspect of the NOE fracture before placement of an anteriorly based pericranial flap, to allow access to this region.

The goal of modern panfacial fracture repair and reconstruction is achievement of the preinjury level of both function and cosmesis. The treatment of these complex fractures mandates knowledge of facial bony anatomy and facial cosmetic surgery.

Bibliography

Bagheri SC, Dierks EJ, Kademani D, et al: Comparison of the severity of bilateral Le Fort injuries in isolated midface trauma, *J Oral Maxillofac Surg* 63:1123-1129, 2005.

Bagheri SC, Dierks EJ, Kademani D, et al: Application of a Facial Injury Severity Scale in craniomaxillofacial trauma, *J Oral Maxillofac Surg* 64:404-414, 2006.

Bähr W, Stoll P: Nasal intubation in the presence of frontobasal fractures: a retrospective study, *J Oral Maxillofac Surg* 50:445-447, 1992.

Bell RB, Dierks EJ, Homer L, Potter BE: Management of cerebrospinal fluid leak associated with craniomaxillofacial trauma, *J Oral Maxillofac Surg* 62(6):676-684, 2004.

Bouma GJ, Muizelaar JP: Relationship between cardiac output and cerebral blood flow in patients with intact and with impaired autoregulation, *J Neurosurg* 73:368-374, 1990.

Bouma GJ, Muizelaar JP, Bandoh K, et al: Blood pressure and intracranial pressure-volume dynamics in severe head injury: relationship with cerebral blood flow, *J Neurosurg* 77:15-19, 1992.

Buehler JA, Tannyhill RJ: Complications in the treatment of midfacial fractures, *Oral Maxillofacial Surg Clin N Am* 15:195-212, 2003.

Changaris DG, McGraw CP, Richardson JD, et al: Correlation of cerebral perfusion pressure and Glasgow Coma Scale to outcome, *J Trauma* 27:1007-1013, 1987.

Haug RH, Wible RT, Likavek MJ, et al: Cervical spine fractures and maxillofacial trauma, *J Oral Maxillofac Surg* 49:725, 1991.

Horellou MF, Mathe D, Feisse P: A hazard of naso-tracheal intubation, *Anaesthesia* 33:73-74, 1978.

Kreiner B, Stevens MR, Bankston S, Piecuch JF: Management of panfacial fractures, *Oral Maxillofac Surg Knowledge Update* 3:63-81, 2001.

Le Fort R: Experimental study of fractures of the upper jaw. Pars I, II and II. *Rev Chir De Paris* 23:208-227, 360-379, 479-507, 1901; translated by Tessier P: *Plast Reconstr Surg* 50:600-607, 497-506, 1972.

Manson PN, Clark N, Robertson B, Crawley WA: Comprehensive management of pan-facial fractures, *J Craniomaxillofac Trauma* 1(1):43-56, 1995.

Manson PN, Hoopes JE, Su CT: Structural pillars of the facial skeleton: an approach to the management of Le Fort fractures, *Plast Reconstr Surg* 66:53-61, 1980.

Marion DW, Darby J, Yonas H: Acute regional cerebral blood flow changes caused by severe head injuries, *J Neurosurg* 74:407-414, 1991.

Marlow TJ, Goltra DD, Schabel SI: Intracranial placement of a nasotracheal tube after facial fracture: a rare complication, *J Emerg Med* 15:187-191, 1997.

Marmarou A, Anderson RL, Ward JD, et al: Impact of intracranial pressure instability and hypotension on outcome in patients with severe head trauma, *J Neurosurg* 75:S59-S66, 1991.

Ng M, Saadat D, Sinha UK: Managing the emergency airway in Le Fort fractures, *J Craniomaxillofac Trauma* 4:38, 1998.

Rosner MJ, Daughton S: Cerebral perfusion pressure management in head injury, *J Trauma* 30:933-941, 1990.

8 Orthognathic Surgery

Shahrokh C. Bagheri, DMD, MD, and Chris Jo, DMD

This chapter addresses:
- Mandibular Orthognathic Surgery
- Maxillary Orthognathic Surgery
- Maxillomandibular Surgery for Apertognathia
- Distraction Osteogenesis: Mandibular Advancement in Conjunction With Traditional Orthognathic Surgery

---

Correction of dentofacial deformities using combined orthodontic and surgical treatment can provide dramatic changes in both the cosmetic and functional aspects of the face. Patient commitment to an extended period of treatment, along with a close working relationship with the orthodontist, is essential to a successful outcome.

An important component of the management of patients planning for orthognathic surgery is the correct diagnosis of both dental and skeletal abnormalities. Dental compensation can frequently mask an underlying skeletal deformity. Assessment of the maxilla and mandible should consider the three dimensions: anteroposterior, vertical, and transverse. Evaluation at each dimension should account for cosmetic factors (e.g., amount of tooth/gingival show, or size of chin), growth abnormalities (hypoplasia or hyperplasia), and asymmetries.

Treatment is tailored at each patient based on the procedure that would achieve the best result while minimizing morbidity. Patient education about the procedure, postoperative healing, and potential complications of orthognathic surgery is by far the most important factor toward ensuring patient satisfaction.

In this chapter, we provide four teaching cases that address maxillary, mandibular, and bimaxillary surgery. In addition, we present a case of severe mandibular horizontal hypoplasia that is treated using distraction osteogenesis surgery.

Mandibular Orthognathic Surgery

Shahrokh C. Bagheri, DMD, MD, Timothy M. Osborn, DDS, and Brett A. Ueeck, DMD, MD

CC

A 21-year-old man presents for consultation regarding his abnormal bite.

HPI

The patient is referred by his orthodontist for combined surgical orthodontic correction of his skeletal Class II deformity. He explains that he has difficulty eating foods with the front teeth and has become very self-aware of his small lower jaw and chin (both functional and cosmetic complaint). He does not have any symptoms of temporomandibular joint (TMJ) dysfunction (TMD) (although a relationship between malocclusion and TMD has been suggested, the scientific evidence is not clear).

PMHX/PSHX/MEDICATIONS/ALLERGIES/SH/FH

Noncontributory.

EXAMINATION

The examination of a patient for orthognathic surgery can be divided into four components: TMJ, skeletal, dental, and soft tissue components. Skeletal discrepancies (hypoplasia or hyperplasia) should be assessed in three dimensions: transverse (horizontal), anteroposterior, and vertical.

- **Maxillofacial.**
  - **TMJ.** There are no abnormalities (no muscle tenderness, click, or pops).

    The maximal interincisal opening is 42 mm with good lateral excursions.
  - **Skeletal.** There is no facial asymmetry.
    - **Transverse.**
      - Maxillary dental midline is coincident with the facial midline.
      - Mandibular dental midline is coincident with the maxillary dental midline.
      - Chin point is coincident with the maxillary and mandibular midlines.
      - Maxillary occlusal plane is canted down 1 mm on the right.
      - Mandibular angles are level.
      - Maxillary and mandibular arch widths are adequate (evaluated by handheld models or by having the patient posture the mandible forward into a Class I relationship).

      - **Vertical.** Within normal limits
        - **Anteroposterior.**
          - Nasolabial angle is 110° (normal is 100° ± 10°).
          - There is a convex facial profile.
          - Chin is microgenic.
          - Labiomental angle is deep (consistent with mandibular hypoplasia).
      - **Dental.** Occlusion and dentition
        - Class II relationship is present at first molars and canines.
        - Overjet is 10 mm (Figure 8-1).
        - There is no crossbite.
        - The arch form is level with no crowding.
      - **Soft tissue.**
        - Upper lip has adequate thickness and length.

IMAGING

The panoramic and lateral cephalogram are the minimum preoperative radiographs necessary for mandibular orthognathic surgery. The panoramic radiograph allows evaluation of the dentition, the mandibular bony anatomy, and the position of any impacted third molars. Most surgeons recommend surgical removal of the mandibular third molars at least 9 months prior to a sagittal split osteotomy (alternatively, third molars can be removed during the procedure).

The lateral cephalogram is the best film for evaluation of the anteroposterior position of the soft and hard tissue. Measurements of cephalometric norms are used for evaluation of the mandible (and maxilla) in the vertical and anteroposterior dimensions. Most current cephalometric analysis involves comparing the position of the mandible in reference the cranial base (SNB) and the maxilla (ANB). A variety of other measurements are used to assess the vertical or horizontal abnormalities of the maxillomandibular complex (including teeth). Lateral cephalometric analysis does not assess mediolateral facial parameters.

For this patient, the following cephalometric measurements were obtained (Figure 8-2). Normal parameters for Caucasians are given in parentheses.

- **Assessment of the relationship of the maxilla and mandible to the cranial base and to each other.**
  - SNB: 71° (80° ± 3°) (suggestive of mandibular hypoplasia)
  - ANB: 10° (2° ± 2°) (maxillomandibular discrepancy due to mandibular hypoplasia)
  - SNA: 81° (82° ± 3°)

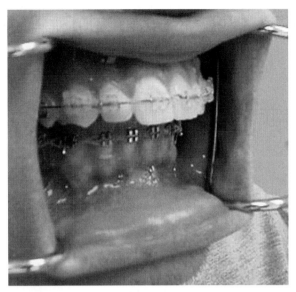

Figure 8-1. Preoperative occlusion demonstrating an overjet of 10 mm.

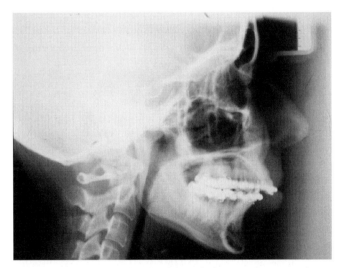

Figure 8-2. Preoperative lateral cephalogram demonstrating a severe Class II molar relationship.

- **Vertical facial measurements.**
  - Nasion to anterior nasal spine (N-ANS): 57 mm (female: 53 mm, male: 58 mm)
  - ANS-Me: 70 mm (female: 74 mm, male: 67 mm)
- **Relationship of the teeth to the skeletal base.**
  - Upper 1 to SN: 104° (102° to 104°)
  - Lower 1 to mandibular plane (MP): 105° (90° to 95°) (suggestive of dental compensation for mandibular hypoplasia)

The lateral cephalometric analysis (taken during early orthodontic treatment) is consistent with mandibular hypoplasia with dental compensation of the mandibular teeth.

LABS

A baseline hemoglobin and hematocrit are the minimum preoperative laboratory values necessary for orthognathic surgery in the otherwise healthy patient.

Before and after orthodontic treatment, maxillary and mandibular dental casts are obtained for treatment planning and construction of an occlusal splint.

ASSESSMENT

Mandibular hypoplasia most pronounced in the anteroposterior dimension, resulting in a Class II skeletal malocclusion

TREATMENT

Treatment of mandibular hypoplasia or hyperplasia is dependent on any coexisting maxillary dentofacial abnormalities. If the position of the maxilla is deemed to be appropriate (clinical and radiographic analysis), mandibular surgery alone can be considered, since the final position of the mandible will be dictated by the occlusion and the position of the maxilla. If the maxilla is abnormally positioned, then maxillomandibular surgery is indicated. Setting the mandible anteriorly or posteriorly in the ideal occlusion may produce an unaesthetic chin position. Therefore the need for adjunctive surgical procedures (advancement/reduction genioplasty/submental liposuction) should be considered, especially in mandibular setbacks.

The basic method of the sagittal split osteotomy remains unchanged since its original description; however, individual surgeons have developed different instrumentations and drilling sequences to complete the surgery. Similarly, practitioners differ on the preference for fixation ranging form using bicortical position screws, lag screws, or rigid fixation plate(s).

Patients with mandibular asymmetry require special consideration related to correction of the deformity. Surgical implications include the uneven overlap of the osteotomized distal and proximal segments. Similarly, the end position of the chin and the mandibular angles have to be anticipated for optimal results. Bony recontouring, genioplasty, or augmentation at the angles or chin may be required.

The overlying soft tissue response to mandibular osteotomies can be predicted. In general, the soft tissue (chin/lip) response for mandibular advancement or setback is about 90% of the skeletal move (i.e., advancing the mandible 10 mm will advance the chin and lip about 9 mm). The status of facial growth also needs to be determined in younger patients. The gold standard for evaluation of facial growth is superimposition of interval (6 months apart) standard lateral cephalograms.

This patient underwent a bilateral sagittal split osteotomy (Figure 8-3, *A*) resulting in an 8-mm advancement. The proximal and distal segments were fixated using three bicortical position screws at the superior border (Figure 8-3, *B*) on each side. Figure 8-4 demonstrates the occlusion 9 months after

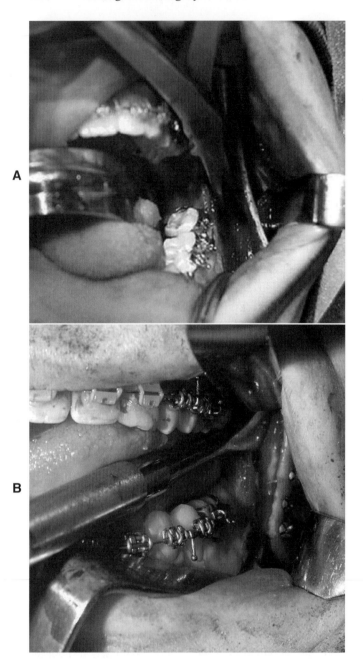

Figure 8-3. **A,** Intraoperative view immediately after completion of the left sagittal split osteotomy. **B,** Intraoperative view demonstrating placement of three bicortical position screws placed above the inferior alveolar canal.

completion of surgery and 1 month after removal of the orthodontic appliances.

COMPLICATIONS

Complications of mandibular orthognathic surgery can be categorized into intraoperative, early, and late. The complications related to the sagittal split osteotomy are emphasized next:

Intraoperative. The most common intraoperative complication is an undesirable split or fracture of the segments,

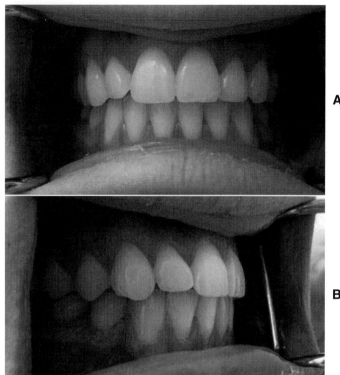

Figure 8-4. **A** and **B,** Postoperative occlusion after completion of the postoperative orthodontics.

reported in 3% to 20% of cases. A common cause of proximal segment fractures is failure to complete the osteotomy at the inferior border, resulting in free segment. Some proximal segment fractures can lead to fracture propagation up to the condylar head. Confirmation of the continuity of the condyle with the proximal segment will detect this fracture. Undesirable fractures can be treated with rigid fixation or a period of 6 to 8 weeks of intermaxillary fixation.

Damage to the interior alveolar nerve is a known complication of the sagittal split osteotomy. When possible, intraoperative transection of the nerve is best treated by immediate epineural repair. Retention of the neurovascular bundle in the proximal segment as the mandible is split is a common cause of injury to the nerve. If the nerve is observed to be in the proximal segment as the mandible is split, it should be gently dissected and positioned along the canal in the distal segment.

Uncontrollable intraoperative hemorrhage is uncommon for mandibular orthognathic surgery in an otherwise healthy patient. However, it can be seen in patients with vascular anomalies or undiagnosed coagulopathies. Damage to the facial artery or retromandibular vein is uncommon but can be caused by inadvertent laceration of the periosteal envelope.

Early. Early complications include malocclusion, wound infection, hardware failure, periodontal defects (more common with interdental osteotomies), and injury to teeth. Early postoperative neurosensory deficit (inferior alveolar nerve) is not considered a complication because the majority of cases (over 85%) demonstrate some degree of paresthesia. Progressive improvement can be observed up to 9 to 12 months postoperatively.

The presence of immediate postoperative malocclusion can be indicative of hardware failure or intersegmental shifting. If this is not detected clinically or radiographically, it is most likely due to proximal (condylar) segment malpositioning during fixation (e.g., if the condyle is not seated in the fossa as it is fixated to the distal segment, upon release of intermaxillary fixation, the condyles will reposition resulting in a anterior open bite).

Infection is a rare complication (less than 3%) in otherwise healthy patients. Hardware removal commonly allows rapid resolution of a draining fistula or ongoing acute infection. Antibiotics may be used to hasten the recovery. Bone fragments that form a sequestrum (frequently a segment of the inferior border) should also be considered in the differential diagnosis of a nonhealing wound.

Late. Permanent neurosensory abnormalities (beyond 12 months) are seen in less than 10% of bilateral sagittal split osteotomies. Intraoperative nerve transection, placement of a screw through the nerve, and neurovascular encroachment by bony segments are possible etiologies of permanent nerve injury. Given the high incidence of prolonged postoperative hypoesthesia, the diagnosis of a permanent nerve injury is often very difficult. Due to the spontaneous recovery of the majority of cases, surgeons are generally inclined to observe postoperative hypoesthesia/anesthesia for extended periods of time. This may lead to permanent neurosensory deficits in a small number of patients that may benefit from early postoperative nerve exploration.

Relapse refers to late postoperative occlusal changes toward the preoperative occlusion. The etiology of relapse is not entirely clear; however, it is hypothesized to be related to postoperative changes in the mandibular bony architecture (e.g., condylar resorption) or to failure of the neuromuscular system to adjust to the new mandibular position resulting in an unfavorable muscle pull. Relapse is seen in approximately 20% of mandibular advancements and is usually limited to about 15% of the total surgical advancement. It has been shown that larger surgical moves (greater than 7 mm) have a greater possibility of relapse, supporting the neuromuscular adaptation/pull etiology for relapse.

DISCUSSION

The first description of mandibular osteotomy dates to Hullihen in 1849 (mandibular subapical osteotomy). Subsequently, several techniques and modifications were described, including the Blair ramus osteotomy, Limberg oblique ramus osteotomy C-osteotomy, inverted L-osteotomy, and the vertical ramus osteotomy. The vertical ramus osteotomy procedure is still used by many surgeons via an intraoral approach (intraoral vertical ramus osteotomy). Mandibular orthognathic surgery was revolutionized by the development of the bilateral sagittal split osteotomy by Obegwesser in 1955 in

Germany. The procedure has since undergone several modifications by Obegwesser, Dalpont, Hunsuck, and others. Today, the bilateral sagittal split osteotomy remains the most commonly used osteotomy for advancement or setback of the mandible. The Dalpont modification was one of the earlier changes that introduced the vertical cut through the cortex. Hunsuck suggested a shorter medial osteotomy posteriorly, resulting in a shorter split and allowing reduced soft tissue trauma and improved posterior mandibular contour, especially with larger setbacks.

Successful orthognathic surgery requires good communication between the surgeon and orthodontist, as well as patient commitment toward a long treatment period. The main goals of preoperative orthodontic treatment include leveling and aligning of the arches, positioning of the teeth over the basal bone, and proper inclination of the teeth (dental decompensation), especially the incisors. Placement of molar bands and adequate orthodontic hardware is important for intraoperative maxillomandibular fixation.

Augmentation or reduction genioplasty is frequently used in conjunction with mandibular orthognathic surgery. Similarly, some patients may elect to defer orthognathic surgery and only undergo chin surgery. A patient with mandibular hypolasia may elect to "camouflage" the abnormality by an advancement genioplasty alone. Although this does not alter the dental relationship, it can improve the aesthetic outcome.

The preoperative work-up is a combination of clinical and radiographic planning. The decision for the surgical movements should be predominantly determined from the patient and not the radiographs, leading to the adage, "Treat the patient, not the radiograph." Once the clinical and cephalometric plans are in place, preoperative dental casts should be made and mounted on an articulator with facebow transfer and occlusal registration. The casts should be trimmed anatomically so that measurements and moves on the casts can be accurately transferred to the operating room. Once the model surgery has been performed based on the cephalometric predictions and clinical examination, the acrylic splint can be made. Measurements should be recorded and verified on the films and surgical casts.

There are several adjuncts used clinically during the operative period to enhance both the surgical field and the patient's recovery. The use of hypotensive anesthesia at the time of the osteotomy helps to minimize the amount of blood loss and increase the surgeon's visibility, allowing for more precise and timely surgery. In general, an increase of up to 500 ml of blood loss can be expected in patients not undergoing hypotensive anesthesia. While the exact amount of blood loss and increase in visibility are still debated, several studies have shown this method to be effective. A reverse Trendelenburg (head-up) position will also aid in reduction of venous congestion in the head and neck.

The use of antibiotics and steroids has been debated. A single preoperative prophylactic dose of antibiotic is probably useful in reducing the infection risk without undo adverse sequelae. Studies have shown an infection rate of less than

5% with a single preoperative antibiotic dose. Some surgeons suggest continuing antibiotics for 5 to 7 days postoperatively, but this practice is not supported by clinical studies. To continue antibiotics beyond the preoperative dose is probably unwarranted in an otherwise healthy patient. Corticosteroids have been shown to decrease the total amount and length of time of postsurgical edema. They are also beneficial antinausea medications.

Despite the decreasing reimbursement and insurance coverage, orthognathic surgery continues to be a viable tool for treatment of a variety of clinical diagnoses, with significant impact on both function and cosmetisis. The skills required to successfully perform these operations is challenging and requires continuing refinement and education.

Bibliography

Baqain ZH, Hyde N, Patrikidou A, Harris M: Antibiotic prophylaxis for orthognathic surgery: a prospective, randomised clinical trial, *Br J Oral Maxillofac Surg* 42(6):506-510, 2004.

Bays RA: Complications of orthognathic surgery. In Kaban LB, Perrot DH, Pogrel MA, eds: *Complications of oral and maxillofacial surgery,* Philadelphia, 1997, WB Saunders.

Dalpont G: Retromolar osteotomy for the correction of prognathism, *J Oral Surg Anesth Hosp D Serv* 19:42, 1961.

Hullihen SP: Case of elongation if the under jaw and distortion of the face and neck, caused by a burn, successfully treated, *Am J Dent Sci* 9:157, 1849.

Hunsuk EE: Modified intraoral sagittal splitting technique for correction of mandibular prognathism, *J Oral Surg* 26:250, 1968.

Obwegeser H: The indications for surgical correction of mandibular deformity by the sagittal split technique, *Br J Oral Surg* 1:157, 1962.

Praveen K, Narayanan V, Muthusekhar MR, Baig MF: Hypotensive anaesthesia and blood loss in orthognathic surgery: a clinical study, *Br J Oral Maxillofac Surg* 39(2):138-140, 2001.

Shepherd J: Hypotensive anaesthesia and blood loss in orthognathic surgery, *Evid Based Dent* 5(1):16, 2004.

Zijderveld SA, Smeele LE, Kostense PJ, Tuinzing DB: Preoperative antibiotic prophylaxis in orthognathic surgery: a randomized, double-blind, and placebo-controlled clinical study, *J Oral Maxillofac Surg* 57(12):1403-1406, discussion 1406-1407, 1999.

Maxillary Orthognathic Surgery

Chris Jo DMD, Brett A. Ueeck, DMD, MD, and Timothy M. Osborn, DDS

CC

A 19-year-old woman is referred by her orthodontist for combined surgical-orthodontic management of her Class III skeletal malocclusion and maxillary hypoplasia. She complains that, "My face looks sunken in and looks too short."

For the treatment planning of patients presenting for orthognathic surgery, it is essential to differentiate the degree of cosmetic versus functional complaints. For elective surgical procedures, a successful outcome requires this distinction to be well integrated in the surgical plan. Although this patient's functional impairments are obvious, she focuses mostly on her appearance.

HPI

The patient admits to some difficulty and discomfort when chewing certain foods, but her main concern is her appearance. She presents to your office after finishing 3 years of orthodontic therapy. She was being monitored for cessation of mandibular growth and possible development of mandibular hyperplasia in conjunction with maxillary hypoplasia. Serial 1-year-interval lateral cephalograms showed that her mandibular growth was complete (interval superimposition of standard lateral cephalogram is a reliable way to monitor facial growth). Her occlusion has been aligned and leveled for a single-piece Le Fort I osteotomy (if the curve of Spee cannot be leveled in the mandibular arch preoperatively, then postoperative tripod occlusion and postoperative leveling are planned). There is no history or symptoms of TMDs (preexisting TMD should be recognized and addressed before orthognathic surgery. It is possible that orthognathic surgery may exacerbate preexisting TMD. Although some surgeons recommend simultaneous orthognathic and TMJ surgery in select cases of preexisting anterior disc displacement, this issue is highly controversial).

PMHX/PSHX/MEDICATIONS/ALLERGIES/SH/FH

Noncontributory.

Elective orthognathic surgery should be avoided on patients who are of classified as ASA III or greater.

EXAMINATION

The examination of a patient for orthognathic surgery can be divided into four components: TMJ, skeletal, dental, and soft tissue. Skeletal discrepancies (hypoplasia or hyperplasia) should be assessed in three dimensions: transverse (horizontal), anteroposterior, and vertical. As for all surgical patients, the airway, cardiopulmonary, neurological, and other organ systems should be assessed in anticipation of general anesthesia.

- **Maxillofacial.**
  - **TMJ.** The muscles of mastication and the TMJ capsule are nontender, with no evidence of clicking, or crepitus (seen with disc perforation). The maximal interincisal opening is 45 mm with good excursive movements and no deviation upon opening or closing (normal TMJ examination).
  - **Skeletal.** There is no vertical orbital dystopia. The intercanthal distance is 31 mm (normal). The nose is straight and coincident with the midline. Malar eminences are within norm.
    - **Transverse.**
      - Maxillary dental midline is 1 mm right of the facial midline.
      - Mandibular dental midline is 1 mm left of the maxillary dental midline and coincident with the facial midline.
      - Chin point is coincident with the facial midline.
      - Maxillary occlusal plane is canted down 1 mm on the left at the canine.
      - Mandibular occlusal plane and angles are level.
      - Maxillary arch width is adequate (evaluated by handheld models).
    - **Vertical.**
      - The lower facial third is deficient (normal nasion-ANS–to–ANS-menton ratio is 7:8).
      - Maxillary incisor length is 10 mm.
      - Upper incisor show is 0 mm at rest (ideally, 2- to 4-mm tooth show at rest) and 6 mm in full smile (in an aesthetically pleasing smile line, the gingival papilla or 1 mm of gingival margin is visible at full smile).
  - **Anteroposterior.**
    - Overjet is −6 mm.
    - Nasolabial angle is 45° (normal is 100° ± 10°).
    - Labiomental fold is within normal limits.
    - Chin is relatively prognathic.
    - Profile is brachycephalic (Figure 8-5, *A*).
  - **Dental.** Occlusion and dentition
    - There is deep bite (Figure 8-5, *B*).
    - Overjet is −6 mm (normal is +3.5 mm ± 2.5 mm).
    - Class III relationship is present at the first molars and canines bilaterally.

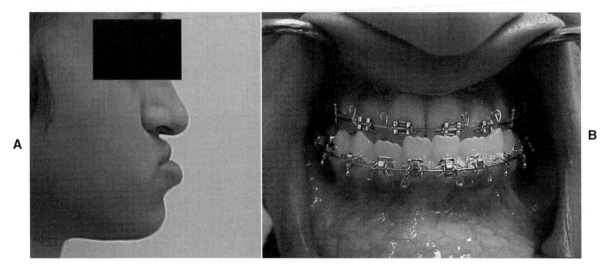

Figure 8-5. **A,** Preoperative profile view showing shortened lower facial third height and midface hypoplasia. **B,** Preoperative intraoral view showing Class III skeletal malocclusion.

- Arch width is adequate on hand-held models (transverse maxillary deficiencies may require a segmental Le Fort I osteotomy or surgically assisted rapid palatal expansion).
- Curve of Spee has been appropriately leveled, and additional postoperative leveling will be required (1 to 1.5 mm of arch space is required for each 1 mm of curve of Spee leveled).
- The maxillary and mandibular arch forms are ideal.
- Dental compensations have been adequately decompensated without the need for bicuspid extractions (retracting proclined incisors require 0.8 mm of arch space for each 1° retracted; proclining incisors 1.25° gains 1 mm of arch space).
- The dentition is in good repair with no missing teeth (except for third molars).
  ○ **Soft tissue.**
    - Upper lip has adequate thickness and length.
    - Nasolabial angle is 40° (normal is 100° ± 10°).
    - Downward rotation of the nasal tip.

IMAGING

The panoramic radiograph and a lateral cephalometric radiograph are the minimum imaging modalities necessary for orthognathic surgery. Preoperative profile, frontal (upon smiling and rest), and occlusal photographs should be obtained.

For this patient, the panoramic radiograph shows normal bony architecture of the condylar head and no other pathology. The right and left maxillary and mandibular third molars (teeth Nos. 1, 16, 17, and 32) are full bony impacted with minimal root formation.

An initial lateral cephalogram was obtained with the patient in centric relation and lips in a relaxed/reposed position (Figure 8-6). Cephalometric analysis reveals anteropos-

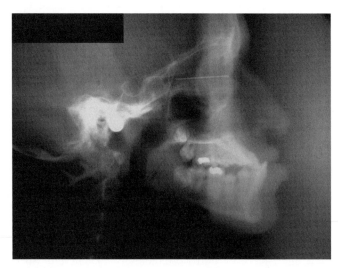

Figure 8-6. Preoperative lateral cephalogram showing maxillary hypoplasia and severe compensation of the maxillary incisors.

terior maxillary hypoplasia. This preorthodontic lateral cephalogram illustrates the degree of skeletal discrepancies, as well as the degree of dental compensations (proclined maxillary incisors), that are important considerations when calculating the adequacy of the existing arch space and determining the need for extractions (decompensating or retroclining flared incisors require 0.8 mm of arch space for each 1° of retraction). It is important to note that measurements differ betwecn Caucasians, Asians and African Americans (Caucasian normal values are listed in Box 8-1).

LABS

Baseline hemoglobin and hematocrit values are the minimum preoperative laboratory values necessary for orthognathic surgery in the otherwise healthy patient. This patient had

---

Box 8-1. Cephalometric Analysis (Normal Caucasian Measurements)

- Cranial base angle is normal (nasion-sella [SN]-basion angle norm is 129° ± 4° and sella-nasion [SN] to Frankfurt horizontal [FH] normal value is 7° ± 4°).
- SNA 79° (suggestive of a maxillary anteroposterior deficiency relative to the cranial base. Normal value is 82° ± 3°).
- SNB 88° (suggestive of an excessive anteroposterior position of the mandible relative to cranial base. Normal value is 80° ± 3°).
- Harvold difference (distance from condylion to pogonion minus distance from condylion to A point) is excessive (suggestive of maxillary hypoplasia or mandibular hyperplasia. Normal value in females is 27 mm and 29 mm in males).
- Mandibular plane (MP) is flat (SN-MP normal value is 32° ± 10° and FH-MP normal value is 22° ± 6°).
- Long axis of upper incisor to SN angle is 134° (severely compensated maxillary incisors. Normal value is 104° ± 4°).
- Long axis of lower incisor to MP angle is 100° (normal value is 90° ± 5°).
- Upper lip to E-plane is −5 mm (normal value is −3 mm ± 2 mm).
- Lower lip to E-plane is +3 mm (shows retrusive soft tissue chin and concave profile. Normal value is −2 mm).

---

normal values (hemoglobin of 13.1 mg/dL and hematocrit of 40.2%).

A pregnancy test (urine pregnancy test or serum beta-hCG) is also warranted for females of childbearing age. The need for transfusion of blood products is rare, so a type and screen is generally not warranted.

ASSESSMENT

Maxillary hypoplasia resulting in a Class III skeletal facial deformity

TREATMENT

Treatment of maxillary hypoplasia involves a combined orthodontic and surgical approach for stable results. A coordinated approach between orthodontist and oral and maxillofacial surgeon requires a close working relationship to meet the needs of the patient. The goals of presurgical orthodontic therapy are to:

- Align and level the occlusion
- Coordinate the maxillary and mandibular arches (progress is monitored with hand-held models)
- Eliminate dental compensations in preparation for surgical correction of the skeletal deformities
- Diverge the roots of adjacent teeth for planned segmental osteotomies (only the roots should be diverged while the crowns retain interproximal contact).

During the treatment-planning phase, the need for dental extractions is determined. The surgeon should be aware of the rationale for arch space management during the presurgical orthodontic phase. It is important to avoid any unstable orthodontic movement (closing anterior open bites by extruding maxillary or mandibular anterior teeth or widening the posterior maxillary horizontal dimension by tipping the molars) that would later result in relapse. Postsurgical orthodontic is aimed at creating a final stable occlusion and closure of any posterior open bites that resulted from the surgical correction. Frequently, the orthodontist is not able to level the mandibular curve of Spee presurgically and sets up a tripod occlusion. The curve is leveled and spaces are closed postoperatively. Most orthodontists use a retainer for maintenance of the final occlusal relationship and alignment.

The orthognathic surgical treatment options/plan for maxillary hypoplasia is case specific but may include a Le Fort I osteotomy and advancement (single piece versus multiple piece) or bimaxillary surgery. During maxillary advancement, the surgeon can also control the vertical position of the maxilla and incisors, as the mandibular arc of rotation and model setup will determine the final position of both the maxilla and mandible (mounted model surgery is paramount to determine anteroposterior position of the maxillomandibular unit when it is set at the desired vertical position). A Le Fort I osteotomy alone can be considered when:

- The mandible is in good position (dental midline and chin midline coincident with the facial midline)
- There is no mandibular occlusal cant
- The mandible is aligned with the face (symmetrical)
- The mandibular arc of rotation positions the maxilla into a good anteroposterior position, while maintaining an appropriate chin projection

A segmental Le Fort I osteotomy is indicated when a transverse deficiency or when a dual occlusal plane exists. Bimaxillary (maxillomandibular) surgery (Le Fort I and sagittal split or vertical ramus osteotomies) may be warranted when deformities exist in both the maxilla and mandible, and the mandibular position and arc of rotation cannot be used to position the maxilla (see the section on maxillomandibular surgery for Apertognathia later in this chapter). Surgically assisted rapid palatal expansion should be considered when there is a maxillary transverse discrepancy or arch length discrepancy with no other vertical or anteroposterior discrepancies.

Once the surgical treatment plan has been developed, the surgeon can proceed with model surgery to fabricate surgical splint(s) on mounted models. If the open bite is to be closed with maxillary surgery alone, then the maxillary cast is set to the ideal occlusion with the opposing mounted mandibular cast (occlusion set with a small posterior open bite will maximize the amount of incisor overlap and reduce relapse). Small posterior open bites can be easily closed orthodontically, especially in young patients (surgically created posterior open bites allow maximal overlap of the anterior teeth, reducing the risk of relapse). A thin interocclusal acrylic wafer (splint) is made to stabilize the occlusion intraoperatively during rigid fixation of the maxilla. If a segmental osteotomy is performed, then the splint is made with a palatal strap and wired to the maxillary dentition during the healing phase to prevent horizontal collapse and relapse of the open bite. The maxilla is generally fixated with four-point fixation (at piriform rim and zygomaticomaxillary buttress bilaterally) using 1.5- or 2.0-mm plates.

When performing maxillary osteotomy, surgeons should communicate with the anesthesiologist the need for hypotensive anesthesia to reduce intraoperative bleeding. When feasible, hypotension induced with beta-blockers rather than "deep anesthesia" with anesthetic gases is preferred, as the former is more effective and easily titrated. After nasotracheal intubation, Marcaine (bupivacaine) with epinephrine is infiltrated in the maxillary buccal vestibule (injection of vasoconstrictor in the palate should be avoided). Incision design is a critical portion of the surgery, and the vascular perfusion of the hard and soft tissues is the most important factor in healing. The most common incision used during Le Fort I osteotomy is a horizontal incision through the mucosa well above the level of the keratinized gingiva (1 cm past the buccal sulcus) from first molar to first molar with scalpel or electrocautery (the parotid papilla should be identified and protected before the incision). Incision is then carried down through the periosteum to bone. Keeping the periosteal incision perpendicular to the bone prevents extrusion of the buccal fat pad. Subperiosteal dissection is performed on the superior aspect of the incision, preserving the cuff of mucogingival tissue. Dissection is to the piriform rim, up to the infraorbital foramen with exposure of the zygomaticomaxillary buttress. Dissection is then carried posteriorly with subperiosteal tunneling to the pterygomaxillary fissure. Attention is then turned to elevation of the nasal mucosa from the medial portion of the lateral wall and floor. After the maxilla is exposed, vertical reference points can be established (both internal and external references have been used).

A curved retractor is then placed at the pterygomaxillary junction, and a Freer or other retractor is placed under the nasal mucosa for protection during the osteotomy. The osteotomy is then made by using a reciprocating saw, with care taken to remain 5 to 6 mm above the root apices. A nasal septal osteotome is then used to free the septal cartilage and vomer from the nasal floor. A spatula osteotome can be used to complete the lateral nasal osteotomies. A pterygoid osteotome is then placed and angled slightly inferiorly so as to avoid inadvertently lacerating the internal maxillary artery, which is approximately 25 mm superior to the pterygomaxillary junction. The pterygomaxillary junction is then separated with the osteotome. Gentle pressure can be applied to the anterior maxilla as the nasal mucosa is elevated. With continuing downfracture, the descending palatine neurovascular bundle will come into view, and care should be taken to prevent injury to the vessels (some surgeons elect to ligate and section the descending palatine neurovascular bundle). Any areas of incomplete osteotomy can be identified and mobilized to completely free the mobilized segment. The maxilla should be completely mobilized so that it can be repositioned and stabilized as planned. If a multiple-piece Le Fort is planned, the interdental osteotomy is made before downfracture of the maxilla and parasagittal (thinner bone and thicker soft tissue compared with the midline) osteotomies are made after the downfracture. Also, inferior turbinate reduction should be considered when performing maxillary impactions.

Next, the surgical splint is inserted and secured to the dental arch. The maxillomandibular complex is then passively seated, and any bony interferences are selectively removed until the desired vertical height is achieved (complete paralysis should be verified with train of four twitches by the anesthesiologist). If there are any large defects in the walls of the maxilla, bone grafts can be used. Rigid fixation techniques with plates at the buttress and piriform region is the most commonly used method of stabilizing the maxilla. Once rigidly fixed, the maxillomandibular fixation can be removed so that the occlusion can be checked. The mandible should seat passively into the splint, verifying proper stabilization as planned. Some surgeons place deep sutures into the muscular layer to reapproximate the facial and labial musculature, prior to mucosal closure. The mucosal layer is closed with a running suture in a V-Y pattern to help maintain lip length. A completion of the procedure, the occlusion is verified, and light elastics are used as needed to guide the occlusion.

The final results of the patient described above can be seen in Figure 8-7.

COMPLICATIONS

An important aspect of orthognathic surgery is management of complications. A well-informed patient and attention to detail cannot be overemphasized. The most important complications of maxillary orthognathic surgery are as follows (see Box 8-2 for more details):

- Hemorrhage
- Vascular compromise and maxillary necrosis
- Relapse and malpositioning
- Neurosensory deficits (greater and lesser palatine, nasopalatine, infraorbital nerves)
- Damage to the dentition (maxillary roots) and periodontal defects
- Postoperative nasal deformity

Other complications of maxillary orthognathic surgery include infection, hardware failure, malunion, fibrous union, and pulpal necrosis (devitalization of the teeth, is generally prevented if osteotomy is at least 5 to 6 mm superior to the root apices).

DISCUSSION

The success of maxillary orthognathic surgery owns its origin to recognition of the blood supply to the maxilla first investigated by Bell. The main blood supply is based on branches of the external carotid system including the ascending palatine, ascending pharyngeal, palatine, nasopalatine, posterior

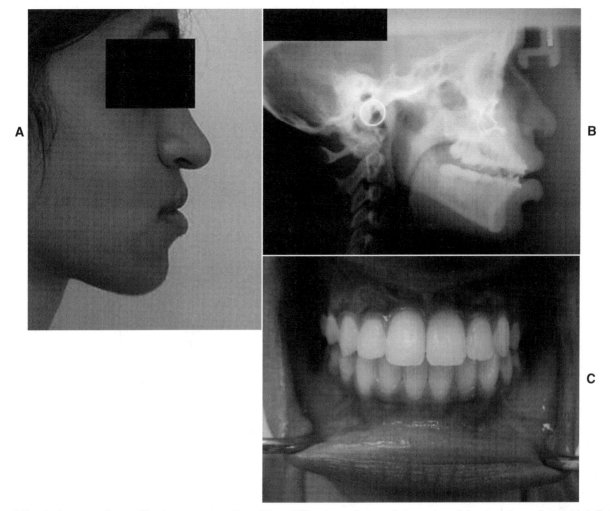

Figure 8-7. **A,** Postoperative profile showing correction of the midface hypoplasia and elongation of the short lower facial third. **B,** Postoperative lateral cephalogram showing correction of the maxillary hypoplasia and aesthetically pleasing facial profile. **C,** Postoperative intraoral view revealing the final occlusion.

superior, and infraorbital arteries. With the maxillary oste-otomy, it has been shown that the buccal gingival and muco-periosteal pedicle and the palatal soft tissue pedicle allow for the preserved blood supply and proper wound healing for the maxillary osteotomy. Proper incision design and minimal dissection of the palatal soft tissues will ensure an adequate blood supply.

Traditional methods of stabilizing the maxillary with wires and prolonged periods of maxillomandibular fixation have been replaced with rigid internal fixation using titanium plates and screws. Resorbable fixation materials have been studied successfully for orthognathic surgery, but they are not routinely applied by most surgeons. Direct bony contact, especially at the zygomaticomaxillary buttresses, is needed to improve immediate and long-term stability. When there are bony gaps, bone grafts may be warranted (especially with large advancements or widening or downgrafting procedures). In those undergoing maxillary advancement, Egbert looked at horizontal and vertical relapse and demonstrated improved stability with rigid fixation compared with wire fixation and maxillomandibular fixation.

The soft tissue changes associated with maxillary surgery are predominantly observed in the nasal and labial struc-tures. The nasal changes depend on the type of movement; anterior repositioning results in widening of the nasal base and increase in the supratip break, superior repositioning leads to elevation of the nasal tip and widening of the nasal base, inferior repositioning results in loss of tip support, while posterior movement results in loss of tip support because of posterior movement of the ANS with minimal change at the alar base. The labial changes include upper lip widening and lengthening of the philtral columns. With V-Y closure, shortening of the upper lip and loss of vermillion are minimized.

Hierarchy of stability in orthognathic surgery has been classically described by Profitt and associates (modifications to original description are given in parentheses) as follows, from most to least stable:

- Maxilla up (non–open bite cases are more stable than open bite cases)
- Mandible forward (low mandibular plane angle is better)
- Maxilla forward

Box 8-2.   Most Important Complications of Maxillary Orthognathic Surgery

- **Hemorrhage.** Intraoperative or postoperative hemorrhage can be life threatening (although rare). Hypotensive anesthesia (mean arterial pressure maintained at around 60 mm Hg) is used by most surgeons to reduce the amount of intraoperative bleeding and to improve visualization of the surgical field. Vascular injury to the pterygoid plexus of veins (most common) can result in a significant amount of blood loss (usually easy to control by packing the wound). An arterial injury (descending palatine artery most common) is more difficult to control and can result in a significant amount of blood loss in a short period of time (internal maxillary artery and its terminal branches are most susceptible during the osteotomy and downfracture of the maxilla). Typically, arterial bleeding can be controlled by controlling the blood pressure, proper visualization, pressure/packing, and electrocautery or hemoclips. Uncontrollable arterial hemorrhage warrants emergent angiography and embolization (a carotid cutdown and ligation of the external carotid artery can be performed but is less efficacious due to collateral arterial supply). Turvey and associates have shown the internal maxillary artery is located 25 mm superior to the to the most inferior junction of the maxilla and pterygoid plate, leaving a 1-mm margin of safety if a 15-mm-wide curved osteotome is used. A late bleed (usually preceded by a sentinel bleed) can arise from undetected injury to the descending palatine artery (most common source of postoperative bleeding), pseudoaneurysm formation, or ischemic necrosis of the descending palatine artery due to excessive stretching (especially if the descending palatine artery was not ligated and sectioned during the procedure) and warrants immediate angiography. When required, selective arterial embolization should be cautiously performed to avoid compromising the blood supply to the maxilla. Self-donated blood banking was previously advocated by some groups, but this practice is no longer used (severe bleeding that requires transfusion of packed red blood cells is very rare when following appropriate transfusion thresholds). The patient should be informed that intermittent small amounts of dark blood may drain from the nose, which may mimic epistaxis, as the blood collection is emptied from the maxillary sinuses.
- **Vascular compromise and maxillary necrosis.** Avascular necrosis of the maxilla is the most feared complication after maxillary orthognathic surgery (higher risk for segmental osteotomies and large advancements). The vascular supply to the maxilla arises from branches of the external carotid artery (ascending palatine artery from the facial artery, and the ascending pharyngeal, greater and lesser palatines, descending palatine, and nasopalatine artery all from the internal maxillary artery). Some surgeons elect to ligate and section the descending palatine neurovascular bundle, which has been shown to not significantly affect labial gingival perfusion. Vascular insult results from not only the incisions and osteotomies/downfracture but also from repositioning of the maxilla. If signs of serious hypoperfusion (pale gingival or palatal mucosa with no capillary refill are early signs and mucosal sloughing is a late sign) is noted intraoperatively, then the procedure should be aborted and the maxilla positioned and rigidly fixed into its original position. If poor perfusion is observed postoperatively, then removal of splints (if wired to the maxilla for postoperative stability) and removal of rigid fixation to allow the maxilla back into its presurgical position may be required. Maxillary splints with a palatal strap should

be constructed with caution; because if they are impinging on the palatal mucosa, they can result in vascular compromise. Hyperbaric oxygen should be considered postoperatively for maxillary hypoperfusion. Smoking has also been implicated in increasing the risk of avascular necrosis.
- **Relapse and malpositioning.** Long-term stability is one of the main goals of orthognathic surgery. Closing anterior open bites with posterior impaction of the maxilla is more stable than a mandibular osteotomy with surgical counterclockwise rotation of the mandible. However, more recent studies suggest that counterclockwise surgical rotation of the mandible is very stable, especially with the advent of rigid fixation. If anterior open bite occurs in the immediate postoperative period, it is likely due to incomplete seating of the condyles intraoperatively. This can be minimized by inducing complete paralysis during fixation and upward manual pressure at the angles of the mandible when positioning the maxillomandibular unit (the maxilla can pivot around a posterior bony prematurity, which will pull the condyle out of the glenoid fossa during positioning of the maxillomandibular complex). Bays introduced the Rigid Adjustable Pin (RAP) system, which allows for postoperative three-dimensional adjustability. If relapse of the open bite occurs several weeks to months after surgery or release of maxillomandibular fixation, the most common cause is collapse of the horizontal dimension of the posterior maxilla (bony horizontal relapse for segmental Le Fort osteotomies or dental relapse of molars inappropriately tipped laterally). The RAP system can also be used when there is inadequate bone for miniplate fixation. Aggressive mobilization of the maxilla and passive repositioning with rigid internal fixation is also important for improved long-term stability. Widening and downward moves are the most unstable moves in maxillary surgery.
- **Neurosensory deficits (greater and lesser palatine, nasopalatine, infraorbital nerves).** Although not severed, traction and compression injury to the infraorbital nerve result in a reported 6% incidence of infraorbital nerve neurosensory deficits at 1 year postoperatively. Nasopalatine and superior alveolar nerves (posterior, middle, and anterior) are severed during surgery (some surgeons also ligate and section the descending palatine neurovascular bundle). Sensory recovery of the palate is much slower and less complete and is likely due to collateral reinnervation. Neurosensory disturbances of the palate are generally well tolerated.
- **Damage to the dentition (maxillary roots) and periodontal defects.** This is especially a concern for segmental Le Fort I osteotomies (although there are no studies to suggest a higher incidence of periodontal defects in segmental osteotomies). The majority of these complications can be avoided by careful presurgical orthodontic preparation (diverging the roots at the interdental osteotomy sites) and careful surgical technique.
- **Postoperative nasal deformity.** Buckling of the cartilaginous nasal septum (quadrangular cartilage) can cause a nasal deformity (deviation of the nasal tip and buckling of the upper lateral cartilages). The nasal septum and the nasal spine of the maxilla and palatine bones should be appropriately trimmed (especially during maxillary impaction), and the caudal portion of the quadrangular cartilage should be trimmed during maxillary advancement. The nasal septum should be secured to the anterior nasal spine with a heavy resorbable suture to prevent displacement during the recovery phase.

- Maxilla up-mandible forward
- Maxilla forward-mandible back
- Mandible back
- Maxilla down
- Maxilla wider

Bibliography

Bays RA: Descending palatine artery ligation in LeFort osteotomies, *J Oral Maxillofac Surg* 8:142, 1993.

Bays RA: Maxillary osteotomies utilizing the Rigid Adjustable Pin (RAP) system: a review of 31 clinical cases, *Int J Adult Orthod Orthognath Surg* 1:275, 1986.

Bays RA, Bouloux GF: Complications of orthognatic surgery, *Oral Maxillofac Surg Clin N Am* 15:229-242, 2003.

Bell WH: Revascularization and bone healing after anterior maxillary osteotomy: a study using adult rhesus monkeys, *J Oral Surg* 27(4):110-115, 1969.

Bell WH, Proffit WR: Esthetic effects of maxillary osteotomy. In Bell WH, Proffit WR, White RP, eds: *Surgical correction of dentofacial deformities,* Philadelphia, 1980, WB Saunders, pp 368-370.

Betts NJ: Techniques to control nasal features, *Atlas Oral Maxillofac Surg Clin N Am* 8(2):53-69, 2000.

Betts NJ, Dowd KF: Soft tissue changes associated with orthognathic surgery, *Atlas Oral Maxillofac Surg Clin N Am* 8(2):1-11, 2000.

Betts NJ, Fonseca RJ, Vig P, et al: Changes in nasal and labial soft tissues after surgical repositioning of the maxilla, *Int J Adult Orthod Orthognath Surg* 8:7, 1993.

Dodson TB, Bays RA, Neuenschwander MC: Maxillary perfusion during Le Fort I osteotomy after ligation of the descending palatine artery, *J Oral Maxillofac Surg* 55:51-55, 1997.

Egbert M, Hepworth B, Myall R, West R: Stability of Le Fort I osteotomy with maxillary advancement: a comparison of combined wire fixation and rigid fixation, *J Oral Maxillofac Surg* 53:243, 1995.

Guymon M, Crosby DR, Wolford LM: The alar base cinch suture to control nasal width in maxillary osteotomies, *Int J Adult Orthod Orthognath Surg* 3:89, 1988.

Ingersoll SK, Peterson LJ, Weinstein S: Influence of horizontal incision on upper lip morphology, *J Dent Res* 61:218, 1982.

Lanigan DT: Vascular complications associated with orthognathic surgery, *Oral Maxillofac Surg Clin N Am* 9(2):231-250, 1997.

Milles M, Betts NJ: Techniques to preserve or modify lip form during orthognathic surgery, *Atlas Oral Maxillofac Surg Clin N Am* 8(2):71-79, 2000.

O'Ryan F, Schendel S: Nasal anatomy and maxillary surgery, I. Esthetic and anatomic principles, *Int J Adult Orthod Orthognath Surg* 4:75, 1989.

O'Ryan F, Schendel S: Nasal anatomy and maxillary surgery, II. Unfavorable nasolabial esthetics following LeFort I osteotomy, *Int J Adult Orthod Orthognath Surg* 4:157, 1989.

Proffit WR, Turvey TA, Phillips C: Orthognathic surgery: a hierarchy of stability, *Int J Adult Orthod Orthognath Surg* 11:191, 1996.

Quejada JG, Kawamura H, Finn RA, et al: Wound healing associated with segmental total maxillary osteotomy, *J Oral Maxillofac Surg* 44:366, 1986.

Radney LJ, Jacobs JD: Soft tissue changes associated with surgical total maxillary intrusion, *Am J Orthod* 80:191, 1981.

Tiner BD, Van Sickels IE, Schmitz JP: Life threatening delayed hemorrhage after LeFort I osteotomy requiring surgical intervention: report of two cases, *J Oral Maxillofac Surg* 49:571, 1997.

Turvey TA, Fonseca RJ: The anatomy of the internal maxillary artery in the pterygopalatine fossa: its relationship to maxillary surgery, *J Oral Surg* 38:92-95, 1980.

Van Sickels JE: Treatment of skeletal open bite deformities, *OMFS Knowledge Update* 2:45-56, 1998.

Wolford ME: Management of transverse maxillary deficiency, *OMFS Knowledge Update* 1:15-20, 1995.

Zweig BE: Esthetic analysis of the cervicofacial region, *Atlas Oral Maxillofac Surg Clin N Am* 8(2):1-11, 2000.

Maxillomandibular Surgery for Apertognathia

Chris Jo, DMD, and Shahrokh C. Bagheri, DMD, MD

CC

A 17-year-old girl is referred by her orthodontist for combined surgical-orthodontic management of her anterior open bite (apertognathia) and mandibular hypoplasia. She complains that, "I have difficulty eating and would like to have my open bite fixed."

For the treatment planning of patients presenting for orthognathic surgery, it is essential to differentiate the degree of cosmetic versus functional complaints. For elective surgical procedures, a successful outcome requires this distinction to be well integrated in the surgical plan.

HPI

The patient reports difficulty chewing certain foods due to the anterior open bite and is also concerned about her facial profile and her retrusive chin. She completed extensive orthodontic therapy as a teenager to close her anterior open bite, which has progressively relapsed (orthodontic closure of an anterior open bite has a high relapse rate). One week before this consultation, she had orthodontic appliances placed by her orthodontist. She admits to a history of a thumb-sucking habit from childhood into her early teen years (thumb- or finger-sucking habits can cause apertognathia). There is no history of tongue thrusting (although this is a difficult parameter to rule out, an unrecognized tongue-thrusting habit can cause future relapse of surgical and orthodontic treatment. Macroglossia should be recognized and treated as needed by tongue reduction procedures). She is congenitally missing the right maxillary third molar, but the remaining third molars are full bony impactions (most surgeons prefer that impacted mandibular third molars be extracted at least 6 to 9 months before mandibular sagittal split osteotomy procedures, to avoid complications related to fixation. Maxillary molars do not need to be removed in advance). There is no history or symptoms of TMDs (preexisting TMD should be recognized and addressed before orthognathic surgery. It is possible that orthognathic surgery may exacerbate preexisting TMD. Although some prominent surgeons recommend simultaneous orthognathic and TMJ surgery in select cases of preexisting anterior disc displacement, this issue is highly controversial).

PMHX/PSHX/MEDICATIONS/ALLERGIES/SH/FH

Noncontributory.

Elective orthognathic surgery should be avoided on patients who are ASA Class III or greater.

EXAMINATION

The examination of a patient for orthognathic surgery can be divided to four components: TMJ, skeletal, dental, and soft tissue. Skeletal discrepancies (hypoplasia or hyperplasia) should be assessed in three dimensions: transverse (horizontal), anteroposterior, and vertical. As for all surgical patients, the airway, cardiopulmonary, neurological, and other organ systems should be fully assessed in anticipation for general anesthesia.

- **Maxillofacial.**
  - **TMJ.** The muscles of mastication and the TMJ capsule are nontender, with no evidence of clicking, or crepitus (seen with disc perforation). The maximal interincisal opening is 45 mm with good excursive movements and no deviation upon opening or closing (normal TMJ examination).
  - **Skeletal.** There is no vertical orbital dystopia. The intercanthal distance is 31 mm (normal). The nose is straight and coincident with the midline. Malar eminences are within normal limits.
    - **Transverse.**
      - Maxillary dental midline is coincident with the facial midline.
      - Mandibular dental midline is 1 mm right of the maxillary dental midline.
      - Chin point is 2 mm right of the maxillary midline.
      - Maxillary occlusal plane is canted down 1 mm on the right at the canine.
      - Mandibular angles are level.
      - Maxillary arch width is adequate.
    - **Vertical.**
      - Maxillary incisor length is 10 mm.
      - Upper incisor show is 3 mm at rest (ideally, 2 to 4 mm tooth show at rest) and 8 mm in full smile (in an aesthetically pleasing smile line, the gingival papilla or up to 1 mm of gingival margin is visible at full smile).
      - Anterior open bite is 7 mm.
    - **Anteroposterior.**
      - Overjet is 6 mm.
      - Nasolabial angle is 110° (normal is 100° ± 10°).
      - Labiomental fold is deep.
      - Chin is retrognathic.
      - Profile is brachycephalic.

○ **Dental.** Occlusion and dentition
  ▪ Open bite is 7 mm at incisors and 3 mm at canines, with single divergent occlusal planes (Figure 8-8).
  ▪ Overjet is 6 mm (normal is +3.5 ± 2.5 mm).
  ▪ Class II relationship is present at first molars and canines bilaterally.

▪ Arch width is adequate on hand-held models.
▪ Curve of Spee has been leveled.
▪ The dentition is in good repair with no missing teeth (except for third molars).
▪ Mandibular arch form is good. There is no mandibular occlusal cant.
○ **Soft tissue.**
  ▪ Upper lip has adequate thickness and length.
  ▪ Nasolabial angle is 85° (normal is 100° ± 10°).
  ▪ Nasal contour is within normal limits (dorsum, alar base, tip).

IMAGING

The panoramic radiograph and a lateral cephalometric radiograph are the minimum imaging modalities necessary for orthognathic surgery. Preoperative profile, frontal (upon smiling and rest), and occlusal photographs should be obtained.

For this patient, the panoramic radiograph shows normal bony architecture of the condylar head and no other pathology. The right left maxillary third molar is missing, and the left maxillary and left and right mandibular third molars are full bony impacted with minimal root formation (Figure 8-9, *A*).

A lateral cephalogram was obtained with the patient in centric relation and lips in a relaxed/reposed position (Figure 8-9, *B*). Cephalometric analysis reveals anteroposterior

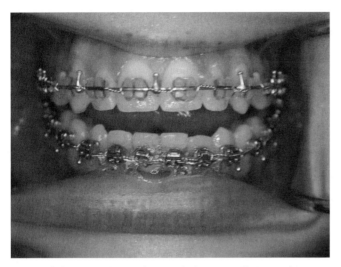

Figure 8-8. Preoperative intraoral view revealing anterior open bite. *(Courtesy Dr. Vincent J. Perciaccante.)*

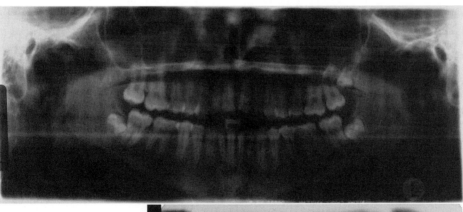

A

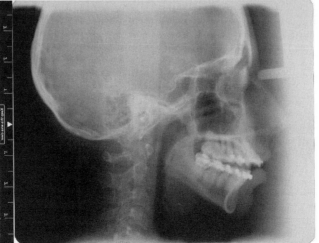

B

Figure 8-9. A, Preoperative panoramic radiograph, demonstrating impacted left maxillary and mandibular third molars and an anterior open bite. **B,** Preoperative lateral cephalogram showing the apertognathia and degree of mandibular hypoplasia. *(Courtesy Dr. Vincent J. Perciaccante.)*

Box 8-3.   **Cephalometric Analysis (Normal Caucasian Measurements)**

- Cranial base angle is normal (nasion-sella [SN]-basion angle norm is 129° ± 4° and sella-nasion [SN] to Frankfurt horizontal [FH] normal value is 7° ± 4°).
- SNA 74° (suggestive of a maxillary anteroposterior deficiency relative to the cranial base. Normal value is 82° ± 3°).
- SNB 72° (suggestive of a deficiency in the anteroposterior position of the mandible relative to cranial base. Normal value is 80° ± 3°).
- Harvold difference (distance from condylion to pogonion minus distance from condylion to A point) is 18 mm (suggestive of mandibular hypoplasia. Normal value in females is 27 mm and 29 mm in males).
- Mandibular plane (MP) is steep, with SN-MP of 47° and FH-MP of 33.5° (SN-MP normal value is 32° ± 10° and FH-MP norm is 22° ± 6°).
- Long axis of upper incisor to SN angle is 102° (normal value is 104° ± 4°).
- Long axis of lower incisor to MP angle is 95° (normal value is 90° ± 5°).
- Upper lip to E-plane is −2 mm (normal value is −3 mm ± 2 mm).
- Lower lip to E-plane is +2.5 mm (shows retrusive soft tissue chin and concave profile. Normal value is −2 mm).

---

maxillary hypoplasia. It is important to note that measurements differ between Caucasians, Asians and African Americans (Caucasian normal values are listed in Box 8-3).

LABS

Baseline hemoglobin and hematocrit are the minimum preoperative laboratory values necessary for orthognathic surgery in the otherwise healthy patient. Although blood loss requiring transfusion therapy is uncommon for orthognathic surgery, baseline hemoglobin and hematocrit values are helpful in cases of excessive blood loss to determine the need for transfusion or guide fluid resuscitation. This patient had normal values (hemoglobin of 13.1 mg/dl and hematocrit of 40.2%).

A pregnancy test (urine pregnancy test or serum beta-hCG) is also warranted for females of childbearing age. The need for transfusion of blood products is rare, so a type and screen is generally not warranted.

ASSESSMENT

Maxillary and mandibular hypopalsia resulting in apertognathia and a Class II skeletal facial deformity

TREATMENT

Treatment of a significant anterior open bite typically involves a combined orthodontic and surgical approach for stable results. A coordinated approach between orthodontist and oral and maxillofacial surgeon requires a close working relationship to meet the needs of the patient. The goals of presurgical orthodontic therapy are to:
- Align and level the occlusion
- Coordinate the maxillary and mandibular arches (progress is monitored with hand-held models)
- Eliminate dental compensations in preparation for surgical correction of the skeletal deformities

It is important to avoid any unstable orthodontic movement (closing anterior open bites by extruding maxillary or mandibular anterior teeth or widening the posterior maxillary horizontal dimension by tipping the molars) that would later result in relapse. Postsurgical orthodontic is aimed at creating a final stable occlusion and closure of any posterior open bites that resulted from the surgical correction. Most orthodontists use a retainer for maintenance of the final occlusal relationship and alignment.

Orthognathic surgical treatment options/plan for closure of an anterior open bite include Le Fort I osteotomy with posterior impaction and anterior advancement (clockwise rotation), allowing the mandibular arc of rotation to close the anterior open bite (determined by mounted model surgery). The surgeon can control the vertical position of the maxilla and incisors, as the mandibular arc of rotation and model setup will determine the final position of both the maxilla and mandible (mounted model surgery is important to determine anteroposterior position of the maxillomandibular unit when it is set at the desired vertical position). A Le Fort I osteotomy alone can be considered when:
- The mandible is in good position (dental midline and chin midline coincident with the facial midline)
- There is no mandibular occlusal cant
- The mandible is aligned with the face (symmetrical)
- The mandibular arc of rotation positions the maxilla into a good anteroposterior position, while maintaining an appropriate chin projection

A segmental Le Fort I osteotomy is indicated when a transverse deficiency or when a dual occlusal plane exists.
- Bimaxillary (maxillomandibular) surgery (Le Fort I and sagittal split or vertical ramus osteotomies) may be warranted when deformities exist in both the maxilla and mandible, and the mandibular position and arc of rotation cannot be used to position the maxilla (see Discussion).
- Although controversial and historically considered as an unstable move (especially before the advent of rigid fixation), mandibular osteotomies with surgical counterclockwise rotation of the dentate mandibular segment can be used in select clinical situations to close anterior open bites. Frequently, occlusal equilibration is required to remove any prematurities that can cause an unstable occlusion.

Once the surgical treatment plan has been developed, the surgeon can proceed with model surgery to fabricate surgical splint(s) on mounted models. If the open bite is to be closed with maxillary surgery alone, then the maxillary cast is set to the ideal occlusion with the opposing mounted mandibular cast (occlusion set with a small posterior open bite will maximize the amount of incisor overlap and reduce relapse). Small posterior open bites can be easily closed orthodontically, especially in young patients (surgically created posterior open bites allow maximal overlap of the anterior teeth, reducing the risk of relapse). A thin interocclusal acrylic wafer (splint) is made to stabilize the occlusion intraoperatively during rigid fixation of the maxilla. If a segmental osteotomy is performed, then the splint is made with a palatal strap and wired to the maxillary dentition during the healing phase to prevent horizontal collapse and relapse of the open bite. Various fixation techniques can be used, depending on the clinical situation and surgeon's preference. The maxilla is generally fixated with four-point fixation (at piriform rim and zygomaticomaxillary buttress bilaterally) using 1.5- or 2.0-mm plates. The mandible can be fixated using position screws (lag screws are contraindicated because of its tendency to torque the condylar head) and/or rigid fixation plates.

In this patient, a Le Fort I osteotomy and bilateral sagittal split osteotomies were used to correct the anterior open bite and to advance the hypoplastic mandible forward (Figure 8-10). The maxilla was advanced 2 mm at the incisors and 2.5 mm at the anterior nasal spine. The posterior maxilla was impacted 3 mm and the anterior maxilla was impacted 0.5 mm. The mandible was allowed to autorotate and was surgically advanced (it is important to realize the difference between net move [total change in position] and surgical

move [surgical change in position after autorotation is accounted for]). The patient underwent postoperative orthodontic treatment, and the orthodontic appliances were removed 6 months following surgery. Figure 8-11 shows the final occlusion.

COMPLICATIONS

Complications of maxillary and mandibular surgery are discussed in teaching cases elsewhere in this book. However, an important complication related to orthognathic surgery for closure of an anterior open bite is long-term stability of the final occlusion (relapse). Several measures can be taken to minimize this outcome:
- Sound orthodontic therapy
- Patient compliance with postoperative retainers
- Avoidance of unstable maxillary or mandibular surgical movements

Immediate postoperative malocclusion or anterior open bite usually results from either failure of fixation, inadequate mandibular positioning (condyles not seated during fixation), or inadequate maxillary impaction causing condyles to be malpositioned. It is generally recommended to correct any postsurgical malocclusion promptly once the diagnosis is confirmed, because maintaining the patient in intermaxillary fixation to treat the problem is simply delaying and complicating the future treatment.

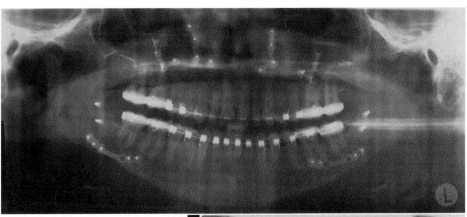

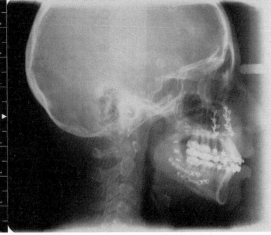

Figure 8-10. A, Postoperative panoramic radiograph showing the rigid fixation hardware. **B,** Postoperative lateral cephalogram showing correction of the apertognathia and esthetically pleasing facial profile. *(Courtesy Dr. Vincent J. Perciaccante.)*

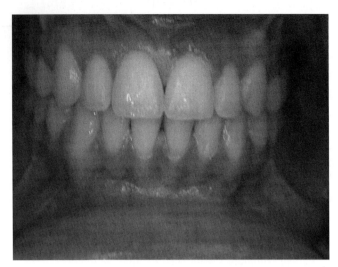

Figure 8-11. Postoperative intraoral view revealing the final occlusion. *(Courtesy Dr. Vincent J. Perciaccante.)*

DISCUSSION

An anterior open bite can be categorized based on etiology as either predominantly of dental origin without a skeletal component (seen with thumb or finger sucking, or abnormal tongue habits) or skeletal abnormality (most commonly, posterior maxillary hyperplasia) with or without a dental component. The skeletal deformity in skeletal open bite can be in the maxilla only (elongated poster maxilla), mandible only (steep mandibular plane angle), or both maxilla and mandible.

Closing a large anterior open with orthodontic therapy alone is frequently complicated by relapse. A combined orthodontic and surgical modality will offer the most stable results. Preoperative and postoperative orthodontic therapy is mandatory for most orthognathic surgical procedures (except for some cases of sleep apnea surgery). During the preoperative orthodontic phase, the maxillary and mandibular arch form is idealized. The occlusion is leveled by eliminating the curve of Spee. Dental compensations are reduced or eliminated by correcting proclined or retroclined incisors. Arch space is evaluated to predict if it will allow for these changes, as leveling the curve of Spee, aligning the teeth to proper arch form, and retracting proclined incisors require more arch space. This can be accomplished by interproximal stripping or bicuspid extractions, when crowding is an issue.

The Le Fort I osteotomy alone (without mandibular surgery) for correction of an anterior open bite is indicated when the mandible is in an ideal position (the mandibular midline is coincident with the facial midline, there is no mandibular occlusal cant, and its anteroposterior position is within normal limits) or it demonstrates only a mild anteroposterior hypoplasia (because posterior maxillary impaction will allow autorotation of the mandible forward, increasing

the anteroposterior projection). Closure of the open bite cannot be esthetically successful with maxillary surgery alone if the mandible is in an asymmetrical position. Setting the maxilla to an asymmetrical mandible will have poor esthetic results, especially if there is a maxillary anteroposterior discrepancy. In cases where the mandible has a significant midline discrepancy or occlusal cant, a double jaw procedure will be necessary to correct the mandibular discrepancies. Also, the anteroposterior position of the mandible must allow autorotation of the maxilla to a possible and acceptable anteroposterior position, which can be verified only by mounted model surgery.

In case of anterior open bite where the maxilla is deficient in the anteroposterior dimension, advancing the maxilla forward and impacting it posteriorly will close the open bite with improved long-term stability. The posterior teeth may need to be positioned in slight infraocclusion to allow for overcorrection of the overlap. When performing maxillary surgery alone, the final maxillary position and occlusion are dictated by the position of the mandible and its arc of rotation. The desired tooth show at rest and during full smile will dictate the anterior vertical position of the maxilla and the amount of impaction or disimpaction, using the mandible's arc of rotation. Closing an open bite with mandibular surgery alone is generally considered a less stable move and not recommended by most surgeons, although it has been recently described for cases with a smaller open bite.

Bibliography

Bays RA: Maxillary osteotomies utilizing the Rigid Adjustable Pin (RAP) system: a review of 31 clinical cases, *Int J Adult Orthod Orthognath Surg* 1:275, 1986.

Bays RA, Bouloux GF: Complications of orthognatic surgery, *Oral Maxillofac Surg Clin N Am* 15:229-242, 2003.

Betts NJ: Techniques to control nasal features, *Atlas Oral Maxillofac Surg Clin N Am* 8(2):53-69, 2000.

Betts NJ, Dowd KF: Soft tissue changes associated with orthognathic surgery, *Atlas Oral Maxillofac Surg Clin N Am* 8(2):1-11, 2000.

Dodson TB, Bays RA, Neuenschwander MC: Maxillary perfusion during Le Fort I osteotomy after ligation of the descending palatine artery, *J Oral Maxillofac Surg* 55:51-55, 1997.

Lanigan DT: Vascular complications associated with orthognathic surgery, *Oral Maxillofac Surg Clin N Am* 9(2):231-250, 1997.

Milles M, Betts NJ: Techniques to preserve or modify lip form during orthognathic surgery, *Atlas Oral Maxillofac Surg Clin N Am* 8(2):71-79, 2000.

Turvey TA, Fonseca RJ: The anatomy of the internal maxillary artery in the pterygopalatine fossa: its relationship to maxillary surgery, *J Oral Surg* 38:92-95, 1980.

Van Sickels JE: Treatment of skeletal open bite deformities, *OMFS Knowledge Update* 2:45-56, 1998.

Wolford ME: Management of transverse maxillary deficiency, *OMFS Knowledge Update* 1:15-20, 1995.

Zweig BE: Esthetic analysis of the cervicofacial region, *Atlas Oral Maxillofac Surg Clin N Am* 8(2):1-11, 2000.

Distraction Osteogenesis: Mandibular Advancement in Conjunction With Traditional Orthognathic Surgery

Lee M. Whitesides, DMD, MMSc, and Shahrokh C. Bagheri, DMD, MD

CC

A 26-year-old woman is referred by her orthodontist for consultation regarding the correction of her maxillofacial skeletal deformity. She complains about the excessive amount of maxillary anterior gingiva visible upon smiling ("gummy smile"), and she is not pleased with the amount of overbite.

HPI

The patient has had her "gummy smile" (secondary to vertical maxillary excess) and excessive over bite (secondary to mandibular hypoplasia) since puberty. She explains that this has significantly influenced her appearance during adolescence and adulthood. In addition, she has difficulty biting into food with her front teeth. More recently, she has decided to pursue possible treatment options for her cosmetic and functional deformity. Her orthodontist has recommended a combined surgical/orthodontic correction of the dentofacial deformity.

It is not uncommon for patients with maxillofacial skeletal deformities to have both a cosmetic and functional component related to the maxillofacial abnormality.

PMHX/PDHX/MEDICATIONS/ALLERGIES/SH/FH

Noncontributory.

EXAMINATION

The patient is a well-developed and well-nourished woman in no apparent distress. She appears to have realistic expectations regarding possible surgical interventions.

- **Maxillofacial.** Evaluation of patients for dentofacial deformities should be done in three dimensions (transverse, vertical, and anteroposterior) for the maxilla and the mandible. The dentition is evaluated for occlusion, alignment, and the status of the periodontal tissue.
  - **Transverse dimension.**
    - Maxillary midline to facial midline: coincident
    - Mandible midline to maxillary midline: mandible is to the left 1 mm.
    - Chin to maxillary midline: chin is to the left 2 mm.
    - Occlusal plane is level with no cant and no curve of Spee or Wilson.
    - Mandibular angles are level with no visible cant.
    - Arch width is adequate (as determined by examination of models).
  - **Vertical dimension.**
    - Upper central teeth show at rest is 8 mm (normal for females is 3 to 4 mm).
    - Upper central teeth show with speech is 7 to 9 mm (excessive).
    - Upper central teeth show with smiling is 5 mm of gingival show (gummy smile).
    - Open bite is Class II occlusion.
  - **Anteroposterior dimension**
    - Overjet is −12 mm.
    - Nasolabial angle is 125° (normal is about 100° to 110°).
    - Labiomental fold is deep (abnormal).
    - Chin is microgenic.

Examination of the TMJ reveals no abnormalities.

IMAGING

A lateral cephalogram, panoramic radiograph, and standard facial and dental photographs are the minimal imaging studies necessary in preparation for distraction osteogenesis in combination with orthognathic surgery. A three-dimensional actual-size stereolithographic model can be reconstructed using high-resolution computed tomography (CT) scans. These models can be used in preparation for distraction osteogenesis to demonstrate the quantity and topography of the bone in the distraction site. They also assist the surgeon by delineating pertinent anatomical structures in the bone such as the inferior alveolar nerve. This information is extremely helpful.

The lateral cephalogram is used for analysis of cephalometric norms. By comparing a patient's values with normal values, an appropriate diagnosis and prediction of anticipated surgical movements in the anteroposterior and vertical dimensions can be made. It also allows for evaluation of the facial soft tissue profile.

The preoperative lateral cephalogram for this patient is shown in Figure 8-12. Cephalometric analysis was performed using the COGS analysis (as described by Burnstone in 1978) prior to orthodontic therapy. Pertinent values are as follows (normal ranges are given in parentheses):

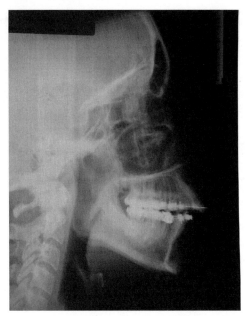

Figure 8-12. Preoperative lateral cephalogram demonstrating significant anteroposterior mandibular hypoplasia

- **Horizontal skeletal profile.**
  - Nasion perpendicular to B point: −15 mm (−5.3 ± 6.7)
  - Nasion perpendicular to pogonion: −17 mm (−4.3 ± 8.5)
- **Vertical Skeletal Profile**
  - N-ANS: 60 mm (54.7 ± 3.2)
  - Posterior nasal spine (PNS) to nasion: 77 mm (53.9 ± 1.7)
  - Maxillary central incisor edge to nasal floor: 41 mm (30.5 ± 2.1)
  - Maxillary molar cusp tip to nasal floor: 40 mm (26.2 ± 2.0)
  - ANS to gnathion: 81 mm (68.6 ± 3.8)
  - Mandibular central incisor edge to MP: 50 mm (45 ± 2.1)
  - MP : horizontal plane: 34° (23 ± 5.9)

The two abnormal measurements from the horizontal skeletal profile are indicative of mandibular hypoplasia in the anteroposterior dimension. The first four values of the vertical skeletal profile indicate that the patient has an increased facial height (vertical maxillary excess). The ANS to gnathion, and the distance of the mandibular plane indicate that the patient has a "long face." The high mandibular plane angle (34°) is typical of patients with vertical maxillary excess and long facial height.

The panoramic radiograph reveals no osseous or dental pathological processes.

LABS

Baseline hemoglobin and hematocrit is the minimum laboratory test necessary in anticipation for orthognathic surgery. Although significant blood loss requiring transfusion therapy is highly unlikely with the modern practice of maxillary and mandibular orthognathic surgery, the hemoglobin and hematocrit is important as a baseline marker for all major surgical procedures. Other laboratory tests are indicated based on the medical history. A pregnancy test is highly recommended in all women of childbearing age.

This patient had a hemoglobin of 13.0 mg/dl and a hematocrit of 39.5 percent. Her urine pregnancy test was negative.

ASSESSMENT

A healthy 26-year-old woman with maxillary hyperplasia, mandibular hypoplasia (anteroposterior), mild mandibular asymmetry, and microgenia

TREATMENT

The goals of combined surgical/orthodontic treatment are to establish a functional and cosmetic improvement in the dentofacial structures. Several surgical modalities are available for advancement of the mandible to correct the anteroposterior deficiency. Techniques of distraction osteogenesis are usually considered in cases where a large mandibular advancement would be necessary to treat the mandibular hypoplasia.

The two most common methods for mandible advancement are the bilateral sagittal split osteotomy as first described by Obwgeser, and mandibular osteotomy with application of bilateral distraction devices as described by Guerreo. The sagittal split osteotomy has been used by surgeons for more than 30 years and is described elsewhere in this text. Distraction osteogenesis surgery has been used for at least 10 years to treat deformities of the maxillofacial and craniofacial skeleton.

Distraction osteogenesis surgery can be divided into five phases:
1. Surgery: the sectioning of hard and soft tissue and application of a distraction device
2. Latency: the healing time between surgery and device activation
3. Activation: the process of gradually separating the tissue to increase length and mass
4. Consolidation: the primary healing of the distracted tissue and formation of the bony callus
5. Remodeling: the secondary healing of soft tissue and the change of immature bone into mature bone in the distraction gap

For this patient, the left mandibular cuspid and the right mandibular first bicuspid (teeth Nos. 22 and 28) were extracted per the orthodontist to permit her to level and align the mandibular teeth before orthognathic/distraction osteogenesis surgery. The initial amount of overjet increased to 15 mm after the presurgical orthodontics, correcting the dental compensation. Additionally, surgical impaction of the maxilla will increase the mandibular arc of rotation, therefore farther increasing the distance for mandibular advancement.

It was decided to address the skeletal deformity in two stages. First, correction of the maxillary hyperplasia, fol-

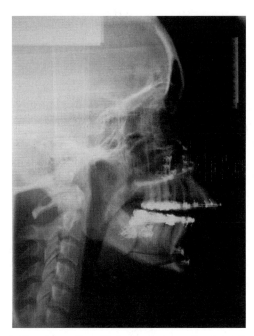

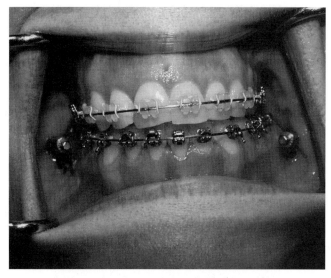

Figure 8-14. Intraoral view demonstrating the position of the bilateral distraction near completion of the active phase.

Figure 8-13. Immediate (2 days) postoperative lateral cephalogram after a mandibular osteotomy and placement of bilateral mandibular distraction device, Le Fort I osteotomy, and sliding genioplasty. The distraction device has not been activated.

lowed by distraction osteogenesis for mandibular advancement. In correcting the maxillary hyperplasia, a Le Fort I osteotomy is used to separate the maxilla from the cranial base for correction of the vertical dimension. Bilateral distraction osteogenesis devices are placed in the posterior mandible after mandibular sagittal split osteotomy, for forward distraction of the mandible.

While the patient was under general anesthesia, she underwent a standard Le Fort I osteotomy with reduction of the vertical height of the maxilla of approximately 5 mm. The maxilla was appropriately positioned on the cranial base and then rigidly fixed with plates and screws. Subsequently, mandibular sagittal split osteotomy was performed bilaterally and a distraction device was applied across each osteotomy site. An advancement sliding genioplasty was also preformed to correct for microgenia. The patient recovered uneventfully from the surgery and was discharged from the hospital 2 days later with oral analgesics and antibiotics. Figure 8-13 shows the postoperative lateral cephalogram.

After 6 days of latency, the distraction devices were activated at the rate of 1 mm per day until the patient's mandible had advanced into a Class I occlusion. During the activation process, the patient was permitted to activate the device herself unless she was seen in the clinic. She was monitored at least every 4 days at the office visit, where the surgeon activated the device to obtain a "feel" for how well the devices were working. The patient was maintained in Class II elastics bilaterally during the activation period and allowed to eat a soft diet. Figure 8-14 shows the distraction devices in position close to completion of the activation phase.

After 5 days of consecutive activation, the patient was permitted a day when the devices were not activated. Total

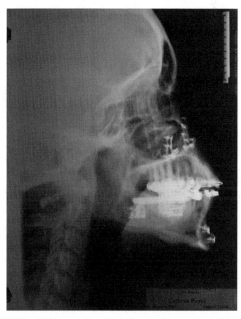

Figure 8-15. Postoperative lateral cephalogram at 5 weeks after completion of anterior mandibular distraction osteogenesis and before completion of postsurgical orthodontics.

time of the active phase of distraction was approximately 1 month.

At the end of distraction, the patient's mandible had advanced into a Class I occlusion. The total advancement measured at 18 mm. Figure 8-15 demonstrates the postoperative lateral cephalogram after completion of the activation phase.

Six months after cessation of distraction, the patient underwent removal of bilateral distraction devices under intravenous sedation. Removal of the distraction devices was predicated on radiographic demonstration of adequate bone mass in the distraction gap and clinical confirmation of adequate healing.

COMPLICATIONS

Complications of mandibular advancement with traditional sagittal split osteotomies are discussed elsewhere in this text (see section on mandibular orthognathic surgery earlier in this chapter).

Potential complications of mandibular advancement with distraction osteogenesis should include those discussed for traditional mandibular osteotomies, as well as failure of the device, infected hardware, and patient noncompliance. A complication unique to distraction osteogenesis surgery is placement of the device along the improper vector. When this occurs, the surgeon must either replace the device at a second surgery or use elastic traction to gradually influence the direction of the advancing segment. Such use of elastics is commonly called "molding the regenerate."

DISCUSSION

The history of distraction osteogenesis surgery dates to the late 1800s; however, Dr. Gavril Ilizarov is considered the "father" of modern distraction osteogenesis surgery. More recently in the 1990s, McCarthy, Guerrero, Chin, Molina, and many others pioneered the use of distraction osteogenesis surgery to treat selected deformities of the maxillofacial and craniofacial skeletal. Since then, distraction osteogenesis surgery has gained popularity as a predictable method to treat selected deformities of the facial skeleton as the technology has improved and more surgeons have learned the technique.

The process of distracting a healing wound to grow tissue takes advantage of the body's natural healing mechanisms. During the active distraction process, as the segments of bone are gradually separated, and the body sends massive amounts of growth factors, bone morphogenic proteins, and precursor cells to the wound. These cells, which are the building blocks for new tissue, work to regenerate the missing hard and soft tissue in the gap created by the distraction.

Like any other surgical technique, distraction osteogenesis surgery has certain principles that must be respected if the surgeon is to be successful. The basic surgical principles of maintaining excellent blood supply and conserving soft tissue in the area to be distracted are paramount for success. If either of these axioms is ignored, the body will not be capable of regenerating new tissue in the distraction gap and/or the wound will undergo a dehiscence.

Close attention to the wound as it heals is very important. Because the distraction device protrudes out of the soft tissue mucosa, these wounds are at an increased risk for infection.

Last, the surgeon must be diligent in critically evaluating how the distraction process is proceeding. Frequent evaluations, both clinical and radiological, must be done to examine the device, the vector of distraction, and the response of the soft tissue. This diligence permits anticipation of potential complications.

The advantages and disadvantages of each method should be considered in the presurgical planning phase. A bilateral sagittal split osteotomy with rigid fixation offers the patient an acute lengthening of the mandible into the desired position at the time of surgery. Drawbacks of this method in this particular case include the likely need of a bone graft and/or maxillomandibular fixation in association with rigid fixation for large mandibular advancements. Additionally, the acute, severe stretching of the inferior alveolar nerve has been reported to cause damage to the inferior alveolar nerve. Furthermore, large mandibular advancements are associated with a greater propensity for relapse.

Mandibular osteotomy, sagittal or vertical, with application of distraction devices can potentially produces less acute trauma, eliminates the need of a bone graft, and produces less damage to the inferior alveolar nerve. Additionally, mandibular advancement with distraction osteogenesis surgery allows the surgeon to fine-tune the advancement by gradually molding the regenerate with elastic forces as the patient's mandible is advanced. Long-term stability of the distracted mandible is considered to be stable and predictable.

Bibliography

Burstone CJ, James RB, Legan H, et al: Cephalometrics for orthognathic surgery, *J Oral Surg* 36:269-277, 1978.

Chin M, Toth BA: Distraction osteogenesis in the maxillofacial surgery using internal devices: review of five cases, *J Oral Maxillofac Surg* 54:485-453, 1996.

Choy JY, Hwang KG, Baek SH, et al: Original sagittal split osteotomy revisited for mandibular distraction, *J Craniomaxillofac Surg* 29:165-173, 2001.

Diner TA, Tomatt C, Soupre V, et al: Intraoral mandibular distraction: indications, technique, and long term results, *Ann Acad Med* 28:634-643, 1999.

Garey TM, Klotch DW, Sasse J, et al: Basement membrane of blood vessels during distraction osteogenesis, *Clin Orthop Relat Res* 301:132-138, 1994.

Guerrero CA, Bell WH, Gonzalez M, Mesa LS: Intraoral distraction osteogenesis. In *Fonseca oral and maxillofacial surgery,* Philadelphia, 2000, WB Saunders, pp 359-402.

Ilizarov GA: The tension-stress effect on the genesis and growth of tissues: Part I. the influence of stability and fixation and soft tissue preservation, *Clin Orthop Relat Res* 238:249, 1989.

Ilizarov GA, Ledyaev VI: The replacement of long tubular bone defects by lengthening distraction osteotomy of defragments, *Clin Orthop Res* 238:7, 1992.

Ilizarov GA: The tension-stress effect on the genesis and growth of tissues: Part II. The influence of rate and frequency of distraction, *Clin Orthop Rel Res* 239:263, 1989.

McCarthy JG: The role of distraction osteogenesis in the reconstruction of the mandible in unilateral craniofacial microsomia, *Clin Plast Surg* 21:625, 1994.

Molina F, Ortis-Monasterio F: Mandibular elongation and remodeling by distraction: a farewell to major osteotomies, *Plast Reconstr Surg* 96:825, 1995.

Robiony M, Polini F, Costa F, et al.: Osteogenesis distraction and platelet rich plasma for bone restoration of the severely atrophic mandible: preliminary results, *J Oral Maxillofac Surg* 60(6):630-635, 2002.

Whitesides LM, Meyer RA: Effect of distraction osteogenesis on the severely hypoplastic mandible and inferior alveolar nerve function, *J Oral Maxillofac Surg* 62(3):292-297, 2004.

9 Temporomandibular Joint Disorders

Chris Jo, DMD

This chapter addresses:

- Myofascial Pain Dysfunction
- Internal Derangement of the Temporomandibular Joint
- Degenerative Joint Disease of the Temporomandibular Joint
- Ankylosis of the Temporomandibular Joint

"FIRST DO NO HARM."

Disorders of the temporomandibular joint (TMJ) can result in debilitating pain and limited function. Although TMJ dysfunction (TMD) includes a broad spectrum of disease states, it can be categorized into two general categories: intracapsular (internal derangement, ankylosis, and degenerative joint disease) and extracapsular (myofascial pain dysfunction [MPD]) disease. Most cases of TMD can be managed nonsurgically with conservative therapy. Accurate diagnosis of the etiology of TMD is paramount for avoiding unwarranted invasive treatment.

The teaching cases in this chapter cover the identification and management strategies of internal derangement, MPD, degenerative joint disease (DJD), and ankylosis of the TMJ. The distinction between intracapsular and extracapsular TMD is emphasized. As in many complex disorders, the majority of information is obtained from the patient's presenting complaint and history of symptoms. In these cases, the key features of the chief complaint and history of present illness are emphasized. The significant findings in the physical examination are highlighted along with the explanation of the findings.

Although nonsurgical management strategies are more consistent between individual practitioners, various surgical strategies have been used based on surgeons' preference and clinical presentation. Some of the advantages and disadvantages of different treatment modalities are outlined. The surgical options are discussed, along with the rationale for treatment and relative success rates. Reconstructive strategies for advanced disease states are also presented.

Myofascial Pain Dysfunction

Gary F. Bouloux, MD, DDS, MDSc, FRACDS, FRACDS(OMS), and Chris Jo, DMD

CC

A 43-year-old white woman presents with a 6-month history of daily bitemporal headaches that exacerbate as the day progresses.

TMDs, including MPD, have a very high predilection for Caucasian women in the second to fifth decades of life.

HPI

The patient reports that the pain is dull and, while often present upon awakening, it continues to worsen throughout the day (characteristic of MPD). When asked to point to the regions of pain, she readily identifies the areas over her temporalis and masseter muscles. She has difficulty falling asleep and wakes up frequently throughout the night. The pain is worse when eating food, especially when chewing tough foods like steak (increasing pain and muscle fatigue during mastication are typical findings in MPD). She has modified her diet by excluding hard and chewy foods to reduce the pain and discomfort associated with eating. She reports no history of migraines but admits to a high level of stress at work (work- or home-related stress can exacerbate MPD). She denies any history of TMJ dysfunction and is not aware of any parafunctional habits such as bruxism (grinding of teeth; many patients may be unaware of nocturnal bruxism, unless reported by their bed partner. Also, patients with nocturnal bruxism are characteristically worse on waking and improve over the course of the day).

PMHX/PDHX/MEDICATIONS/ALLERGIES/SH/FH

Her medical and dental histories are unremarkable. She is happily married with one child. She denies any history of depression (depression is a risk factor for MPD). She works at a regional bank and was recently promoted to vice president, which she finds quite stressful (stress is a risk factor for MPD).

EXAMINATION

General. The patient is a well-developed and well-nourished anxious woman.

Maxillofacial. There is no facial swelling or asymmetry. On palpation, there is tenderness of the temporalis, masseter, and sternocleidomastoid muscles bilaterally (temporalis and masseter muscles are most commonly involved in MPD). Intraoral palpation of the medial pterygoid muscles also elicits dull pain. There is no TMJ capsular tenderness and no clicks or crepitus (making an intracapsular source of pain less likely). She has a maximal incisal opening of 28 mm (less than normal) with a soft end feel, which can be stretched to 39 mm with pain (limited opening due to muscle guarding that can be slowly stretched to a normal opening is consistent with MPD). Her left and right lateral excursions are 9 and 8 mm, respectively (normal condylar translation makes TMJ internal derangement less likely). The remainder of her physical examination is noncontributory.

IMAGING

A panoramic radiograph is the initial screening examination of choice. Although it cannot diagnose MPD, it provides a general overview of the teeth and related bony structures to rule out other sources of pain. Magnetic resonance imaging (MRI) and computed tomography (CT) scans are ordered based on the clinical suspicions of pathology in conjunction with MPD (see the section on internal derangement). However, MRI and CT are not indicated when MPD is the sole clinical diagnosis.

The panoramic radiograph in this patient reveals no odontogenic or osseous pathology.

LABS

Laboratory tests are not indicated in the work up of MPD, unless associated with other suspected or diagnosed comorbidities (such as rheumatoid arthritis or neuromuscular disorders). The suspicion of temporal arteritis would warrant further laboratory testing (erythrocyte sedimentation rate and C-reactive protein as markers of inflammation) and biopsy of the superficial temporal artery.

ASSESSMENT

MPD syndrome

The diagnosis of MPD is largely based on the patient history, which is confirmed with a thorough clinical examination. MPD can occur alone (as in this patient) or in association with internal derangement of the TMJ (see the section on internal derangement later in this chapter).

TREATMENT

The treatment of MPD begins with the correct diagnosis. The etiology of MPD is multifactorial, and therefore the management of MPD requires a multimodal approach. Initially, the patient should be reassured that the pain is purely myofascial and likely to be the result of increased muscle activity secondary to any of a number of entities. Many cases of MPD are acute exacerbations associated with other conditions that may resolve without treatment or may require only supportive measures. These may include stress, anxiety, bruxism, clenching, malocclusion, parafunctional oral habits, TMDs, rheumatological diseases, and vasculitis (e.g., temporal arteritis). Treatment must address the contributing etiology but, given the difficulty associated with correct diagnosis, the approach is often generic.

Conservative therapy is generally the first-line treatment, unless other identifiable associated diagnosis (tumors, infections, severe internal derangements, DJD) are present that are thought to exacerbate the symptoms of MPD. Treatment options include reassurance, stress management (relaxation exercises, biofeedback), occlusal splint therapy, physical therapy, application of heat to affected muscles, nonsteroidal antiinflammatory drugs (NSAIDs), muscle relaxants, and anxiolytics (anxiolytics should be prescribed with caution due to abuse potential). Conservative treatment will often result in significant improvement or resolution of the MPD.

Patients who do respond to conservative therapy with an occlusal splint and have a significant malocclusion may be considered for occlusal equilibration, orthodontic treatment, or orthognathic surgery (there is some evidence for malocclusion to be the cause of MPD, but the evidence is not strong). These modalities may offer a long-term solution to MPD, but they are invasive and not without complications.

Triggerpoint injections may be beneficial is a select group of patients with MPD who are refractory to all conservative approaches. Typically, a local anesthetic (with or without a steroid) is injected directly into tender areas within the muscles. This can be repeated as often as necessary. It may also be possible to improve MPD with injection of botulinum toxin into the muscle to reduce contractions. This may need to be repeated every 3 to 6 months, due to the temporary effect of the botulinum toxin. Regeneration of the nerve endings at the motor end plate of the neuromuscular junction is responsible for cessation of the clinical effects. Intraarticular procedures including arthrocentesis, arthroscopy, and arthroplasty have no place in the management of isolated MPD.

In this case, the patient was encouraged to manage her life stressors more effectively by taking stress management classes and using biofeedback to reduce muscle tension. She was instructed to avoid hard-to-chew foods and to apply moist heat (using a warm moist towel) to the affected muscles as often as necessary for symptomatic relief. A short course of ibuprofen 800 mg three times a day was prescribed (a muscle relaxant can also be added to this regimen). A hard, flat plane maxillary occlusal splint was constructed. This was worn at all times except while eating and brushing her teeth. The splint was adjusted weekly to ensure good contacts in centric relation and no interferences during lateral excursions. Splint adjustments became less frequent as the occlusion stabilized, and by 2 months, she was wearing the splint only at night and

was able to open to 44 mm with complete resolution of her pain.

COMPLICATIONS

With conservative (nonsurgical) approaches to the treatment of MPD, complications are relatively uncommon and are mostly related to the failure of available treatments to alleviate pain, the side effects of medications, or difficulties with occlusal splint therapy.

NSAIDs are often helpful and carry no risk of physiological dependence, although gastrointestinal irritation/bleeding, platelet dysfunction, and decreased renal function are potential complications. The use of muscle relaxants and anxiolytics can be associated with dependence and abuse. The frequently chronic and recurrent nature of MPD can lead to the long-term use of these medications and therefore carry the inherent risk of dependence and abuse.

Occlusal splint therapy is not without complications (especially when inappropriately designed). Several different types of splints are used by prescribing clinicians, and unfortunately, there are no clear evidence-based guidelines for splint therapy. Different splints include maxillary, mandibular, flat plane, anterior repositioning, and pivotal splints. Flat plane occlusal splints, whether maxillary or mandibular, are the most popular and technically the least demanding. Although complications related to conservative splint therapy are uncommon, an incorrectly adjusted splint can result in the exacerbation of the preexisting TMJ dysfunction, tooth movement, and/or the development of new symptoms. Anterior repositioning splints are occasionally useful in patients with Class II malocclusions and function by holding the mandible in a forward position, thus unloading the richly innervated retrodiscal tissue and helping to reestablish a more normal disc–condyle relationship. These splints are likely to be associated with permanent occlusal changes and require considerable experience in their use. Pivotal splints are rarely used and are thought to function by decreasing masticatory muscle forces (via periodontally mediated biofeedback). Following splint therapy, changes in the occlusion are not uncommon. Before splint therapy, most patients have a centric occlusion–centric relation discrepancy. A flat plane occlusal splint may eliminate this discrepancy over time, resulting in a less-than-ideal occlusion when the splint is removed or discontinued. This may necessitate continued splint therapy, occlusal adjustment, orthodontics, or orthognathic surgery.

DISCUSSION

The main muscles of mastication are the temporalis, masseter, lateral pterygoid, and medial pterygoid muscles. They all function harmoniously during speech and deglutination. As with any group of muscles, they are susceptible to inflammation, which may in turn cause pain. This is commonly due to excessive activity of these muscles, but the exact pathophysiology has not been clearly defined. Increased muscle activity has a multifactorial etiology that includes malocclusion, parafunctional habits, TMJ internal derangements, and psychological stressors. The management of the acute symptoms of MPD is generally similar regardless of the etiology, but long-term treatment and success need to address any known precipitating or etiologic factors. As is often the case, no definitive factors can be identified, and subsequently a generic approach using several modalities must be adopted.

Bibliography

Auerbach SM, Laskin DM, Frantsve LME, et al: Depression, pain, exposure to stressful life events, and long-term outcomes in temporomandibular disorder patients, *J Oral Maxillofac Surg* 59:628-633, 2001.

Kraus SL: Physical therapy management of temporomandibular disorders. In Bays RA, Quinn P, eds: *Oral and maxillofacial surgery: temporomandibular disorders,* Philadelphia, 2000, WB Saunders, pp 161-193.

Roth R: Orthognathics and the temporomandibular joint. In Bays RA, Quinn P, eds: *Oral and maxillofacial surgery: temporomandibular disorders,* Philadelphia, 2000, WB Saunders, pp 238-252.

Sollecito T: Role of splint therapy in treatment of temporomandibular disorders. In Bays RA, Quinn P, eds: *Oral and maxillofacial surgery: temporomandibular disorders,* Philadelphia, 2000, WB Saunders, pp 145-160.

Tallents R, Stein S, Moss M: The role of occlusion in temporomandibular disorders. In Bays RA, Quinn P, eds: *Oral and maxillofacial surgery: temporomandibular disorders,* Philadelphia, 2000, WB Saunders, pp 194-237.

Internal Derangement of the Temporomandibular Joint

Gary F. Bouloux, MD, DDS, MDSc, FRACDS, FRACDS(OMS), and Chris Jo, DMD

CC

A 22-year-old female college student presents with several months of a painless "pop" in front of her right ear while eating (TMDs are more commonly diagnosed in females).

HPI

The patient first noted a "popping" sound in her right ear soon after she had her annual visit to her dentist 4 months earlier. The sound is noticeable with chewing, yawning, and brushing of her teeth. The click is not associated with pain. She denies any history of trauma (which may precipitate internal derangement) and has never had any symptoms of TMD (popping, clicking, pain, open lock, closed lock, or limited range of motion) before her annual dental visit.

PMHX/PDHX/MEDICATIONS/ALLERGIES/SH/FH

Her past medical and dental history is noncontributory. She is in her final year of college.

EXAMINATION

General. The patient is a well-developed and well-nourished woman in no apparent distress.

Maxillofacial. The right external auditory meatus is patent without evidence of erythema or exudate. The tympanic membrane is normal. There is no TMJ capsular tenderness. An opening click (caused by the condyle translating and recapturing a normal position beneath the disc) and reciprocal click (a second click that occurs during closure of the mandible with anterior displacement of the disc) are evident within the right TMJ to both lateral capsular and endaural palpation. Auscultation over the TMJ reveals a harsh opening click and a softer closing click. No crepitation is present (crepitus would be suggestive of disc perforation with degeneration of the condyle and glenoid fossa). The left TMJ clinical examination is within normal limits. There is no evidence of masticatory muscle tenderness (masseter, temporalis, and medial pterygoid muscles). She has a maximal interincisal opening of 43 mm (normal), although there is an initial right-sided deviation on opening (due to restricted right condylar translation), followed by a right TMJ click at about 30 mm (as the anteriorly displaced disc is recaptured) and subsequent realignment toward the end of opening. She is noted to have a Class II division II malocclusion (may be associated with increased incidence

of TMDs). The remainder of her clinical examination is unremarkable.

IMAGING

The panoramic radiograph is the initial screening study of choice for assessment of TMDs, especially when pain is present (to rule out pain of odontogenic origin). It provides a general overview of the bony morphology of the mandible and condyle. MRI, in open and closed mouth positions, is considered the standard when evaluating for TMJ internal derangement. It provides the most information regarding the soft tissue structures and disc position in the open and closed mouth positions (some patients may not be able to open sufficiently due to pain). A TMJ arthrogram (fluoroscopy with dye injected into the superior joint space) is an invasive procedure that shows the disc in dynamic function and is the study of choice for evaluation of disc perforations. Arthrograms can also be used to evaluate disc position, but the study is technique sensitive and is not readily available in most institutions. Bony window CT scans are indicated when bony or fibrous ankylosis of the TMJ or other bony pathology is suspected.

In this patient, no osseous or dental abnormalities were seen on the panoramic radiograph. Sagittal and coronal MRI scans illustrate an anteromedially displaced (most frequent location of a dislocated disc) right TMJ disc in the closed mouth position (Figure 9-1, *A*), which reduces to a normal anatomical relationship in the open mouth position (Figure 9-1, *B*). The disc demonstrates a normal morphology (anatomy best seen with T1-weighted images). No joint effusion is seen (inflammation and effusions are best evaluated with T2-weighted images).

LABS

No routine laboratory tests are indicated for the work-up of anterior disc displacement (ADD) of the TMJ. Clinical suspicion of systemic arthropathy (e.g., rheumatoid arthritis, systemic lupus erythematosus, psoriatic arthritis, and gout) would dictate further laboratory testing.

ASSESSMENT

Internal derangement of the right TMJ; in this case, a non-painful ADD with reduction of the right TMJ

Patients with ADD with or without reduction may present with or without pain originating from the joint itself or from

231

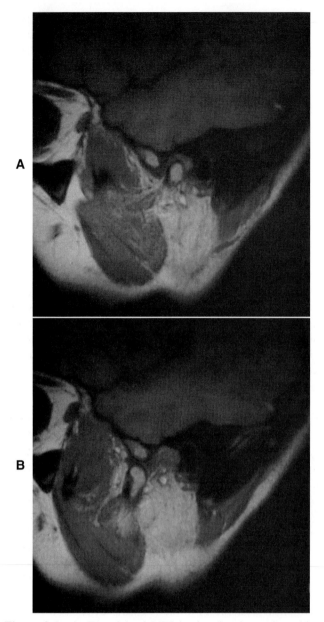

Figure 9-1 **A,** T1-weighted MRI in the closed mouth position showing anterior disc displacement. **B,** T1-weighted MRI in the open mouth position showing recapture or reduction of the disc.

the muscles of mastication (MPD). ADD without reduction would present with different clinical findings, showing no evidence of an opening or closing click and with restricted condylar translation on the affected side (reduced lateral excursion to the contralateral side). The MRI would demonstrate anterior displacement of the disc with no evidence of reduction in the open mouth position. It is not uncommon for MPD to accompany internal derangement of the TMJ. It is important to distinguish between internal derangement and MPD, because treatments are very different. MPD may also present as the sole source of pain, which warrants proper diagnosis to avoid unnecessary and inappropriate surgical management (see the section Myofascial Pain Dysfunction earlier in this chapter).

The Wilkes staging classification for internal derangement of the TMJ characterizes the progressive nature of the disease process into five stages (early, early/intermediate, intermediate, intermediate/late, and late, stages I through V, respectively), based on the clinical, radiographic, anatomical, and pathological features.

TREATMENT

Treatment of TMD is generally guided by the presence of pain and/or limited function. In the absence of symptoms, active treatment may be avoided or minimized, given that adequate patient education and reassurance and follow-up are provided.

Conservative (reversible or nonsurgical) treatment is generally the first line of therapy in symptomatic patients, including splint therapy, soft nonchew diet, elimination of parafunctional habits (bruxism), limited oral function, warm moist compresses and ice packs, physical therapy, NSAIDs, and muscle relaxants. These measures should also be used during the postoperative rehabilitation phase of the surgical patient. However, protocol-driven treatment should be avoided, and individualized patient assessment is necessary. Undo delay with conservative therapy when an effective surgical solution is indicated can be counterproductive, resulting in delay and further frustration of the patient and clinician.

Patients who are unresponsive to conservative therapy or present with advanced disease are candidates for various invasive (surgical) interventions. Surgical options include arthrocentesis, arthroscopy, arthroplasty with disc plication, meniscectomy (with or without autogenous, allogeneic, or alloplastic graft/replacement), and modified condylotomy.

Arthrocentesis is accomplished by irrigating and distending the superior joint space with lactated Ringer's solution, removing inflammatory mediators, and improving joint mobility by lysis of adhesions. A steroid or hyaluronic acid injection may follow, particularly if pain is a significant component of the patient's complaint. Arthroscopy is a more invasive procedure, requiring general anesthesia, but enables the surgeon to visualize, irrigate, and lyse adhesions within the superior joint space. Arthroscopy is reported to have a success rate approaching 80% to 90%. Holmium:YAG laser can be used during arthroscopy for lysis of adhesions and partial synovectomy of the inflamed synovium.

Open joint arthroplasty with disc plication is the most conservative open technique, which involves mobilizing the anteriorly displaced disc and plicating it posteriorly (with sutures or staples) to ensure that it rests in the correct anatomical position on the mandibular condyle. Success rates approaching 90% have been reported. Meniscectomy involves removal of the disc, and although it readily eliminates the disc displacement, it may be associated with significant DJD unless it is replaced with some type of graft (cartilage, fat, and dermis grafts have been used) or flap (temporalis muscle–fascia flap). The modified condylotomy is an extraarticular procedure that spares the TMJ itself but involves allowing the mandibular condyle to reposition inferiorly and anteriorly in order to facilitate a more normal relationship between the condyle and disc. This procedure is associated with significant postoperative occlusal changes that can be difficult to manage in the long term, especially when done bilaterally.

In this patient, although ADD with reduction was present within the right TMJ, no symptoms were present. The patient did not require any treatment, she was reassured that her clinical findings are not uncommon, and in the absence of pain or limited function, observation is all that is necessary.

COMPLICATIONS

Although not a complication, the sequelae of observational treatment include progression to symptomatic disease and the development of ADD without reduction or DJD. Progression of disease may warrant further noninvasive and/or invasive surgical treatment (see Discussion), each with its associated potential complications.

Complications associated with arthrocentesis are rare and mostly related to traumatic needle placement. Arthroscopy is more invasive and therefore is associated with several complications, including facial nerve injury, penetration into the middle cranial fossa, damage to the joint structures, laceration or edema of the external auditory canal, otological injury resulting in hearing loss, infection, and instrument failure. Increased joint noise is common after athrocentesis or arthroscopy, especially in patients with ADD without reduction.

Open joint procedures are the most invasive and are associated with the most potential complications, which include those mentioned for arthroscopy. Preauricular or endaural incisions are most commonly used to access the joint, which may result in sensory and motor nerve injuries. Injury to the auricular temporal nerve (most common sensory nerve injury) usually results in altered sensation to the skin overlying the preauricular region (although this is usually temporary). Frey syndrome (auriculotemporal nerve syndrome or gustatory sweating) may result from injury to the auriculotemporal nerve, which carries parasympathetic fibers to parotid gland and sympathetic fibers to the sweat glands of the skin. Misdirected nerve regeneration may cross the sympathetic and parasympathetic pathways, causing the ipsilateral facial sweating when tasting or smelling food. Gustatory neuralgia (much less common) is similar to Frey syndrome but results in electric shock and/or pain in the preauricular region when tasting or smelling food. Injury to the temporal (frontal) branch (most common motor nerve injury) of the facial nerve (crosses the zygomatic arch 8 to 35 mm, 20 mm on average, anterior to the external auditory meatus), results in weakness or paralysis of the frontalis (resulting in eyebrow ptosis) or orbicularis oculi muscles (resulting in lagophthalmos). Other branches or the main trunk of the facial nerve may be injured when more complex reconstructive joint procedures are performed, due to the need for wider access and multiple incisions. There is a higher incidence of motor nerve injury in the multiply operated TMJ patient.

Temporary postoperative malocclusion (ipsilateral posterior open bite) is common after any invasive joint procedure. This may result from surgical anatomic changes and edema in the joint. Modified condylotomy (extracapsular procedure) is associated with temporary or permanent postoperative malocclusion (anterior open bite and increased overjet), especially when performed bilaterally. This may result from condylar sag and loss of posterior vertical height or from condylar dislocation. Most cases of malocclusion may be treated with elastics, but surgical correction may be required.

Progression to DJD may occur in the operated or unoperated patient. The literature is inconsistent concerning the need for disc replacement after discectomy. There is concern that discectomy without replacement has a higher incidence of progression to DJD or ankylosis. Heterotopic bone formation may occur after any open joint procedure and may result in bony ankylosis.

DISCUSSION

Asymptomatic ADD with reduction is present in a significant proportion of the general population. The criteria for treatment are based on the degree of pain and functional impairment. Surgical intervention should be reserved for those with significant impairment and/or those for whom conservative therapy has failed. Disc displacement with reduction, whether symptomatic or not, may progress to disc displacement without reduction, which bears a worse prognosis. This is suggested to be the natural progression of the disease toward a more complex pathologic process that is more difficult to treat. The natural progression of disc displacement has been classically described by Wilkes, although a simpler functional description with ADD with or without reduction is more frequently used.

For those patients with disc displacement with reduction who are asymptomatic, reassurance is often all that is needed. The potential for progressing to disc displacement without reduction should be discussed. For patients desiring treatment, conservative splint therapy should be offered. While flat plane occlusal splints are most popular, an anterior repositioning splint that holds the mandible in a protruded position may help recapture the anteriorly displaced disc. An anterior repositioning splint is much more likely to result in occlusal changes that will necessitate further treatment including occlusal equilibration, orthodontics, or orthognathic surgery.

Bibliography

Bays R: Surgery for internal derangement. In Bays RA, Quinn P, eds: *Oral and maxillofacial surgery: temporomandibular disorders*, Philadelphia, 2000, WB Saunders, pp 275-300.

Katzberg RW, Westesson PL: Pathology. In *Diagnosis of the temporomandibular joint,* Philadelphia, 1993, WB Saunders, pp 25-43.

Laskin D, editor: Current controversies in surgery for internal derangements of the temporomandibular joint, *Oral Maxillofac Surg Clin North Am* 6:223-355, 1994.

Quinn P: Surgery for internal derangements. In *Color atlas of temporomandibular joint surgery,* Philadelphia, 1998, WB Saunders, pp 55-99.

Wilkes CH: Internal derangement of the temporomandibular joint. Pathological variations, *Arch Otolaryngol Head Neck Surg* 115:469-477, 1989.

Degenerative Joint Disease of the Temporomandibular Joint

Chris Jo, DMD, and Shahrokh C. Bagheri, DMD, MD

CC

A 56-year-old woman (DJD has a higher prevalence with advancing age and in females) presents to your office with a long history of TMD, complaining that, "I've been through several TMJ surgeries and now my right joint is very painful and makes grinding noises."

HPI

The patient reports several months of anxiety and stress that she relates to the pain centered around her right TMJ that is most pronounced upon opening her mouth or talking. She has a long, progressive history of TMJ problems. In her late teens, she developed bilateral TMJ click/pop (suggestive of ADD with reduction), which was confirmed by an arthrogram (before the development of MRI, this was a more commonly used modality to diagnose TMDs) with intermittent right-sided precapsular pain and bilateral myofascial pain. She was treated conservatively with occlusal splint therapy and NSAIDs. She reported mild improvement and did not pursue further treatment as she tolerated her discomfort by minimizing masticatory function. In her mid-20s, the right side stopped clicking, and she developed an acute closed lock with severe right-sided pain and restricted left lateral excursive movements of her mandible (consistent with the progression of ADD with reduction to ADD without reduction on the right). She underwent right-sided arthrocentesis, which provided 8 months of relief, followed by a second arthrocentesis procedure that provided only short-term relief. Subsequent MRI studies showed evidence of DJD (displaced, deformed, nonreducing disc with evidence of perforation of the posterior band and degenerative bony changes) of the right TMJ and ADD without reduction on the left side with degenerative bony changes. Her surgeon elected to treat her with a discectomy (removal of the disc) without disc replacement, with an excellent outcome for several years. She now presents with a 2-year history of loud grinding noises or crepitus (pathognomonic sign of advanced arthrosis) in the right with increasing levels of debilitating pain localized to the TMJ.

PMHX/PDHX/MEDICATIONS/ALLERGIES/SH/FH

Noncontributory, except for arthritic changes diagnosed in her cervical spine and proximal interphalangeal joints. She has taken NSAIDs as needed for pain over the past several years.

Patients with arthritic degeneration of the TMJ frequently have involvement of other joints that precede the TMJ. It is, however, possible to have DJD of the TMJ with no evidence of arthritis in any other joints.

EXAMINATION

General. The patient is a well-developed and well-nourished woman in moderate distress due to right-sided TMJ pain.

Maxillofacial. The patient has no facial swelling or asymmetry. The right TMJ is exquisitely tender to palpation (both precapsular and endaural palpation). The left TMJ is nontender. She has limited opening (20 mm) due to pain and a loud bony crepitance of the right TMJ that is easily heard without a stethoscope. Lateral excursive movements are limited (3 mm to the left and 6 mm to the right). She has a Class I occlusion without an open bite (advanced condylar degeneration and loss of posterior mandibular height can lead to an anterior open bite). Her external auditory canals are clear and the tympanic membranes appear normal. Her preauricular surgical scar is well healed and cranial nerve VII is intact (multiple open joint procedures increase the risk of cranial nerve VII injury, especially the frontal or temporal branch).

IMAGING

The panoramic radiograph is the initial imaging study of choice for evaluation of TMDs. It provides a general overview of the bony morphology of the mandible and condyle. MRI, in open and closed mouth positions, is considered the standard when evaluating for TMJ internal derangement. It provides the most information regarding the soft tissue structures (disc morphology) and disc position in the open and closed mouth positions (some patients may not be able to open sufficiently due to pain). A TMJ arthrogram (fluoroscopy with dye injected into the superior joint space) is an invasive procedure that shows the disc in dynamic function and is the best study to detect disc perforations. Bony window CT is indicated when bony or fibrous ankylosis of the TMJ or other bony pathology is suspected. A CT scan can be used to better delineate the bony anatomy of the TMJ and demonstrate any degenerative changes.

In this patient, the panoramic radiograph demonstrates radiographic evidence of bilateral osteoarthrosis (breakdown and remodeling of bony structures, likely due to joint overloading), which includes flattening of the condylar head, subchondral eburnation (sclerosis), and osteophyte

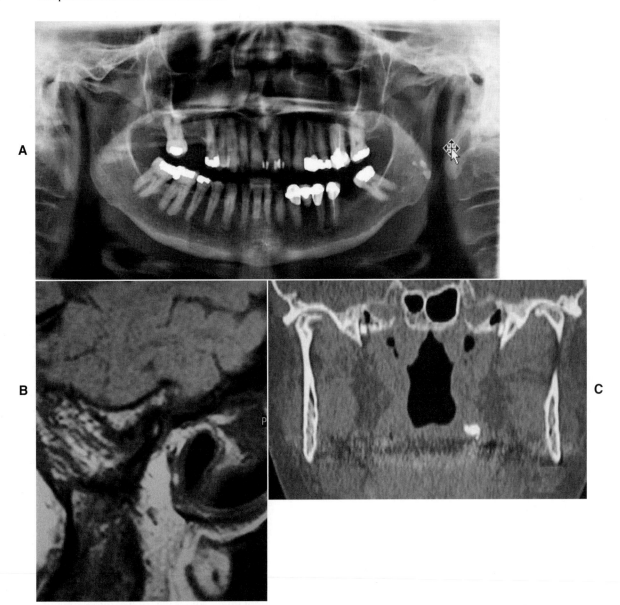

Figure 9-2 **A,** Panoramic radiograph revealing severe degenerative bony changes of the bilateral (right greater than left) condylar heads including loss of normal architecture and loss of smooth cortical outline. **B,** T1-weighted MRI revealing remnants of the anterior portion of a displaced disc from a previous discectomy and significant degenerative changes of the condylar head. **C,** Direct coronal CT showing degenerative bony changes of the bilateral mandibular condylar heads (right greater than left).

formation. The right condylar head (Figure 9-2, *A*) has a greater loss of normal anatomy, is significantly smaller with sharp edges, and has lost its cortical definition (signs of advanced degeneration). Sagittal and coronal MRI scans illustrate an anteromedially displaced (most frequent location of a dislocated disc) left TMJ disc in the closed mouth position that does not reduce in the open mouth position, with moderate degenerative changes (anatomy is best seen with T1-weighted images). T1-weighted MRI images of the right TMJ (Figure 9-2, *B*) reveals remnants of the anterior portion of the displaced disc (consistent with previous discectomy) and evidence of severe degenerative changes of the condylar head and inflammatory changes (inflammation and effusions are best seen with T2-weighted

images). CT scan was also obtained revealing bilateral bony degenerative changes that are more severe on the right (Figure 9-2, *C*).

LABS

No routine laboratory testing is indicated for the work-up of DJD. Clinical suspicion of systemic arthropathies (e.g., rheumatoid arthritis, systemic lupus erythematosus, psoriatic arthritis, and gout) would dictate further laboratory testing. Other laboratory values are obtained based on the medical history. Baseline preoperative hemoglobin and hematocrit levels are recommended for patients undergoing an open joint or total joint reconstruction.

ASSESSMENT

DJD of bilateral TMJs, with localized pain on the multiply operated right side

TREATMENT

Treatment of TMJ DJD can be difficult, especially in the multiply operated patient. Patients may present with a history of previous attempts at arthrocentesis, arthroscopic surgery, and/or open joint procedures. Some patients may present with no previous history of TMD or prior treatments. Individualized treatment plans, based on the presenting history, signs, and symptoms, are warranted. Attempts at minimally invasive procedures such as arthrocentesis and arthroscopic surgery may be adequate to relieve the pain and potentially halt or slow the disease process. However, with progression of the degenerative process, more invasive procedures may be indicated.

Advanced DJD is frequently treated with open joint surgery. The surgical procedure of will be based on the surgeon's preference, training, and clinical diagnosis. TMJ arthroplasty can be performed with either disc repair, or disc plication, and osseous recontouring of the condylar head. Alternatively, TMJ arthroplasty with discectomy can be performed. After the disc or disc remnant is removed, the disc can be replaced with an autogenous fat graft, dermal graft, alloplastic graft, cadaveric graft, temporalis muscle-fascia flap, ear cartilage, or nothing. Osseous recontouring of the condylar head is performed as needed. In end-stage DJD, total joint replacement or reconstruction may be warranted. Various alloplastic total joint implants are available for TMJ reconstruction, either one-stage or two-staged (see the section on TMJ ankylosis). Alternatively, the condylar remnants can be resected and replaced with an autogenous bone graft (costochondral or full-thickness calvarial bone graft) and a temporalis muscle-fascia flap to separate the glenoid fossa from the graft. Vascularized free-flaps have also been described but are not widely used. Adjunctive orthognathic surgery may be warranted in select cases, performed either during TMJ reconstruction or in a secondary phase. In the postoperative rehabilitative phase, physical therapy and adequate pain control are paramount.

In this patient, total joint replacement using a custom prefabricated condylar head and fossa alloplastic implants were used. This required a two-stage approach. In the first stage, a gap arthroplasty was performed with a discectomy and condylectomy, to provide adequate space for the TMJ implant (a Silastic block can be left in situ to preserve the surgically created space). The TMJ fossa and condylar prosthesis were implanted in stage II surgery via a preauricular approach and two stab incisions (in addition, a retromandibular approach can be used to facilitate fixation of the condylar component).

Long-term outcome regarding the success of TMJ implants has yet to be determined. However, the initial results have been encouraging.

COMPLICATIONS

TMJ surgery for treatment of DJD shares similar complications as surgery for internal derangement or TMJ ankylosis. Refer to the respective sections on ankylosis and internal derangement for discussion of surgical complications.

DISCUSSION

Osteoarthrosis of the TMJ is defined as breakdown or degeneration of articular bone and soft tissues due to "excessive joint loading" or normal "wear and tear." The breakdown products, including inflammatory mediators and lysozymes, lead to a secondary synovitis and capsulitis resulting in joint pain and tenderness. DJD encompasses the entire degenerative process or spectrum, but the term is mostly applied in clinically advanced degenerative joint changes accompanied by limited function and/or the presence of pain.

The Wilkes staging classification for internal derangement of the TMJ characterizes the progressive nature of the disease process into five stages (early, early/intermediate, intermediate, intermediate/late, and late) based on the clinical, radiographic, anatomical, and pathological features.

The treatment of DJD had challenged clinicians for many years. Optimal treatment and reconstructive modalities are yet to be determined. Understanding of the pathology and molecular biology of arthritis and advances in material science will be the key to prevention and treatment of this debilitating condition.

Bibliography

Auerbach SM, Laskin DM, Frantsve LME, et al: Depression, pain, exposure to stressful life events, and long-term outcomes in temporomandibular disorder patients, *J Oral Maxillofac Surg* 59:628-633, 2001.

Bays RA: Temporomandibular joint disc preservation, *Atlas Oral Maxillofac Surg Clin N Am* 4:33-50, 1996.

Bertolami CN, Gay T, Clark GT, et al: Use of sodium hyaluronate in treating temporomandibular joint disorders: a randomized, double-blind, placebo-controlled clinical trial, *J Oral Maxillofac Surg* 51:232-242, 1993.

Bjornland T, Larheim TA: Discectomy of the temoromandibular joint: 3-year follow-up as a predictor of the 10-year outcome, *J Oral Maxillofac Surg* 61:55-60, 2003.

Carvajal WA, Laskin DM: Long-term evaluation of arthrocentesis for the treatment of internal derangements of the temporomandibular joint, *J Oral Maxillofac Surg* 58:852-855, 2000.

Dimitroulis G: A review of 56 cases of chronic closed lock treated with temporomandibular joint arthroscopy, *J Oral Maxillofac Surg* 60:519-524, 2002.

Dimitroulis G: The use of dermis grafts after discectomy for internal derangement of the temporomandibular joint, *J Oral Maxillofac Surg* 63:173-178, 2005.

Dolwick MF: Disc preservation surgery for the treatment of internal derangements of the temporomandibular joint, *J Oral Maxillofac Surg* 59:1047-1050, 2001.

Edwards SP, Feinber SE: The temporalis muscle flap in contemporary oral and maxillofacial surgery, *Oral Maxillofac Surg Clin N Am* 15:513-535, 2003.

Emschoff R, Rudisch A: Are internal derangement and osteoarthrosis linked to changes in clinical outcome measures of arthrocentesis of the temporomandibular joint? *J Oral Maxillofac Surg* 61:1162-1167, 2003.

Emschoff R, Rudisch A: Determining predictor variables for treatment outcomes of arthrocentesis and hydraulic distention of the temporomandibular joint, *J Oral Maxillofac Surg* 62:816-823, 2004.

Eriksson L, Westesson PL: Long-term evaluation of meniscectomy of the temporomandibular joint, *J Oral Maxillofac Surg* 43:263-269, 1985.

Eriksson L, Westesson PL: Discectomy as an effective treatment for painful temporomandibular joint internal derangement: a 5-year clinical and radiographic follow-up, *J Oral Maxillofac Surg* 59:750-758, 2001.

Feinberg SE: Use of local tissues for temporomandibular joint surgery disc replacement, *Atlas Oral Maxillofac Surg Clin N Am* 4:51-74, 1996.

Fricton JR, Look JO, Schiffman E, et al: Long-term study of temporomandibular joint surgery with alloplastic implants compared with nonimplant surgery and nonsurgical rehabilitation for painful temporomandibular joint disc displacement, *J Oral Maxillofac Surg* 60:1400-1411, 2002.

Hendler BH, Gateno J, Mooar P, et al: Holmium : YAG laser arthroscopy of the temporomandibular joint, *J Oral Maxillofac Surg* 50:931-934, 1992.

Indresano AT: Surgical arthroscopy as the preferred treatment for internal derangements of the temporomandibular joint, *J Oral Maxillofac Surg* 59:308-312, 2001.

Israel HA, Ward JD, Horrell B, et al: Oral and maxillofacial surgery in patients with chronic orofacial pain, *J Oral Maxillofac Surg* 61:662-667, 2003.

Iwase H, Sasaki T, Asakura S, et al: Characterization of patients with disc displacement without reduction unresponsive to nonsurgical treatment: a preliminary study, *J Oral Maxillofac Surg* 63:1115-1122, 2005.

Keith DA: Complications of temporomandibular joint surgery, *Oral Maxillofac Surg Clin N Am* 15:187-194, 2003.

Mazzonetto R, Spagnoli DB: Long-term evaluation of arthroscopic discectomy of the temporomandibular joint using the holium YAG laser, *J Oral Maxillofac Surg* 59:1018-1023, 2001.

McKenna SJ: Discectomy for the treatment of internal derangements of the temporomandibular joint, *J Oral Maxillofac Surg* 59:1051-1056, 2001.

Milam SB: Chronic temporomandibular joint arthralgia, *Oral Maxillofac Surg Clin N Am* 5-26, 2000.

Nitzan DW, Price A: The use of arthrocentesis for the treatment of osteoarthritic temporomandibular joints, *J Oral Maxillofac Surg* 59:1154-1159, 2001.

Park J, Keller EE, Reid KI: Surgical management of advanced degenerative arthritis of temporomandibular joint with metal fossa-eminence hemijoint replacement prosthesis: an 8-year retrospective pilot study, *J Oral Maxillofac Surg* 62:320-328, 2004.

Reston JT, Turkelson CM: Meta-analysis of surgical treatments for temporomandibular articular disorders, *J Oral Maxillofac Surg* 61:3-10, 2003.

Tucker MR, Spagnoli DB: Autogenous dermal and auricular cartilage grafts for temporomandibular joint repair, *Atlas Oral Maxillofac Surg Clin N Am* 4:75-92, 1996.

Umeda H, Kaban LB, Pogrel MA, Stern M: Long-term viability of the temporalis muscle/fascia flap used for temporomandibular joint reconstruction, *J Oral Maxillofac Surg* 51:530-533, 1993.

White RD: Arthroscopic lysis and lavage as the preferred treatment for internal derangement of the temporomandibular joint, *J Oral Maxillofac Surg* 59:313-316, 2001.

Yun PY, Kim YK: The role of facial trauma as a possible etiologic factor in temporomandibular joint disorder, *J Oral Maxillofac Surg* 63:1576-1583, 2005.

Zingg M, Iizuka T, Geering AH, et al: Degenerative temporomandibular joint disease: surgical treatment and long-term results, *J Oral Maxillofac Surg* 52:1149-1158, 1994.

Ankylosis of the Temporomandibular Joint

Vincent J. Perciaccante, DDS, and Deepak G. Krishnan, BDS

CC

A 64-year-old woman presents to your office complaining of progressively worsening inability to open her mouth.

While there is no predilection for gender in ankylosis, there is a correlation with age and geographic distribution. Ankylosis in children is more common in developing countries.

HPI

The patient has a protracted history of bilateral TMD and multiple attempts at nonsurgical and surgical management (see the sections on internal derangement and myofascial pain dysfunction) to alleviate the pain associated with her TMJs. The multimodality treatment included splint therapy, physical therapy, NSAIDs, multiple arthrocentesis procedures (resulted in transient relief of pain), and TMJ arthroplasties with bilateral disc plication, followed by bilateral discectomies and abdominal fat grafting (see the previous section, Degenerative Joint Disease). With unresolved symptoms, which included painful crepitus, and findings of atrophic failure of these grafts, she underwent bilateral temporalis muscle fascia interpositioning surgery 2 years earlier. She admits to being noncompliant with postoperative jaw opening exercises due to pain. However, following her last surgery, the patient's mouth opening has progressively decreased, and the associated TMJ pain has reduced considerably.

PMHX/PDHX/MEDICATIONS/ALLERGIES/SH/FH

This patient has chronic pain associated with her cervical spine and TMJ (osteoarthritis, chronic neck pain status post cervical-spine fusion of C4-5).

Osteoarthritis can be an initiating factor in the cascade of events that lead to the ankylosis of an adult TMJ. Patients with chronic TMJ pain and associated MPD may also present with significant chronic neck pain.

EXAMINATION

General. The patient is a well-developed and well-nourished woman in mild distress due to chronic neck pain and inability to open her mouth.

Maxillofacial. She has limited range of motion of her cervical spine, especially with flexion and extension (increases the difficulty of intubation). Her maximal incisal opening is 2 mm with a hard stop and no lateral excursive movements (consistent with mechanical obstruction). Upon palpation of the TMJs, a bony mass is present, and no condylar movement is palpable. The temporal (frontal) branch of the right facial nerve (cranial VII) is weak (there is an increase in the incidence of facial nerve injury with each open joint procedure in the multiply operated TMJ). Bilateral preauricular surgical scars are well healed. She is in Class I occlusion. There is tenderness of the masseter, temporalis, and sternocleidomastoid muscles upon palpation. There is mild masseteric hypertrophy (the muscles of mastication will attempt to open an ankylosed joint constantly; this effect is more profound in ankylosis seen in children, where masseteric hyperactivity also causes formation of a prominent antegonial notch).

IMAGING

A panoramic film is the initial screening study of choice when dealing with TMDs, especially when pain is present (to evaluate for odontogenic causes of pain). It provides a general overview of the bony morphology of the mandible and condyle, as well as the glenoid fossa. When suspecting bony or fibrous ankylosis of the TMJ, bony window CT scans without contrast in the axial and coronal views is the study of choice. It provides the most diagnostic information on the bony architecture (anatomical and pathological) of the TMJ, including the presence of heterotopic bone formation. MRI is indicated when internal derangement is suspected (see the section on internal derangement earlier in this chapter), but it has little diagnostic value in the case of ankylosis.

In this patient, the panoramic radiograph shows normal adult dentition with multiple previous dental restorations. In addition, it shows some evidence of heterotopic bone formation in the bilateral TMJ areas with obliteration of normal joint space and distortion of condylar articular anatomy. Coronal bony CT scans (Figure 9-3) clearly demonstrate obliteration of the bilateral TMJ space. The heterotopic bone appears "mushroom shaped" and appears to distort the entire TMJ anatomy. No evidence of any remnants of normal discs or previously attempted grafts or flaps is visible.

LABS

In the case of TMJ ankylosis, no laboratory values are needed in the initial work-up unless dictated by the patient's medical history. A preoperative hemoglobin and hematocrit is needed during the surgical phase of treatment because of potential intraoperative blood loss. Clinical suspicion of systemic arthropathy (e.g., rheumatoid arthritis, systemic lupus

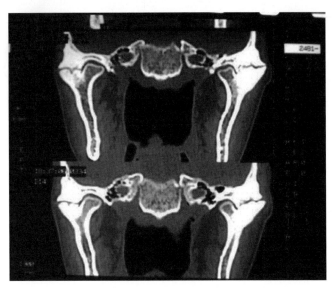

Figure 9-3   Bony window, direct coronal CT scans showing bilateral TMJ bony ankylosis.

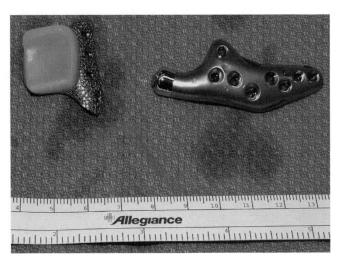

Figure 9-4   Total TMJ prosthesis (TMJ Concepts is shown).

erythematosus, psoriatic arthritis, and gout) would dictate further laboratory work-up.

This patient had a hemoglobin of 12 mg/dl and a hematocrit of 35.6%.

ASSESSMENT

Bony ankylosis of the bilateral TMJs and associated MPD

Ankylosis of TMJ is a condition that results from a variety of etiologies but eventually results in a fusion of the mandibular condylar head to the glenoid fossa. These etiologies are all insults and invasions of the joint space in one form or another, from a traumatic event, surgery, or infection (infectious etiology mostly occurs via direct spread from mastoiditis or otitis but rarely via the hematogenous route). Ankylosis can be bony or fibrous, complete or partial. Reference to fibrous ankylosis is made clinically and radiographically when the limitation in motion of the joint is caused by fibrous adhesions or scar tissues rather than actual bone formation. Fibrous ankylosis often precedes bony ankylosis.

TREATMENT

The goals of treatment for TMJ ankylosis are to release the ankylotic joint(s) and to reconstruct a functional joint. This can be done as simultaneous procedures or as staged procedures, depending on the elected reconstructive modality (stock or custom fabricated alloplastic TMJ prosthesis or autogenous costochondral, cranial, or vascularized bone grafts). Postoperative pain management, aggressive physical therapy, and prevention of reankylosis are also paramount during the rehabilitation phase.

Release of ankylotic joint(s). In the adult with TMJ ankylosis, the procedure of choice to release the ankylosis will depend on the type and severity of the condition. In fibrous ankylosis, often detachment of the fibrous scars and a coro-

noidectomy (or coronoidotomy) provide good mouth opening. If there is bony ankylosis, a gap arthroplasty is warranted. Gap arthroplasty involves osseous recontouring of the deformed glenoid fossa and condylar head (condylectomy may be performed depending on the reconstruction modality), removal of heterotopic bone, and creation of adequate space to accommodate the reconstructive plans. Ipsilateral coronoidectomy or coronoidotomy is indicated if mouth opening is restricted after releasing the ankylotic joint, followed by contralateral coronoidectomy or coronoidotomy if opening is still restricted.

Reconstruction of TMJ. There is mounting evidence on the safety, utility, and longevity of alloplastic prosthetic reconstruction of the TMJ. While in the growing child, this is not a valid option, in adults this may have a valuable role. Alloplastic TMJ prostheses may be custom-made or stock. If one intends to reconstruct the joint with a custom CAD-CAM–generated joint, the surgery is usually done in two stages—gap arthroplasty and maxillomandibular fixation to stabilize the occlusion and retain the gap—followed by CT for custom fabrication of the TMJ prosthesis (Figure 9-4) and surgical implantation of the prosthesis. The stock prostheses eliminate this two-stage treatment plan.

Before the advent of the total TMJ reconstruction systems, the costochondral graft was the workhorse of TMJ reconstruction. It is still the graft of choice for growing children. The most-cited disadvantage of the costochondral graft is its nonreliable growth pattern, especially in children. Other autogenous bone grafts, including calvarial strips, metatarsal joints and sternoclavicular junction, and vascularized grafts from the fibula, the second toe, and iliac crest, have been reported. In using autogenous grafting for reconstruction of the TMJ complex, the fossa is most often aligned and interpositioned by a pedicled temporalis muscle–fascia flap.

Rehabilitation and prevention of reankylosis. The importance of postoperative pain management and physical therapy is paramount in the success of TMJ ankylosis surgery. Reluctance and noncompliance from the patient in following a thorough physical therapy regimen are often cited as the most contributing factors for reankylosis or failure to achieve good mouth opening. There is also some evidence that low-dose radiation can prevent heterotropic bone formation after joint surgery (see Discussion).

COMPLICATIONS

TMJ ankylosis surgery shares all the potential complications associated with any open TMJ surgery, which may include scar formation, facial nerve damage, Frey syndrome or gustatory sweating, external auditory meatus perforations, infections, and reankylosis (see the section on internal derangement earlier in this chapter).

There are also the potential complications associated with anesthesia related to the hypomobility of the mandible causing a difficult airway that potentially requires advanced intubation techniques. In addition, there are complications associated with concomitant procedures, including the morbidities from a graft procurement (donor and recipient site), orthognathic surgery, or distraction osteogenesis procedures.

The greatest challenge for the surgeon is the probability of reankylosis. Sometimes despite aggressive resection, interpositioning, and aggressive physiotherapy, the intrinsic ability of a young adult to form heterotopic bone overcomes all obstacles and lead to reankylosis. The same low-dose radiation protocol—10 Gy fractionated in five doses used in prevention of heterotopic bone formation after hip arthroplasties—can be replicated to potentially prevent TMJ heterotopic bone formation. This has been suggested to be effective in preventing TMJ reankylosis after release and reconstruction.

Complications associated with surgical techniques can include perforation into the middle cranial fossa from the gap arthroplasty. Dural exposure through the glenoid area should be carefully examined to ensure that the dura is intact. If a dural tear is seen or suspected, neurosurgical consultation is warranted.

Severe bleeding may be encountered from the medial infratemporal fossa. Peoples and associates reported management of an iatrogenic tear of the internal maxillary artery during TMJ arthroplasty via selective embolization. Their review of literature shows that arguments against a carotid cutdown and ligation arise from the suspicion that continued bleeding could arise from the collateral vessels distal to the bleeding site. Transantral ligation has also been documented as somewhat unreliable due to documented cases of continued postligation bleeding. Their choice of management is selective embolization to obtain proximal control. The location of the middle meningeal artery, the internal jugular vein, and the main trunk of the third division of the trigeminal nerve can vary greatly, and this can make surgery more dangerous than may be anticipated. When resecting the medial aspect of the ankylosed TMJ, excessive bleeding can be attributed to the internal maxillary artery. This arterial bleeding can have the potential to cause serious morbidity. Navigation-aided resection of an ankylosis of the mandible has been

reported as a safe technique that may become a routine part of craniomaxillofacial surgery

DISCUSSION

Ankylosis alters the normal anatomy of the TMJ to varying degrees and can be classified according to the tissues involved and the extent of involvement. It can also be based on the location of the ankylosis. Consolidation and fibro-osseous restructuring of hemarthrosis form the basic pattern of the pathogenesis of ankylosis of the TMJ. The destruction of a growing joint may directly affect the mandible and has secondary effects on the growing facial skeleton and soft tissues.

The objectives of TMJ ankylosis surgery can be summarized as follows:
- Restoring mouth opening and joint function
- Allowing for adequate condylar growth
- Correction of the facial profile
- Relief of any upper airway obstruction.

The basic principles of ankylosis release should be followed, regardless of the patient's age and type of ankylosis. These include:
- Gap arthroplasty for resection of the ankylotic mass
- The interpositioning of a material or structure of choice to prevent recurrence of ankylosis correction of secondary deformities

The joint can be reconstructed in several ways. Advantages of autogenous grafting include:
- Ease of adaptation to the host site and remodeling over time
- Associated low morbidity from graft harvest
- Infrequent rate of infections
- Reduced relative cost and time for preparation compared to allografts

A disadvantage of costochondral grafts is the unpredictable growth pattern, which may lead to progressive dental midline shifts, occlusal changes, chin deviation, and modification of the graft itself.

Advantages of alloplastic grafting include:
- Ability to begin physical therapy immediately after surgery
- Avoidance of a secondary surgical site
- Ability to mimic normal anatomy

Contraindications for alloplastic grafting include:
- Growth requirements of the graft and a finite life span
- Uncontrolled systemic diseases
- Active infection at the implantation site
- Allergies to the materials used in the implant

Today's technology allows adult patients with severe TMJ ankylosis the option of complete TMJ prostho-rehabilitation. However, the consensus for treatment options for children with ankylosis is variable and unclear.

Bibliography

De Bont LGM, van Loon JP: The Groningen temporomandibular joint prosthesis, *Oral Maxillofac Surg Clin N Am* 12:125-132, 2000.

Dierks EJ, Buehler MJ: Complete replacement of the temporomandibular joint with a microvascular transfer of the second metatarsal-phalangeal joint, *Oral Maxillofac Surg Clin N Am* 12:139-147, 2000.

Donlon WC: Nonprosthetic reconstructive options, *Oral Maxillofac Surg Clin N Am* 12:133-137, 2000.

Edwards SP, Feinber SE: The temporalis muscle flap in contemporary oral and maxillofacial surgery, *Oral Maxillofac Surg Clin N Am* 15:513-535, 2003.

Gerard DA, Hudson JW: The Christensen temporomandibular joint prosthesis system, *Oral Maxillofac Surg Clin N Am* 12:61-72, 2000.

Guyuron B, Lasa CI: Unpredictable growth pattern of costochondral graft, *Plast Reconstr Surg* 90:880-889, 1991.

Hoffman DC, Pappas MJ: Hoffman-Pappas prosthesis, *Oral Maxillofac Surg Clin N Am* 12:105-124, 2000.

Kaban LB, Perrott DH, Fisher K: A protocol for management of temporomandibular joint ankylosis, *J Oral Maxillofac Surg* 48:1145-1151, 1990.

Mercuri LG: The TMJ Concepts patient fitted total temporomandibular joint reconstruction prosthesis, *Oral Maxillofac Surg Clin N Am* 12:73-91, 2000.

Milam SB: Chronic temporomandibular joint arthralgia, *Oral Maxillofac Surg Clin N Am* 5-26, 2000.

Pellegrini G: Preoperative irradiation for prevention of heterotopic ossification following total hip arthroplasty, *J Bone Joint Surg* 78-A(6):870-881, 1996.

Peoples JR, Herbosa EG, Dion J: Management of internal maxillary artery hemorrhage from temporomandibular joint surgery via selective embolization, *J Oral Maxillofac Surg* 46:1005-1007, 1988.

Quinn PD: Lorenz prosthesis, *Oral Maxillofac Surg Clin N Am* 12:93-104, 2000.

Schmelzeisen R, Gellrich N, Schramm A, et al: Navigation guided resection of temporomandibular joint ankylosis promotes safety in skull base surgery, *J Oral Maxillofac Surg* 60:1275-1283, 2002.

Shah FR, Sharma RK, Hilloowalla RN, Karandikar AD. Anesthetic considerations of temporomandibular joint ankylosis with obstructive sleep apnea: a case report, *J Indian Soc Pedod Prev Dent* 20(1):16-20, 2002.

10 Oral Cancer

Deepak Kademani, DMD, MD, FACS, and Shahrokh C. Bagheri, DMD, MD

This chapter addresses:
- Squamous Cell Carcinoma
- Verrucous Carcinoma
- Mucoepidermoid Carcinoma
- Adenoid Cystic Carcinoma
- Acinic Cell Carcinoma

Malignant diseases of the oral cavity include a spectrum of neoplastic disorders that can emerge from the cellular structures present in the oral cavity to, less frequently, metastatic disease to the area. Primary oral squamous cell carcinoma (SSCa) comprises more than 90% of all head and neck malignancies. Malignant diseases of the salivary glands and ductal epithelium account for the majority of the remaining cases. A greater proportion of oral cancer is diagnosed and referred for treatment by dental professionals than by general medical practitioners. Therefore, recognition and knowledge of the diagnostic tools necessary to identify these disorders are the minimum required by general dental practitioners and oral and maxillofacial surgeons. There are an increasing number of oral and maxillofacial surgeons who are also trained in the treatment of head and neck malignancies. The primary modality of treatment for head and neck cancer remains surgical.

In this chapter, we present five cases representing the most commonly encountered oral cavity malignancies — two cancers originating from the epithelium (oral squamous cell and verrucous carcinoma) and three salivary gland malignancies (acinic cell, adenoid cystic, and mucoepidermoid carcinoma).

Box 10-1 outlines the TNM staging used for staging of oral cancer, and Box 10-2 provides the staging classification that is correlated with survival, using the TNM system.

Box 10-1. TNM Staging for Lip and Oral Cavity Cancers According to the American Joint Committee on Cancer

Primary Tumor (T)

TX	Primary tumor cannot be assessed
T0	No evidence of primary tumor
Tis	Carcinoma in situ
T1	Tumor 2 cm or less in greatest dimension
T2	Tumor more than 2 cm but not more than 4 cm in greatest dimension
T3	Tumor more than 4 cm in greatest dimension
T4 (lip)	Tumor invades through cortical bone, inferior alveolar nerve, floor of mouth, or skin of face, i.e., chin or nose
T4a (oral cavity)	Tumor invades adjacent structures (e.g., through cortical bone, into deep [extrinsic] muscle of tongue [genioglossus, hyoglossus, palatoglossus, and styloglossus], maxillary sinus, skin of face)
T4b	Tumor invades masticator space, pterygoid plates, or skull base and/or encases internal carotid canal

Note: Superficial erosion of bone/tooth socket by gingival primary is not sufficient to classify a tumor as T4.

Regional Lymph Nodes (N)

NX	Regional lymph nodes cannot be assessed
N0	No regional lymph node metastasis
N1	Metastasis in a single ipsilateral lymph node, 3 cm or less in greatest dimension
N2a	Metastasis in single ipsilateral lymph node more than 3 cm but not more than 6 cm in greatest dimension
N2b	Metastasis in multiple ipsilateral lymph nodes, none more than 6 cm in greatest dimension
N2c	Metastasis in bilateral or contralateral lymph nodes, none more than 6 cm in greatest dimension
N3	Metastasis in a lymph node more than 6 cm in greatest dimension

Distant Metastasis (M)

MX	Distant metastasis cannot be assessed
M0	No distant metastasis
M1	Distant metastasis

From Sobin LH, Wittekind CH, editors: *International Union Against Cancer (UICC) TNM classification of malignant tumors*, ed 6, Hoboken, NJ, 2002, John Wiley and Sons.

| Box 10-2. | Staging of Oral Squamous Cell Carcinoma |

Stage 0
Tis, N0, M0

Stage I
T1, N0, M0

Stage II
T2, N0, M0

Stage III
T3, N0, M0
T1, N1, M0
T2, N1, M0
T3, N1, M0

Stage IVA
T4a, N0, M0
T4a, N1, M0
T1, N2, M0
T2, N2, M0
T3, N2, M0
T4a, N2, M0

Stage IVB
Any T, N3, M0
T4b, any N, M0

Stage IVC
Any T, any N, M1

From Sobin LH, Wittekind CH, editors: *International Union Against Cancer (UICC) TNM classification of malignant tumors,* ed 6, Hoboken, NJ, 2002, John Wiley and Sons.
is, Carcinoma in situ.

Squamous Cell Carcinoma

David C. Swiderski, DDS, MD, and Deepak Kademani, DMD, MD, FACS

CC

A 55-year-old African-American man presents to your office stating that, "there is something wrong with my tongue, and my dentist said I need to have it checked" (African Americans have a higher incidence and double the mortality rates from SCCa).

HPI

The patient recently visited his general dentist for evaluation of his loose upper dentures. Upon examination, a red and white, fungating mass of the right lateral border of his tongue was noted (SCCa until proved otherwise). The patient was otherwise asymptomatic (early mucosal lesions of oral cancer are usually asymptomatic). Painful ulcers would be more suggestive of an inflammatory/infectious etiology). Within 2 weeks he had an incisional biopsy of the lesion by a local oral surgeon, with a subsequent diagnosis of an invasive SCCa.

The biopsy report from the previous surgeon was requested and reviewed (it is important to confirm the diagnosis before definitive treatment). The histopathology report described a loss of normal maturation of the epithelial cells, with invasion of abnormal cells beyond the basement membrane into the underlying subcutaneous tissues and muscle layers (indicative of invasive tumor). Stranding and islands of keratin-like material are also noted (keratin is indicative of greater cellular differentiation). The abnormal cells appeared pleomorphic (many different shapes) with increased nuclear-to-cytoplasmic ratio and occasional mitotic figures (signs of cellular malignant transformation). Generalized inflammatory infiltration was noted at the deepest portion of the specimen. The diagnosis of a grade III (see later), invasive SCCa was made.

PMHX/PDHX/MEDICATIONS/ALLERGIES/SH/FH

The patient has a 45 pack-year history of tobacco use. In addition, he regularly consumes alcoholic beverages on weekends and occasionally on weekdays (tobacco and alcohol are both risk factors for the development of oral SCCa; see Discussion). He does not receive routine medical or dental treatment.

The strong association between SCCa and tobacco use is well established. The risk for developing SCCa in a smoker is approximately 5 to 9 times greater than that for a nonsmoker. It is also postulated that smoking is responsible for approximately 90% of oral cavity tumors in men and 61%

of those in women. Chewing tobacco is associated with an increased risk of oral SCCa. Alcohol alone and in conjunction with tobacco has been shown to have an increased risk of oral SCCa. In studies controlled for smoking, those who consumed moderate to heavy amounts of alcohol were found to have a 3 to 9 times greater risk of the development of SCCa. When alcohol and smoking are combined, alcohol is considered to be a promoter and a possible co-carcinogen to tobacco, with some studies showing a 100-fold increased risk.

EXAMINATION

The examination of a patient with the diagnosis of SCCa should entail a complete head and neck examination to search for neck metastasis (the most common areas of distant metastasis are the lungs), synchronous primary tumors, or, in cases of presenting neck disease, occult primary tumors. Particular attention is given to the status of the lymph nodes and the size of the presenting lesion. Previous studies have shown that on initial examination of a known primary tumor, there is a 3% to 7% incidence of a synchronous tumor in the upper aerodigestive tract. A nasopharyngoscopic examination is indicated to evaluate the subepiglottic and supraepiglottic regions, posterior oropharynx, and nasopharynx.

General. The patient is a well-developed and well-nourished white man who appears his stated age, with no signs of cachexia (seen with advanced disease).

Maxillofacial. There is a 3.5-cm red and white, fungating mass on the right lateral border of tongue with central ulceration (a nonhealing ulcer within the oral cavity is considered to be SCCa until proved otherwise) (Figure 10-1). There is no pain or bleeding noted on palpation of the lesion (although ulcers from SCCa may occasionally bleed, they are usually painless). Examination of the remaining oral cavity, including the buccal mucosa, hard and soft palate, parotid and submandibular glands, oropharynx, and nasopharynx, revealed no other abnormalities. Nasopharyngoscopy was performed, revealing no abnormal tissues in the posterior oropharynx, subglottic or supraglottic regions, or nasopharynx (nasopharyngoscopy should be performed as part of the head and neck evaluation of tongue SCCa).

Neck. No cervical or submandibular lymphadenopathy was noted (cancers of the tongue usually metastasize to the level I and II nodes). There was no pain upon palpation of the neck (lymphadenopathy form cancer is usually painless).

The presence of occult neck disease in the N0 neck is related to the tumor stage, size and depth invasion, perineural

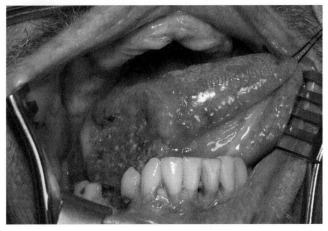

Figure 10-1　Ulcerating fungating mass of the right lateral border of the tongue, diagnosed as SCCa.

invasion, and histological grade. Lesions greater than 4 mm in depth along with a high-grade histology, have a greater than 20% risk of neck disease in the N0 neck.

IMAGING

The initial imaging modalities for the evaluation of patients with SCCa begin with a panoramic radiograph. This is a useful screening tool to evaluate the presence of bony infiltration associated with the tumor. It also provides valuable information regarding the long-term prognosis of the remaining dentition as some patients may require extraction of carious or periodontally involved teeth before radiotherapy.

A computed tomography (CT) scan of the head and neck is the commonly used imaging study of choice to delineate the lesion and assess the neck for cervical lymphadenopathy (nodes greater than 1.5 cm, with central necrosis, ovoid shape, and fat stranding are indicative of nodal metastasis). Additional tests such as magnetic resonance imaging (MRI) and ultrasonography can be used to assess the status of the cervical nodes.

Anteroposterior and lateral chest radiographs are used to screen for underlying pulmonary disease and evaluate for pulmonary metastasis because the lungs are the most common areas of metastasis for this tumor. Positron emission tomography (PET) scans are becoming a common modality for the evaluation of distant metastasis. This technology uses a ^{18}F-fluorodeoxyglucose (FDG) marker to examine sites of increased glucose uptake that are seen with metabolically active cancer cells.

In this patient, axial and coronal CT images of the head and neck with and without contrast revealed a 3.5-cm well-circumscribed lesion of the right lateral border of the tongue musculature. No evidence of cervical lymphadenopathy was noted. The PET scan performed with ^{18}F-FDG showed a hypermetabolic area in the right tongue coinciding with the clinical lesion. The panoramic and chest radiographs revealed no abnormalities.

LABS

A complete metabolic panel (CMP), complete blood count (CBC), and coagulation profile (PT, PTT, and INR) are mandatory laboratory studies in the cancer patient because of metabolic, electrolyte, and nutritional derangements that may accompany malignant disease. Liver function tests are obtained as part of the complete metabolic panel and are important screening tests for liver metastasis. Other laboratory studies can be ordered based on the patient's medical history.

In this patient, the CBC, CMP, liver function tests, and coagulation studies were within normal limits.

ASSESSMENT

A T2, N0, M0 (tumor greater than 2 cm but less than 4 cm, with no positive nodes and no distant metastasis) stage II, oral SCCa of the right lateral border of the tongue with a Broders histological grade of III

TREATMENT

Treatment of SCCa of the tongue begins first with a complete history and physical examination including nasopharyngoscopy. This is followed by appropriate tests including CBC with differentials, electrolytes, liver function tests, chest radiographs, and CT with contrast. The role of PET scanning for occult metastasis continues to evolve.

The treatment of SCCa is site specific; surgical ablation with minimum 1- to 1.5-cm margins is the main modality of treatment. Most oral cavity tumors are approached intraorally, however some tumors may need to be accessed extraorally via a transfacial approach. When the tumor is located in the mandible, the inferior border can be preserved (marginal mandibulectomy), depending on the degree of infiltration. However, when the cancellous portion of the mandible is invaded, segmental resection is required to maintain oncological safety.

A common procedure that accompanies the removal of the tumor is the removal of the fibrofatty contents of the neck, for treatment of cervical lymphatic metastases as well as complete staging of the cancerous process. This procedure is called a neck dissection and was first described by Crile in 1906, with several subsequent modifications. The neck is divided into anatomical divisions for purposes of neck dissection. The system most widely used today was adopted at the Memorial Sloan-Kettering Cancer Center. Researchers at that institution divide the neck into seven regions denoted as levels I through VII (Figure 10-2 and Box 10-3).

Radical neck dissection. This is the standard procedure for the removal of the entire cervical lymphatic chain from the unilateral neck, encompassing levels I through V, the spinal accessory nerve, the internal jugular vein and the sternocleidomastoid muscle. Indications include advanced neck disease with multiple-level positive lymph nodes with gross extracapsular spread, infiltration of the spinal accessory nerve, sternocleidomastoid muscle, or the internal jugular vein.

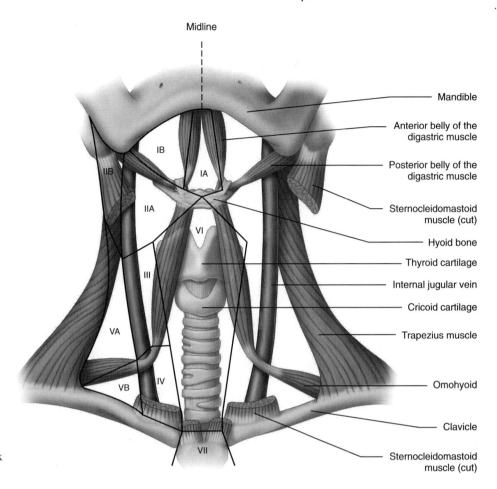

Figure 10-2 The levels of the neck for oncologic surgery.

Box 10-3. **Seven Levels of the Neck**

Level I: Submental and submandibular. This level contains the submental and submandibular triangles, which are bounded by the posterior belly of the digastric muscle, the midline, the body of the mandible superiorly, and the hyoid bone inferiorly. Level I can be further subdivided into Ia (submental triangle) and Ib (submandibular triangle).

Level II: Upper jugular. Contains the upper jugular lymph nodes and extends from the skull base superiorly to the hyoid bone inferiorly. Anterior landmarks are the midline strap muscles, and posteriorly, it is bound by the anterior border of the trapezius muscle. The spinal accessory nerve (XI) travels obliquely across this area and can be used to subdivide this area into IIa (anteriorly) and IIb (posteriorly).

Level III: Midjugular. Contains the middle jugular lymph nodes from the hyoid bone superiorly to the level of the lower border of the cricoid cartilage inferiorly.

Level IV: Lower jugular. Contains the lower jugular lymph nodes from the level of the cricoid cartilage superiorly to the

clavicle inferiorly. Nodes that are deep to the sternal head of the sternocleidomastoid are subdivided into IVa, and those deep to the clavicular are denoted as IVb.

Level V: Posterior triangle. Contains the lymph nodes in the posterior triangle bounded by the anterior border of the trapezius muscle posteriorly, the posterior border of the sternocleidomastoid muscle anteriorly, and the clavicle inferiorly. It may be further classified into the upper, middle, and lower levels corresponding to the superior and inferior planes that define levels II, III, and IV.

Level VI: Prelaryngeal (delphian), pretracheal, and paratracheal. Contains the lymph nodes of the anterior central compartment from the hyoid bone superiorly to the suprasternal notch inferiorly. On each side, the lateral boundary is formed by the medial border of the carotid sheath.

Level VII: Upper mediastinal. Contains the lymph nodes inferior to the suprasternal notch in the superior mediastinum.

Modified radical neck dissection. This procedure involves the removal of lymph nodes from levels I through V but requires the preservation of one or more of the nonlymphatic structures that are included in a radical neck dissection (the spinal accessory nerve, internal jugular vein, or the sternocleidomastoid muscle).

Selective neck dissection. This is an umbrella term encompassing several procedures where neck nodes of certain ("selected") levels are removed while other areas are preserved.

- **Supraomohyoid neck dissection.** The selective removal of levels I through III, its main indication is for the N0 neck in cases of oral cavity SCCa where there exists a 20% or greater chance of occult neck disease. The guiding parameters include an aggressive high-grade tumor (characterized histopathologically), invasion of greater than 4 mm (if discussing oral SCCa), and perineural invasion. This is performed on the ipsilateral side as the primary tumor, except in the cases of primary tumors arising from midline structures such as the floor of the mouth, which are known to metastasize bilaterally.

- **Anterior compartment neck dissection.** The selective removal of level VI nodes, the primary indications for this procedure are primary tumors of the thyroid gland, hypopharynx, cervical trachea, cervical esophagus, and subglottic larynx.
- **Posterolateral neck dissection.** Removal of lymph nodes II through V, it is indicated for scalp and auricular tumors.
- **Lateral neck dissection.** Selective removal of levels II through IV, its main indication is for primary cancers of the oropharynx, hypopharynx, and larynx.

Extended neck dissection. This involves removal of structures not routinely involved with radical neck dissections. These structures can include retropharyngeal lymph nodes, hypoglossal nerve, prevertebral musculature, or the carotid artery. Indications include advanced neck disease with difficulty in obtaining negative margins.

Reconstruction and rehabilitation. Depending on the defect, the reconstructive surgery can be divided into soft tissue and/or bony reconstruction. Closing the defect primarily is ideal if it can be accomplished. Soft tissue surgical procedures include closure by secondary intention, skin grafts, local flaps, or microvascular free flaps. Simultaneous bony reconstruction can be accomplished using vascularized free flaps from the iliac crest, scapula, or fibula when needed. When performing large ablative and reconstructive procedures, these procedures can be performed simultaneously (see also sections in Chapter 11). Depending on the amount of healing and dysfunction anticipated, a percutaneous endoscopic gastrostomy tube and elective tracheostomy can be performed to secure the airway and aid in the nutritional support of the patient during the postoperative period.

Radiation therapy. Radiation therapy can be used as a primary or an adjuvant therapy. Primary radiotherapy is usually reserved for those patients with significant comorbidities or in situations where the primary tumor or patient is not amenable to surgery. This is not a primary indication for early-stage SCCa because of the associated morbidity including dysphagia and xerostomia. Another significant risk is the occurrence of metachronous lesions arising after radiation therapy.

Postoperative radiation therapy is commonly used as a part of the comprehensive treatment. The indications for its use include positive or near margins, significant perineural or perivascular invasion, bone involvement, multiple nodal involvement, extracapsular spread, or stage III or IV disease. Typically, about 6,000 cGy in divided doses is administered and is initiated soon after the healing from the initial surgery is complete. Surgery combined with radiation and chemo-

therapy has increased the 5-year survival rates of stage III and IV cancers by 10%.

For this patient, a right partial glossectomy via a transoral approach was performed with 1.5-cm margins. The status of the margins was evaluated using frozen section microscopy, demonstrating negative margins. An ipsilateral supraomohyoid neck dissection (levels I through III) was completed for staging, which revealed no positive lymph nodes. The tongue defect was reconstructed with a radial forearm free flap, anastomosing with the facial artery and vein. An elective tracheostomy was performed.

Following complete healing, the patient was then followed closely for signs of recurrence (85% of recurrences occur in the first 3 years after initial treatment).

COMPLICATIONS

Complications are best categorized into intraoperative, postoperative (within 1 month), and long term (after 1 month).

Intraoperative complications. The main intraoperative concerns associated with oncological ablative and reconstructive surgery include the control of hemorrhage, and anesthetic complications. When simultaneous neck dissection is performed, additional complications such as nerve palsies (facial and spinal accessory nerves); vascular injury to the carotid artery or internal jugular vein; and, more rarely, pneumothorax, air embolism, and formation of a chylous fistula (especially on the left side) can be seen.

Postoperative complications. Postoperative complications include wound infection, hematoma, skin necrosis, flap failure, orocutaneous fistula, poor speech, and swallowing dysfunction. Complications after bony reconstruction include malunion, nonunion, contour irregularities, resorption of bone, osteomyelitis, and hardware failure.

Long-term complications. The gravest long-term complications are recurrence of the primary tumor and death (85% of the recurrences occur in the first 3 years). The lifetime risk of development of a second primary tumor is 2% to 3% per year, and the 5-year survival rate is 56% for all tumor stages. Routine diagnostic tests are performed based on the clinical suspicion of recurrence. Imaging studies can be difficult to assess in the postoperative setting due to the difficulty of separating recurrent tumors from postoperative anatomical changes. Recurrent disease usually occurs at the surgical wound margin. Other complications include facial nerve weakness, shoulder drop from spinal accessory nerve weakness, and flap failure. Dysphagia, xerostomia, mucositis, and the risk of osteoradionecrosis are associated with radiation therapy. The most common causes of death in patients with oral cancer are related to locoregional disease, distant metastasis, or cardiopulmonary failure. Metastases of SCCa tend to involve the lung, bones, liver, and brain.

DISCUSSION

SCCa accounts for roughly 90% of neoplastic cases in the head and neck. It has a 3:1 male predilection with the median

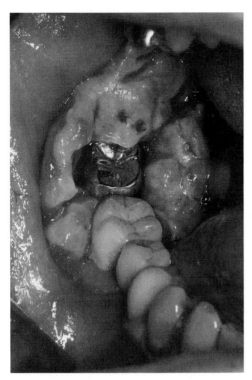

Figure 10-3 Squamous cell carcinoma of the right retromolar area (different patient than the patient shown in Figures 10-1 and 10-2).

age of onset (diagnosis) in the sixth decade of life (recently there has been an increasing prevalence in the third decade). The overall 5-year survival rate for SCCa is over 50%. African Americans are reported to have significantly lower survival rates, approaching 35%. In 2005, an estimated 29,370 new cases were diagnosed, with 7320 patients dying from their disease. Roughly two thirds of these cases can be prevented with cessation of known risk factors (tobacco and alcohol). From an epidemiological and clinicopathological standpoint, carcinomas in the head and neck region can be divided into three anatomical areas:

1. Carcinomas arising in the oral cavity, which includes the tongue, gingiva, floor of mouth, hard palate, buccal mucosa, and retromolar area
2. Carcinomas of the lip vermilion
3. Carcinomas of the oropharynx, including the base of the tongue, lingual tonsil, soft palate, and uvula

Figure 10-3 demonstrates a different patient with a large fungating SCCa of the right retromolar area.

In addition to alcohol and tobacco, the use of *betel quid* or *Paan,* popular in India and southeast Asia, has been associated with an increased risk for developing SCCa. The *quid* consists of a betel leaf wrapped around a mixture of areca nut and slaked lime, commonly in combination with tobacco. The slaked lime releases an alkaloid from the areca nut, causing a feeling of euphoria. Chronic use of the quid can lead to a debilitating condition known as submucous fibrosis, which is a premalignant condition.

Human papillomavirus (HPV) types 16 and 18 have been shown to increase the risk of SCCa. Data from recent studies show that HPV 16 and 18 increase the ratio of SCCa by approximately 3- to 5-fold. When examined, tonsillar SCCa has the highest rate of HPV infection, with approximately 50% testing positive.

Other known risks factors include chronic sun exposure leading to cutaneous SCCa of the lip. Several studies have suggested that oral lichen planus, particularly the erosive form, is associated with a increased risk for SCCa. Severe iron deficiency presenting as Plummer-Vinson syndrome is associated with an increased risk for pharyngeal and esophageal SCCa. Previous radiation exposure is linked to an increased risk for developing SCCa.

Premalignant conditions. There are several well-known entities pathologically that have a distinct association with SCCa: leukoplakia, erythroplakia, and lichen planus.

Leukoplakia is a white patch or plaque that cannot be characterized clinically or pathologically as any other disease. Erythroplakia is defined as a red lesion of the oral cavity that cannot be classified clinically or pathologically as any other lesion (see the section on Oral Leukoplakia in Chapter 6).

Oral lichen planus has been a subject of controversy in the literature concerning its possible role as a premalignant condition. Several recent studies have shown that the transformation rate of oral lichen planus to SCCa is approximately 0.04% to 1.74%.

Early oral SCCa usually presents as one of the premalignant conditions discussed — a white, red, or a mixed red and white lesion. As the lesion matures, it can become centrally ulcerated, and the borders become less distinct. The surface can become exophytic with papillary projections or endophytic with raised rolled borders.

The tongue is the most common site for SCCa (30%), followed closely by the floor of the mouth (28%). These sites are at the higher risk, probably due to carcinogens that pool with saliva in these areas, contributing to a greater exposure. The thin nonkeratinized layer of epithelium in these areas may contribute to the greater susceptibility. The other areas of prevalence, in descending order, are the upper and lower alveolar ridges (including the hard palate), the retromolar trigone, buccal mucosa, and the lips.

Broders classification is an index of malignancy based on the fact that less differentiation is proportionally related to greater malignancy of the tumor.

Grade 1 contains greater than 75% differentiated cells; grade 2, 25% to 75% differentiated cells; grade 3, less than 25% differentiated cells; and, grade 4, anaplastic with no cells differentiated. Differentiation is defined as the degree of keratinization. Histopathological factors correlating with a poorer outcome include depth of invasion, perineural invasion, and extracapsular spread.

The 5-year survival rates remain around 50% and are related to the stage at diagnosis (Table 10-1). Unfortunately, there has been only a modest improvement in survival during the past several decades.

Table 10-1. Survival Rates by Stage

Relative survival by stage	Year 1	Year 2	Year 3	Year 4	Year 5
Stage I	93.9	84.4	77.5	73.0	68.1
Stage II	88.1	72.7	64.2	58.6	52.9
Stage III	77.5	60.9	52.5	46.0	41.3
Stage IV	60.3	40.6	33.5	29.3	26.5

Modified from National Cancer Institute, *U.S. National Institutes of Health: Surveillance Epidemiology and End Results (SEER)*, http://seer.cancer.gov/publicdata/access.html.

Bibliography

Braakhuis BJM, Tabor MP, Kummer JA, et al: A genetic explanation of Slaughter's concept of field cancerization: evidence and clinical implications, *Cancer Res* 63:1727-1730, 2003.

Broders AC: Carcinomas of the mouth: types and degrees of malignancy, *Am J Roentgenol Red Ther Nucl Med* 17:90-93, 1927.

Funk FF, Karnell LH, Robinson RA, et al: Presentation, treatment, and outcome of oral cavity cancer: a national cancer data base report, *Head Neck* 24:165-180, 2002.

Kademani D, Bell RB, Bagheri SC, et al: Prognostic factors for intraoral squamous cell carcinoma: the influence of histologic grade, *J Oral Maxillofac Surg* 63:1599-1605, 2005.

Neville BW, Day TA: Oral cancer and precancerous lesions, *CA Cancer J Clin* 52:195-215, 2002.

Oliver AJ, Helfrick JF, Gard D: Primary oral squamous cell carcinoma, *J Oral Maxillofac Surg* 54:949-954, 1996.

Reichart PA, Philipsen HP: Oral erythroplakia: a review, *Oral Oncol* 41:551-561, 2005.

Schmidt BL, Dierks EJ, Homer L, et al: Tobacco smoking history and presentation of oral squamous cell carcinoma, *J Oral Maxillofac Surg* 62:1005-1058, 2004.

Schwartz LH, Ozsahin M, Zhang GN, et al: Synchronous and metachronous head and neck carcinomas, *Cancer* 74:1933-1938, 1994.

Shafer WG, Waldron CA: Erythroplakia of the oral cavity, *Cancer* 36:1021-1028, 1975.

Smith GI, O'Brien CJ, Clark J, et al: Management of the neck in patients with T1 and T2 cancer in the mouth, *Br J Oral Maxillofac Surg* 42:494-500, 2004.

Syrjanen S: Human papillomavirus (HPV) in head and neck cancer, *J Clin Virol* 32S:S59-S66, 2005.

Todd R, Donoff RB, Wong DTW: The molecular biology of oral carcinogenesis: toward a tumor progression model, *J Oral Maxillofac Surg* 55:613-623, 1997.

Van der Meij EHDDS, Schepman KP Van der Waal I: The possible premalignant character of oral lichen planus and oral lichenoid lesions: a prospective study, *Oral Surg Oral Med Oral Pathol Oral Radiol Endod* 96:164-171, 2003.

Waldron CA, Shafer WG: Leukoplakia revisited: a clinicopathological study of 3,256 oral leukoplakias, *Cancer* 36:1386-1392, 1975.

Wooglar JA: Histological distribution of cervical lymph node metastases from intraoral/oropharyngeal squamous cell carcinomas, *Br J Oral Maxillofac Surg* 37:175-180, 1999.

Verrucous Carcinoma

Scott D. Van Dam, DDS, MD, and Deepak Kademani, DMD, MD, FACS

CC

A 68-year-old white male farmer is referred to you complaining that; "I'm worried about this growth on my gums. It just won't seem to go away" (verrucous carcinoma is more commonly seen in the elderly male population, generally over 60 years of age).

HPI

The patient reports a 6-month history of a rough, corrugated area on his anterior maxillary gingiva. He was seen by his dentist and was referred to you for evaluation of possible "oral cancer" (verrucous carcinoma cannot be distinguished clinically from SCCa). The area has not been painful but has recently become more irritated (pain is not characteristically seen with neoplastic processes). He has been inadvertently chewing on the area with occasional bleeding. He denies any weight loss or constitutional symptoms (may be seen with metastatic disease).

PMHX/PDHX/MEDICATIONS/ALLERGIES/SH/FH

The patient has a positive history of chronic obstructive pulmonary disease (secondary to chronic tobacco use). He sees his local dentist only when he develops a problem (does not have routine oral cancer screening). He has used smokeless tobacco for 30 years and consumes three or four alcoholic beverages per week.

Many patients with verrucous carcinoma are reported to chew tobacco, but this association is not consistent. Both tobacco use and chronic alcohol consumption are risk factors for the development of SCCa. The association with verrucous carcinoma is uncertain.

EXAMINATION

General. The patient is a thin white elderly man who appears older than his stated age, most apparent by his sun-damaged skin and extensive facial rhytids (chronic tobacco and sun exposure both contribute to early signs of aging secondary to changes in collagen synthesis).

Maxillofacial. He has deeply tanned skin with many rhytids (secondary to prolonged sun exposure). There are no skin lesions in the sun-exposed areas (important to look for early signs of basal cell carcinoma and actinic keratosis), and there is no facial or cervical lymphadenopathy (enlarged lymph nodes would be suggestive of a malignant disease process).

Intraoral. The patient has multiple restored teeth, significant enamel staining (secondary to smokeless tobacco use), and moderate generalized periodontal disease. There is an exophytic grayish and white cauliflower-like growth involving the edentulous anterior maxillary ridge (most common site for verrucous carcinoma is the buccal mucosa), measuring 2 × 3.5 cm (Figure 10-4). The lesion has areas of surrounding erythema with dispersed white patches that appear traumatized. It is firm to palpation with rolled margins. The keratotic surface is covered with pink-red pebbly papules that do not rub off. The surrounding mucosa appears normal and does not feel indurated. (Ulceration is typically not seen with verrucous carcinoma.)

IMAGING

A panoramic radiograph should be obtained to screen for any bony erosion or infiltration and to evaluate the dentition. Although verrucous carcinoma has a low tendency to metastasize, it does represent a malignancy and therefore formal oncological staging should be considered. Routine oncological work-up includes an assessment of the extent of locoregional disease using clinical and radiographic modalities (panoramic radiograph, CT scan of the head and neck, nasopharyngeal laryngoscopy, and chest radiograph or CT). The likelihood of distant disease is remote and can be addressed based on system-driven findings.

In this case, a panoramic radiograph demonstrated normal bony anatomy of the jaws. The maxillary sinuses appear clear and have no evidence of widening of the periodontal ligaments or localized resorption of teeth (signs of infiltrative disease processes).

A contrast-enhanced CT scan (contrast enhances visualization of soft tissue) of the head and neck was obtained. This showed focal thickening of the oral soft tissues in the area of the anterior maxilla. There was no evidence of infiltration or extension of the lesion and no enlarged lymph nodes (signs of metastatic disease). Due to the risk of occult malignancy, a nasopharyngoscopy was performed. No abnormalities where detected.

An anteroposterior chest radiograph revealed mild cardiomegaly and lung hyperinflation (secondary to chronic obstructive pulmonary disease) but no focal lung lesions indicative of metastatic disease.

LABS

Routine laboratory tests are indicated in the routine work-up of verrucous carcinoma as dictated by the medical history. A

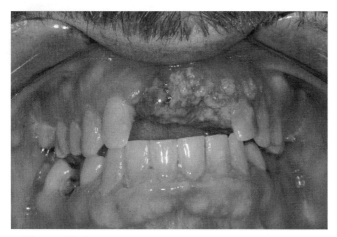

Figure 10-4 Verrucous carcinoma of the anterior maxilla.

hemoglobin level may be obtained before the removal of larger lesions. Liver function tests are typically not required, as the risk of liver metastasis is extremely low.

DIFFERENTIAL DIAGNOSIS

Based on history and clinical examination, verrucous carcinoma can be confused with a number of white lesions. These different lesions may represent a spectrum of similar diseases. Proliferative verrucous leukoplakia is a diagnosis for lesions that begin as simple hyperkeratosis and spread to other sites, become multifocal, and progress slowly through a spectrum of dysplasia to frank invasive carcinoma. Histologically, the associated dense inflammatory infiltrate may contribute to the occasional misdiagnosis as pseudoepitheliomatous hyperplasia or chronic hyperplastic candidiasis.

BIOPSY

When a diagnosis of verrucous carcinoma is considered, a full-thickness biopsy sample down to the periosteum or submucosa must be taken to minimize the possibility of misdiagnosis. Appropriate treatment relies on a good biopsy technique with attention to include the base of the lesion as part of the specimen. The key in differentiating between benign and malignant lesions is to take a biopsy sample that is both deep (full thickness) and large enough to allow examination of the relationship between the tumor and the underlying connective tissue. On occasion, multiple biopsies may be necessary to diagnose verrucous carcinoma.

ASSESSMENT

Verrucous carcinoma and a low-grade SCCa

For this patient, under local anesthesia, a full-thickness wedge biopsy sample was taken from the periphery of the lesion that included normal tissue. The tissue was sent for permanent hematoxylin and eosin staining, which showed a thick surface layer of orthokeratinized squamous epithelium with occasional parakeratosis. There were exaggerated blunt rete pegs extending into the lamina propria, with an intact, well-polarized basal layer and a "pushing border" appearance. The suprabasilar cells were well differentiated. Lymphocytic inflammation was seen throughout the lamina propria with a high degree of keratinization and minimal pleomorphism.

TREATMENT

Surgical resection is the mainstay of management of verrucous carcinoma of the oral cavity. For treatment planning purposes, preexisting comorbidities, site, grade and stage of the tumor, and the effectiveness of the particular therapy and its associated complications should be taken into account.

Due to its superficial, cohesive growth pattern and sharply demarcated margins, a number of authors recommend surgical excision as the treatment of choice. Surgery involves wide excision of the primary lesion and surrounding tissues, including bone and muscle when invasion is suspected. Wide surgical excision with 0.5- to 1-cm margins is the recommended treatment for verrucous carcinoma. With adequately treated tumors, the recurrence rate is low. It should be noted that any oral cancer that invades beyond 4 mm carries an increased risk of cervical lymph node metastasis.

Radiation therapy can be used as an adjunctive procedure and offers the advantage of treating a wide field, especially in cases where extensive surgery would cause significant morbidity. Patients should be aware of the risks of mucositis, xerostomia, radiation caries, and osteoradionecrosis of the jaws.

For this patient, under general anesthesia with nasal endotracheal intubation and local anesthesia injections, the lesion was excised with wide margins (0.5 to 1 cm) of uninvolved surrounding tissue. The specimen measured 2.5×4 cm. The depth of specimen measured less than 2 mm relative to the surrounding normal mucosa, which included excision to the level of the buccinator fascia. After complete hemostasis was obtained, the wound bed was covered with a 0.015-inch split-thickness skin graft harvested from the thigh.

COMPLICATIONS

The prognosis is excellent following adequate excision. Complications relate mainly to local destructive effects from the tumor itself and its surgical removal. Large lesions can be locally destructive with invasion or erosion of adjacent tissue and bone. Metastasis is rare. Focal areas of invasive SCCa are sometimes found within an excised specimen. Those with hybrid features (verrucoid SCCa) should be treated similar to conventional SCCa.

DISCUSSION

The terms *verrucous carcinoma of Ackerman* and *oral florid papillomatosis* have been used to describe verrucous carcinomas occurring within the aerodigestive tract. This is an uncommon tumor, diagnosed in 1 to 3 of 1 million persons each year, accounting for 2% to 9% of oral cancers. Most patients with verrucous carcinoma are older than 50, with an average age of 65 years at the time of diagnosis. Males are affected more often than females. Verrucous carcinoma is typically associated with a favorable prognosis, with 5-year survival rates up to 85% (compared to slightly over 50% for SCCa).

The most common site for verrucous carcinoma is the oral cavity. Verrucous carcinoma most commonly involves the buccal mucosa and the mandibular gingiva alveolar ridge, or palate. It typically presents as a nonulcerated, slow-growing, exophytic, "papulonodular" or "warty," fungating gray or white mass. Less frequently, the roughened, pebbly surface can be inconspicuous and the tumor can present as a flattened white lesion. It can vary in size from a small patch to a confluent, extensive mass. Verrucous carcinoma can superficially invade the soft tissues and underlying bone structures, becoming fixed to the periosteum. Distant metastasis is exceedingly rare.

The etiology of verrucous carcinoma remains unclear, but tobacco is thought to play a significant role for lesions of the aerodigestive tract. Tobacco smoking and excess alcohol are known risk factors for development of SCCa of the mouth, and they may play a role in the pathogenesis of verrucous carcinoma. Similarities between morphological features of verrucous carcinoma and virally infected epithelial lesions suggest a possible etiologic link with HPV infection. HPV types 6, 11, 16, and 18 have been detected to varying degrees in verrucous carcinoma of the oral cavity.

The hallmark of this tumor is the discrepancy between histological pattern and clinical behavior. Microscopically, verrucous carcinoma appears as a papillary or verrucous low-grade (i.e., well-differentiated) SCCa. Squamous cells display minimal or no dysplasia with infrequent mitoses localized to the invading (pushing) front. There is an overlying hyperorthokeratosis or parakeratosis, resulting in keratin-filled clefts of the surface epithelium with prominent, bulbous rete processes extending to a uniform distance into the underlying connective tissue—this creates a "pushing border" rather than an infiltrating quality at the base of this tumor. The basement membrane is intact, with little evidence of connective tissue invasion. An intense mixed inflammatory infiltrate may surround and blend with the tumor, sometimes obscuring the epithelium–connective tissue interface.

Verrucous carcinoma is an uncommon tumor that can be seen in the oral cavity. Excision of the tumor should be followed by frequent follow-up evaluations for recurrence as well as for new-onset SCCas of the upper aerodigestive tract.

Bibliography

Batsakis JG, Suarez P, El-Naggar AK: Proliferative verrucous leukoplakia and its related lesions, *Oral Oncol* 35:354-359, 1999.

Bouquot JE: Oral verrucous carcinoma. Incidence in two US populations, *Oral Surg Oral Med Oral Pathol Oral Radiol Endod* 86(3):318-324, 1998.

Charles S: The man behind the eponym: Lauren V. Ackerman and verrucous carcinoma of Ackerman. *Am J Dermatopathol* 26(4): 334-341, 2004.

Jordan RC: Verrucous carcinoma of the mouth, *J Canad Dent Assoc* 61(9):797-801, 1995.

Jyothirmayi R, Sankaranarayanan R, Varghese C, et al: Radiotherapy in the treatment of verrucous carcinoma of the oral cavity, *Oral Oncol* 33(2):124-128, 1997.

Mirbod S, Ahing S: Lesions of the oral cavity: part II. Malignant lesions, *J Can Dent Assoc* 66:308-311, 2000.

Schwartz RA: Verrucous carcinoma of the skin ad mucosa, *J Am Acad Dermatol* 32(1):1-21, 1995.

Paleri V, Orvidas LJ, Wight RG, et al: Verrucous carcinoma of the paranasal sinuses: a case report and clinical update, *Head Neck* 26(2):184-189, 2004.

Mucoepidermoid Carcinoma

Deepak Kademani, DMD, MD, FACS, David Rallis, DDS, and Chris Jo, DMD

CC

The patient is a 64-year-old woman who is referred for evaluation of a mass on the right posterior hard palate.

Mucoepidermoid carcinoma occurs in a wide age range with a slight female predilection.

HPI

The patient first noticed a lump on her hard palate approximately 6 months earlier (while the parotid gland is the most common site for mucoepidermoid carcinoma, minor salivary glands, especially from the palate, are the second most common). The patient is asymptomatic, although the mass has been slowly increasing in size (mucoepidermoid carcinoma usually presents as progressively enlarging asymptomatic swelling). She denies pain, fever, chills, night sweats, nausea, vomiting, weight loss, or other constitutional symptoms. She also denies any history of dental pain or sinus congestion.

PMHX/PDHX/MEDICATIONS/ALLERGIES/SH/FH

The patient denies tobacco or alcohol use (tobacco and alcohol use has not been shown to increase the risk of mucoepidermoid carcinoma).

EXAMINATION

General. The patient is a well-developed and well-nourished white woman who appears her stated age and is in no apparent distress. She is noncachexic (possible sign of advanced disease).

Maxillofacial. The face is symmetrical without any extraoral swelling. She has no proptosis (maxillary sinus malignancies can invade both the palate and orbit). The infraorbital nerves are intact (low-grade mucoepidermoid carcinoma typically does not display perineural invasion).

Intraoral. A 2×2 cm submucosal swelling is present on the right posterior hard palate (Figure 10-5). The mass is firm, nonmobile, nonpulsatile, and nontender to palpation (highly suggestive of a neoplastic process). The overlying mucosa is pink (may present with a bluish or reddish color) and nonulcerated. The greater and lesser palatine nerves are intact. The dentition is in good repair, and all teeth are vital without pain upon percussion. There are no other intraoral lesions or masses.

Neck. There is no lymphadenopathy (regional lymph node metastasis is uncommon, especially for low-grade lesions, but may occur in high-grade or advanced disease).

IMAGING

The work-up for a biopsy-proved mucoepidermoid carcinoma involves a complete head and neck physical examination, CT scan of the head and neck (with intravenous contrast) for delineation of the primary tumors and regional metastasis, a panoramic radiograph (initial screening examination), and a chest radiograph for evaluation of pulmonary metastasis. Newer imaging modalities such as PET scanning have become a powerful tool for evaluation of cancer patients for delineation of local and distant disease. Most PET studies are performed using the glucose analog ^{18}F-FDG, which has been shown to accumulate into areas of higher metabolic activity.

For this case, no abnormalities of the dentition and surrounding bony structures where identified on the panoramic radiograph. The CT scan of the head and neck performed with intravenous contrast (for improved delineation of soft tissue) using axial and coronal views demonstrated a 2×1 cm enhancing soft tissue mass of the right posterior hard palate, which does not appear to involve the underlying bone. No cervical lymphadenopathy was noted. The chest radiograph was normal.

LABS

For the biopsy procedure, routine laboratory studies are not indicated in an otherwise healthy patient. CBC, electrolyte studies, and coagulation studies may be performed to establish a baseline before the definitive surgery. Liver function tests are not routinely obtained, because liver metastasis is rare.

DIFFERENTIAL DIAGNOSIS

The differential diagnosis in the case of a submucosal mass of the posterior hard palate should include benign (pleomorphic adenoma, monomorphic adenoma, canicular adenoma) versus malignant minor salivary gland tumors (mucoepidermoid carcinoma, adenoid cystic carcinoma, polymorphous low-grade adenocarcinoma, acinic cell carcinoma, and adenocarcinoma). Lesions of infectious etiology should be considered but are unlikely given the presentation. An incisional biopsy is indicated.

BIOPSY

Mucoepidermoid carcinoma is graded on a scale of I to III (low, intermediate, and high grade, respectively) with features

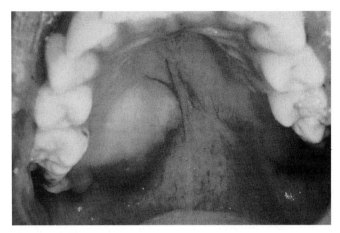

Figure 10-5 A submucosal swelling on the right posterior hard palate. *(From Ibsen OAC, Phelan JA: Oral pathology for the dental hygienist, ed 4, Philadelphia, 2004, WB Saunders.)*

such as nuclear atypia, necrosis, perineural spread, mitoses, bony invasion, lymphatic and vascular invasion, intracystic component, and tumor front invading in small nests and islands being features of high grade. The grading system for mucoepidermoid carcinoma is subjectively assessed based on the degree of epidermoid versus mucinous cellular components. High-grade tumors have a relatively higher proportion of epidermoid cells (squamous and intermediate cells) and few mucus-producing cells, while low-grade tumors have a high proportion of mucus cells.

In this patient, an incisional biopsy of the central portion of the palatal mass was performed under local anesthesia. Histopathology of the specimen confirmed a low-grade mucoepidermoid carcinoma (high proportion of mucus cells with minimal cellular atypia). It is important to obtain a tissue sample from the center of the lesion in cases of suspected salivary gland neoplasms. A biopsy from the periphery may result in a nondiagnostic specimen due to inadequate depth.

ASSESSMENT

A T1, N0, M0 (a tumor 2 cm or less in diameter, with no lymphadenopathy and no evidence of distant metastases) low-grade mucoepidermoid carcinoma of the right posterior hard palate

TREATMENT

Once a biopsy-proved diagnosis of low-grade mucoepidermoid carcinoma is made, the lesion is definitively treated by wide local excision with 1-cm margins. High-grade lesions may require more extensive resection with surgical management of the neck to limit the potential for locoregional recurrence. A right partial maxillectomy with a split-thickness skin graft and immediate placement of a prosthetic obturator form the treatment of choice for this patient. Adjuvant radiation therapy is not indicated for low-grade lesions that are completely excised.

This patient was placed under general anesthesia and underwent a formal right partial maxillectomy with 1-cm tumor-free margins via a transoral approach (a Weber-Ferguson incision may be indicated for larger tumors that require a more extensive ablative surgery). A split-thickness skin graft (0.015 inch) was harvested from the right thigh and used to line the ablative defect. This was bolstered using xeroform gauze packing (Coe-Soft [GC America] denture liner can also be used) and a preformed surgical stent, which was secured to the maxilla with a midpalatal screw. The stent was removed after 2 weeks, and an impression was taken for fabrication of a temporary maxillary obturator.

COMPLICATIONS

Complications associated with a partial maxillectomy include bleeding due to vascular injury of the terminal branches of the internal maxillary artery (greater and lesser palatine vessels) or the internal maxillary artery itself.

Hemorrhage can be controlled with direct pressure, hemostatic agents, electrocautery, or vessel ligation. Uncontrollable arterial bleeding may require angiography and embolization of the feeding vessels to obtain proximal control. The use of a maxillary stent will help promote hemostasis and improve patient comfort and speech in the healing period.

Local recurrence or regional metastases, although uncommon, is a major concern (see Discussion). Complications associated with the rehabilitation and reconstruction of the defect can also have significant impacts on the patient's quality of life.

DISCUSSION

Salivary gland neoplasms exhibit an approximate distribution of 85% in the major and 15% in the minor salivary glands. Of the major glands, the parotid accounts for 90%, followed by the submandibular at 5% to 10% (rare in the sublingual gland). For minor salivary glands, the palate is involved in 60% of cases, followed by the lips in 15%. Other less common sites include the tongue, retromolar trigone, floor of the mouth, and buccal mucosa. In general, the size of the salivary gland is inversely related to the likelihood of tumor malignancy. Approximately 10% of parotid, 30% of submandi-bular, and 50% of intraoral salivary gland lesions are malignant.

Mucoepidermoid carcinoma is the most common malignancy originating from both the major and minor salivary glands and is comprised of epidermoid, mucus-producing, and intermediate cells. It has been shown to involve approximately 3% to 15.5% of salivary gland tumors with 12% to 34% being malignant. The parotid gland, followed by the palate and submandibular glands, are the most common sites of primary tumors, representing 42%, 15%, and 10% of cases, respectively. The disease is seen most often within the third to fifth decades of life and has a slight female predilection. Tumor grade, stage, and negative margin status have correlated with disease-free survival. In studies involving mucoepidermoid carcinoma of both major and minor salivary glands, 5- and 10-year survival rates have ranged from 61% to 92% and 51% to 90%, respectively.

Low-grade mucoepidermoid carcinoma is a low-grade malignant process with a low risk of locoregional recurrence. Surgical extirpation is typically all that is required along with long-term follow-up. High-grade mucoepidermoid carcinoma is an aggressive malignancy with affinity for regional lymphatic spread and has the potential for distant metastasis (the lungs are the most common site).

The primary goal in surgical treatment of mucoepidermoid carcinoma is to obtain widely negative margins at the primary location, but additional factors must be evaluated to determine the need for adjunctive therapy. Low-grade lesions, such as in this case, are typically resected with a 1-cm margin without adjunctive treatment. High-grade lesions typically require more extensive resection with additional management of the neck. When surgical margins are positive, radiotherapy has been effective in improving local control.

Mucoepidermoid carcinoma of the parotid gland (most common site) typically presents with a unilateral preauricular mass and facial swelling. These findings are nonspecific to parotid tumors. Although the majority of parotid tumors are benign and occur in the superficial pole of the gland, approximately 20% of parotid tumors may be malignant, with mucoepidermoid carcinoma being the most common. When a lesion of the parotid is suspected and properly imaged with CT or MRI, fine needle aspiration is performed to establish a preoperative diagnosis. Treatment consists of a parotidectomy with facial nerve dissection and preservation (the facial nerve is typically spared, except in high-grade lesions with direct involvement of the facial nerve). A margin of normal salivary gland tissue should be resected around the lesion.

High-grade lesions may require multimodality treatments with a more extensive resection.

Bibliography

Beckhardt RN, Weber RS, Zane R, et al: Minor salivary gland tumors of the palate: Clinical and pathologic correlates of outcome, *Laryngoscope* 105:1155-1160, 1995.

Bhattacharyya N: Factors affecting survival in maxillary sinus cancer, *J Oral Maxillofac Surg* 61(9):1016-1021, 2003.

Boahene DK, Olsen KD, et al: Mucoepidermoid carcinoma of the parotid gland: the Mayo Clinic experience, *Arch Otolaryngol Head Neck Surg* 130(7):849-856, 2004.

Brandwein MS, Ivanov K, et al: Mucoepidermoid carcinoma: a clinicopathologic study of 80 patients with special reference to histological grading, *Am J Surg Pathol* 25(7):835-845, 2001.

Carlson ER, Schimmele SR: The management of minor salivary gland tumors of the oral cavity, *Atlas Oral Maxillofacial Surg Clin N Am* 6:1, 1998.

Goode R, Auclair P, Ellis G: Mucoepidermoid carcinoma of the major salivary glands: clinical and histopathological analysis of 234 with evaluation and grading criteria, *Cancer* 82:7, 1997.

Guzzo M, Andreola S, et al: Mucoepidermoid carcinoma of the salivary glands: clinicopathologic review of 108 patients treated at the National Cancer Institute of Milan, *Ann Surg Oncol* 9(7):688-695, 2002.

Hosokawa Y, Shirato H, et al: Role of radiotherapy for mucoepidermoid carcinoma of salivary gland, *Oral Oncol* 35:105-111, 1999.

Mullins JE, Ogle O, et al: Painless mass in the parotid region, *J Oral Maxillofac Surg* 58(3):316-319, 2000.

Plambeck K, Friedrich RE, Schmelzle R: Mucoepidermoid carcinoma of salivary gland origin: classification, clinical-pathological correlation, treatment results and long-term follow-up in 55 patients, *J Craniomaxillofac Surg* 24:133-139, 1996.

Pogrel MA: The management of salivary gland tumors of the palate, *J Oral Maxillofac Surg* 52:454-459, 1994.

Schramm VL, Imola MJ: Management of nasopharyngeal salivary gland malignancy, *Laryngoscope* 111(9):1533-1544, 2001.

Adenoid Cystic Carcinoma

David C. Swiderski, DDS, MD, and Deepak Kademani, DMD, MD, FACS

CC

A 53-year-old white woman presents to the office with the complaint of "swelling and numbness in my lip" (adenoid cystic carcinoma has a relatively equal male-to-female distribution and is most commonly seen in the elderly population).

HPI

Over the past several months, the patient had noticed a slowly enlarging mass in her lower left lip (the most common location for minor salivary gland tumors is in the palate and the lip). In addition, she has noticed that her left lower lip has become progressively anesthetic (indicative of perineural invasion of the mental nerve). There are no other oral or constitutional complaints.

Most patients report a slow-growing (months) mass at the primary site. Some patients present with pain (30% of cases), most likely due to perineural invasion.

PMHX/PDHX/MEDICATIONS/ALLERGIES/SH/FH

Noncontributory.

Although exposure to ionizing radiation has been implicated as a cause of salivary gland cancer, the etiology of most salivary gland cancers cannot be determined. Occupations that may be associated with an increased risk for salivary gland cancers include rubber product manufacturing, asbestos mining, plumbing, and some types of woodworking. Tobacco and alcohol consumption do not seem to have a causal relationship with adenoid cystic carcinoma.

EXAMINATION

General. The patient is a well-developed and well-nourished white woman who appears her stated age and in no acute distress.

Maxillofacial. There is a 2×1-cm indurated lesion of the left lower lip with central ulceration. No pain or tenderness is elicited upon palpation of the lip. The lip is anesthetic to light touch and painful stimuli in the distribution of the left mental nerve (suggestive of perineural invasion).

Neck. There is no lymphadenopathy (adenoid cystic carcinoma can metastasize via the hematogenous route leading to pulmonary lesions, which are the most common sites for distant metastasis). Salivary gland malignancies tend to spread via the hematogeneous route, so distant metastasis can occur early.

Intraoral. Dentition appears in good repair. There are no other intraoral lesions or masses.

Pulmonary. Chest is clear to auscultation bilaterally.

IMAGING

The work-up for adenoid cystic carcinoma involves a complete head and neck physical examination, CT scan of the head and neck (with intravenous contrast) for delineation of the primary tumors and regional metastasis, a panoramic radiograph, and a chest radiograph to evaluate for pulmonary metastasis. Newer imaging modalities such as PET scanning have become a powerful tool in the evaluation of patients with cancer for delineation of local and distant disease. Most PET studies are performed using the glucose analog ^{18}F-FDG, which has been shown to accumulate in many tumors (uptake into areas of higher metabolic activity).

Panoramic radiograph. There are no abnormalities of the dentition and surrounding structures, and no periapical radiolucent lesions are noted around the teeth or the body of the mandible (important to rule out any acute or chronic sources of infection, especially if radiation therapy is to be administered).

CT scan (head and neck). CT is performed with intravenous contrast (for improved delineation of soft tissue). Axial and coronal views demonstrate a 2×1 cm mass in the area of the lip with poorly differentiated margins. No cervical lymphadenopathy is seen.

Chest radiograph. Lung fields are clear bilaterally, and the mediastinum in not enlarged. The heart shadow appears to be of normal size (important to evaluate for pulmonary lesions, which may indicate metastasis).

PET scan (whole body scan). The PET scan performed with ^{18}F-FDG shows a hypermetabolic area in the left lip; no other abnormalities are noted. (This test is good for evaluation of distant disease, given the tendency for early metastasis. It is also useful for surveillance imaging during treatment to determine tumor response to nonsurgical interventions.)

LABS

Routine laboratory studies such as CBC, electrolyte studies, and coagulation studies may be performed to establish baseline levels preoperatively.

CBC and electrolyte panel results were within normal limits for this patient.

BIOPSY

Three major forms of adenoid cystic carcinoma are recognized histopathologically—the cribiform, tubular, and solid variants. Microscopically, adenoid cystic carcinoma is composed of small cells arranged in groups that form glandular spaces filled with mucoid material or a hyaline plug. Of the three types, the most common is the cribiform type.

In this patient, an incisional biopsy, with local anesthesia, of the lip mass was performed, confirming the diagnosis of adenoid cystic carcinoma with perineural invasion.

ASSESSMENT

A T1, N0, M0 (a tumor less than 2 cm, with no lymphadenopathy and no metastatic disease), stage I, adenoid cystic carcinoma (cribiform type) of the left lip with associated perineural invasion involving the branches of the mental nerve (perineural invasion is a common finding with adenoid cystic carcinoma)

TREATMENT

Radical surgery with wide surgical margins (minimum of 1 to 1.5 cm) is the treatment of choice. Despite good local control, in the long term, many patients die from their disease. The 5-year survival rate is 75%, falling to 20% at 10 years with pulmonary metastasis. By 20 years, the mortality rate is almost 100%. Adjunctive treatments such as postoperative radiotherapy are indicated in the majority of patients for improvement of locoregional control.

This patient was placed under general anesthesia and underwent a wide local excision with 1.0- to 1.5-cm margins. Frozen sections revealed positive margins and perineural invasion; further resection followed by frozen section confirmed negative margins. The surgical defect was primarily reconstructed using an Abbe-Estlander flap from the upper lip. Following adequate time for surgical healing (6 weeks), the patient underwent external beam radiation therapy.

COMPLICATIONS

Major complications associated with adenoid cystic carcinoma are its propensity toward high locoregional recurrence regardless of surgical margin as well as a poor 20-year survival rate. Functional and aesthetic complications from tumor surgery depend on the size and involvement of anatomical structures in the resection and subsequent reconstruction.

DISCUSSION

Adenoid cystic carcinoma is a salivary gland malignancy of myoepithelial and ductal cells. It is well known for its indolent course and propensity for perineural invasion (Figure 10-6), wide local metastasis, and locoregional recurrence. Locoregional recurrence is thought to occur via skip lesions along nerve fibers. This implies that although the nerve may be without

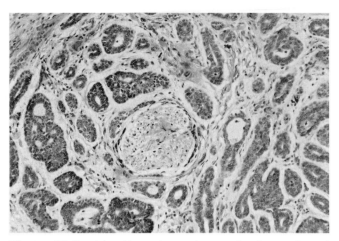

Figure 10-6 Adenoid cystic carcinoma showing perineural invasion. *(From Regezi JA, Sciubba JJ, Jordan RCK:* Oral pathology: clinical pathologic correlations, *ed 4, St Louis, 2003, Elsevier.)*

disease at the surgical margins, tumor cells may be present farther along the nerve sheath ("skip lesions"). For this reason, it is not uncommon that during resection the nerve is sacrificed as far proximally as possible, often to the skull base.

The tumor was first described by Bilroth in 1856 and was given the name cylindroma, secondary to its unique histological appearance. This term has fallen out of favor because of the confusion with the benign adnexal tumor that bears the same name.

Overall, tumors of the salivary glands are relatively rare, usually accounting for less than 5% of all head and neck neoplasms, with approximately 10% to 15% occurring in the submandibular glands and 85% to 90% occurring in the parotid glands and with the sublingual gland constituting only 1%. Of all submandibular malignancies, adenoid cystic carcinoma accounts for 35% of occurrences.

Adenoid cystic carcinoma usually occurs in the fourth through sixth decades of life with its peak incidence in the fifth decade, although there are cases reported in the early third and eighth decades of life. There is no gender predilection, although the reviewed literature is not entirely clear on this subject. Seventy percent of lesions appear in the minor salivary glands, with the most common locations being the hard and soft palates and the lip. The other 30% occur in the parotid and submandibular glands in equal distribution. Differentiation between a minor gland tumor and that of the sublingual gland may be difficult.

There appears to be no predisposing factors for the development of adenoid cystic carcinoma. The tumor is very slow growing and takes many months to be noticed clinically. If treated at an early stage, there is a high 5-year survival rate. Unfortunately, there is a high rate of locoregional recurrence regardless of negative margin status. Adenoid cystic carcinoma also has a high rate of distant metastasis, with some studies reporting a rate as high as 50%. The lungs are the main organ of metastasis, followed by bone and liver. These lesions are classically described as "coin" lesions on chest radiographs. The survival rate continues to fall until the

20-year mark, when the survival rate is less than 5%. The mean survival rate is well equated to the stage at diagnosis based on the American Joint Commission on Cancer guidelines for major salivary gland pathology.

Bibliography

Avery CME, Moody AB, McKinna FE, et al: Combined treatment of adenoid cystic carcinoma of the salivary glands, *Int J Oral Maxillofac Surg* 29:277-279, 2000.

Darling MR, Schneider JW, Phillips VM: Polymorphous low-grade adenocarcinoma and adenoid cystic carcinoma: a review and comparison of immunohistochemical markers, *Oral Oncol* 38:641-645, 2002.

Enamorado I, Lakhani R, Korkmaz H, et al: Correlation of histopathological variants, cellular DNA content, and clinical outcome in adenoid cystic carcinoma of the salivary glands, *Otolaryngol Head Neck Surg* 131:646-650, 2004.

Kokemueller H, Eckardt, Brachvogel P, et al: Adenoid cystic carcinoma of the head and neck—a 20 year experience, *Int J Oral Maxillofac Surg* 33:25-31, 2004.

Nascimento AG, Amaral ALP, Prado LAF, et al: Adenoid cystic carcinoma of the salivary glands: a study of 61 cases with clinicopathological correlation, *Cancer* 57:312-319, 1985.

Prokopakis EP, Snyderman CH, Hanna EY, et al: Risk factors for local recurrence of adenoid cystic carcinomas, *Am J Otolaryngol* 20:281-286, 1999.

Rapidis AD, Givolas N, Gakiopoulou H, et al: Adenoid cystic carcinoma of the head and neck. Clinicopathological analysis of 23 patients and review of the literature, *Oral Oncol* 41:428-435, 2005.

Spiro RH: Distant metastasis in adenoid cystic carcinoma of salivary origin, *Am J Surg* 174:495-498, 1997.

Spiro RH, Huvos AG, Strong EW: Adenoid cystic carcinoma of salivary origin: a clinicopathologic study of 242 cases, *Am J Surg* 128:512-520, 1974.

Acinic Cell Carcinoma

David Rallis, DDS, and Deepak Kademani, DMD, MD, FACS

CC

A 58-year-old woman (acinic cell carcinoma is commonly seen in the fifth and sixth decades of life, with a female predominance) is referred by her general dentist for evaluation of a painful mass in the area of the right parotid gland (painful parotid mass is the most common presentation).

HPI

The patient has noticed a persistent progressively enlarging painful mass in the area of her right parotid gland for approximately 8 months. She does not report any facial nerve deficits (indicative of perineurial spread and more advanced disease). She denies constitutional symptoms such as fever, malaise, weight loss, or dysphagia (these symptoms may indicate the presence of metastatic disease).

PMHX/PDHX/MEDICATIONS/ALLERGIES/SH/FH

The patient has a 10 pack-year history of smoking and denies alcohol use (although associated with the development of epidermoid tumors in the head and neck, tobacco and alcohol consumption do not seem to have a causal relationship with acinic cell carcinoma).

EXAMINATION

General. The patient is a well-developed and well-nourished woman who appears her stated age and is in no apparent distress.

Maxillofacial. A 2-cm well-circumscribed indurated and freely mobile mass is present anterior to the right tragus. The mass is painful to palpation (acinic cell carcinoma is usually not fixed, particularly in the early stages).

Ears. The ears are grossly normal externally with intact tympanic membranes (it is important to document an ear examination with parotid lesions to evaluate for gross invasion of the external auditory canal).

Neck. The neck is bilaterally supple with no palpable lymphadenopathy (important prognostic factor, because presence of lymphadenopathy would be suggestive of regional metastatic disease). The trachea is midline and stable.

Neurological. Cranial nerves II through XII are intact, and there is no evidence of facial nerve deficit (perineurial invasion may cause facial nerve deficit).

Pulmonary. Lungs are clear to auscultation bilaterally. (The most common site of metastases of acinic cell carcinoma is the lungs. Patients with pulmonary metastases may do well in the near term, but almost all die from their disease within 20 years.)

IMAGING

Adequate imaging studies need to be obtained to determine the extent of the disease process at the primary site, to detect regional lymphadenopathy, and to identify any distant metastasis. Evaluation of the lungs and the skeleton is important because they are the most common sites of distant metastasis.

MRI (with intravenous contrast) is the imaging study of choice to localize the lesion within the parotid gland. MRI provides better resolution for soft tissue lesions than CT. PET scan uses radiolabeled glucose (^{18}F-FDG) to detect areas of increased hypermetabolism that may be indicative of local, regional, or distant disease.

In this patient, MRI with intravenous contrast shows an enhancing mass within the superficial lobe of the parotid gland measuring $18 \times 17 \times 15$ mm, with no evidence of lymphadenopathy.

A PET scan outlines a hypermetabolic region in the area of the right parotid gland.

The chest radiograph is negative. (The lung is the most common site of distant metastasis, which may present as a coin lesion on the chest film.)

LABS

The patient's CBC and basic metabolic panel were within normal limits.

Liver metastasis is very rare, therefore liver function tests are not routinely obtained for the work-up of acinic cell carcinoma.

Cytology. Fine needle aspiration involves the cytological examination of cells obtained from the specimen; this is performed by an experienced cytopathologist. For additional accuracy, the fine needle aspiration may be performed under CT or ultrasonographic guidance. This is an effective tool to distinguish between benign and malignant salivary gland tumors with a reported sensitivity and specificity of 80% and 92%, respectively.

In this patient, the fine needle aspiration showed the presence of glandular cells with increased nuclear pleomorphism and cytotypic features consistent with acinic cell carcinoma.

ASSESSMENT

A T1, N0, M0 (a tumor less than 2 cm, with no lymphade-nopathy and no metastatic disease) stage I, acinic cell carcinoma located within the superficial lobe of the right parotid gland

TREATMENT

Acinic cell carcinoma is a primary salivary gland malignancy originating within the serous acinar cells. The treatment for acinic cell carcinoma consists of surgical excision. For tumors involving the parotid gland, a parotidectomy with facial nerve preservation is recommended. In the absence of facial paralysis (uncommon with acinic cell carcinoma), the facial nerve should be preserved.

This patient was treated in the operating room and under general anesthesia. The surgical field was draped to allow exposure of the right ear, lateral canthus, and corner of the mouth. A modified Blair incision (preauricular crease curving around the mandibular angle with anterior extension approximately 3 cm beneath the inferior border) was marked. The incision extends through the skin into subcutaneous tissue. An anterior and posterior skin flap was raised at the level of the parotid fascia that was extended to the periphery of the gland. The greater auricular nerve was identified and preserved as it crosses superficial to the sternocleidomastoid muscle. The parotid gland was then elevated from the muscle and dissected from the external auditory canal until the tragal pointer was identified. This is approximately 1 cm inferior to the tympanomastoid suture. The gland was then dissected from the posterior belly of the digastric. Three landmarks should be identified: the tragal pointer, the superior aspect of the posterior digastric, and the tympanomastoid suture.

These landmarks along with their predictable anatomy are used to identify the main trunk of the facial nerve as follows:
- The main trunk of the facial nerve courses 1 cm medial and inferior to the tragal pointer
- The stylomastoid foramen is 6 to 8 mm deep to the tympanomastoid suture
- The facial nerve is superior and posterior to the cephalic margin of the posterior digastric or midway to the tympanomastoid suture

Subsequently, gentle dissection was carried out through fascia and gland until the facial nerve was visualized. Dissection continues along the main trunk until the division of cervical facial and temporal facial branches (pes anserinus) is identified. The gland was palpated, and the tumor found to be well circumscribed within the superficial lobe. Dissection was carried out following the branches of the facial nerve to the periphery of the gland. Figure 10-7 shows the specimen being removed from the superficial lobe of the parotid gland.

Frozen histopathological specimens identified a low-grade acinic cell carcinoma within the specimen and widely nega-

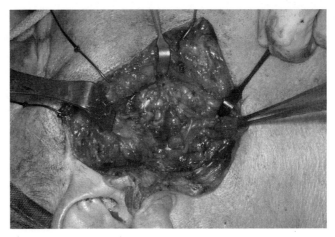

Figure 10-7 Intraoperative view of the specimen being removed after identification of the facial nerve.

tive margins (frozen section analysis is on occasion not precise for salivary gland disease, but it can provide information regarding benign versus malignant disease processes and can still be helpful in guiding intraoperative decision making). No perineural or angiolymphatic invasion was identified. A drain was inserted, and a layered closure was obtained with deep 4-0 monofilament resorbable and skin 5-0 nylon suture.

COMPLICATIONS

Surgical treatment of acinic cell carcinoma varies greatly depending on location as well as a number of additional factors. In the case described, superficial parotidectomy was the sole surgical procedure necessary. Despite careful dissection and correct technique, several significant complications may occur.

Facial nerve deficit may be encountered as a result of skeletonization of the nerve. Studies have shown that early transient facial nerve paresis follows parotidectomy in 9.3% to 64.6% of cases, with permanent total paralysis occurring in 0% to 0.9%. With paralysis of the orbicularis occuli muscle, impairing closure of the upper eye lid, desiccation of the eye and keratoconjunctivitis are the major concerns. Ophthalmic eye drops and ointment should be used as needed. Placement of a gold weight posterior to the tarsal plate of the upper lid is one popular method to regain upper lid closure in patients with persistent deficit of the temporozygomatic branches of the facial nerve.

The other nerve at risk during this surgery is the greater auricular nerve (sensory branch of the third division of the trigeminal nerve). Paresthesia (altered sensation) of the ipsilateral ear may occur as result of division or skeletonization of this nerve.

Postoperative sialocele formation presents in a minority of patients and will usually occur within the first 2 weeks after surgery. This presents as a soft mobile nonerythematous swelling within the gland. Untreated significant swelling, skin necrosis, and cutaneous fistula formation may result.

Management of a sialocele involves needle aspiration/drainage with placement of a pressure dressing. The use of antisialogues can also be considered.

Frey syndrome or recurring gustatory sweating may arise as a result of aberrant regeneration of the postganglionic parasympathetic nerve fibers reinnervating the sweat glands. An incidence ranging from 5% to 100% of patients undergoing parotidectomy has been reported. A number of surgical procedures have been used to treat this condition, including ligation of the auriculotemporal and chorda tympani nerves, temporal fascia grafting, placement of synthetic materials into the surgical site, anticholinergic agents (pilocarpine), and, more recently, injection of *Clostridium* botulinum toxin (Botox) into the involved area. Treatment is not always necessary unless the condition is particularly bothersome to the patient.

Aesthetic concerns may arise from the facial depression created by removal of the superficial lobe. Autogenous fat grafting may be performed for reconstruction of the area.

DISCUSSION

Acinic cell carcinoma is rare malignancy that accounts for about 6% of all salivary gland tumors. This tumor most commonly presents in females and is usually seen in the fifth and sixth decades of life. The parotid gland is the most common location, with painful swelling being seen in 18% to 71% of patients and facial paresis being reported in 11%. Survival rate has been reported at 76%, 63%, and 55% at 5, 10, and 15 years, respectively, although there is significant variation in the literature.

Acinic cell carcinoma is considered a low-risk tumor for regional and distant metastasis, with a 12% and 16% metastatic rate being reported, respectively. The lungs represent the most common site of distant metastasis, followed by bone. Staging is the primary determinate of treatment, but histological grade, facial paralysis, age, pain, and extraglandular spread are prognostic factors that must be considered. Higher histological grade or lack of cellular differentiation has been associated with a poorer prognosis.

The use of postoperative radiotherapy may be used to improve local control.

As with any oncological surgical procedure, the goal in treating acinic cell carcinoma is to obtain wide negative margins at the primary location. Equally important, the clinician must use diagnostic tools to accurately stage the malignancy and determine the need for adjunctive therapy.

Bibliography

Abrams AM, Cornysn J, Scofield HH, et al: Acinic cell adenocarcinoma of the major salivary glands: a clinicopathologic study of 77 cases, *Cancer* 18:1145-1162, 1965.

Canosa A, Cohen MA: Post-traumatic parotid sialocele: report of two cases, *J Oral Maxillofac Surg* 57:742-745, 1999.

Dulguerov P, Marchal F, Lehmann W: Postparotidectomy facial nerve paralysis: possible etiologic factors and results with routine facial nerve monitoring, *Laryngoscope* 109:754-761, 1999.

Ellis GL, Corio FL: Acinic cell adenocarcinoma: a clinico-pathologic analysis of 294 cases, *Cancer* 52:542, 1983.

Enoroth CM, Jakosson PA, Blanck C: Acinic cell carcinoma of the parotid gland, *Cancer* 19:1761, 1976.

Gold DR, Annino DJ: Management of the neck in salivary gland carcinoma, *Otolaryngol Clin N Am* 38:99-105, 2005.

Haberal I, Gocmen H, Safak MA, et al: The value of fine-needle aspiration biopsy in salivary gland tumors, *Int Fed Otorhinolaryngol Soc Int Congr Series* 1240:629-634, 2003.

Huber PE, Debus J, Latz D, et al: Radiotherapy for advanced adenoid cystic carcinoma: neutrons, photons or mixed beam? *Radiat Oncol* 59:161-167, 2001.

Jozefowicz-Korczynska M, Debniak E, Lukomski M: Treatment of parotid glands cancer, *Int Fed Otorhinolaryngol Soc Int Congr Series* 1240:635-639, 2003.

Laskawi R, Rodel R, Zirk A, et al: Retrospective analysis of 35 patients with acinic cell carcinoma of the parotid gland, *J Oral Maxillofac Surg* 56:440-443, 1998.

Lewis J, Olsen K, Weilan L: Acinic cell carcinoma: clinicopathologic review, *Cancer* 67:172-179, 1991.

Licitra L, Grandi C, Prott FJ, et al: Major and minor salivary glands tumors, *Crit Rev Oncol Hematol* 45:215-225, 2003.

Luna-Ortiz K, Sanson-RioFrio JA, Mosqueda-Taylor A: Frey syndrome. A proposal for evaluating severity, *Oral Oncol* 40:501-505, 2004.

Olsen KD: Superficial parotidectomy, *Oper Techn Gen Surg* 6:102-114, 2004.

Raine C, Saliba K, Chippindale AJ, et al: Radiological imaging in the primary parotid malignancy, *Br J Plast Surg* 56:637-643, 2003.

Reilly J, Myssiorek D: Facial nerve stimulation and postparotidectomy facial paresis, *Otolaryngol Head Neck Surg* 128:530-533, 2003.

Spiro RH, Huvos AG, Strong EW: Acinic cell carcinoma of salivary origin: a clinicopathologic study of 67 cases, *Cancer* 41:924-935, 1978.

Terhaard CHJ, Lubsen H, Rasch CRN, et al: The role of radiotherapy in the treatment of malignant salivary gland tumors, *Int J Radiat Oncol Biol Phys* 61(1):103-111, 2005.

11 Reconstructive Oral and Maxillofacial Surgery

Shahrokh C. Bagheri, DMD, MD

This chapter addresses:
- Mandibular Implants
- Maxillary Posterior Fixed Partial Denture
- Sinus Lift for Implants
- Mandibular Vestibuloplasty
- Radial Forearm Free Flap
- Pectoralis Major Myocutaneous Flap
- Free Fibula Flap for Mandibular Reconstruction
- Mandibular Reconstruction With Iliac Crest Bone Graft

Reconstructive maxillofacial surgery refers to the wide range of procedures designed to rebuild or enhance soft or hard tissue structures of the maxillofacial region. Ablative tumor surgery (benign or malignant) and traumatic injuries (especially avulsive) commonly demand reconstructive procedures to restore the functional and cosmetic deficit. Loss of soft or hard tissue secondary to infectious processes (e.g., osteomyelitis), or tissue injury due to radiation (e.g., osteoradionecrosis) may also require reconstructive measures. In addition, the decrease in quantity and quality of maxillomandibular structures with age (that may be accelerated by other processes such as early teeth loss), can be addressed with reconstructive measures to augment the tissue for restoration using dental implants.

In the past two decades, three developments have revolutionized the reconstruction of the maxillofacial structures. First, the understanding of bone biology has allowed advanced bone grafting procedures in a variety of circumstances (e.g., sinus lift procedures, mandibular augmentation/reconstruction). Second, the advent of microvascular free flap techniques allows the transfer of tissue to reconstruct large soft and/or hard tissue defects (e.g., radial forearm fasciocutaneous or fibula osteocutaneous free flaps). Third, the development of and advances in dental implant techniques allow for successful dental rehabilitation. More recently, purification and identification of bone morphogenic proteins (BMPs) and other chemicals that induce new tissue (bone) formation are becoming available but remain to be fully elucidated. Future research may reveal methods of regenerating neural and muscle tissue. Molecular biology techniques using gene therapy may reveal further knowledge that can be applied to maxillofacial reconstruction.

In this chapter, we present eight important teaching cases that describe some of the main issues in maxillofacial reconstruction. Mandibular reconstruction remains to be one of the greatest challenges in maxillofacial surgery. We present cases of mandibular reconstruction using corticocancellous bone grafts with implants and using the free fibula osteocutaneous flap.

Mandibular Implants

Sam E. Farish, DMD, and Shahrokh C. Bagheri, DMD, MD

CC

A 30-year-old woman who is missing the lower right first and second molars (teeth Nos. 30 and 31) and second premolar (tooth No. 29) presents to the office via a referral from her general dentist who suggested restoration using mandibular implants.

HPI

The patient lost the mandibular right posterior teeth after failed endodontic and restorative therapy. The patient was offered a removable partial denture or mandibular posterior implants, and she chose the latter.

PMHX/PDHX/MEDICATIONS/ALLERGIES/SH/FH

The patient has maintained excellent general and oral health. She is allergic to penicillin. She is not currently taking any medications and specifically denies a history of type 1 diabetes mellitus.

There is literature support for placing implants in type 2 diabetics but none for placing implants in type 1 diabetics. In working up patients for dental implants, several risk factors should be considered. Early studies showed a marked increase in failure of osseointegration of implants in smokers. More recent work has not shown a significant difference between smokers and nonsmokers regarding osseointegration. Most believe that closure of the gap between failure rates is due to surface modifications in more recently manufactured implants. Bruxers place greater stresses on implants, so such patients should have overengineered prostheses. Radiation therapy in jaw structures where implants will be placed is considered a relative contraindication. Hyperbaric oxygen therapy and skillful conservative surgical techniques minimize these risks. Patients with severe mental illness are not usually considered good implant candidates. Immunosuppression, hemophilia, organ transplantation, osteomalacia, Paget disease, and osteogenesis imperfecta are other possible contraindications to implants to be considered. In such patients, informed consent with shared liability can prevent misunderstanding should failures occur.

EXAMINATION

Examination of both the quality and quantity of bone is essential in successful implant placement.

Intraoral. Clinical examination reveals that the mandibular ridge form is rounded and wide (6 to 7 mm) in the buccal lingual aspect at the edentulous posterior right mandible. The anteroposterior ridge space is adequate for placement of three implants posterior to the first bicuspid (the minimum amount of bone between an implant and adjacent natural tooth is 1.25 mm).

The interarch space between the edentulous mandibular ridge and the opposing dentition is adequate for the restoration and its attachment to the implant. No soft tissue or bony abnormalities are noted in the oral examination. The patient has a maximum incisal opening of 50 mm (restricted mouth opening can pose a problem for implant placement).

IMAGING

The panoramic radiographic is an essential imaging modality for placement of mandibular implants. In this patient, the panoramic radiograph reveals an edentulous space in the posterior right lower jaw 6 weeks after multiple extractions (Figure 11-1). The bone appears to be Type II (Box 11-1), and there is more than 15 mm of available bone above the inferior alveolar nerve and mental foramen. The surgical planning template reveals that implants of 4.5-mm diameter and 11.5 mm long would be an appropriate selection for the case. In certain cases, detailed computed tomography (CT) scanning is helpful in planning implant surgery (such as to determine the position of the inferior alveolar nerve or the maxillary sinus), but CT is not indicated for all cases. Bone density and quality are determined by radiography and by tactile sense on drilling.

LABS

There is no routine laboratory testing is indicated for implant placement unless dictated by the medical history.

ASSESSMENT

A healthy 30-year-old woman who desires three mandibular posterior implants

Her work-up reveals that 11.5-mm implants would be appropriate with no contraindications to the planned procedure under intravenous sedation with local anesthesia in the office.

A minimum distance of 2 mm from the mandibular canal is recommended to avoid injury to the inferior alveolar neurovascular bundle.

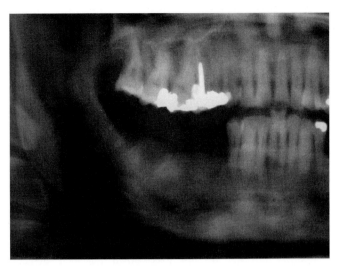

Figure 11-1 Preoperative panoramic radiograph demonstrating the position of the mandibular canal demonstrating adequate height of bone for implant placement.

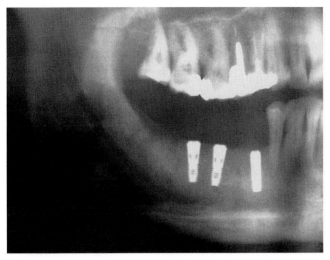

Figure 11-2 Postoperative panoramic radiograph demonstrating the final position of three endosseous implants.

Box 11-1.	Bone Classification Based on Radiographic and Clinical Parameters

Type I: Entire jaw composed of homogenous compact bone. Has the tactile sense of drilling into oak or maple wood.
Type II: A thick layer of compact bone surrounding a core of dense trabecular bone. Has the tactile sense of drilling into white pine or spruce.
Type III: A thin layer of cortical bone surrounding a core of dense trabecular bone of favorable strength. Has the tactile sense of drilling into balsa wood.
Type IV: A thin layer of cortical bone surrounding a core of low-density trabecular bone Has the tactile sense of drilling into styrofoam.

TREATMENT

The planned treatment was discussed in detail with the patient and the restorative dentist. A surgical guide was prepared by the restorative dentist, indicating the ideal position for the implants in his planned restorative schema (although a surgical guide is not essential in the planning of dental implants, they are useful in guiding the ideal position of the implant. However, the underlying bony anatomy dictates the implant position). Chlorhexidine mouth rinse was used before surgery, and 600 mg of clindamycin (patient is allergic to penicillin) was given intravenously immediately before surgery. A bite block was used to maintain an adequate oral opening (and to protect the temporomandibular joint). Under intravenous sedation and local anesthesia, implant placement surgery was performed according to the system protocol. The wound was sutured and a gauze sponge was placed to achieve hemostasis. The patient recovered and was discharged with instructions for home care, analgesics, and a return appointment in 1 week for suture removal. Postoperative panoramic radiograph revealed satisfactory placement of three implants well above the mandibular canal (Figure 11-2). A final restoration was placed 4 months later and a very satisfactory cosmetic and functional result was obtained. The crown placed is similar in contour and emergence to a natural tooth. Such design minimizes maintenance.

Although there is research indicating good results with immediate placement of healing caps and even immediate loading, fewer problems can be expected from implants submerged and unloaded (two-stage) for 4 months in the mandible and 6 months in the maxilla and in grafts.

COMPLICATIONS

Implant procedures are associated with a high rate of success and minimal complications, but patients should be well informed of the possible associated risks.

The primary limiting factor for lower molar single-implant placement is the bone height above the inferior alveolar canal. If it is determined that a lower molar implant has been placed in contact with the inferior alveolar nerve, causing postoperative hypoesthesia or anesthesia (Figure 11-3), the implant should be backed out, if possible, or removed. Radiographic superimposition of the implant versus direct contact of the nerve with the implant cannot be determined on a panoramic radiograph alone. In the presence of symptoms (paresthesia), a CT scan may be helpful before removing the implant. If the CT shows that the implant is not in contact with the nerve, removal of the implant is unlikely to resolve the paresthesia, and only interval neurosensory testing will determine whether expectant or microneurosurgical exploration is indicated.

Perforation of the lingual cortex with implant drills and implants or direct injury to the nerve is possible (Figure 11-4). Bleeding, salivary gland involvement, painful impingement of implants on the lingual surface of the mandible, and associated buccal/lingual misalignment have been reported. Such problems can be minimized by paying attention to the anatomy of the lower jaw. Implants in the posterior mandible must be

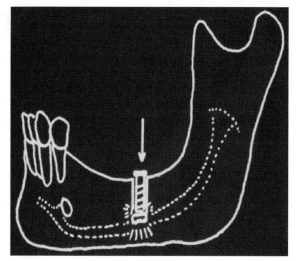

Figure 11-3   Direct injury to or contact of the inferior alveolar nerve by the implant drill.

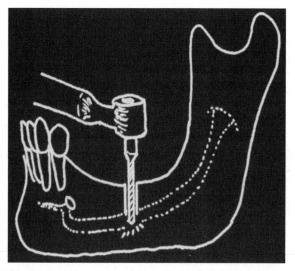

Figure 11-4   Direct injury to the inferior alveolar nerve by the implant drill.

placed with a slight buccal-to-lingual inclination to avoid perforation through the mandible.

Infection in implant surgery is a rare event. In a study by Dent and associates of the 2641 implants placed, preoperative prophylactic antibiotic at any level resulted in a failure rate between 1.2% and 1.5%, whereas failure to use antibiotics at an appropriate dose or the use of none at all resulted in a failure rate between 3.3% and 4.0%. There is strong support in the literature regarding the use of preoperative antibiotics (however, the routine use of postoperative antibiotics is not supported). Should infection occur, conservative management, including antibiotics, debridement, and incision and drainage, is indicated with implant removal as a last resort. Occasionally, inflammation and the development of a fistula can result from a loose cover screw. In this case, the implant site should be exposed, the screw is removed, the site is debrided, and the screw is replaced. A satisfactory replacement is a new screw or the screw that was removed after it is

sterilized in an autoclave. The benefit of the routine use of preoperative rinsing with chlorhexidine is not clear.

Other complications with implant surgery include aspiration of instruments or implant components. This may be prevented by paying attention to positioning, using a well-placed gauze curtain, and attaching a 12- to 16-inch floss cord to screw drivers so retrieval is possible should the instrument be dropped.

DISCUSSION

There is a wide range of implant designs, materials, and surfaces for the implant surgeon to choose, although a detailed analysis of such implant variables is beyond the scope of this discussion. At the present, a textured-surface titanium alloy implant is indicated because it is known that such surfaces are better receptors for fibrin strands forming the initial attachments of implants to bone in the microgap. Immediate loading, one-stage placement, or traditional two-stage implant surgery all have their proponents. In posterior mandibular molars, two-stage placement seems ideal as no cosmetic considerations come into play. The placement of two standard platform implants to replace a missing lower molar where the mesiodistal space is wide (greater than 12 mm) increases the biomechanical resistance of the restoration but may compromise oral hygiene practices.

There are several techniques that increase inadequate bone volume above the inferior alveolar canal: onlay or particulate grafting, guided tissue regeneration, distraction, and nerve repositioning are documented. When any technique is used other than standard implant surgery, there are tradeoffs, with additional potential complications associated with the technique used.

Bibliography

Bain CA: Smoking and implant failure: benefits of a smoking cessation protocol, *Int J Oral Maxillofac Implants* 11:756-759, 1996.

Bain CA, Moy PK: The association between failure of dental implants and cigarette smoking, *Int J Oral Maxillofac Implants* 8:609-615, 1993.

Dent CD, Olson JW, Farish SE, et al: The influence of preoperative antibiotics on success of endosseous implants up to and including stage II surgery: a study of 2,641 implants, *J Oral Maxillofac Surg* 55(suppl 5):19-24, 1997.

Engelman MJ: *Clinical decision making and treatment planning in osseointegration,* Chicago, 1996, Quintessence.

Lekholm U, Zarb GA: Patient selection and preparation. In Branemark PI, Zarb GA, Albrektsson T, editors: *Tissue-integrated prostheses: osseointegration in clinical dentistry,* Chicago, 1985, Quintessence, pp 199-209.

Marx RE, Garg AK: *Dental and craniofacial applications of platelet-rich plasma,* Chicago, 2005, Quintessence.

Misch CE: Density of bone: effect on treatment plans, surgical approach, healing and progressive bone loading, *Int J Oral Implantol* 6:23-31, 1990.

Nevins M, Mellonig JT, editors: *Implant therapy: clinical approaches and evidence of success, volume 2,* Chicago, 1998, Quintessence.

Renouard F, Rangert B: *Risk factors in implant dentistry,* Chicago, 1999, Quintessence.

Maxillary Posterior Fixed Partial Denture

Sam E. Farish, DMD

CC

A 58-year-old man presents complaining of missing teeth in the left maxilla between the cuspid (tooth No. 11) and second molar. He was referred by his general dentist for evaluation for an implant-based fixed partial denture.

HPI

The patient states he lost the three teeth due to failed endodontics of the first bicuspid, which was the anterior pontic of a three-unit bridge. Shortly after the bridge was cut from the posterior pontic and the anterior abutment was removed, the first molar split and required removal. He has been wearing a removable partial denture for 2 years and is very unhappy with it. The patient has otherwise well-restored functional arches with porcelain baked onto gold posteriors and natural restoration-free anterior teeth.

PMHX/PDHX/MEDICATIONS/ ALLERGIES/SH/FH

The patient reports that he had three-vessel bypass surgery 2 years earlier. He denies chest pain or exercise intolerance and works as a structural engineer on outdoor jobs where he is engaged in regular physical exertion. He is taking simvastatin (HMG-CoA reductase inhibitor) for hyperlipidemia and clopidogrel, along with 81 mg of aspirin for reduction of thromboembolic events. He has no known drug allergies and no other medical problems. He is a nonsmoker and has excellent oral hygiene.

Clopidogrel reduces atherosclerotic events by blocking adenosine diphosphate receptors, which prevent fibrinogen binding at that site and reduce the possibility of platelet adhesion and aggregation. Aspirin irreversibly inhibits platelet-dependent cyclooxygenase (COX), which decreases platelet-aggregation for the life of the platelet, thereby reducing the risk of thrombotic vascular events. Aspirin is a much more potent inhibitor of COX-1 than COX-2. Higher doses inhibit endothelial cell synthesis of prostacyclin, which is a vasodilator and inhibitor of platelet aggregation (therefore, higher aspirin doses may be deleterious, although the ideal dosing regimen remains to be determined). It is suggested that clopidogrel be discontinued 5 days before elective surgery. Low-dose aspirin (81 mg) should have no clinically significant effect on bleeding and can be continued.

EXAMINATION

Quality and quantity of bone must be adequate for successful implant restorations.

General. The patient is a cooperative, well-developed and well-nourished man in no apparent distress.

Vital signs. His vital signs are normal.

Intraoral. Clinical examination of the posterior right maxilla reveals that the ridge form is rounded and greater than 10 mm in width but that there is a slight undercut on the facial aspect of this area. Caution will need to be exercised to avoid buccal perforation in placement, but augmentation is not indicated due to the minimal amount of undercut. The mesiodistal space is 24 mm, and thus three 3.75- or 4.0-mm implants can be placed. The center of a 3.75- or 4.0-mm implant should be 4 mm from an adjacent tooth, and 3.75- or 4.0-mm implants are ideally placed on 7-mm centers from implant to implant (i.e., the distance between implants will ideally be 3 to 3.5 mm). The interarch space between the mandibular dentition and the maxilla is adequate for the restoration and its attachment to the implant. No bone or soft tissue abnormalities are noted, and the patient can open his mouth 52 mm.

IMAGING

The panoramic radiograph reveals a 24-mm edentulous space in the posterior left maxilla. The bone quality is judged to be type II. Bone quality is determined by radiographic appearance and by the tactile feeling upon drilling (see Box 11-1). A tracing is made of the area of interest, and using the implant manufacturer's template at 25% larger than normal size (due to magnification factor of 1.25 on the panoramic radiograph), it is determined that 3.75×13-mm implants can be placed in the most anterior and middle sites and a 3.75×11.5 mm implant can be placed in the most posterior site. The implants can be placed below the floor of the left maxillary sinus. There are cases where detailed CT scanning is helpful in maxillary posterior implant planning because it can accurately determine the position of the floor of the maxillary sinus and clarify the need for sinus augmentation and the ability to place the implants in a single stage or as a two-stage procedure with preemptive sinus grafting followed by implants 4 to 6 months after the graft. Most surgeons agree that if 4 to 5 mm of bone is present between the edentulous ridge and the floor of the sinus, a one-stage surgery is possible because initial implant stability is ensured. In a straightforward case, the use of CT is not indicated.

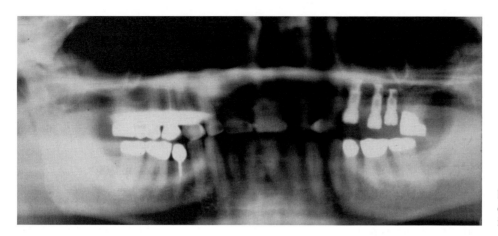

Figure 11-5 Postoperative panoramic radiograph showing ideal implant placement.

LABS

No routine laboratory studies are indicated for implant placement, unless dictated by the medical history.

For this patient, the most recent total body cholesterol level was 165 mg/dl (a total cholesterol level of less than 200 mg/dl is associated with a relatively low risk of myocardial infarction, unless other risk factors are present).

ASSESSMENT

A 58-year-old man with controlled hyperlipidemia and asymptomatic atherosclerotic heart disease who desires an implant-based fixed partial denture in the left posterior maxilla

Work-up reveals that two 3.75 × 13-mm and one 3.75 × 11.5-mm implants are indicated. There are no contraindications to the planned procedure in the office setting with intravenous sedation and local anesthesia.

TREATMENT

The planned implant surgery is discussed in detail with the restorative dentist, who has shown the patient on a diagnostic wax-up what the final restoration will look like and has provided a surgical guide indicating the ideal position and angulation for the implants. The patient has been off of clopidogrel for 6 days on presentation. He is given amoxicillin 2 g by mouth 1 hour before surgery, and chlorhexadine oral rinse is used immediately before surgery. Under intravenous sedation and local anesthesia, the implant placement surgery was performed according to the manufacturer's protocol. After all the osteotomies were completed, the sites were probed with a blunt probe and the sinus floor was found to be intact at all sites. Implants were placed and wound closure was obtained with 4-0 polyglactin (Vicryl) sutures. The patient recovered and was discharged with instructions in home care, analgesics, and a return appointment in 1 week. Postoperative panoramic radiograph revealed satisfactory implant placement (Figure 11-5). A final restoration was placed 6 months later, and a very satisfactory cosmetic and functional result was obtained. The crown placed is similar in contour and emer-

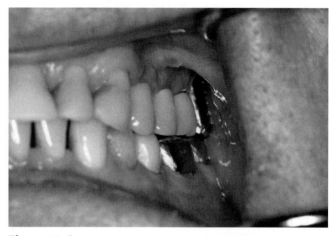

Figure 11-6 Postoperative view showing the final prosthesis in place.

gence to a natural tooth, and such design minimizes maintenance (Figure 11-6).

Although there is research indicating good results with immediate placement of healing caps and even immediate loading, fewer problems can be expected from implants submerged and unloaded (two-stage) for 4 months in the mandible and 6 months in the maxilla and in grafts.

COMPLICATIONS

Success rates for fixed partial dentures in the posterior maxilla are reported at 99.0%, while implant fixture survival is reported at 95.2% in a long-term retrospective study (1 to 8 years) by Nevins and Langer. In that same study, when the 6- to 8-year group is studied in isolation from the larger group, 90.9% of the implants in the maxilla were still functional. In a prospective study with 5-year data, Lekholm and colleagues report a 92% success rate for maxillary fixtures in posterior partially edentulous applications. Patients should be informed of the possible associated risks, such as sinus penetration, buccal perforation, infection, and failure to integrate, even though survival data suggest an adequate success rate for this application of dental implants. The most common lost implants are shorter fixtures, while wide fixtures show the lowest failure rates. Other complications associated with implants used to treat partial edentulism are fractures of the occlusal surface of restorations and loose anchorage components.

DISCUSSION

There is a wide range of implant designs, materials, and surfaces for the implant surgeon to choose, although detailed analysis of such implant variables is beyond the scope of this discussion. At the present, a textured-surface titanium alloy implant is indicated because it is known that such surfaces are better receptors for fibrin strands forming the initial attachments of implants to bone in the microgap. Immediate loading, one-stage placement, or traditional two-stage implant surgery all have their proponents. In posterior maxilla, two-stage placement seems ideal as no cosmetic considerations come into play. There are several techniques that will increase inadequate bone volume below the maxillary sinus or decrease buccal undercuts: onlay or particulate grafting, guided tissue regeneration, distraction, and sinus grafting are documented. When any technique is used other than standard implant surgery, there are tradeoffs, with additional potential complications associated with the technique used.

Bibliography

Engelman MJ: *Clinical decision making and treatment planning in osseointegration,* Chicago, 1996, Quintessence.

Lekholm U, et al: Osseointegrated implants in the treatment of partially edentulous jaws. A prospective 5-year multicenter study, *Int J Oral Maxillofac Implants* 9:627-635, 1996.

Nevins M, Langer B: The successful application of osseointegrated implants to the posterior jaw: a long-term retrospective study, *Int J Oral Maxillofac Implants* 8:428-432, 1993.

Nevins M, Mellonig JT, editors: *Implant therapy: clinical approaches and evidence of success, volume 2,* Chicago, 1998, Quintessence.

Renouard F, Rangert B: *Risk factors in implant dentistry,* Chicago, 1999, Quintessence.

Sinus Lift for Implants

John M. Allen, DMD, and Sam E. Farish, DMD

CC

A 49-year-old woman is referred by a restorative dentist for evaluation of her edentulous posterior maxilla. The patient requests restoration of her maxillary posterior quadrants using implant-based fixed partial dentures.

HPI

The patient had lost most of her posterior teeth at a younger age due to decay and failed endodontic therapy (early loss of teeth will cause bone resorption and pneumatization of the maxillary sinus). She has now decided to follow her general dentist's recommendation for full mouth rehabilitation and presents to your office for evaluation and placement of endosseous implants. Her general dentist informed her that she may require a "sinus lift" procedure due to the amount of bone resorption and pneumatization of the maxillary sinuses.

PMHX/PDHX/MEDICATIONS/ALLERGIES/SH/FH

The medical history is significant for untreated chronic sinusitis. She currently smokes one half pack of cigarettes per day, with a 10 pack-year history.

Cigarette smoking decreases tissue perfusion and oxygen delivery to tissues. Previous studies have linked smoking to failure of osseointegration with dental implants. However, more recent work has not shown a significant difference in osseointegration rates between smokers and nonsmokers. Some surgeons advise patients to stop smoking at least 1 week before surgery and up to 2 months postoperatively to permit reversal of the high levels of platelet adhesions and blood viscosity associated with nicotine intake.

A history of acute or chronic sinusitis may be problematic for a sinus lift procedure. Prolonged inflammation and/or infection of the sinus membrane will create an inappropriate environment for the procedure. Bacterial sinusitis results from secondary bacterial infection of an obstructed sinus. This results in mucosal edema, increased mucus production with accumulation of bacteria and inflammatory debris, and creation of an unfavorable environment for surgery and subsequent healing. The two most common bacteria involved in acute bacterial sinusitis are *Haemophilus influenzae* and *Streptococcus pneumoniae*. *Staphylococcus aureus*, α-hemolytic *Streptococcus*, *Bacteroides* species, and *Pseudomonas* species are most frequently found in chronic bacterial sinusitis. Any form of sinus infection should be treated with decongestants and antibiotics (some may require functional endoscopic sinus surgery) before performance of a sinus lift procedure. A broad-spectrum antibiotic such as amoxicillin with clavulanic acid (Augmentin) is often the initial antibiotic used in the management of infections caused by nasal or sinus flora.

EXAMINATION

General. The patient is a well-developed and well-nourished woman in no apparent distress.

Intraoral. The patient is missing multiple teeth, including the right maxillary molars. In the maxilla, the ridge form is rounded, without undercuts, and is greater than 10 mm in width (adequate ridge width and shape are important to accommodate an implant without dehiscence or fenestration). The patient's maximal interincisal opening is 48 mm (limited opening may prevent ideal placement and angulation of posterior implants). There is adequate interarch spacing to allow placement of the implant-borne restorations. There are no bony exostosis or irregularities with either ridge and no evidence of soft tissue pathology.

IMAGING

A panoramic radiograph provides the most accurate diagnostic information when treatment planning for placement of endosseous implants. It provides an excellent overview of the bony architecture of the maxilla and mandible (including alveolar bone height, location of the inferior alveolar canal, and maxillary sinus floor position), as well as the status of the existing teeth (caries and horizontal and vertical bone loss). It is important to remember that a conventional panoramic radiograph has an approximate magnification factor of 1.25 when calculating the implant length. Reformatted CT can be used to further evaluate the bony architecture when adequate alveolar bone height, width, or shape is in question. It can provide the exact locations of vital structures (antral floor and inferior alveolar canal) to prevent unplanned injury or disruption, as well as volume rendering (a nonpneumatized maxillary sinus is normally 25 to 30 ml in volume). A DentaScan is routinely used by many surgeons when treatment planning dental implants. More recently, CT has been used to place implants (incisionless technique) and deliver a fixed appliance simultaneously, in select patients. Despite the available technology, the use of advanced imaging modalities (CT) is not absolutely necessary in the placement of dental implants in uncomplicated cases.

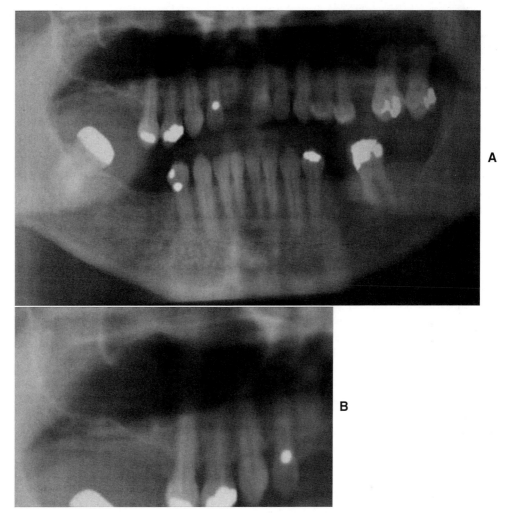

Figure 11-7 A, Preoperative panoramic radiograph showing multiple missing teeth and severe pneumatization of the right maxillary sinus. **B,** Close-up panoramic view showing the degree of pneumatization of the right maxillary sinus. There is 3 to 5 mm of residual alveolar bone, which is insufficient for implant placement.

The panoramic radiograph for this patient reveals pneumatization of the right maxillary sinus and no evidence of bony pathology (Figure 11-7, *A*). A 26-mm edentulous space is present in the right posterior maxilla (spacing is important when planning the number of implants to be placed). Within this region, there is approximately 5 mm of subantral bone at the first molar region and approximately 3 mm of subantral/residual alveolar bone at the second molar region (Figure 11-7, *B*).

LABS

No routine laboratory testing is necessary for sinus lift procedures unless dictated by the medical history.

ASSESSMENT

Resorbed edentulous right posterior maxilla with pneumatization of the maxillary sinus and insufficient bone height for implant placement

TREATMENT

Treatment for dental implants begins with a thorough physical and radiographic examination and a coordinated treatment plan with the restorative dentist. Numerous reconstructive modalities for the management of the atrophic maxilla are available to the oral and maxillofacial surgeon (maxillary sinus augmentation, zygomaticus implants, Le Fort I downgraft osteotomy, distraction osteogenesis, onlay cortical block, or cancellous marrow grafting) for different clinical situations. Maxillary sinus floor augmentation has become the most popular strategy among surgeons due to its predictability, low morbidity, and technical simplicity. Various methods can be used to augment the pneumatized maxillary sinus to accommodate a 10-mm or longer endosseous implant(s) in the posterior maxilla. A lateral sinus wall antrostomy, or window, is the most common technique to access the maxillary sinus floor. Alternatively, the Sumner osteotome technique can be used for select cases (when less than 4 mm of sinus floor elevation or augmentation is needed). Next, the grafting material(s) is selected based on surgeon preference, clinical situation, and available resources (tibial plateau bone harvesting technique is discussed later). Finally, the decision for simultaneous or staged augmentation and implant placement is made based on the quality and quantity of host bone and implant stability.

There are four primary types of bone graft material available for sinus augmentation:

1. Autogenous bone (gold standard)
2. Allogenic
3. Alloplastic
4. Xenogenic

These can be used alone or in combination (composite graft) for sinus augmentation. Autogenous bone (cancellous marrow or cortical shavings) represents the most popular and predictable material. Donor sites for bone harvest include intraoral sites (maxillary tuberosity, zygomaticomaxillary buttress, mandibular ramus, posterior body and symphysis), and extraoral sites (tibial plateau or anterior iliac crest are the most common). Donor site selection is based on the clinical situation and the amount and type of bone needed. Intraoral sites provide a limited source of cancellous marrow but are a good source of surface-derived autogenous bone (cortical shavings). Extraoral sites can provide sufficient autogenous cancellous marrow to perform large bilateral augmentations. Some surgeons prefer to make a composite graft by mixing autogenous bone with either allogenic, alloplastic, or xenogenic graft material, especially when an insufficient quantity of autogenous bone is available. The graft can be enhanced with platelet-rich plasma, which has been shown to improve bone formation and hasten bone graft consolidation.

Another alternative modality for maxillary sinus floor augmentation is recombinant human BMP 2 (rhBMP-2), which has been shown to induce de novo bone formation. The rhBMP-2 is absorbed onto a collagen sponge and is placed onto the sinus floor in a similar fashion to a bone graft augmentation, and it acts as an osteoinductive factor that stimulates undifferentiated mesenchymal cells to transform into osteoprogenitor cells. De novo bone formation for sinus augmentation and placement of functional dental implants has been shown to be predictable and comparable to autogenous bone grafting.

The maxillary sinus wall (in the area just below the zygomaticomaxillary buttress) is exposed with a crestal incision and a vertical releasing incision. An antrostomy, or window, to access the maxillary sinus can be created through the use of several different techniques. A round carbide or diamond bur can be used to outline the bony window (rounded corners are recommended to prevent tearing the sinus membrane), which can be completely feathered away, infractured, and reflected inward with the attached sinus membrane, or completely removed. The sinus membrane (Schneiderian membrane) is carefully elevated off the antral floor and positioned medially and superiorly. Occasionally, the maxillary sinus may have a septum in the area in need of augmentation (increases the difficulty of membrane elevation and increases the risk of perforation). If the sinus membrane is torn during the procedure, a collagen or platelet-rich plasma membrane is placed to cover the opening (suturing is not practical and not necessary) and act as a barrier while the sinus membrane remucosalizes. It is suggested that scraping the antral floor and walls with an instrument will promote revascularization and endosteal osteoblast migration into the graft. The graft material(s) of choice is packed into the sinus floor. The antral window that is now packed with graft material can be covered with a sheet of platelet-rich plasma gel, resorbable collagen membrane, or left alone. The periosteum is scored as needed to allow for primary closure. The patient is placed on "sinus precautions" postoperatively. The bone graft is allowed to consolidate for 4 to 6 months before placement of endosseous implants; alternatively, if the maxillary sinus augmentation was done simultaneously with implant(s), a period of 6 months should be allowed before implant uncovering.

The cancellous bone marrow of the tibial plateau can be accessed via a medial or lateral approach depending on surgeon's preference (lateral approach will be discussed here). The proximal tibia can provide up to 20 to 40 ml of uncompressed cancellous marrow, depending on the amount needed. The knee is placed into a flexed position with a bolster beneath. The landmarks are identified (fibular head, patella, and Gerdy's tubercle) and marked. The proximal head of the fibula is palpated and identified laterally just below the knee joint. Medial to this is the bony prominence of the tibial plateau called Gerdy's tubercle (Figure 11-8). A 1.5- to 2-cm

Knee

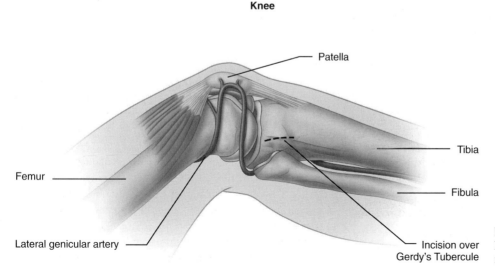

Patella

Tibia

Fibula

Femur

Lateral genicular artery

Incision over Gerdy's Tubercule

Figure 11-8 Tibial plateau harvest. Note Gerdy's tubercle, which is the landmark used for the lateral approach.

oblique incision is made through skin and subcutaneous tissue to the level of the insertion of the iliotibial tract (Gerdy's tubercle). The periosteum is incised between the insertions of the iliotibial tract superiorly and anterior tibialis muscle inferiorly. Minimal refection of the anterior tibialis muscle is needed to expose a 1-cm circular area of cortex. A dime-sized corticotomy (cortex can be morselized and incorporated into the graft) is performed with a fissured bur to access the cancellous bone marrow. Curettes (directed medially and inferiorly to prevent entry into the joint space) are used to harvest the marrow (20 to 40 ml of uncompressed cancellous marrow). Microfibrillar collagen (Avitene) or activated platelet-poor plasma can be placed into the bony defect (alternatively, it can be left alone) to assist in hemostasis. The wound is closed in layers and a pressure dressing is applied.

Simultaneous maxillary sinus augmentation and implant placement are traditionally recommended when a minimum of 4-5 mm of residual alveolar bone height is present, because less than 4 mm of alveolar bone may not provide sufficient support to stabilize the implant during bone graft consolidation. Some surgeons perform simultaneous procedures despite having less than 4 mm of bone height, relying on the compaction of bone graft around the implant to provide stabilization. In either case, the implants are placed by direct visualization and the graft material is firmly packed around the implants. Cover screws are placed on the implant(s) and the wound is closed primarily.

This patient underwent a right maxillary sinus augmentation with autogenous bone harvested from the tibial plateau and simultaneous placement of endosseous implants while under intravenous sedation in the office. The graft and implants were allowed to consolidate for 6 months. Following this period, the implants were uncovered, and maxillary posterior dental prostheses were fabricated (Figure 11-9).

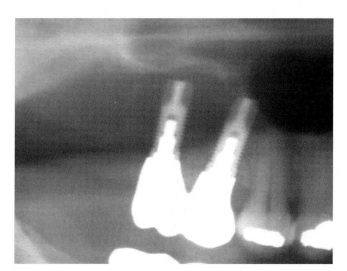

Figure 11-9 Postoperative panoramic radiograph showing restored endosseous implants after simultaneous sinus augmentation and implant placement.

COMPLICATIONS

The complications associated with maxillary sinus augmentation are uncommon but include postoperative wound infection, bony sequestrum formation, hematoma, maxillary sinusitis, oroantral fistula, wound dehiscence, loss of bone graft, loss of implant, implant migration, obstruction of the ostium, and damage to adjacent teeth. A high success rate of osseointegration in the grafted sinus has been reported (higher when autogenous bone is used). Perforation of the sinus membrane during elevation of the antral floor is the most common "complication" or unwanted intraoperative event (20% to 60% occurrence rate). However, several studies suggest that the complication rate and successful osseointegration are not compromised compared with cases where no perforation was encountered. Ardekian and associates in 2006 reviewed 110 maxillary sinus augmentations and simultaneous implant placement and found 35 perforations (all less than 10 mm) that were sealed using a resorbable collagen membrane. There was no statistically significant difference in the success rate for implants placed between the perforated and nonperforated groups (94.4% and 93.9% success rates, respectively). Residual bone of 3 mm or less correlated with a higher incidence of perforation (85% of cases).

The complication rate associated with tibial bone graft harvest is very low and may include local wound infection, wound breakdown, seroma, hypertrophic scar, prolonged pain, gait disturbance (limp), tibial plateau fracture, and compartment syndrome (anterior compartment during lateral approach). In 1991, O'Keeffe reviewed 230 cases and found only three complications (1.3% complication rate): one patient had a nondisplaced tibial eminence fracture and two patients had local wound complications (one hematoma and one infection). All three complications were managed conservatively and had no long-term sequelae. Catone and associates in 1992 presented 21 cases with no donor site complications. Kalaaji and colleagues in 2001 reviewed 140 tibial bone grafts and found no major donor site complications and several minor complications (three wound infections, one partial wound breakdown, one hypertrophic scar, and one consisting of pain that lasted 2 weeks). Alt and colleagues in 2003 showed that there was no increased risk of postoperative tibial plateau fracture in a cadaveric study.

Many surgeons use prophylactic antibiotics after a sinus lift procedure (preoperative antibiotic dose improves osseointegration rate). Complications usually result from introduction and proliferation of microbes from the sinus into the graft site. Sinus flora that could produce infection include *S. pneumoniae, Streptococcus pyogenes, H. influenzae, Moraxella cararrhalis, Staphylococcus proteus,* and *Bacteroides* species. The development of sinusitis (higher incidence when the maxillary sinus is overfilled with graft material) usually involves a mixture of aerobic and anaerobic organisms. The prophylactic antibiotic regimen should include one preoperative dose and postoperative course of 5 to 14 days (although there are no data to suggest the duration of antibiotic coverage, revascularization of the graft is complete at 2 weeks and antibiotic coverage during that time may be prudent) to prevent graft infection and loss of graft volume. Penicillins, or clindamycin for the penicillin-allergic patient, remain the antibiotics of choice.

DISCUSSION

Partial or total edentulism is generally treated by fabrication of dentures in order to restore function and aesthetics and to improve the quality of life. Following the loss of teeth, alveolar bone undergoes both vertical and horizontal resorption. The rate of resorption is accelerated through the use of dentures, which transmit traumatic occlusal forces against the edentulous areas. The edentulous posterior maxilla provides an additional concern in that its volume can be reduced over time by pneumatization of the maxillary sinus.

An alternative to dentures as a replacement for missing teeth is dentoalveolar implants. There must be adequate bone volume to support the implants structurally. The sinus lift procedure serves to increase the amount of available bone, to allow placement and retention of dental implants. Patient selection represents the most important factor in determining the success for sinus lift and dentoalveolar implant procedures. The amount of available bone, medical history, and patient compliance all contribute to the prognosis following treatment.

Before the placement of implants, it is critical to determine the amount of vertical alveolar bone present. If there is less than 3 mm of natural bone height, the placement of the implants should be delayed for 4 to 6 months to allow consolidation of the graft and sufficient bone volume to support the implants. If there is a minimum of 4 to 5 mm of natural bone height, implants can be placed at the time of the sinus lift procedure because there is sufficient bone volume to immediately support the implant.

A consensus on sinus grafts in 1999 showed a 5-year survival rate of 85% for implants placed immediately and of 89% for implants placed 4 to 6 months after sinus grafting. There was no significant difference in cumulative success rates between these two groups. More recently, overall higher success rates are being reported, although not all studies provide 5 or more years of follow-up.

Bibliography

Alt V, et al: The proximal tibia metaphysis: a reliable donor site for bone grafting? *Clin Orthop Relat Res* 414:315-321, 2003.

Ardekian L, Oved-Peleg E, Mactei EE, et al: The clinical significance of sinus membrane perforation during augmentation of the maxillary sinus, *J Oral Maxillofac Surg* 67:277-282, 2006.

Bain CA, Moy PK: The association between the failure of dental implants and cigarette smoking, *Int J Oral Maxillofac Implants* 8:609, 1993.

Boyne PJ, Lilly LC, Marx RE, et al: De novo bone induction by recombinant human bone morphogenetic protein-2 (rhBMP-2) in maxillary sinus floor augmentation, *J Oral Maxillofac Surg* 63:1693-1707, 2005.

Catone GA, Reimer BL, McNeir D, et al: Tibial autogenous cancellous bone as an alternative donor site in maxillofacial surgery: a preliminary report, *J Oral Maxillofac Surg* 50:1258-1263, 1992.

Clayman L: Implant reconstruction of the bone-grafted maxilla: review of the literature and presentation of 8 cases, *J Oral Maxillofac Surg* 64:674-682, 2006.

Ewers R: Maxilla sinus grafting with marine algae derived bone forming material: a clinical report of long-term results. *J Oral Maxillofac Surg* 63:1712-1723, 2005.

Fattahi T: Perioperative laboratory and diagnostic testing — what is needed and when? In Perioperative management of the oral and maxillofacial surgery patient, part I, *Oral Maxillofac Surg Clin N Am* 18(1):1-6, 2006.

Garg AK: *Bone-biology, harvesting, grafting for dental implants — rationale and clinical applications,* St Louis, 2004, Quintessence.

Hallman M, Hedin M, Sennerby L, et al: A prospective 1-year clinical and radiographic study of implants placed after maxillary sinus floor augmentation with bovine hydroxyapatite and autogenous bone, *J Oral Maxillofac Surg* 60:277-284, 2002.

Herford AS, King BJ, Audia F, et al: Medial approach for the tibial bone graft: anatomic study and clinical technique, *J Oral Maxillofac Surg* 61:358-363, 2003.

Jarvis B: Clopidegrel: a review of its use in the prevention of atherothrombosis, *Drug* 60(2):347-377, 2000.

Jensen OT, Greer R: Immediate placement of osseointegrated implants into the maxillary sinus augmented with mineralized cancellous allograft and Gore-Tex: second stage surgical and histological findings. In Laney WR, Tolman DE, editors: *Tissue integration in oral, orthopedic, and maxillofacial reconstruction,* Chicago, 1992, Quintessence, pp 47-51.

Jensen OT, et al: Report of the Sinus Consensus Conference of 1996, *Int J Oral Maxillofac Implants* 13(11):323, 1998.

Kalaaji A, et al: Tibia as donor site for alveolar bone grafting in patients with cleft lip and palate: long term experience, *Scand J Plast Reconstr Hand Surg* 35:35-42, 2001.

O'Keeffe RM, et al: Harvesting of autogenous cancellous bone graft from the proximal tibial metaphysis, *J Orthop Trauma* 5:469-474, 1991.

Peleg M, Garg AK, Misch CM, et al: Maxillary sinus and ridge augmentations using surface-derived autogenous bone graft, *J Oral Maxillofac Surg* 62:1535-1544, 2004.

Renouard F, Rangert B: *Risk factors in implant dentistry,* Chicago, 1999, Quintessence.

Rodriguez A, Anastassov GE, Lee H, et al: Maxillary sinus augmentation with deproteinated bovine bone and platelet-rich plasma with simultaneous insertion of endosseous implants, *J Oral Maxillofac Surg* 61:157-163, 2003.

Shulman LB, et al: A consensus conference on the sinus graft. In Jensen OT, editor: *The sinus bone graft,* Chicago, 1999, Quintessence.

Silva FMS, Albergaria-Barbosa JR, Mazzonetto R: Clinical evaluation of association of bovine organic osseous matrix and bovine bone morphogenetic protein versus autogenous bone graft in sinus floor augmentation, *J Oral Maxillofac Surg* 64:931-935, 2006.

Timmenga NM, Ragboebar GM, van Weissenbruch R, et al: Maxillary sinusitis after augmentation of the maxillary sinus floor: a report of 2 cases, *J Oral Maxillofac Surg* 59:200-204, 2001.

Ziccardi VB, Betts NJ: Complications of maxillary sinus augmentation. In Jenson OT, editor: *The sinus bone graft,* Chicago, 1999, Quintessence.

Mandibular Vestibuloplasty

Sam E. Farish, DMD, and Shahrokh C. Bagheri, DMD, MD

CC

A 64-year-old man was referred from a general dentist for difficulty in wearing his lower denture.

HPI

The patient had been edentulous since age 34 and had marked alveolar atrophy. He stated he had a family member who had a "major problem" with implants and he refused implant surgery, but asked if anything else could be done to help him wear his dentures better. He has been wearing the current set of dentures for 6 years with frequent relinings and occlusal adjustments.

PMHX/PDHX/MEDICATIONS/ALLERGIES/SH/FH

Noncontributory.

EXAMINATION

General. The patient is a well-developed white man in no acute distress who appears younger than his stated age. He is examined with and without the dentures in place. Moderate overclosure with overlap and downward tilting of the lateral commissures is noted with the dentures in place and is accentuated with the dentures removed.

Intraoral. His mandibular range of motion is adequate and without signs of temporomandibular joint dysfunction. The mucosa is moist and pink without lesions. The lower denture is held in with adhesive but displaces from the lower arch with opening, speaking, and chewing. High muscle attachments are noted buccally and lingually, which contribute to the denture instability. The upper denture appears very stable and easily retained without adhesive.

IMAGING

A panoramic radiograph is the minimal imaging modality needed for evaluation of the mandible before planned vestibuloplasty procedures.

In this patient, the panoramic radiograph reveals approximately 24 mm of mandibular thickness in the anterior region. In general, 15 mm or more of body height will provide good vestibular depth after a vestibuloplasty and lowering the floor of the mouth with a split-thickness skin graft procedure. In cases where the atrophy is more severe, vestibuloplasty and lowering the floor of the mouth with split-thickness skin graft

will produce only minimal vestibular deepening. Some improvement in even markedly atrophic ridges can be expected from increasing the area of immobile stress-bearing tissue.

LABS

Hemoglobin and hematocrit levels, along with an electrocardiogram, were ordered for preoperative baseline assessment. No other routine laboratory tests are indicated unless dictated by the medical history.

ASSESSMENT

Marked mandibular alveolar atrophy with high muscle attachments

TREATMENT

A classic description of a vestibuloplasty procedure for this patient is as follows. Under general anesthetic via a nasoendotracheal intubation, a local anesthetic with epinephrine was infiltrated in the mandibular structures. Next, an incision was made slightly buccal to the crestal attached mucosa from the area of the first molar on the right to the first molar on the left. A careful superperiosteal dissection was carried out to expose an additional 12 mm of mandibular height buccally (Figure 11-10). The lingual sulcus depth was also lowered several millimeters in a similar manner. The buccal dissection was feathered out distally over the mental nerve area bilaterally, sutured with 3-0 gut to the periosteum at the depth of the sulcus anteriorly, and then tapered up as the dissection progressed posteriorly. The lingual tissues did not require suturing and were held inferiorly by the stents extension. All muscle attachments that were lacerated in the initial dissection were carefully removed from the buccal periosteum with Metzenbaum scissors. At this time the patient's lower denture was modified by drilling holes in the lateral flange to help retain compound. Green dental compound was molded in water warmed in a microwave oven and adapted to the denture flange and border molded in the base of the surgically created sulcus. Subsequently, soft reline was placed in the modified denture and an impression of the surgically created ridge was made. Bilateral circummandibular wires of 26-gauge stainless steel were passed in the midbody portion of the mandible. Attention was then turned to the right lateral thigh, where a split-thickness skin graft was obtained with a dermatome. The skin graft site was dressed with an

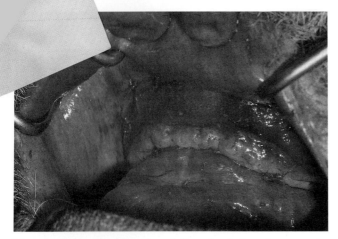

Figure 11-10 A supraperiosteal dissection before placement of a split-thickness skin graft.

occlusive dressing. The area of the graft site in the surgical stent was coated with dermatome glue, and the graft was placed in the splint with the surface side against the soft reline material (alternatively, the graft can be sutured to the graft bed with 3-0 gut sutures, and the stent placed on the sutured graft and secured). The excess margins were trimmed. The stent was then carried carefully to the mouth and fixated with the two circummandibular wires. The graft take was excellent at stent removal in 10 days, and marked improvement in ridge height, flange extension, and denture stability was obtained (Figure 11-11).

COMPLICATIONS

Among the possible complications from vestibuloplasty and lowering the floor of the mouth with split-thickness skin graft are failure of the graft to take, infection at the surgical or graft donor site, mental nerve damage, and excessive swelling in the floor of the mouth (particularly if lowering the floor of the mouth is included in the surgery). Skin graft take can be optimized by careful dissection to prevent exposure of bone by periosteal perforation and adequate splint stability. Infections are usually managed easily by local wound care measures. There is emerging evidence that platelet-rich plasma application will speed healing at split-thickness skin graft sites. A fair number of infections are associated with removal of the circummandibular wire. This can be minimized by careful preparation of the mouth before removal and cutting the wires as close to the mucosal surface as possible to minimize introducing oral flora to the anatomical spaces through which the wires pass. A stent or denture can also be secured to the ridge in the maxilla or mandible with the use of bone screws. If screws are used, it is a good idea to reinforce the holes in the stent or denture with washers so that the possibility of fracture of the acrylic is reduced with tightening of the screws (Figure 11-12). When the stent is removed in 7 to 10 days, the patient's existing denture, an interim denture, or even the surgical stent itself should be

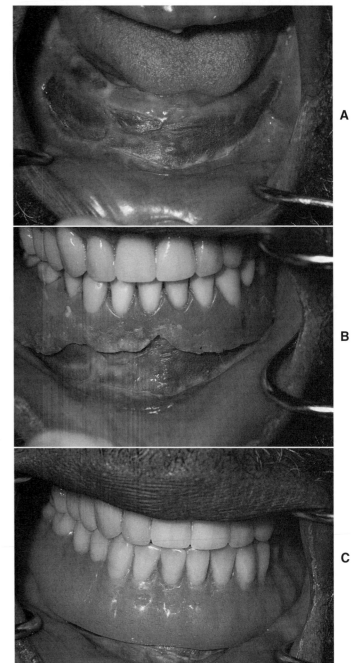

Figure 11-11 **A,** Split-thickness skin graft before fabrication of the new prosthesis demonstrating excellent graft take. **B,** Patient's existing denture in place, which demonstrates the amount of extension provided by the myotomy and split-thickness skin graft procedure. **C,** New denture in place demonstrating greatly increased extension of the buccal flange and associated increased stability.

modified just a little short of the full extension and relined with soft denture liner. The patient is instructed to wear it constantly with frequent saline rinses. There is little tendency for shrinkage or scar contraction with the vestibuloplasty and lowering the floor of the mouth and split-thickness skin graft.

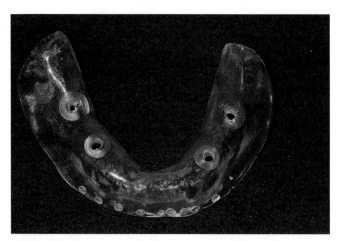

Figure 11-12 Surgical stent can be fashioned from study models taken in the surgical work-up phase. Note perforations in the flange to retain compound during border molding. The washers are placed to reinforce screw holes drilled in the stent for screw retention of the surgical stent.

DISCUSSION

The various techniques of vestibuloplasty are much less frequently used that implant retained removable prosthetics are commonplace. The importance of keeping these techniques in one's armamentarium is the frequent need for the reconstruction of sulcus depth in patients who have had resections for malignant or benign tumors or bone grafts to continuity defects. To prevent donor site morbidity, many surgeons choose human allograft tissue for the graft in vestibuloplasty procedures; palatal or buccal mucosa grafts can also be used. A lip-switch myotomy is a simpler vestibuloplasty procedure in which no graft or stent is needed. The crestal and inner lip mucosa are excised in a super-periosteal plane and pedicled from the lingual. The periosteum on the buccal aspect of the mandible is excised horizontally at the crest of the ridge, elevated anteriorly, excised again horizontally at the depth of the sulcus, and sutured to the denuded inner lip. The lingually pedicled mucosal flap is then positioned in the newly created sulcus and sutured to the periosteal tag left on the buccal surface of the mandible. A genioplasty type dressing is applied for 5 to 7 days.

Bibliography

Davis WH, Davis CL: Surgical management of soft tissue problems. In Fonseca RJ, Davis WH, editors: *Reconstructive preprosthetic oral and maxillofacial surgery,* Philadelphia, 1986, WB Saunders.

Fonseca WH, Davis WH: *Reconstructive preprosthetic oral and maxillofacial surgery,* Philadelphia, 1995, WB Saunders.

Marx RE, Garg AK: *Dental and craniofacial applications of platelet-rich plasma,* Chicago, 2005, Quintessence.

Radial Forearm Free Flap

Samuel L. Bobek, DMD, and R. Bryan Bell, DDS, MD, FACS

CC

A 70-year-old edentulous man is referred by his general dentist for evaluation of a tongue mass. The patients states, "My tongue hurts."

HPI

The patient is referred by his general dentist for evaluation of an ulcerative tongue lesion. Approximately 8 months earlier, he developed pain while wearing his dentures and noticed an ulcer on the side of his tongue. He did not seek medical or dental attention until he recently experienced several weeks of rapid growth of the ulcer and precipitous worsening of his pain. His dentist noted a large ulcerative lesion involving the right posterior tongue, and the patient was referred for further evaluation and treatment. An incisional biopsy (under local anesthesia) of the tongue mass was performed, revealing the diagnosis of a poorly differentiated, invasive squamous cell carcinoma.

PMHX/PDHX/MEDICATIONS/ALLERGIES/SH/FH

The patient has a 70 pack-year history of cigarette smoking and has drank alcohol regularly for more than 40 years (risk factors for oral cancer).

EXAMINATION

General. The patient is a well-developed and well-nourished, pleasant white man who appears his stated age.

Intraoral. The patient is noted to be edentulous. A prominent ulceration that measures 3 cm in length, 2 cm in width, and 1.5 cm in depth is located at the right dorsolateral junction of the posterior and middle thirds of the tongue. The lesion has a grayish, necrotic center at its depth and everted, erythematous, firm edges at its periphery (Figure 11-13). Palpation elicits pain, but no hemorrhage. The tongue is freely mobile. There appears to be no extension into the floor of the mouth.

Neck. There is no lymphadenopathy (the lack of cervical lymph nodes is an important positive prognostic factor).

Extremity. Peripheral pulses are 2+ for all extremities, and there is no cyanosis, clubbing, or edema. Bilateral Allen's test revealed good collateral circulation to the hands.

Allen's test is a test used to determine the integrity of the blood supply to the hand and is absolutely essential before the performance of a radial forearm free flap. The examination is performed by elevating the intended hand (usually the nondominant hand) and digitally occluding both the ulnar and the radial arteries, which leads to blanching of the hand. Releasing the pressure on the ulnar artery should result in the resolution of the physiological color of the hand (and nail beds) in less than 15 seconds. If there are areas that do not regain their original color, the Allen test is negative and consideration should be made for an alternate harvest location, as this may indicate that the hand is dependent on the radial artery for perfusion. Radial artery dependence is the only absolute contraindication to the radial forearm free flap.

IMAGING

In general, if the patient has a normal Allen test, no imaging is necessary prior to radial forearm free flap harvest. In the presence of a positive Allen test, magnetic resonance angiography or conventional angiography is indicated to confirm vascular perfusion of the hand.

The work-up of squamous cell carcinoma of the tongue includes CT scanning of the head and neck with intravenous contrast (for improved delineation of soft tissue) and a chest radiograph (see the section on oral squamous cell carcinoma in the Oral Cancer chapter). In this patient, axial and coronal CT scans demonstrate a 3 × 2-cm mass in the area of the tongue with poorly differentiated margins. No cervical lymphadenopathy was noted. The results of the chest radiograph were within normal limits.

LABS

Routine laboratory studies such as complete blood count (CBC), electrolyte studies, and coagulation studies may be obtained to establish a baseline preoperatively. Liver function tests are obtained as part of the complete metabolic panel (CMP) and are important screening tests for liver metastasis. No specific laboratory tests are essential before radial forearm free flap harvest.

For this patient, results for all the laboratory studies mentioned were within normal limits.

ASSESSMENT

A T2, N0, M0 (tumor between 2 and 4 cm, with no regional nodal metastasis, and no distant metastasis) stage II, squamous cell carcinoma of the right lateral tongue

TREATMENT

Treatment of oral squamous cell carcinoma remains primarily surgical. The lesion in this patient is amenable to transoral resection. Primary closure of the ablative tongue defect, however, will result in significantly impaired speech and swallowing. The primary goals of tongue reconstruction are to restore bulk and mobility necessary for proper deglutition and intelligible speech. The reconstructive options in this patient include a split-thickness skin graft, various local or regional pedicled rotational flaps, or microvascular free tissue transfer. The latter approach is currently considered state of the art.

The radial forearm fasciocutaneous flap is the soft tissue flap of choice for reconstructing small- to medium-sized oral and oropharyngeal defects. Based on the radial artery and cephalic vein or venae comitantes, it consists of thin, pliable skin with minimal soft tissue and a very long pedicle, which make it well-suited for use in the oral cavity. It can be designed to include tendons, muscle, or a vascularized segment of bone up to 12 cm in length, making it also useful for composite maxillary and mandibular defects.

Other soft tissue free flaps that are useful for reconstruction of partial glossectomy defects include the lateral arm flap and anterolateral thigh flap. Total or subtotal glossectomy defects require flaps with more soft tissue bulk, such as the rectus abdominis or latissimus dorsi flap.

Sequence of treatment for this patient. The patient was placed under general anesthesia and underwent a tracheostomy to secure his airway. A marking pen was used to delineate the planned resection edges, and a paper template was used to approximate the size and shape of the resection. A right hemiglossectomy was performed, with care taken to obtain 1.0- to 1.5-cm tumor-free margins, confirmed with frozen sections (Figure 11-14).

A right modified radical neck dissection was then performed to clear lymph nodes from levels I through V, as well as to expose the great vessels (Figure 11-15). Care was taken to protect and preserve the internal jugular vein, the internal and external carotid arteries (and its branches), the sternocleidomastoid muscle, and the hypoglossal, spinal accessory and lingual nerves.

Simultaneous harvest of the radial forearm free flap was performed on the nondominant hand (Figure 11-16). The tem-

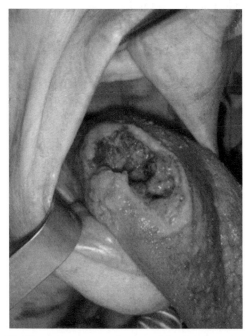

Figure 11-13 Squamous carcinoma of the right lateral and dorsal tongue.

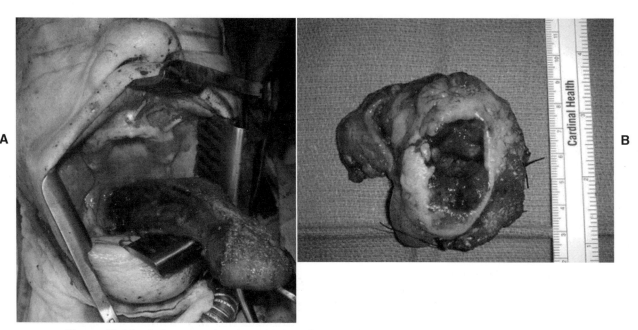

Figure 11-14 **A,** Intraoperative view of defect after resection of the lesion. **B,** The resected specimen.

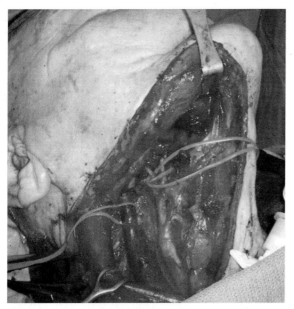

Figure 11-15 The sternocleidomastoid is retracted laterally following completion of the neck dissection to reveal the internal jugular, common carotid, carotid bulb, and first five branches of the external carotid artery. Coursing horizontally and lateral to the facial and lingual arteries is the hypoglossal nerve.

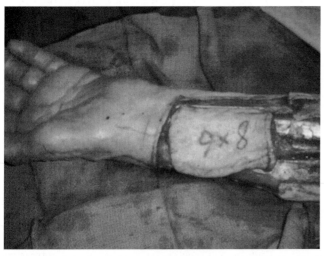

Figure 11-16 An 8 × 6-cm skin flap is raised on the distal forearm. Note the marking of the radial artery distal to the skin harvest site.

plate was used to approximate the area of skin needed for the fasciocutaneous flap. A distal skin site was used to take advantage of both the thinner skin in this area and the ability to harvest a longer vascular pedicle. The main disadvantage of choosing this location is the exposure of tendons of the distal forearm, which make a poor recipient bed for skin grafting. This is in contrast to the more proximal forearm skin, which overlies robust forearm muscles but is generally too thick for use in the oral cavity. The proximal forearm can be used if a large, bulky flap is needed.

Before the incision, the Allen test was performed again, to verify sufficient collateral circulation to the hand. A tourni-

quet, which was placed proximal to the elbow, was then inflated to 250 mm Hg. An incision was made proximal to the skin paddle, beginning at the antecubital fossa. The skin was reflected, along with the deep fascia, exposing the brachioradialis, pronator teres, and flexor carpi radialis muscles. As the skin is reflected distally, the brachioradialis tendon and flexor carpi radialis tendon are exposed. If one were to continue the dissection along the tendons, the radial artery, which lies between them, would be encountered. The periphery of the skin paddle is then dissected. Proximally, the paddle is dissected below the dermis, while on all other aspects it is dissected below the fascia. As the lateral aspect of the paddle is dissected, care is taken not to damage the cephalic vein, which lies just laterally. If brachioradialis were to be incorporated into the flap (e.g., to provide bulk to the paddle), it would be done so on the lateral dissection. On the medial side of this lateral dissection, the vascular pedicle (radial artery and venae comitantes) is preserved.

On the medial aspect of the skin flap, care is taken to not damage the ulnar artery during dissection (deep between the flexor digitorum superficialis and flexor carpi ulnaris muscles). The lateral aspect of this dissection can be done so as to include the tendon of the palmaris longus muscle in the skin flap. This tendon is sometimes used for lower lip reconstruction to provide support for and maintain the lower lip height.

At this point, the radial artery and venae comitantes are ligated distally and the elevation of the skin flap and vascular pedicle is done subfascially. The pedicle is raised proximally until you have sufficient pedicle length. The superficial branch of the lateral cutaneous nerve of the forearm (radial nerve) runs with the radial artery beneath the distal belly of the brachioradialis. At approximately midbelly, the nerve continues laterally, while the radial artery courses medially. For this reason, it is often not included in the raised pedicle, thus relying on the antebrachial cutaneous nerve to supply the paddle. During the dissection of the deep vascular pedicle, the superficial pedicle is also raised; this consists of the cephalic vein and lateral antebrachial cutaneous nerve. As a side note, if the flap were to include radial bone, you would expose the bone after approximately 1 to 2 cm of reflection proximally.

Once the flap and its pedicle were mobilized, the proximal vessels were ligated, and the flap was set into the intraoral defect (Figure 11-17). With care taken to not kink the vessels, the pedicle is carried through a tunnel proximal to the right mandibular body and up against the great vessels. Excess skin was removed to achieve desired bulk; the flap was completely sutured intraorally prior to the vessel anastomosis.

Following flap harvest, the tourniquet was released, hemostasis was confirmed, and a split-thickness skin graft was harvested from the left thigh and grafted to the radial forearm free flap donor site.

Meanwhile, the arterial anastomosis was performed in an end-to-end fashion into the facial artery, and the venous anas-

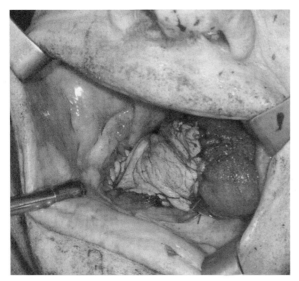

Figure 11-17 The inset skin flap.

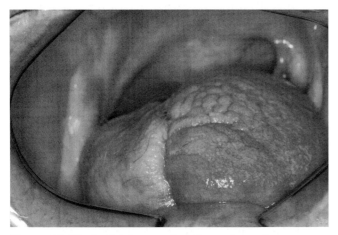

Figure 11-18 Radial forearm free flap at 3 months postoperatively with good coloration and adequate contour.

tomosis was performed in end-to-side fashion into the internal jugular vein. Some surgeons prefer double venous anastomoses, but we generally use the larger of the cephalic and venae comitantes. Good perfusion of the flap was confirmed visually and acoustically (Doppler). The neck was closed over a suction drain.

The donor site wound was dressed with wound vacuum-assisted closure, and the arm was immobilized for a period of 1 week. The flap remained viable at the recipient site and healed without complications (Figure 11-18).

COMPLICATIONS

While the complication rate for radial forearm free flap has been estimated to be 25% to 30%, the overall flap loss rate is 2.3% to 3.6%. To put this in perspective, the success rate of all head and neck free flap reconstructions has been estimated to be 92% to 98%, putting the radial forearm free flap

at the high range of success for free flaps to the head and neck.

The complication risk is increased with increasing medical comorbidities and may also be increased by an anesthesia time of greater than 10 hours and prior radiation therapy. Complications are few in number but may be substantial. The most common at the donor site is partial or full failure of the split-thickness skin graft at the harvest site. Other complications include radial fracture (as an osteocutaneous free flap), abnormal sensation, decreased grip strength, infection, and poor aesthetic outcome. Complications may also arise at the site of anastomosis, including thrombus formation, hematoma formation, and infection, potentially leading to reexploration of the initial surgical site.

The use of the radial forearm flap as an osteocutaneous flap is associated with significant complications when used for bony reconstructions. However, with the popularization of the free fibula osteocutaneous flap, the radial forearm free flap is predominantly used for soft tissue reconstructions, which have a significantly lower complication rate.

DISCUSSION

There are many applications of the radial forearm free flap in head and neck reconstruction. Here we used the radial forearm free flap to reconstruct the tongue and floor of the mouth, which is its most common application but certainly not the only one. Dual skin flaps have been used to reconstruct through-and-through defects in the cheek and lip. The skin flap can be folded onto itself to form the lip or soft palate. Radial bone can be used as a portion of the flap to reconstruct the mandible, but the amount of bone may be more appropriate in the maxilla.

Taylor first described a flap based on the radial artery in 1976. He reported the transfer of the superficial branch of the radial nerve as a component of a neurofascial free flap. In 1981, Yang and associates published a report on a series of 56 patients (60 flaps) who received a free fasciocutaneous flap based on their radial artery and reported a 98.3% success rate. Soutar subsequently popularized the use of the radial forearm free flap for intraoral reconstruction.

The anatomy of the lower forearm lends itself well to a harvest site for free grafting to the head and neck. It is easily accessible, and it has a widely anastomosing blood supply from lengthy vessels and thin, pliable skin. The area allows access to any and all components of an osteocutaneous flap: bone (radius), tendon (palmaris longus), muscle (brachioradialis), sensory innervation (antebrachial cutaneous nerve), vessels, and skin.

The radius is situated laterally to the ulna and articulates with the humerus and ulna proximally and with the ulna, scaphoid, and lunate bones distally. It averages 23 cm in length, and in cross section, the radial shaft appears triangular. While the radius plays only a small (but important) role in the elbow, it forms the radiocarpal joint at its distal end, which is the majority of the wrist. Its proximal head allows the hand to pronate, and its distal head plays a role in hand flexion, extension, adduction, and abduction.

The brachioradialis, one of nine muscles that attach to the radius, is used to provide bulk to a fasciocutaneous or an osteocutaneous flap. It can also be used for intraoral reconstruction without a skin paddle (as a fascial flap), with the idea that secondary mucosalization of the muscle may result in a better match of intraoral mucosa than forearm skin. The insertion of the brachioradialis forms the distal limit of radial bone harvesting, while the pronator teres insertion defines the proximal extension. This distance ranges from 9 to 13 cm. These muscles play an important role in the stability of the forearm, and their attachments must not be removed.

Harvesting radial bone may result in fracture of the radius if certain guidelines are not followed. Current suggestions include plating the radius prophylactically at time of harvest, using bevel bone cuts, and limiting the amount of harvested bone. Urken and colleagues suggested that no more than 40% of the circumference of the radius be harvested, to minimize the risk of fracture. An easy way to conceptualize this is to look at the minimum diameter of the radius from its medial-to-lateral border on a plain forearm film. According to Collyer and Goodger, this approximates 40% of the circumference of the radius (with an average margin of safety of 1 to 3 mm). A preoperative anteroposterior forearm film can be taken to evaluate this width and thus estimate the maximum height of the desired bone graft.

A major consideration of any free flap harvest site is the vascular sufficiency of the limb. This is evaluated both preoperatively and intraoperatively in the hand by a simple Allen test.

The anatomy behind the Allen test lies in the communications between the deep and superficial palmar arches. The distal end of the radial artery chiefly supplies the deep palmar arch, while the ulnar artery ends in the superficial palmar arch. Proximally, the radial and ulnar arteries begin as the brachial artery, bifurcating in the antecubital fossa. An average length of a radial artery from the antecubital fossa to the wrist is 18 to 20 cm, while its average diameter is 2.0 to 2.5 mm. This available length allows the future pedicle to be tailored to the vessels in the head and neck and enables unlimited neck mobility and even anastomosis to the contralateral neck.

Venous return for the free forearm flap is classified into a deep and superficial venous supply. The deep supply is composed of the venae comitantes, which run in the intermuscular septum along the radial artery. The superficial venous supply consists chiefly of the cephalic vein and other large diameter veins. Thoma and associates classified the pattern of the deep and superficial venous supply into five groups based on their branching pattern, and this may be helpful in deciding on which venous supply will mainly drain the flap.

The skin available to be harvested on the forearm is defined by the radial artery angiosome. It extends from the flexor crease of the wrist to antecubital fossa, with the medial limit being the medial third of the ventral surface, and the lateral being the lateral third of the dorsal surface. If a neurofaciocutaneous flap is considered, the somatosome of the lateral antebrachial cutaneous nerve is used to guide the location of skin flap harvesting. Due to the overlap with the radial artery angiosome, the only modification needed is to situate the flap more laterally, because the medial limit of the somatosome is the midline of the ventral forearm.

Innervated flaps are accomplished by anastomosing (most commonly) the lateral antebrachial cutaneous nerve to the severed lingual nerve. Surprisingly, there is some degree of return in sensation for 80% to 90% of patients who receive a noninnervated flap, although the sensation is unpredictable and variable in its extent.

Functionally, when using the radial forearm free flap to reconstruct a tongue, in comparison to primarily closure of the tongue, the reconstruction provides better swallowing, but the patient may have more speech impairment at 6 months. This is thought to be due to the bulk that is provided by the flap, which aids in sealing the palate when swallowing but limits movement of the native tongue.

The radial forearm free flap is a reliable, versatile flap with physiological characteristics that have made it the "workhorse" soft tissue flap in head and neck reconstruction. Thin pliable skin, a long vascular pedicle, the ability to include bone, muscle, or nerve, and a harvest site that is easily accessible combine to make the radial forearm free flap the first choice in oral tongue reconstruction.

Bibliography

Abraham M, et al: Sensate radial forearm free flaps in tongue reconstruction, *Arch Otolaryngol Head Neck Surg* 127:1463-1466, 2001.

Chen C, et al: Complications of free radial forearm flap transfers for head and neck reconstruction, *Oral Pathol Oral Radiol Oral Surg Endod* 99:671-676, 2005.

Cole R, Robbins K, Cohen J, et al: A predictive model for wound sepsis in oncologic surgery of the head and neck, *Otolaryngol Head Neck Surg* 96:165-167, 1987.

Collyer J, Goodger NM: The composite radial forearm free flap: an anatomical guide to harvesting the radius, *Br J Oral Maxillofac Surg* 43:205-209, 2005.

Disa J, Liew S, Cordeiro P: Soft-tissue reconstruction of the face using the folded/multiple skin island radial forearm free flap, *Ann Plast Surg* 47(6):612-619, 2001.

Eckardt A, Fokas K: Microsurgical reconstruction in the head and neck region and 18-year experience with 500 consecutive cases, *J Craniomaxillofac Surg* 31:197-201, 2005.

Helman J, Blanchaert R: Microvascular free tissue transfer. In *Principles of oral and maxillofacial surgery,* ed 2, 2004, Hamilton, Ontario, Canada, BC Decker, pp 803-818.

Hsiao H, Leu Y, Lin C: Primary closure versus radial forearm flap reconstruction after hemiglossectomy: functional assessment of swallowing and speech, *Ann Plast Surg* 49(6):612-616, 2002.

Lvoff G, et al: Sensory recovery in noninnervated forearm free flaps in oral and oropharyngeal reconstruction, *Arch Otolaryngol Head Neck Surg* 124:1206-1208, 1998.

Sculer D, Scheker L, Tanner N, et al: The radial forearm flap: versatile method for intra-oral reconstruction, *Br J Plast Surg* 36:1-8, 1983.

Shima H, Ohno K, Michi K, et al: An anatomical study of the forearm vascular system, *J Craniomaxillofac Surg* 24:293-299, 1996.

Smith G, et al: Clinical outcome and technical aspects of 263 radial forearm free flaps used in reconstruction of the oral cavity, *Br J Oral Maxillofac Surg* 43:199-204, 2005.

Thoma A, Archibald S, Jackson S, et al: Surgical patterns of venous drainage of the free forearm flap in head and neck reconstruction, *Plast Reconstr Surg* 93:54-59, 1994.

Urken ML, Cheney ML, Sullivan MJ, et al: *Atlas of regional and free flaps for head and neck reconstruction,* Philadelphia, 1994, Lippincott Williams and Wilkins.

Villaret D, Futran N: The indications and outcomes in the use of osteocutaneous radial forearm free flap, *Head Neck* 25:475-481, 2003.

Yang GF, et al: Forearm free skin flap transplantation: a report of 56 cases, *Br J Plast Surg* 50:162-165, 1997.

Pectoralis Major Myocutaneous Flap

Saif S. Al-Bustani, DMD, and R. Bryan Bell, DDS, MD, FACS

CC

A 39-year-old white man with a recent history of T3, N1, M0 squamous cell carcinoma of the right tonsillar fossa presents with the complaint of increasing pain in the throat following chemoradiation.

HPI

The patient is referred by his radiation oncologist for evaluation and consideration for salvage surgery following primary chemoradiation that failed.

Organ-sparing chemoradiation protocols are now standard treatment for advanced-stage squamous cell carcinoma of the oropharynx and base of tongue (stage 3 or 4 disease). Surgery, while acceptable for early-stage lesions, is generally now relegated to salvage therapy in patients for whom chemoradiation has failed. This case represents a "classic example" of a lateral pharyngectomy requiring a pectoralis major flap reconstruction.

PMHX/PDHX/MEDICATIONS/ALLERGIES/SH/FH

The patient has a 15 pack-year history of tobacco use and admits to drinking two to four cans of beer a day (both tobacco and alcohol are risk factors for intraoral squamous cell carcinoma).

There are no absolute contraindications to the pectoralis major myocutaneous flap. However, the flap is more likely to fail in a patient with severe systemic vascular disease, diabetes, or obesity. Additionally, some authors have described problems with skin paddle survival in females.

EXAMINATION

General. The patient is alert, awake, and oriented to time, place, and person.

Oropharyngeal. There is a large, exophytic, firm, indurated mass involving the right tonsillar fossa that extends into the palataloglossal fold, lingual gutter, and base of the tongue (Figure 11-19).

Neck. There is a 2-cm palpable lymph node involving level II of the right neck. Postradiation changes are noted, but the skin turgor remains soft and mobile.

Adequate soft tissue mobility is helpful for unimpeded passage of the pectoralis flap from the chest to the oropharynx. Radiation fibrosis occurs gradually following radiation treatment, but mobilization of the soft tissues becomes significantly more problematic at 1 year after radiation treatment.

Chest. No abnormalities are noted. The pectoralis major muscle is well developed bilaterally.

Inspection and palpation of the chest are necessary to verify the presence of the muscle and to identify previous surgical insults. There have been reports of Poland syndrome in the literature, with an incidence of about 1:30,000. Poland syndrome is characterized by the unilateral absence of the pectoralis major muscle. Inspection of the chest for cutaneous infections or lesions of significance is also performed.

Primary closure of the flap donor site may result in mild restrictive pulmonary disease. While this is generally well tolerated in healthy patients, those with severely impaired pulmonary function may be at increased risk for respiratory compromise postoperatively.

IMAGING

Preoperative imaging should be based on the patient's history and physical examination. Many patients have previously undergone CT of the neck and/or chest as part of a cancer work-up and staging, and even more patients have undergone plain chest radiography. In the absence of pulmonary disease, advanced age, cancer, or previous chest surgery, there is little benefit to obtaining chest imaging before pectoralis major flap harvest.

LABS

Laboratory evaluation should be based on the patient's history and physical examination. In the absence of medical comorbidities, there is no particular laboratory evaluation that is necessary before pectoralis major flap harvest.

BIOPSY

In this patient, before ablative surgery, direct laryngoscopy and reevaluation of the extent of tumor, under general anesthesia with biopsy of the lesion, were performed to confirm the diagnosis of squamous cell carcinoma.

ASSESSMENT

Stage III (T3 N1 M0) squamous cell carcinoma of the right tonsillar fossa, previously treated with chemoradiotherapy with curative intent now with locoregionally recurrent disease

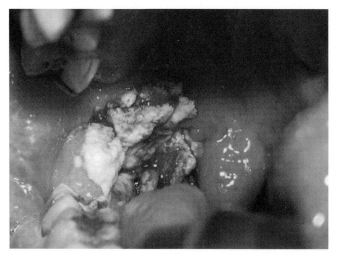

Figure 11-19 Exophytic mass in the right tonsillar fossa.

The patient presents for salvage surgical resection and immediate reconstruction.

TREATMENT

There are several options available to the oncological surgeon for reconstruction of oropharyngeal defects. The most contemporary option is the use of microvascular free tissue transfer — in this case, a radial forearm free flap or anterolateral thigh flap. An excellent fallback flap, however, and one that continues to play an important role in head and neck reconstruction is the pectoralis major myocutaneous flap. The pectoralis major myocutaneous flap is indicated for:

1. Bulky soft tissue defects involving the head and neck, particularly the skin of the face, oral cavity, and oropharynx; while somewhat limited by the vascular pedicle, the arc of rotation generally permits coverage to the level of the zygomatic arch.
2. Carotid coverage in conjunction with neck dissection.

The oncological and reconstructive treatment plan for this patient involved a composite resection of the lesion with a right lateral pharyngectomy, right marginal mandibulectomy, partial maxillectomy, and right partial glossectomy, using a mandibulotomy and lateral swing for access to the oropharynx (Figure 11-20, *A*). The neck was treated with a right modified radical neck dissection. The pectoralis major myocutaneous flap was used for reconstruction of the defect. Figure 11-20, *B* demonstrates the C-shaped flap design and skin paddle marked at the sternal insertion and the vascular pedicle at the lateral clavicular border. Also notes is the tracheostomy performed at the beginning of the procedure for airway control.

Several intraoperative and postoperative considerations are noteworthy:

1. Securing the skin paddle to the underlying muscle during harvest helps prevent shearing injury to perforators (Figure 11-20, *C*).
2. Creating adequate space to tunnel the flap into its final location minimizes compression of flap. At least four fingers should easily fit below the skin flap (Figure 11-20, *D*).
3. Placing a drain in the site of reconstruction is of importance to minimize the formation of a hematoma or seroma.
4. In the female patient, flap design is different, with the skin paddle placed along the inframammary fold to avoid distortion.
5. In the nonirradiated male patient, chest hair growing on the skin paddle can be removed using a CO_2 laser.
6. Physical and occupational therapy consultation is initiated postoperatively to improve shoulder strength and range of motion.

Figure 11-20, *E* demonstrates the flap inset at the recipient site secured with 2-0 Vicryl suture in a horizontal mattress fashion. Figure 11-20, *F* demonstrates the postoperative appearance of the patient following successful reconstruction.

COMPLICATIONS

Complications from the use of the pectoralis major flap as they are reported in the literature include the following:

- Total flap necrosis
- Partial flap necrosis
- Orocutaneous fistulas
- Suture line separation
- Mandibular reconstruction plate exposure
- Wound infection
- Hematoma or seroma formation
- Donor site complications
- Hidden recurrence
- Flap atrophy

Some authors reported complication rates as high as 63%. Although the pectoralis major flap is highly vascular, shortcomings in harvesting technique and the nature of distribution of the vasculature may result in necrosis of the skin paddle, particularly in female patients with poorly developed muscles. Exposure of, formation of fistulas around, or flap necrosis around a mandibular reconstruction plate may necessitate its removal. In their analysis, Shah and associates identified the following risk factors as significant in the development of complications: age over 70, female gender, overweight status, serum albumin less than 4 g/dl, major glossectomy reconstruction, and systemic diseases. Although rare, there has been report of donor site rib osteomyelitis after harvest. Most complications can be managed by conservative means; in only few incidences is a new flap harvest is required.

DISCUSSION

The pectoralis major myocutaneous flap has been used in head and neck reconstruction since its initial description by Ariyan in 1979. Its reliability and versatility made it the "workhorse flap" of the 1980s until the widespread dissemination of microvascular surgeons and techniques relegated

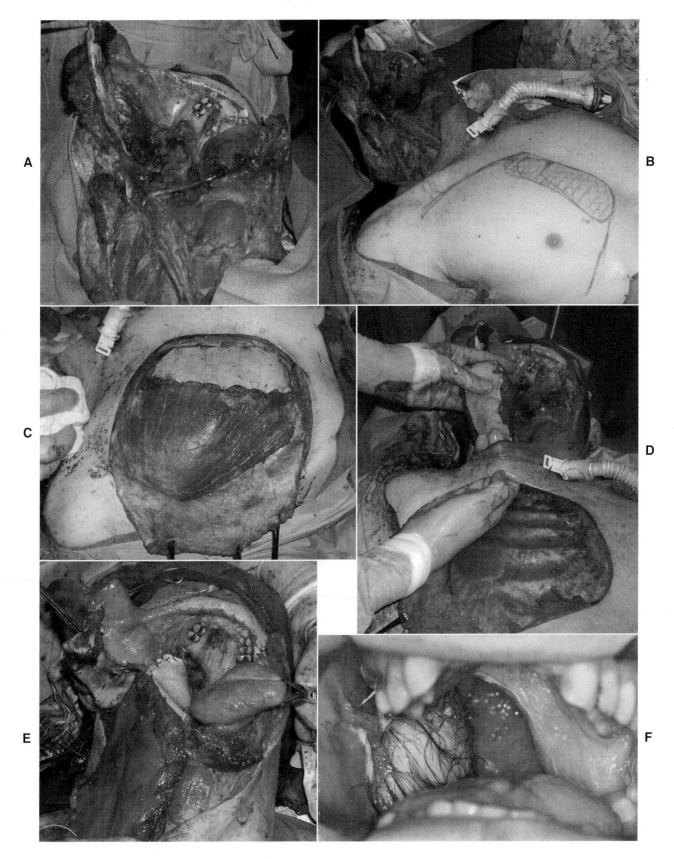

Figure 11-20 **A,** Large soft tissue defect, suitable for reconstruction with pectoralis major myocutaneous flap. **B,** Flap design outlined, demonstrating the skin paddle marked at the sternal insertion (8 × 3 cm), and the vascular pedicle at the lateral clavicular border (PTAT). **C,** The C-type incision carried circumferentially around paddle and full exposure of the pectoralis major muscle (PMM) is seen here. The skin paddle does not extend beyond the PMM. Chromic 3-0 gut suture used to tack skin to muscle (prevents shearing injury to perforators). **D,** Demonstrates the harvest technique. The skin at the neck is elevated superiorly and laterally to expose muscle borders. The PMM is elevated from the underlying pectoralis minor muscle (avascular plane) and underlying rectus abdominis sheath along the intercostal muscles. The humerus insertion divided using GIA staples. The pedicle is identified and verified using a Doppler unit and protected. The clavicular attachment is released (to provide for sufficient arc of rotation without tension), and the skin tunnel is created for passage of the flap. The loose passing of four fingers is sufficient to minimize compression. **E,** Flap is secured in place with interrupted 2-0 Vicryl suture in a horizontal mattress fashion into the defect area. Watertight closure is obtained (to avoid drainage of oral secretions into the neck). **F,** Postoperative appearance of the patient following successful reconstruction. Note chest hair on the skin paddle that is of little concern to most patients.

the "pec flap" to that of a salvage flap for failed or microvascular reconstructions. Based primarily on the pectoral branch of the thoracoacromial artery, numerous modifications have been described in the literature that facilitate the reconstruction of head and neck defects. There is report of longitudinal splitting of the paddle to reconstruct U-shaped intraoral defects, incorporating the medially based deltopectoral flap to raise a bilobed flap, and using the skin overlying the sternum, ipsilateral parasternum, and contralateral parasternum to provide for thinner paddle. Dennis and Kashima introduced the Janus flap to reconstruct through-and-through defects in a two-stage technique with the use of a skin graft to the deep muscle to provide for two immediate epithelial surfaces on transfer. Hypopharyngeal and cervicoesophageal luminal reconstruction has also been reported and widely used. Bilobular flaps with two skin paddles and one or two vascular pedicles have also been described to reconstruct through and through defects. Anterolateral resection of the skullbase has been successfully and reliably reconstructed with this flap. Lee and Lore described using a dermal graft to avoid fully tubing the myocutaneous pectoralis flap in total hypopharyngeal reconstruction. The dermal graft is placed in the posterior, while the muscle flap had an anterior and lateral use. For most applications in the head and neck, however, the development of the pectoralis major myocutaneous flap is now fairly well uniform and widely known. Overall, the pectoralis myocutaneous flap is a reliable and versatile flap that is useful in a number of clinical situations:

- Large soft tissue defects
- Exposure of the great vessels of the neck (radiation, trauma, etc.)
- Skull base reconstruction
- Hypopharyngeal and pharyngoesophageal reconstruction

- Fallback flap if microvascular flap fails or is unavailable
- Poor patient prognosis
- Microvascular surgeon is unavailable

The primary blood supply to the pectoralis myocutaneous flap is the pectoral branch of the thoracoacromial artery, although the specifics of vascular supply to the pectoralis major muscle and associated skin are the subject of debate. The pectoral branch of the thoracoacromial trunk, the lateral thoracic artery, perforators from the internal thoracic artery, and perforators from the intercostal vessels have all been described as nourishing the pectoralis major muscle flap. In their cadaver dissection and aortic arch angiogram analysis, Moloy and Gonzales found that the lateral thoracic artery and the pectoral branch of the thoracoacromial trunk provided pedicles of comparable size to the muscle. In some instances, the lateral thoracic artery was of greater diameter. Yang and colleagues showed that the pectoral branch of the thoracoacromial trunk supplied about 50% of the vascular territory of the muscle. The anterior perforators of the internal thoracic supplied about 43%, while the lateral thoracic artery supplied only about 7%. In their extensive 1984 study, Reid and Taylor demonstrated that the sternocostal and clavicular portions of the muscle have independent sources of blood supply. The former is dominated by the pectoral branch of the thoracoacromial trunk, while the latter is dominated by the deltoid branch of the thoracoacromial trunk. The pectoral branch of the thoracoacromial trunk's supply to the lateral skin arose from fasciocutaneous branches along the free lower border of the muscle. Interestingly, medial and inferior skin paddles, which dominate current clinical practice, derive their blood supply from cutaneous branches belonging to the internal thoracic and superior epigastric system. In a study by Rikimaru and associates in 2005, the importance of the internal thoracic artery in supplying the muscle and skin associated with the pectoralis major myocutaneous flap was demonstrated. Perforating branches from the fourth, fifth, and sixth intercostals anastomose with the pectoral branch of the thoracoacromial trunk to supply the muscle medially and inferiorly. The skin overlying the same area mimics the same distribution. In addition, cutaneous branches from the second and third intercostal perforators and cutaneous branches from the superior epigastric artery demonstrate supply to that same skin.

Bibliography

Ariyan S: Further experiences with the pectoralis major myocutaneous flap for the immediate repair of defects from excisions of head and neck cancers, *Plast Reconstr Surg* 64(5):605-612, 1979.

Ariyan S: The pectoralis major myocutaneous flap. A versatile flap for reconstruction in the head and neck, *Plast Reconstr Surg* 63(1):73-81, 1979.

Baek SM, Lawson W, Biller HF: An analysis of 133 pectoralis major myocutaneous flaps, *Plast Reconstr Surg* 69(3):460-469, 1982.

Deniz O, Tozkoparan E, Gumus S, et al: Poland syndrome (a case report), *Tuberkuloz Toraks* 53(3):275-279, 2005.

Dennis D, Kashima H: Introduction of the Janus flap. A modified pectoralis major myocutaneous flap for cervical esophageal and pharyngeal reconstruction, *Arch Otolaryngol* 107(7):431-435, 1981.

Donegan JO, Gluckman JL: An unusual complication of the pectoralis major myocutaneous flap, *Head Neck Surg* 6(5):982-983, 1984.

Ferraro GA, Perrotta A, Rossano F, et al: Poland syndrome: description of an atypical variant, *Aesthet Plast Surg* 29(1):32-33, 2005.

Freeman JL, Gullane PJ, Rotstein LM: The double paddle pectoralis major myocutaneous flap, *J Otolaryngol* 14(4):237-240, 1985.

Freeman JL, Walker EP, Wilson JS, et al: The vascular anatomy of the pectoralis major myocutaneous flap, *Br J Plast Surg* 34(1):3-10, 1981.

Hodgkinson DJ: The pectoralis major myocutaneous flap for intraoral reconstruction: a word of warning, *Br J Plast Surg* 35(1):80-81, 1982.

Lee KY, Lore JM Jr: Two modifications of pectoralis major myocutaneous flap (PMMF), *Laryngoscope* 96(4):363-367, 1986.

Mehrhof AI Jr, Rosenstock A, Neifeld JP, et al: The pectoralis major myocutaneous flap in head and neck reconstruction. Analysis of complications, *Am J Surg* 146(4):478-482, 1983.

Meyer R, Kelly TP, Abul Failat AS: Single bilobed flap for use in head and neck reconstruction, *Ann Plast Surg* 6(3):203-206, 1981.

Moloy PJ, Gonzales FE: Vascular anatomy of the pectoralis major myocutaneous flap, *Arch Otolaryngol Head Neck Surg* 112(1):66-69, 1986.

Morain WD, Geurkink NA: Split pectoralis major myocutaneous flap, *Ann Plast Surg* 5(5):358-361, 1980.

Ossoff RH, Wurster CF, Berktold RE, et al: Complications after pectoralis major myocutaneous flap reconstruction of head and neck defects, *Arch Otolaryngol* 109(12):812-814, 1983.

Reid CD, Taylor GI: The vascular territory of the acromiothoracic axis, *Br J Plast Surg* 37(2):194-212, 1984.

Rikimaru H, Kiyokawa K, Inoue Y, et al: Three-dimensional anatomical vascular distribution in the pectoralis major myocutaneous flap, *Plast Reconstr Surg* 115(5):1342-1352; discussion 1353-1354, 2005.

Sasaki CT: Pectoralis flap reconstruction in resection of anterior skull base tumors, *Auris Nasus Larynx* 12(suppl 2):S143-S146, 1985.

Shah JP, Haribhakti V, Loree TR, et al: Complications of the pectoralis major myocutaneous flap in head and neck reconstruction, *Am J Surg* 160(4):352-355, 1990.

Sharzer LA, Kalisman M, Silver CE, et al: The parasternal paddle: a modification of the pectoralis major myocutaneous flap, *Plast Reconstr Surg* 67(6):753-762, 1981.

Ueda M, Torii S, Nagayama M, et al: The pectoralis major myocutaneous flap for intraoral reconstruction: surgical complications and their treatment, *J Maxillofac Surg* 13(1):9-13, 1985.

Wadwongtham W, Isipradit P, Supanakorn S: The pectoralis major myocutaneous flap: applications and complications in head and neck reconstruction, *J Med Assoc Thailand* 87 Suppl 2:S95-S99, 2004.

Weaver AW, Vandenberg HJ, Atkinson DP, et al: Modified bilobular ("gemini") pectoralis major myocutaneous flap, *Am J Surg* 144(4):482-488, 1982.

Wei WI, Lam KH, Wong J: The true pectoralis major myocutaneous island flap: an anatomical study, *Br J Plast Surg* 37(4):568-573, 1984.

Withers EH, Franklin JD, Madden JJ, et al: Immediate reconstruction of the pharynx and cervical esophagus with the pectoralis major myocutaneous flap following laryngopharyngectomy, *Plast Reconstr Surg* 68(6):898-904, 1981.

Yang D, Marshall G, Morris SF: Variability in the vascularity of the pectoralis major muscle, *J Otolaryngol* 32(1):12-15, 2003.

Free Fibula Flap for Mandibular Reconstruction

Brian M. Woo, DDS, MD, and R. Bryan Bell, DDS, MD, FACS

CC

A 66-year-old white woman presents to the office with the chief complaint of, "I am having pain in my lower jaw, difficulty eating, and there is drainage from my face."

HPI

The patient sustained a mandible fracture from a motor vehicle accident at age 20. Six years later, she had her remaining teeth extracted but subsequently sustained a pathological fracture of her mandible, which was treated with closed reduction using circummandibular wires fixated to her denture. In the following years, she underwent several preprosthetic procedures in an attempt to restore her dentition. She eventually was restored with implants placed 15 years ago using a Hader bar and overdenture. The patient did well for 10 years, when she developed a pathological fracture and was diagnosed with osteomyelitis. She was treated with intravenous antibiotics, decortication, open reduction and fixation using a reconstruction plate, and hyperbaric oxygen. Several years later, the reconstruction plate was removed after the screws loosened and became infected. She developed lower right facial swelling with a draining orocutaneous fistula over her right anterior mandible. The patient had excision of the orocutaneous fistula, multiple incision and drainage procedures, and debridements of her right mandible. However, the infection and exacerbating osteomyelitis did not respond to treatment. She eventually developed pathological fractures of her right mandibular parasymphysis and left mandibular angle. The patient is referred to your office for definitive treatment.

PMHX/PDHX/MEDICATIONS/ALLERGIES/SH/FH

The patient has hypertension and non–insulin-dependent diabetes mellitus, both of which are well controlled.

Although hypertension and diabetes are not contraindications to microvascular surgery, it is important for both the blood pressure and glucose levels to be strictly controlled in the perioperative period. Severe peripheral vascular disease secondary to advanced atherosclerosis from diabetes may compromise microvascular treatment options.

EXAMINATION

General. The patient is a well-developed and well-nourished alert woman in no acute distress (morbid obesity and severe peripheral vascular disease would be contraindications to microvascular surgery).

Vital signs. Her vital signs are stable and she is afebrile (an elevated temperature is not frequently seen with chronic osteomyelitis).

Maxillofacial. There is a draining orocutaneous fistula exiting the right submental region. The patient has severe mandibular atrophy with gross mobility and pathological fractures of her mandible at the right parasymphysis and left mandibular angle. There is bilateral anesthesia of the third division (V_3) of the trigeminal nerve at the mental nerve distribution.

Intoral. The patient is completely edentulous and, in addition to the pathological fractures, has a functional maxillary subperiosteal implant and a mobile Hader bar in her left anterior mandible.

Extremity. She has 2+ peripheral pulses without claudication or evidence of peripheral vascular insufficiency.

The lower extremities should be examined to evaluate for absence or diminished pulses in the anterior or posterior tibial arteries that could suggest atherosclerosis or vascular insufficiency. Absent or diminished anterior or posterior tibial pulses mandate a preoperative angiogram or magnetic resonance angiogram to define the vascular anatomy.

IMAGING

The panoramic radiograph and CT can be used to help determine the extent of the mandibular resection and aid in predicting the size of the postresection mandibular defect. Stereolithographic models constructed from CT data can also be used to prebend a reconstruction plate, before surgery. For this patient, the panoramic radiograph shows the fractures of her right parasymphysis and left mandibular angle along with a maxillary subperiosteol implant and three mandibular endosteal implants with a Hader bar (Figure 11-21).

Preoperative imaging for the fibula transfer includes angiography/arteriography or magnetic resonance angiography of the lower extremities to evaluate the vascular anatomy for the possible absence or diminished size of the anterior and posterior tibial arteries and for narrowing or occlusion of the vessels secondary to atherosclerosis.

However, some microvascular surgeons order these tests only when dictated by physical examination findings. In about 10% to 20% of cases, the anterotibial or posterotibial artery may become attenuated. In these cases, a communicating branch from the peroneal artery supplies the attenuated

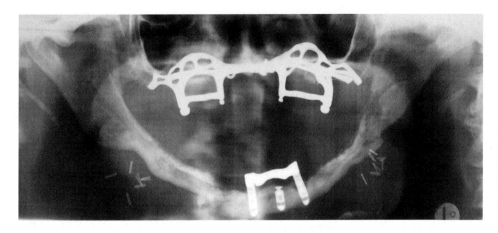

Figure 11-21 A preoperative panoramic radiograph showing the fractures of the patient's right parasymphysis region and left mandibular angle along with a maxillary subperiosteol implant and three mandibular endosteal implants with a Hader bar.

vessel's territory; therefore, sacrifice of the peroneal artery could result in ischemia of the foot.

LABS

Routine laboratory tests such as a CBC and electrolyte and coagulation studies may be performed to establish a baseline preoperatively.

ASSESSMENT

Chronic suppurative osteomyelitis with a draining orocutaneous fistula and nonunion of the mandibular right parasymphysis and left angle

TREATMENT

This is a complex case demonstrating multiple attempts at reconstruction and management of an infected mandible. The goals of mandibular reconstruction include:
- Reestablishment of mandibular continuity and arch form, and maintenance of the existing occlusion and/or taking care that the restored mandible maintains its proper relationship to the maxilla to allow dental rehabilitation
- Provision of soft tissue closure and replacement of resected oral cavity soft tissue
- Dental rehabilitation
- Restoring adequate function (speech, mastication, oral continence) and cosmesis, enabling the patient to enjoy a reasonable quality of life

Several treatment options are available, each associated with specific complications and limitations, that reflect the difficulty in the management of total mandibular reconstruction:
- Reconstruction with only a mandibular reconstruction plate
- Reconstruction with a mandibular reconstruction plate and a pedicled myocutaneous flap (pectoralis major flap)
- Reconstruction with a mandibular reconstruction plate and a soft-tissue free flap
- A nonvascularized bone graft (iliac crest, rib, etc.)

- A vascularized bone flap (fibula, ilium, radial forearm, scapula, etc.)
- Distraction osteogenesis used as alone or in combination to these modalities

This patient was treated with a segmental mandibulectomy, a left neck dissection for vascular access, tracheostomy, and immediate reconstruction with an osseous fibula free flap (Figure 11-22).

COMPLICATIONS

The use of a mandibular reconstruction plate alone for mandibular reconstruction has been reported as having a failure rate ranging from 20% to 80%, with a majority of the failures resulting from plate extrusion. A higher percentage of failures also occurred in patients with segmental defects of the anterior mandible and in patients who received or were receiving radiation therapy. Even with the use of pedicled myocutaneous flaps and soft tissue free flaps to provide coverage of the mandibular reconstruction plate, the failure rate has been reported to range from 7% to 44% (approaching the higher percentage with long-term follow-up). The majority of these failures were also due to plate extrusion. The use of vacularized bone grafts for mandibular reconstruction, however, has been reported as having a success rate of over 90% even in irradiated patients and in patients with segmental defects of the anterior mandible. Vascularized bone grafts also have the advantage of being able to accept endosteal implants for dental rehabilitation, which cannot be done if a mandibular reconstruction plate with or without soft tissue coverage is used.

Despite the reported success rates, perioperative surgical and reconstructive complications and perioperative medical complications of the fibula free flap have been described in the literature (Box 11-2).

DISCUSSION

The application of the fibula free flap for mandibular reconstruction was first described by Hidalgo in 1989. The primary blood supply of the fibula free flap is from the peroneal artery

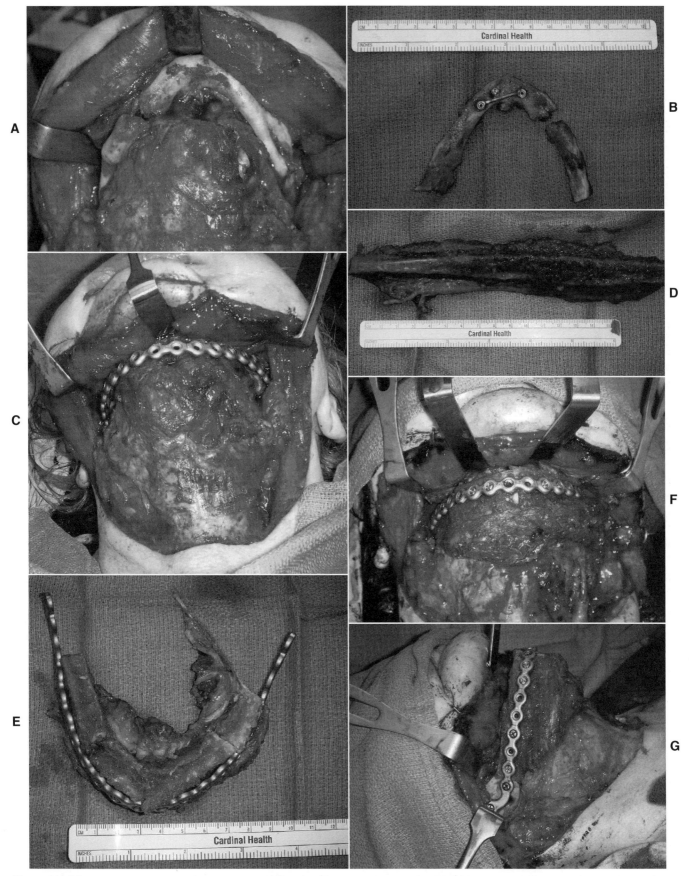

Figure 11-22 **A,** An intraoperative view showing surgical exposure of the mandible and the fracture sites. **B,** The surgical specimen/resected mandible. **C,** The reconstruction plate contoured to the shape of the resected mandible. **D,** The free fibula graft. **E,** The fibula graft after it has been osteotomized and contoured to the shape of the resected mandible. **F,** The free fibula graft after it has been inset and secured in place. **G,** The free fibula graft after it has been inset, from a lateral view.

Continued

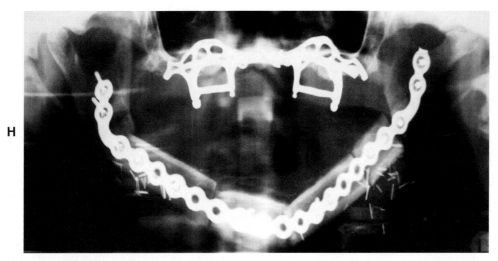

H

Figure 11-22, cont'd   H, The postoperative panoramic radiograph of the free fibula graft in place.

| **Box 11-2.** | **Complication of the Fibular Free Flap** |

Perioperative Surgical/Reconstructive Complications of the Fibula Free Flap
- Venous thrombosis/arterial thrombosis
- Venous congestion
- Wound infection
- Salivary fistula
- Seroma formation
- Cervical hematoma
- Partial free flap necrosis
- Total free flap necrosis
- Hardware extrusion
- Carotid artery rupture
- Donor site complications (infection, skin graft failure, loss of knee and ankle strength, reduced ankle range of motion, damage to the peroneal nerve and its branches)

Perioperative Medical Complications of the Fibula Free Flap
- Myocardial infarction
- Cerebrovascular accidents
- Deep venous thrombosis
- Congestive heart failure/pulmonary edema
- Pneumonia/atelectasis
- Acute respiratory distress syndrome
- Pneumothorax
- Cardiac arrhythmias
- Gastrointestinal hemorrhage/perforation
- Liver failure
- Mental status changes
- Mortality

---

and vein, which supply the fibula bone via endosteal and periosteal vessels. The peroneal artery is classically described as originating from the posterior tibial artery after the popliteal artery branches into the anterior and posterior tibial arteries. The peroneal artery and its two venae comitantes descend in the lower leg between the flexor hallucis longus and the tibialis posterior. The fibula can be transferred as a free osseous or free osteocutaneous flap. The skin is attached to the fibula by the posteriorlateral intermuscular septum and is supplied by the septocutaneous and musculocutaneous perforators arising from the peroneal artery and vein. The anatomical study by Schusterman and associates identified three types of perforators:

1. Septocutaneous
2. Musculocutaneous
3. Septomuscular (which did not run within the muscle substance but is adherent to it)

They also demonstrated that the musculocutaneous perforators were more numerous and proximal, while the septocutaneous perforators were less numerous and more distal. They found that the septocutaneous perforators were not present in 20% of their dissected specimens and that in 6.25% of their dissected specimens there also were no muscular or septomuscular vessels. Eighteen of their clinical cases demonstrated a 33% skin paddle survival when dissected as a septocutaneous flap and a 93% skin paddle survival when dissected as a septomusculocutaneous flap. From these findings, it was recommended that a cuff of soleus and flexor hallucis longus be incorporated into the flap to help ensure flap viability. The lateral sural cutaneous nerve can be harvested and anastomosed to a recipient nerve to restore sensation to the skin component. Harvesting of the peroneal communicating branch as a vascularized nerve graft can be used to bridge the inferior alveolar and mental nerve to restore sensation to the lower lip.

The fibula free flap has several advantages. The fibula has thick cortical bone around its entire circumference, making it suitable to withstand the forces of mastication and for the placement of dental implants. Approximately 22 to 25 cm of bone can be harvested while leaving 6 to 7 cm proximally and distally to maintain adequate stability of the knee and ankle joints. Because of the length of bone that can be harvested, it is suitable for restoration of subtotal and total mandibular defects. The length of the vascular pedicle that can be obtained is also an advantage. Additional length of the pedicle can be obtained by harvesting a more distal segment of bone and skin while discarding the proximal fibula. Hidalgo has described obtaining vascular pedicles as long as 12 cm through this technique. Another advantage is the ability to reconstruct soft tissue defects using the skin paddle (potential for sensory innervation) of the free fibula osteocutaneous flap. The width of the skin paddle is mainly limited only by the ability to achieve primary closure; however, a skin graft can be grafted to the donor site. Multiple osteotomies can be made in the bone for contouring the fibula to the shape of the mandible. These osteotomies are well tolerated if the osteotomized segments are at least 1 cm in length and the overlying periosteum is kept intact. Last, because of the donor site's distance from the head, it has the potential for a two-team approach.

The fibula free flap has been criticized for its use in mandibular reconstruction because of the height discrepancy between the fibula bone and the native mandible and in its use in reconstructing large oral cavity and through-and-through soft tissue defects. To decrease the discrepancy between the fibula bone and the native mandible, a "double-barrel" technique has been described in which a 1-cm segment of the fibula bone is removed and the fibula is folded on itself lengthwise. To reconstruct extensive soft tissue defects, the use of a radial forearm flap in conjunction with the fibula flap has been described. The radial forearm flap can be used to reconstruct the oral cavity, while the free fibula osteocutaneous flap can be used to reconstruct the mandible and the cervical skin. This technique can also be used to reconstruct composite resections of the mandible, tongue, and floor of the mouth or composite resections of the mandible and lower lip. Combined ipsilateral maxillomandibular defects can also be reconstructed using the free fibula flap by removing a central 3-cm segment of the fibula and rotating the distal portion of the fibula upward to reconstruct the maxilla and rotating the proximal portion downward to reconstruct the mandible.

Mandibular reconstruction with the use of nonvascularized bone grafts is well described in the literature. Before the availability of microvascular transfer, immediate bone grafting with nonvacularized grafts had a success rate of only 46%, as opposed to 91% in the delayed setting. Direct comparisons of nonvascularized versus vascularized bone grafts have shown a higher success of bony union with vascularized bone grafts. Pogrel and associates reported a 95% success rate of bony union using vascularized bone grafts and a 76% success rate using nonvascularized bone grafts for primary reconstruction of mandibular defects. Foster and colleagues reported similar results, with a 96% success rate using vascularized bone grafts and a 69% success rate using nonvascularized bone grafts. Pogrel and associates also found that the failure rate for nonvascularized grafts increased for segmental mandibular defects longer than 6 cm and that extreme caution should be used when using nonvascularized grafts for reconstructing segmental mandibular defects longer than 9 cm. The failure rate for nonvascularized grafts of 6 cm or shorter was 17%, increasing to 75% for grafts over 12 cm in length. This correlation of increasing failure rate with increased graft length was not seen with the use of vascularized bone grafts. Foster and colleagues also reported a higher success rate of osseointegration of endosteal implants in vascularized bone grafts (99%) over nonvascularized grafts (82%). In the studies by both groups, the predominant vascularized bone graft used was the fibula free flap.

Various vascularized osteocutaneous free flaps have been used for mandibular reconstruction; available choices include fibula, radius, ilium, scapula, rib, and metatarsal. Rib and metatarsal were among the first to be used for mandibular reconstruction but are rarely used today. The radial forearm flap provides a reliable, thin, and pliable skin flap and is excellent for reconstructing large intraoral defects. However, the radius bone provides only a short segment of unicortical bone (8 to 10 cm), is of poor quality for the reception of endosteal implants, and is easily devascularized with multiple osteotomies. There is also a risk of fracture with using the radial forearm free flap. The scapula can provide a large and excellent skin paddle but with more soft tissue bulk than the radius. The bone of the scapula is thin, is of poor quality, and usually is able to provide only 10 to 14 cm of bone length. The scapula is also easily devascularized with multiple osteotomies and is not adequate for the placement of endosteal implants. Harvesting of the scapula also does not allow a two-team approach. The ilium based on the deep circumflex iliac artery can provide a large amount of bone, and its shape resembles that of the hemimandible. The number of osteotomies that can be made is also limited due to the risk of devascularization, making it more difficult to contour the ilium for anterior mandibular defects. The skin paddle of the ilium is also very bulky, and the donor site can be quite morbid and deforming. In addition, the vascular pedicle of the deep circumflex iliac artery flap is relatively short, making anastomosis into the recipient bed more challenging. Among the remaining choices, the fibula has been the most popular because of its numerous proven advantages (length and quality of bone that can be harvested, segmental blood supply that allows multiple osteotomies for shaping and contouring the fibula, adequate bone height and width to receive endosteal implants, an intermediate-thickness skin paddle, reliable vascular pedicle that can reach 8 to 12 cm in length, low donor site morbidity, and ideal location for a two-team approach).

Bibliography

Anthony J, Rawnsley J, Benhaim P, et al: Donor leg morbidity and function after fibula free flap mandible reconstruction, *Plast Reconstr Surg* 96:146, 1995.

Bahr W: Blood supply of small fibula segments: an experimental study on human cadavers, *J Craniomaxillofac Surg* 26:148, 1998.

Blackwell K: Unsurpassed reliability of free flaps for head and neck reconstruction, *Arch Otolaryngol Head Neck Surg* 125:295, 1999.

Blackwell K, Buchbinder D, Urken M: Lateral mandibular reconstruction using soft-tissue free flaps and plates, *Arch Otolaryngol Head Neck Surg* 122:672, 1996.

Blanchaert R, Harris C: Microvascular free bone flaps, *Atlas Oral Maxillofac Surg Clin N Am* 13:151, 2005.

Boyd J, et al: The free flap and plate in oromandibular reconstruction: long-term review and indications, *Plast Reconstr Surg* 95:1018, 1995.

Buchbinder D: Discussion of "Analysis of reconstruction of mandibular defects using single stainless steel A-O reconstruction plates," *J Oral Maxillofac Surg* 54:862, 1996.

Choi S, et al: Radiation therapy does not impact local complication rates after free flap reconstruction for head and neck cancer, *Arch Otolaryngol Head Neck Surg* 130:1308, 2004.

Cordeiro P, Disa J, Hidalgo D, et al: Reconstruction of the mandible with osseous free flaps: a 10 year experience with 150 consecutive patients, *Plast Reconstr Surg* 104:1314, 1999.

Cordeiro P, Hidalgo D: Soft tissue coverage of mandibular reconstruction plates, *Head Neck* 16:112, 1994.

Fong B, Funk G: Osseous free tissue transfer in head and neck reconstruction, *Fac Plast Surg* 15:45, 1999.

Foster R, Anthony J, Sharma A, et al: Vascularized bone flaps versus nonvascularized bone grafts for mandibular reconstruction: an outcome analysis of primary bony union and endosseous implant success, *Head Neck* 21:66, 1999.

Gilbert R, Dovion D. Near total mandibular reconstruction: the free vascularized fibular transfer, *Oper Tech Otolaryngol Head Neck Surg* 4:145, 1993.

Goodacre T, Walker C, Jawad A, et al: Donor site morbidity following osteocutaneous free fibula transfer, *Br J Plast Surg* 43:410, 1990.

Hayden R, O'Leary M: A neurosensory fibula flap: anatomical description and clinical applications. Presented at the 94th Annual Meeting of the American Academy of Facial Plastic and Reconstructive Surgery, Minneapolis, MN, October 1, 1993.

Hidalgo D: Discussion of "Fibula osteoseptocutaneous flap for reconstruction of composite mandibular defects," *Plast Reconstr Surg* 93:305, 1994.

Hidalgo D: Fibula free flap: a new method of mandible reconstruction, *Plast Reconstr Surg* 84:71, 1989.

Hidalgo D, Pusic A: Free-flap mandibular reconstruction: a 10 year follow-up study, *Plast Reconstr Surg* 110:438, 2002.

Hidalgo D, Rekow A: A review of 60 consecutive fibula free flap mandible reconstructions, *Plast Reconstr Surg* 96:585, 1995.

Horiuchi K, Hattori A, Inada I, et al: Mandibular reconstruction using the double barrel fibular graft, *Microsurgery* 16:450, 1995.

Jones N, Swartz W, Mears D, et al: The "double barrel" free vascularized fibular bone graft, *Plast Reconstr Surg* 81:378, 1998.

Khouri et al: A prospective study of microvascular free-flap surgery and outcome, *Plast Reconstr Surg* 102:711, 1998.

Kroll SS, et al: Choice of flap and incidence of free flap success, *Plast Reconstr Surg* 98:459, 1996.

Lee E, Goh J, Helm R, et al: Donor site morbidity following resection of the fibula, *J Bone Joint Surg* 72:129, 1990.

Myung-Rai K, Donoff RB: Critical analysis of mandibular reconstruction using AO reconstruction plates, *J Oral Maxillofac Surg* 50:1152, 1990.

Pogrel MA, Podlesh S, Anthony J, et al: A comparison of vascularized and nonvascularized bone grafts for reconstruction of mandibular continuity defects, *J Oral Maxillofac Surg* 55:1200, 1997.

Sadove R, Powell L: Simultaneous maxillary and mandibular reconstruction with one free osteocutaneous flap, *Plast Reconstr Surg* 92:141, 1993.

Schusterman M, Reece G, Kroll S, et al: Use of the AO plate for immediate mandibular reconstruction in cancer patients, *Plast Reconstr Surg* 88:588, 1991.

Schusterman M, Reece G, Miller M, et al: The osteocutaneous free fibula flap: is the skin paddle reliable? *Plast Reconstr Surg* 90:787, 1992.

Serletti J, et al: Factors affecting outcome in free-tissue transfer in the elderly, *Plast Reconstr Surg* 106:66, 2000.

Serlitti J, Coniglio J, Tavin E, et al: Simultaneous transfer of free fibula and radial forearm flaps for complex oromandibular reconstruction, *J Reconstr Microsurg* 14:297, 1998.

Shaari CM, et al: Complications of microvascular head and neck surgery in the elderly, *Arch Otolaryngol Head Neck Surg* 124:407, 1998.

Shpitzer T, et al: Oromandibular reconstruction with the fibular free flap: analysis of 50 consecutive flaps, *Arch Otolaryngol Head Neck Surg* 123:939, 1997.

Singh B, et al: Factors associated with complications in microvascular reconstruction of head and neck defects, *Plast Reconstr Surg* 103:403, 1999.

Sphitzer T, et al: The free vascularized flap and the flap plate options: comparative results of reconstruction of lateral mandibular defects, *Laryngoscope* 110:2056, 2000.

Suh JD, et al: Analysis of outcome and complications in 400 cases of microvascular head and neck reconstruction, *Arch Otolaryngol Head Neck Surg* 130:962, 2004.

Ueyama Y, Naitoh R, Yamagata A, et al: Analysis of reconstruction of mandibular defects using single stainless steel A-O reconstruction plates, *J Oral Maxillofac Surg* 54:858, 1996.

Urken ML, et al: Microvascular free flaps in and head and neck reconstruction, *Arch Otolaryngol Head Neck Surg* 120:633, 1994.

Urken ML, Cheney ML, Sullivan MJ, et al: *Atlas of regional and free flaps for head and neck reconstruction,* Philadelphia, 1994, Lippincott Williams and Wilkins.

Mandibular Reconstruction With Iliac Crest Bone Graft

Chris Jo, DMD, and Shahrokh C. Bagheri, DMD, MD

CC

A 28-year-old otherwise healthy man is referred to your office for reconstruction of the left mandible, explaining that, "Now that the tumor is gone, I need my lower jaw reconstructed."

HPI

The patient is now 3 months status post resection of a large, expansile ameloblastoma of the left mandible (with 1.5-cm bony margins) and immediate placement of a locking reconstruction plate (a minimum of 3 months after ablative surgery is recommended to allow sufficient time for soft tissue healing before bone grafting). The tumor was resected via a transoral approach using a previously bent reconstruction plate that was placed to stabilize the mandible and the occlusion (a custom-made three-dimensional stereolithographic model fabricated with the aid of a CT scan is used to prebend the plate, reducing operating time and increasing the accuracy of the reconstruction) (Figure 11-23). In this case, the inferior alveolar nerve was resected with the specimen (on select benign cases, the preservation of the nerve is possible using a nerve pull-out technique). There were no perioperative complications. The patient is now ready for total mandibular reconstruction and functional rehabilitation.

PMHX/PDHX/MEDICATIONS/ALLERGIES/SH/FH

Noncontributory. The patient has no history of cardiac or pulmonary conditions (increased intrathoracic pressure and hemodynamic changes associated with the prone position may not be tolerated well in patients with poor cardiac or respiratory reserves).

EXAMINATION

General. He is a well-developed and well-nourished man in no apparent distress.

Maxillofacial. The patient's examination shows good facial form and symmetry, with a slight loss of left lower lip support (secondary to the resection). There is anesthesia of the left mental nerve distribution. The marginal mandibular branch and the remaining branches of cranial nerve VII are intact.

Intraoral. The occlusion is as planned and reproducible with a good range of motion. There are no traumatic occlusal or soft tissue interferences noted (traumatic occlusion, especially from a supraerupted maxillary third molar, can cause

perforation of the soft tissue overlying the recipient bed). The remaining dentition is in good repair (compromised teeth, especially those adjacent to the recipient bed, should be restored or extracted before reconstruction to prevent graft infection). The soft tissue over the defect has healed well with minimal scar contracture (a qualitative or quantitative soft tissue deficiency may require an alternative reconstructive plan such as a myocutaneous flap [pectoralis major] or reconstruction with a vascularized free flap [free fibula or iliac bone]). There are no signs of infection or exposure of the reconstruction plate (bone grafting into a contaminated field would be contraindicated).

IMAGING

A preoperative panoramic radiograph is the minimum radiographic study necessary to evaluate the size of the defect and to assess the integrity and stability of the hardware. In this patient, the panoramic radiograph revealed an 8-cm continuity defect (10 ml of uncompressed cancellous marrow is needed for each centimeter of continuity defect). The dentition is in good repair, with no supraerupted maxillary teeth and no signs of residual or recurrent pathology.

LABS

The minimum preoperative laboratory studies necessary are hemoglobin and hematocrit levels. Tumor resection can be associated with an unpredictable amount of blood loss. Reconstructive procedures are usually more predictable, but a preoperative baseline measure of hemoglobin and hematocrit should be obtained. Other laboratory tests would be dictated by the past surgical and medical histories.

ASSESSMENT

Continuity defect (8 cm) of the left mandible, status post resection of a benign mandibular tumor (ameloblastoma)

TREATMENT

Reconstruction of the mandible has challenged surgeons for many years, and several techniques are available, all of which have their associated advantages and complications. Treatment is dictated by the surgeon's training, available resources, and patient preferences.

We present the case of a patient with reconstruction of a mandibular continuity defect using a transcutaneous approach

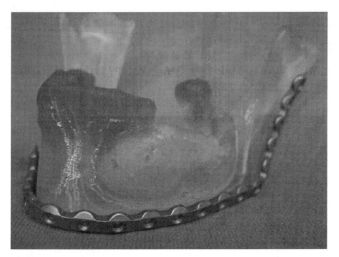

Figure 11-23 A stereolithographic model demonstrating an expanding mass of the left mandible and a well-adapted locking reconstruction plate to be used for surgical adaptation.

Figure 11-24   A, Anatomy of the anterior ilium. It shows the anterior superior iliac spine marked by the "X" with the lateral cutaneous branches of the iliohypogastric nerve, subcostal nerve, and lateral femoral nerves (from posterior to anterior). The incision as shown is made 2 to 3 cm below the crest (to prevent wound dehiscence) and 1 to 2 cm posterior to the anterior superior iliac spine (to prevent injury to the subcostal nerve as it crosses over the anterior superior iliac spine). **B,** Anatomy of the posterior ilium. Note that the posterior superior iliac spine is the bony prominence adjacent to the sacroiliac (SI) joint where the gluteus maximus muscle orginates. The cutaneous branches of the superior cluneal nerves (L1-3) and middle cluneal nerves (S1-3) are shown. The incision is made along the crest and centered over the posterior superior iliac spine, avoiding injury to the superior and middle cluneal nerves.

(to minimize bacterial contamination of the graft) and the (posterior or anterior) iliac crest cancellous marrow graft. The surgical anatomy of the anterior and posterior ilium is shown in Figure 11-24.

Transcutaneous exposure and preparation of the recipient bed. The main advantage of a transoral resection of a benign tumor is the avoidance of a neck incision and its associated scar tissue upon making the transcutaneous exposure in preparation for the bony reconstruction phase. A curvilinear incision is marked at least 2 cm below the inferior border of the mandible with the head in a neutral position (to protect the marginal mandibular branch of the facial nerve) or further inferiorly in a neck crease. The exposure should be sufficient in length to fully expose the proximal and distal segments of the continuity defect. Nerve testing can be carried out to ensure that the dissection is below the marginal mandibular nerve. Dissection is then carried deep to the superficial layer of deep cervical fascia superiorly. The facial artery and vein are identified, ligated, and sectioned. Carrying the dissection deep to these vessels ensures that the facial nerve is protected in the superior flap. The inferior borders of the mandible and reconstruction plate are identified. An incision is made through the periosteum (proximal and distal bony segments) and through the fibrous capsule of the plate. The surgeon must be careful not to perforate into the oral cavity with overzealous dissection (the most common area of mucosal perforation is at the line angles of the distal segment). The fibrous capsule surrounding the reconstruction plate should be carefully excised (excessive scar tissue surrounding the reconstruction plate will prevent capillary diffusion into the graft). Figure 11-25 demonstrates exposure of the recipient site and adaptation of a resorbable crib in preparation for bone graft placement. Some surgeons recommend completely removing the reconstruction plate for recipient bed preparation, then placing the same plate back using the same screw holes (placed with nontapping screws). The graft bed is further prepared with blunt dissection to create a sufficient pocket to accommodate

the bone graft without tension. If an intraoral perforation is noted, the wound should be immediately irrigated and closed in a double-layer fashion, followed by copious irrigation of the bed with an antibiotic solution (to reduce the bacterial load) and redosing the intravenous antibiotic if sufficient time has passed since the preoperative dose.

Posterior iliac crest bone graft harvesting technique. The main advantage of the posterior iliac crest bone graft is the quantity and quality of bone harvested. The main disadvantage is increased operating time due to the change in position and inability to work simultaneously by two teams. The patient is placed in the reverse flex prone position (decreases venous pressure and ooze) with hip and axillary/chest rolls. The posterior superior iliac spine (a bony prominence where the gluteus maximus muscle originates) is palpated and marked (see Figure 11-24, *B*). A 10-cm curvilinear incision (the length of the incision can vary depending on the amount of bone to be harvested), 3 cm from the midline, is made along the crest. Dissection is carried through superficial fat and superficial fascia while the surgeon palpates the posterior iliac crest and posterior superior iliac spine. The lumbodorsal fascia (deep fascia investing the deep muscles of the back and trunk) is identified and sharply incised to expose the posterior iliac crest and spine and its attachments (from medial to lateral: gluteus maximus, latissimus dorsi, and external oblique muscles). Bovie electrocautery can be used to make an incision through these attachments along the posterior crest down to bone. Subperiosteal dissection is carried out to reflect the gluteus maximus off the posterior superior iliac spine and part of the gluteus medius from the lateral aspect of the pelvis. A 5×5 cm corticotomy is made with a reciprocating saw (along the lateral third of the iliac crest and including a portion of the posterior superior iliac spine). The sciatic notch and nerve are located 6 to 8 cm below the crest, which limits the vertical dissection and corticotomy. The corticocancellous window is removed (particulates into approximately 20 ml of uncompressed bone) with a curved osteotome. The cancellous marrow is removed with bone gouges and currettes and stored at room temperature in isotonic normal saline (95% cellular viability for up to 4 hours). The most abundant source of cancellous marrow is

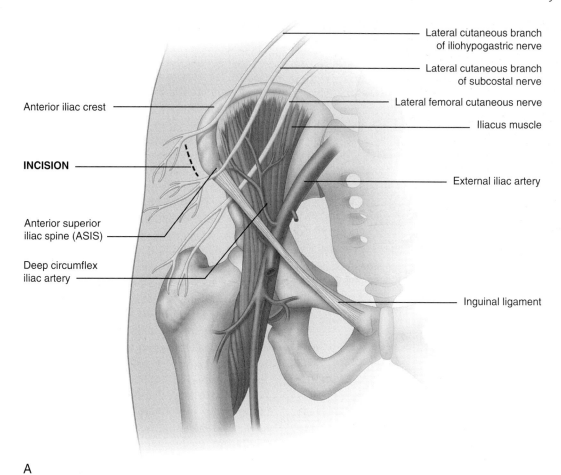

Lateral cutaneous branch of iliohypogastric nerve

Lateral cutaneous branch of subcostal nerve

Lateral femoral cutaneous nerve

Iliacus muscle

Anterior iliac crest

External iliac artery

INCISION

Anterior superior iliac spine (ASIS)

Deep circumflex iliac artery

Inguinal ligament

A

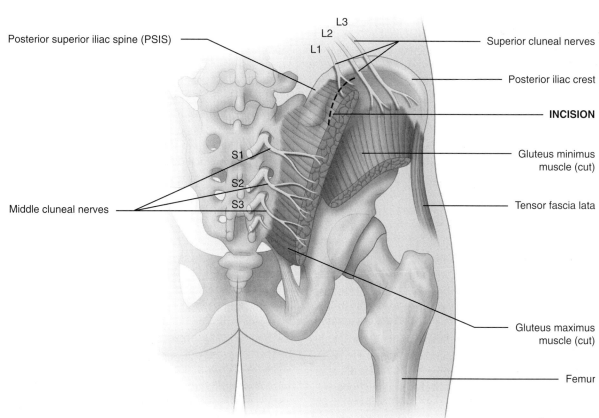

Posterior superior iliac spine (PSIS)

L3
L2
L1

Superior cluneal nerves

Posterior iliac crest

INCISION

Gluteus minimus muscle (cut)

S1

S2

S3

Tensor fascia lata

Middle cluneal nerves

Gluteus maximus muscle (cut)

Femur

B

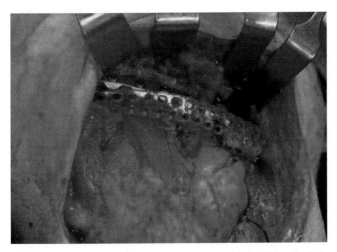

Figure 11-25   Complete exposure of the continuity defect, including the proximal and distal segments, via a transcutaneous approach. In this case, a resorbable alloplastic crib was used to maintain the bone graft from displacing inferiorly. It is important to avoid any intraoral perforations that would contaminate the graft with oral bacteria.

under the gluteus maximus insertion (posterior superior iliac spine), which is a triangular bony prominence near the sacroiliac joint. Approximately 2 to 2.5 times more corticocancellous bone can be harvested from the posterior ilium than from the anterior ilium (anterior iliac crest bone graft provides up to 50 ml of uncompressed bone). Hemostasis is achieved with electrocautery, judicious application of bone wax, and placement of Avitene (microfibrillar collagen) or platelet-poor plasma. Sharp bony edges should be rounded and smoothened. A drain with bulb suction can be placed, although it is not always necessary (Sasso and colleagues showed that there is no advantage to placing drains). Layered closure (periosteum, lumbodorsal fascia, subcutaneous, and skin) and a pressure dressing are applied.

The anterior iliac crest bone graft is an alternative to the posterior iliac crest bone graft when less volume of bone is needed. Its main advantage is the ability to simultaneously prepare the recipient bed and harvest the bone graft when working in two teams.

Anterior iliac crest bone graft (medial approach) harvesting technique (provides up to 50 ml of corticocancellous bone). A hip and knee roll can be placed to externally rotate the hip and to flex the leg respectively. The landmarks (anterior superior iliac spine, crest, and tubercle) and incision site are carefully marked. The incision should be curvilinear and 4 to 6 cm in length, 3 cm lateral to the crest (to prevent wound dehiscence), starting 1 to 2 cm posterior and lateral to the anterior superior iliac spine (to prevent injury to the lateral cutaneous branch of the subcostal nerve) (see Figure 11-24, A). This should not extend beyond the tubercle (which will cause injury to the lateral cutaneous branch of the iliohypogastric nerve). The incision is carried through skin, superficial fat layer, and superficial fascia down to the deep fascia (fascia lata) and the iliotibial tract. The superficial and deep fat layer is bluntly swept superiorly to center the dissection over the

anterior iliac crest. Sharp dissection to bone is conducted, avoiding the musculature by keeping medial to tensor fascia lata and gluteus medius muscles and lateral to iliacus and most of the external abdominal oblique muscles. Once the anterior iliac crest is exposed, various corticotomy techniques can be used to access the cancellous marrow. Both medial and lateral approaches have been described in the literature, but the lateral approach is associated with greater morbidity due to stripping of muscles involved in ambulation and stance. The medial approach strips the iliacus muscle (when a corticocancellous block is needed), which is not a major contributor of gait. The "clamshell" approach (midcrestal greenstick split for small quantities of cancellous marrow), trapdoor approach (midcrestal pedicled osteotomy), Tschapp approach ("decapping" the crest), Tessier's approach (oblique osteotomies to maintain contour of crest), trephine techniques (for small bone grafts), or full-thickness grafts can be used depending on surgeon preference. The authors prefer the technique described by Grillon and colleagues in 1984 (lateral decapping technique with attached superomedial pedicle to access the medial cortex), which allows for minimal dissection of the muscles attached to the anterior iliac crest. The iliacus muscle is dissected off the inner pelvis, and a 5 × 5-cm medial corticotomy can be made using a reciprocating saw and/or curved osteotomes. This block can be morselized with a bone mill (providing up to 20 ml of bone). Bone gouges and curettes are used to harvest the remainder of the cancellous marrow. The cancellous marrow is confined to the area anterior to the tubercle and 2 to 3 cm inferior to the iliac crest (medial and lateral cortices fuse or nearly fuse below this level). Up to 50 ml of uncompressed cancellous bone can be harvested and should be stored in an isotonic solution at room temperature. The anterior superior iliac spine is vulnerable to fracture and avulsion because of muscle attachments (the seven attachments to the anterior superior iliac spine are the fascia lata, inguinal ligament, tensor fascia lata, sartorious, iliacus, internal oblique, and external oblique muscles) and should not be undermined (increases risk of anterior superior iliac spine fracture). The cap should be replaced and stabilized with a wire or suture (to prevent contour deformity). The wound is closed in layers with or without drains.

The harvested bone is milled and compressed into 10- or 12-ml syringes (compaction of the cancellous marrow increases the density of endosteal osteoblasts). The morselized bone is compacted into the prepared recipient bed (Figure 11-26). Various crib techniques can be used (resorbable or titanium mesh, cadaveric cribs, autogenous ribs) to stabilize the graft. The reconstruction plate itself serves as an excellent crib. The deep tissues are sutured to the plate and the bone is packed from above, preventing inferior migration of the bone graft. The wound is closed in layers to further stabilize the graft. Some authors recommend 3 weeks of maxillomandibular fixation to prevent micromovement and shearing of budding capillaries penetrating the graft. Platelet-rich plasma, which has been shown to enhance bone grafting (earlier consolidation into lamellar bone and increased bony density), can be incorporated into the graft. Although there is some doubt regarding the efficacy of platelet-rich plasma in bone grafting, there are no well-controlled human studies to contradict its use.

Figure 11-27 is a panoramic radiograph demonstrating the bony reconstruction at 1 month. Dental implants can be placed into a mature graft (after 4 months) with a very high success rate. Animal studies have shown that implants placed into a cancellous marrow graft have a higher bone-to-metal contact and pull-out resistance than does native mandible.

COMPLICATIONS

Marginal mandibular nerve injury. This can be prevented by keeping the dissection inferior and deep to the nerve, retracting it in the superior flap. Dingman and Grabb studied 100 facial halves and found that the marginal mandibular branch is up to 1 cm below the inferior border of mandible in 19% of cases. Anterior to facial artery, it was found to be superior to the inferior border of mandible. Ziarah and Atkinson studied 76 facial halves and found that 53% of the time the marginal mandibular branch was up to 1.2 cm below the inferior border of the mandible before reaching the facial

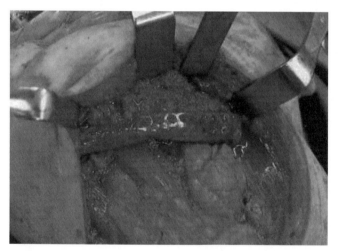

Figure 11-26 Morselized cancellous marrow graft compacted into the prepared recipient bed and alloplastic resorbable crib.

vessels. Six percent remained below the inferior border of the mandible, as far as 1.5 cm anterior to the facial artery.

Pain and gait disturbance. This is more frequently observed with an anterior iliac crest bone graft compared with a posterior iliac crest bone graft (attributed to stripping of the tensor fascia lata muscle along the anterior iliac crest). In a study by Marx and Morales (posterior group, N = 50, and anterior group, N = 50), they reported that 6% of patients were limping at 10 days postoperatively and that no patients were limping at 60 days after posterior iliac crest bone grafting, whereas 42% and 15%, respectively, limped who underwent the lateral approach to the anterior iliac crest bone graft. They also reported a higher pain score for the anterior group at postoperative days 1 and 10. When comparing the medial with the lateral approach for the anterior iliac crest bone graft, Grillon and associates found the lateral approach to be associated with greater morbidity (increased blood loss and number of days requiring a cane or crutch). Others have also found that a lateral approach is associated with more pain, prolonged gait disturbances, and wound hematoma. This is likely due to the stripping of the muscles attached to the lateral aspect of the anterior iliac crest (tensor fascia lata muscle), which is involved in gait and stance.

Infection and delayed wound healing at the donor site. This occurs in fewer than 4%. Delayed wound healing has been reported mostly when the incision was directly over the bony prominence of the iliac crest.

Blood loss. This is directly related to the size of the corticocancellous graft harvested and the operative time. Brazaitis and colleagues reported a case of severe retroperitoneal hemorrhage (Grey-Turner sign or ecchymosis on the flank indicating a retroperitoneal bleed) resulting in death after anterior iliac crest bone grafting.

Hematoma or seroma at the donor site. Some studies have suggested that the incidence of hematoma or seroma formation is less when using drains; however, this has not been consistently shown in the literature. Mazock and associates reported an 8.6% incidence of uncomplicated seromas. Marx and Morales reported a 12% incidence of seroma and a 2% incidence of hematoma formation for the anterolateral approach.

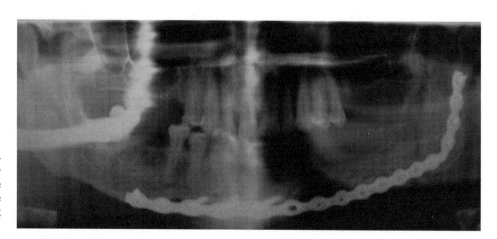

Figure 11-27 Postoperative panoramic radiograph showing an ideally placed reconstruction plate along the inferior and posterior borders of the mandible and a bone graft spanning the defect.

Adynamic ileus (decreased peristalsis due to the lack of smooth muscle contraction). A rarely reported complication, the signs and symptoms include abdominal pain and distention, nausea and vomiting, high-pitched or absent bowel sounds, sentinel loop of gas per abdominal radiograph, and electrolyte abnormalities.

Orthopedic complications. Risk of fractures increases with graft size (2% to 13% incidence of anterior superior iliac spine fracture, which can be avoided by limited undermining of the anterior superior iliac spine). Acetabular fractures and iliac crest subluxations are rare. Pelvic instability in posterior iliac crest bone graft is due to weakening of sacroiliac joint and ligaments and should be avoided with careful dissection.

Contour defects of the anterior ilium. This is seen especially when the anterior iliac crest is removed and stripped from the periosteum. Hypertrophic scarring can also be seen at the incision site.

Sensory nerve injury. Laurie and associates reported a 10% temporary sensory loss after anterior iliac crest bone grafting (lateral cutaneous branches of the iliohypogastric and subcostal nerves). Nkenke and associates report 20% hypoesthesia after anterior iliac crest bone grafting seen exclusively in the lateral femoral cutaneous nerve distribution (all resolved at 1 month). Others report that the lateral cutaneous branch of the iliohypogastric nerve is the most commonly injured nerve in the anterior iliac crest bone graft. Meralgia paresthetica (burning, stabbing pain along the lateral femoral cutaneous nerve distribution) has a reported incidence of 0% to 1.8% (86% of the time the lateral femoral cutaneous nerve runs deep to the inguinal ligament and is protected, while in 2% of patients it runs over the anterior superior iliac spine). The medial branch of the superior cluneal nerves is 6.5 cm from the posterior superior iliac spine and 8 cm from the midline (Mazock and associates reported a less than 3% incidence of superior cluneal nerve injury that resolved at 6 months). Others have reported an incidence of 12% to 20% of temporary sensory loss to the cluneal nerves.

Pain and gait disturbances are rare after 6 months. Hernia, arteriovenous fistula formation, and ureteral injury have been reported but are very rare complications.

DISCUSSION

Mandibular reconstruction using iliac crest bone graft is a three-stage reconstruction:
- Stage I: tumor resection
- Stage II: bony reconstruction
- Stage III: dental implants and rehabilitation

The main goal is to optimize the recipient bed (qualitatively and quantitatively) to improve bone graft survival. Stage I includes resection of the tumor (either malignant or benign) and stabilization of the mandibular segments and occlusion with a reconstruction plate. If there is a soft tissue deficiency at the time of ablative surgery, a soft tissue flap may be used (pectoralis major, latissmus dorsi, or free fibula, iliac crest or radial forearm flaps). If postablative radiation therapy is used

for the treatment of malignant tumors, a hyperbaric oxygen protocol can be used before and after stage II to optimize the quality of the recipient bed (some authors recommend bony reconstruction after 1 year of disease-free state, because 70% of recurrences occur within the first year). Bone grafting can be done 3 months after ablation of a benign tumor or 3 months after the last surgical procedure to optimize the recipient bed (including extractions, vestibuloplasties, scar excisions, or myocutaneous flaps).

Autogenous bone, in the form of a cancellous cellular marrow (formerly called particulate bone and cancellous marrow), is the gold standard for grafting in the maxillofacial region because it possesses osteogenic (new bone formation from osteoprogenitor cells), osteoconductive (new bone formation from host-derived or transplanted osteoprogenitor cells along a biologic or alloplastic framework), and osteoinductive (formation of new bone by guided differentiation of stem cell precursors into secretory osteoblasts by bone inductive proteins) properties.

The ilium provides the highest in cancellous cellular density (posterior ilium > anterior ilium > tibial plateau > mandibular symphysis). Osteocompetent cells (endosteal osteoblasts and cancellous marrow stem cells) are transferred in a viable state to the recipient bed. The transplanted bone is hypoxic (oxygen tension of 3 to 10 mm Hg), acidotic (pH 4 to 6), and rich in lactate, which acts as chemotactic agent to recruit macrophages to secrete angiogenesis factors.

Bone grafting (first 3 to 5 days). Cells survive via diffusion of nutrients from recipient bed. Vascularity of the recipient bed is important for graft survival. This can be optimized with hyperbaric oxygen, especially in previously irradiated patients (quality), added tissue bulk if needed (quantity), removal of scar tissue (to allow diffusion of nutrients into graft), and the absence of any infection. An oxygen gradient greater than 30 mm Hg stimulates macrophage chemotaxis and initiates angiogenesis.

Beginning on day 3, the capillary buds proliferate and begin to penetrate the graft (stimulated by multiple factors, including platelet-derived growth factors, macrophage-derived angiogenesis factors, and macrophage-derived growth factors). These new capillaries bring in nutrients to support mitogenesis and osteoid production.

Bone grafting (days 10 to 14). Completion of revascularization occurs at 2 weeks. An automated shut off mechanism occurs when the oxygen gradient is obliterated. This is a critical period for bone graft survival as small vessels can be easily sheared by micromovement. Two- to 3-week periods of maxillomandibular fixation and empiric antibiotic coverage are recommended during this revascularization phase.

Bone grafting (weeks 3 to 4). Phase I bone (woven bone) regeneration is dependent on the osteocompetent cellular density of the graft (which is increased by compacting the graft). Phase I bone is eventually replaced by phase II bone (mature lamellar bone) because of obligatory resorption of phase I bone by osteoclasts, releasing BMP and linking resorption with new bone formation (capable of self-renewal via the endosteum and periosteum). Ideally, phase II bone replaces phase I bone in a 1:1 ratio over the next several weeks.

Alternatives to a staged cancellous marrow bone graft to reconstruct a continuity defect of the mandible include the vascularized free fibula or deep circumflex iliac artery free flap. These can be used to reconstruct both the soft and hard tissues at the time of tumor ablation (see Free Fibula Flap for Mandibular Reconstruction section in this chapter).

rhBMP can be used as adjunct therapy. rhBMP-soaked gelfoam sponges can be placed into a defect using various cribs (allogeneic split rib is very versatile). rhBMP has been shown to be osteoinductive, creating bone de novo by recruiting circulating mesenchymal cells and initiating their differentiation into functional osteoblasts.

Reconstruction of a severely resorbed mandible is a unique challenge to all reconstructive surgeons (Figure 11-28, *A*). The severely resorbed mandible lacks sufficient bone height to accommodate 10 mm or longer dental implants, and wearing a non–implant-supported lower denture is nearly impossible (insufficient vestibular depth, mental nerve impingement, and lack of retention). These patients are also susceptible to mandibular body fractures (usually the thinnest and weakest

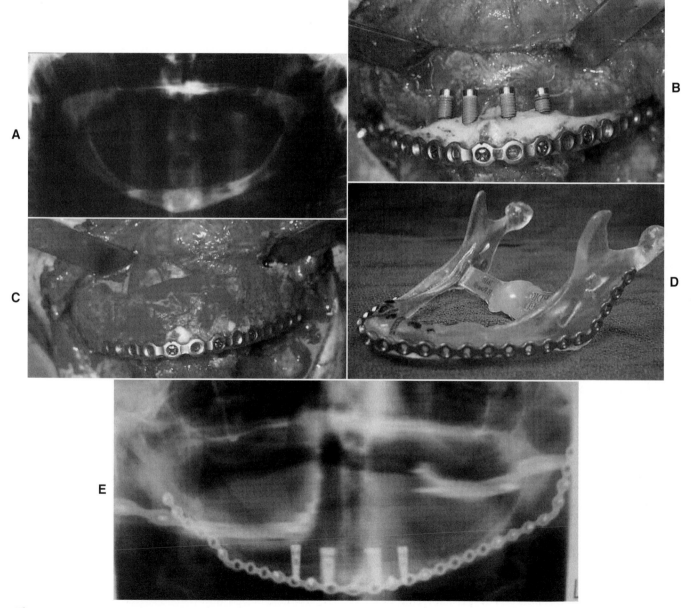

Figure 11-28 **A,** Panoramic radiograph of a severely resorbed edentulous mandible with bilateral body fractures, with severe telescoping on the left side. **B,** Four 15-mm dental implants are placed in the anterior mandible. **C,** Cancellous marrow bone graft from the posterior ilium and platelet-rich plasma is packed from ramus to ramus and around the implants. **D,** A stereolithographic model used to prebend a low-profile 2.3 locking reconstruction plate from angle to angle. The telescoped segment was sectioned on the model and glued together in a reduced position before bending the plate. The position of the condyles were kept the same by fabricating glenoid fossas by impressing the condylar heads into a plastic emesis basin filled with dental stone. **E,** Postoperative panoramic radiograph of the reconstructed mandible using a modification of the tentpole technique.

area). The "tent pole" technique was introduced by Marx and has been found to be a predictable reconstructive modality for the severely resorbed mandible (height of bone is 6 mm or less). It involves placing four to six 15-mm implants in the anterior mandible (Figure 11-28, *B*) (which act to "tent" up or expand the perimandibular soft tissue matrix) and immediate iliac crest bone grafting from ramus to ramus around the implants via a transcutaneous approach (submental omega incision) (Figure 11-28, *C*), to increase the bony dimensions of the mandibular body and reduce the risk of atrophic fractures. Marx presented 64 cases with a mean initial bone height of 4.8 mm. All patients maintained 15 mm of bone height and had an osseointegration rate of 99.5%, with functional rehabilitation of all patients at a mean follow-up of 4.9 years. This concept has been successfully applied to patients with a severely resorbed mandible and bilateral body fractures. In this situation, a visor incision is used and a low-profile locking reconstruction plate is adapted from angle to angle (prebending the plate on a stereolithographic model is advantageous) (Figure 11-28, *D*). The screws are placed in the anterior mandible (anterior to the mental nerve) in every other hole to allow placement of the implants and in the posterior body/ramus region (posterior to the inferior alveolar nerve). Autogenous bone is packed around the fractures and implants from ramus to ramus as previously described. Figure 11-28, *E* shows the postoperative panoramic radiograph.

Bibliography

Brazaitis MP, Mirvis SE, Greenberg J, et al: Severe retroperitoneal hemorrhage complicating anterior iliac bone graft acquisition, *J Oral Maxillofac Surg* 52:314-316, 1994.

Carlson ER: Mandibular bone grafts: techniques, placement, and evaluation, *Oral Maxillofac Surg Knowledge Update* 1, 1994.

Carlson ER, Marx RE: Mandibular reconstruction using cancellous cellular bone grafts, *J Oral Maxillofac Surg* 54:889-897, 1996.

Catone GA, Reimer BL, McNeir D, et al: Tibial autogenous cancellous bone as an alternative donor site in maxillofacial surgery: a preliminary report, *J Oral Maxillofac Surg* 50:1258-1263, 1992.

Dingman RO, Grabb WC: Surgical anatomy of the mandibular ramus of the facial nerve based on dissection of 100 facial halves. *Plast Recon Surg* 29:266-272, 1962.

Grillon GL, Gunther SF, Connole PW: A new technique for obtaining iliac bone grafts, *J Oral Maxillofac Surg* 42:172-176, 1984.

Herford AS, King BJ, Audia F, et al: Medial approach for tibial bone graft: anatomic study and clinical technique, *J Oral Maxillofac Surg* 61:358-363, 2003.

Marx RE: Clinical application of bone biology to mandibular and maxillary reconstruction, *Clin Plast Surg* 21:377-392, 1994.

Marx RE: Mandibular reconstruction, *J Oral Maxillofac Surg* 51:466-479, 1993.

Marx RE: Osteoradionecrosis: a new concept of its pathophysiology, *J Oral Maxillofac Surg* 41:283-288, 1983.

Marx RE: Biology of bone grafts, *Oral Maxillofac Surg Knowledge Update* 1, 1994.

Marx RE: Philosophy and particulars of autogenous bone grafting, *Oral Maxillofac Surg Clin N Am* 5:599-612, 1993.

Marx RE, Ames JR: The use of hyperbaric oxygen therapy in bony reconstruction of the irradiated and tissue-deficient patient, *J Oral Maxillofac Surg* 40:412-420, 1982.

Marx RE, Carlson ER, Eichstaedt RM, et al: Platelet-rich plasma: growth factor enhancement for bone grafts, *Oral Surg Oral Med Oral Pathol* 85:638-646, 1998.

Marx RE, Ehler WJ, Peleg M: Mandibular and facial reconstruction: rehabilitation of the head and neck cancer patient, *Bone* 19(July), 1996.

Marx RE, Ehler WJ, Tayapongsak P, et al: Relationship of oxygen dose to angiogenesis induction in irradiated tissue, *Am J Surg* 160:519-524, 1990.

Marx RE, Johnson RP: Studies in the radiobiology of ORN and their clinical significance, *J Oral Maxillofac Surg* 64:379-390, 1987.

Marx RE, Morales MJ: Morbidity from bone harvest in major jaw reconstruction: a randomized trial comparing the lateral anterior and posterior approaches to the ilium, *J Oral Maxillofac Surg* 48:196-203, 1988.

Marx RE, Shellenberger T, Wimsatt J, et al: Severely resorbed mandible: predictable reconstruction with soft tissue matrix expansion (tent pole) grafts, *J Oral Maxillofac Surg* 60:878-888, 2002.

Marx RE, Smith BR: An improved technique for the development of the pectoralis major myocutaneous flap, *J Oral Maxillofac Surg* 48:1168-1180, 1990.

Marx RE, Snyder RM, Kline SN: Cellular survival of human marrow during placement of marrow cancellous bone grafts, *J Oral Surg* 37:712-718, 1979.

Mazock JB, Schow SR, Triplett RG: Posterior iliac crest bone harvest: review of technique, complications, and use of an epidural catheter for postoperative pain control, *J Oral Maxillofac Surg* 61:1497-1503, 2003.

Nkenke E, et al: Morbidity of harvesting of bone grafts from the iliac crest for preprosthetic augmentation procedures: a prospective study, *Int J Oral Maxillofac Surg* 33:157-163, 2004.

Sasso RC, Williams JL, Dimasi N, et al: Postoperative drains at the donor site of iliac-crest bone grafts: A prospective, randomized study of morbidity at the donor site in patients who had a traumatic injury of the spine, *J Bone Joint Surg Am* 80:631-635, 1998.

Stevens MR: Bone harvesting techniques, *Oral Maxillofac Surg Knowledge Update* 1, 1994.

Ziarah HA, Atkinson ME: The surgical anatomy of the mandibular distribution of the facial nerve, *Br J Oral Surg* 19:159-170, 1981.

12 Facial Cosmetic Surgery

Chris Jo, DMD, and Shahrokh C. Bagheri, DMD, MD

This chapter addresses:
- Lip Augmentation
- Rhinoplasty
- Cervicofacial Rhytidectomy (Facelift)
- Upper and Lower Eyelid Blepharoplasty
- Genioplasty
- Endoscopic Brow-Lift
- Botulinum Toxin A (Botox) Injection for Facial Rejuvenation

---

Facial cosmetic surgery has gained tremendous popularity in the past decade. One reason for this rise in interest is the consumer's increased accessibility to information via television, the Internet, and other media sources. Also, the development of safe and effective surgical techniques with reduced "downtime" and long-lasting natural appearing results has popularized this field. Facial cosmetic surgeons must intimately understand facial anatomy, as well as the anatomy and physiology of the aging process. Although some patients seek to rejuvenate their appearance to "turn back" the hands of time, others are interested in altering their appearance to a more desirable social norm.

In each area of the face, several different surgical techniques have been developed to improve the appearance, each with their own merits. It is the intent of this chapter to introduce readers to the basic concepts of facial cosmetic surgery. Each section is designed to emphasize the key points important in the examination, contrasting the presenting deformity with the ideal, youthful norms. The rationale for surgical techniques to improve outcome and achieve lasting results based on facial anatomy and the process of facial aging is described. Ultimately, the techniques used by facial cosmetic surgeons are based on the surgeon's preference, training, and clinical situation.

Both genetic and extrinsic factors contribute to the aging process. The genetic factors are fixed. Extrinsic factors can be altered and include excess sun damage, smoking, a healthy diet, and exercise. Rejuvenation of the face should be tailored to the individual by improving the overall health of the patient, addressing the health of the skin, and possibly using adjunctive surgical procedures to enhance beauty. For smokers, the single most effective method of improving one's health (including the skin) is to stop smoking. For those "sun lovers," it is old news—excessive sun exposure will damage the skin (burns and dries out the skin). The goal of facial cosmetic surgery is to improve and refresh the appearance of the face without any signs of obvious surgical intervention after the healing is complete.

Oral and maxillofacial surgeons are uniquely trained to recognize and manage facial deformities at all levels. Facial rejuvenation and cosmetic surgery have been described as analogous to building a house. First, the foundation must be established (skeletal surgery). Next, the framing and walls must be built (soft tissue surgery). Finally, the paint must be applied (skin resurfacing). With proper understanding and training, facial cosmetic surgery can be easily incorporated into one's practice.

Lip Augmentation

Shahrokh C. Bagheri, DMD, MD, and Chris Jo, DMD

CC

A 30-year-old healthy white woman presents for consultation for upper lip augmentation. She complains that her upper lip is "thin" and does not match her lower lip. She desires a "mild" augmentation of her upper lip and specifically does not want to have an excessively "pouty" upper lip.

HPI

The patient has no previous history of facial filler for soft tissue augmentation. She has recently gone through a divorce and desires to improve her looks for the new year. She appears to have realistic expectations and is well educated, via the Internet, about the different products available on the market. She has had previous breast augmentation surgery with satisfactory results.

PMHX/PDHX/MEDICATIONS/ALLERGIES/SH/FH

Noncontributory.

EXAMINATION

Maxillofacial. The patient does not have lymphadenopathy. Her facial skin is without any lesions, and her oral mucous membranes are moist. Oral hygiene is excellent. Nasal and maxillary dental midlines are aligned.

Evaluation of *volume* (height, fullness), *projection, vermillion exposure,* and *definition* of the lips is important in preparation for lip augmentation procedures.

Lips. The lips are symmetrical (Figure 12-1). The upper lip to lower lip height ratio is about 1:2 (in general, an aesthetic upper lip is one third of the total lip mass, and the lower lip represents two thirds of the total lip height). The upper lip is relatively deficient in volume compared with the lower lip. Cupid's bow and the vermillion border are well defined with good profile projection. Four millimeters of central incisors is visible at rest (normal range for females 3 to 4 mm, and that for males is 2 to 3 mm), with no gingival show on smiling (no "gummy" smile). She does not exhibit lip incompetence. The nasolabial angle is within normal limits ($100° \pm 10°$).

Normal aesthetic parameters for lips are differently defined among persons of different races and cultures, so "normal" parameters are not well established. As in any cosmetic procedure, patients' desires and expectations along with fashionable trends emphasized by the media and celebrities play a major role in patients' and surgeons' decisions for cosmetic intervention.

IMAGING

Standard frontal facial photographs and close-up views of the lips are routine. Profile and oblique preoperative and postoperative close-up views of the lips may also be helpful.

LABS

Lab tests are not indicated unless there is a known history of coagulopathies (increased risk of hematoma, bruising, and erythema at injection site). Unlike collagen, hyaluronic acid is identical among species, making it highly biocompatible and thus eliminating the need for allergy testing (see Complications).

ASSESSMENT

Patient desires upper lip augmentation to enhance both definition and volume

TREATMENT

Restylane is a stabilized, lower-molecular-weight, partially cross-linked hyaluronic acid that is Food and Drug Administration (FDA) approved for soft tissue augmentation. It is created via bacterial fermentation from streptococci species. This material has been used in Europe before 2000. Hylaform Gel is hyaluronic acid extract that is derived from rooster combs.

Bilateral infraorbital nerve blocks are given to achieve upper lip anesthesia without local infiltration in the areas to be augmented to avoid temporary tissue distortion secondary to the injection. The white roll is augmented on the upper lip, starting at the midline and following the contour of cupid's bow to enhance both definition and projection. The material is injected in a linear threading fashion as the needle is withdrawn away from the midline via two or three injection sites. The upper lips are intermittently massaged to achieve uniform distribution of the filler. The contralateral side is injected in a similar fashion. The body of the lip is also injected in a similar fashion to achieve volume enhancement of the lips. A total of one syringe was used for the upper lip (Figure 12-2).

Many surgeons actively involve the patient by allowing her to occasionally evaluate the lips in a mirror to achieve the

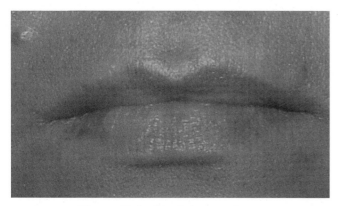

Figure 12-1   Lips before treatment.

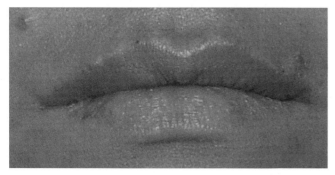

Figure 12-2   Lips after upper lip augmentation with Restylane.

desired effect and to give the patient a sense of participation in the treatment.

Other materials and techniques used for lip augmentation include AlloDerm (cadaveric acellular dermal collagen framework), polytetrafluoroethylene, autologous fat transfer/injection (harvested from periumbilical right medial thigh fat), injectable collagen, or a strip of superficial musculoaponeurotic system (SMAS), when concurrent facelift procedures are performed.

COMPLICATIONS

The ideal facial augmentation material should be inert, biocompatible, and safe and should remain stable over time. Bovine collagen has dominated the facial filler market until recently. The main concern associated with it is the risk of severe allergy, requiring the use of allergy skin testing before injection. The use of autologous collagen harvested from the patient's own skin eliminated the need for allergy testing, but it needs to be harvested, which involves associated morbidity and limited supply. Autologous fat also eliminates the need for skin testing, but it also involves harvesting. This may be desirable if simultaneous liposuction is being performed. Dermalogen (Collagenesis, Beverly, MA) is human collagen prepared from human donor tissue processed from cadavers. This material undergoes extensive screening for infectious agents and is irradiated before use. Skin testing is not required by the FDA.

Several formulations for hyaluronic acid are available for injection into soft tissue, but not all are FDA approved. Olenius conducted the first clinical study to evaluate biodegradable implants. He evaluated 113 subjects after injection with partially cross-linked hyaluronic acid and reported no allergic reactions and infrequent side effects, limited to localized erythema and swelling related to superficial placement of the material, small hematoma formation, and lumpiness secondary to uneven injection. In 2001, Lowe and associates studied 709 patients injected with hyaluronic acid preparations. They reported a 0.42% delayed inflammatory skin reactions that started about 8 weeks postinjection. A review of worldwide data on 144,000 patients treated in 1999 indicated that the major reaction to injectable hyaluronic acid was localized hypersensitivity, occurring in approximately 1 of every 1400 patients treated. This study concluded that hypersensitivity to non–animal-source hyaluronic acid gel is the major adverse event and is most likely secondary to impurities of bacterial fermentation. More recent data indicate that the incidence of hypersensitivity appears to be declining after the introduction of a more purified hyaluronic acid raw material.

Knowledge of vascular anatomy is essential. Case reports have been reported of intraarterial injection of hyaluronic acid causing localized skin changes and autologous fat embolization causing ocular and cerebral ischemia.

DISCUSSION

A common question asked by patients concerns the duration of the augmentation. In the study by Olenius, injection of partially cross-linked hyaluronic acid demonstrated the greatest degree of effectiveness at 2 weeks (98%) with subsequent decline at 3 months (82%), 6 months (69%), and 1 year (66%). Although the effects of this filler are not permanent, repeat injections may require smaller amounts of filler to achieve similar results.

It is essential that surgeons do not apply a single method of augmentation for every patient who presents to the office. Accurate diagnosis of the facial deformity or the desired effect is the key to satisfactory outcomes. Concurrent knowledge of multiple techniques, safety profiles of the existing materials, and their clinical effects is essential for successful soft tissue augmentation.

Bibliography

Danesh-Meyer HV, Savino PJ, Sergott RC: Case reports and small case series: ocular and cerebral ischemia following facial injection of autologous fat, *Arch Ophthalmol* 119(5):777-778, 2001.

Douglas RS, Donsoff I, Cook T, et al: Collagen fillers in facial aesthetic surgery, *Fac Plast Surg* 20(2):117-123, 2004.

Duranti F, Salti G, Bovani B, et al: Injectable hyaluronic acid gel for soft tissue augmentation. A clinical and histological study, *Dermatol Surg* 24(12):1317-1325, 1998.

Fagien S: Facial soft-tissue augmentation with injectable autologous and allogeneic human tissue collagen matrix (autologen and dermalogen), *Plast Reconstr Surg* 105(1):362-373; discussion 374-375, 2000.

Friedman PM, Mafong EA, Kauvar AN, et al: Safety data of injectable nonanimal stabilized hyaluronic acid gel for soft tissue augmentation, *Dermatol Surg* 28(6):491-494, 2002.

Lowe NJ, Maxwell CA, Lowe P, et al: Hyaluronic acid skin fillers: adverse reactions and skin testing, *Am Acad Dermatol* 45(6):930-933, 2001.

Niamtu J: New lip and wrinkle fillers, *Oral Maxillofac Surg Clin N Am* 17(1):17-28, 2005.

Olenius M: The first clinical study using a new biodegradable implant for the treatment of lips, wrinkles, and folds, *Aesthetic Plast Surg* 22(2):97-101, 1998.

Schanz S, Schippert W, Ulmer A, et al: Arterial embolization caused by injection of hyaluronic acid (Restylane), *Br J Dermatol* 146(5):928-929, 2002.

Rhinoplasty

Shahrokh C. Bagheri, DMD, MD, and Chris Jo, DMD

CC

A 24-year-old woman presents for consultation regarding her nose. She explains that it is too bulky and she does not like the "bump" on it.

HPI

The patient works in the beauty industry but has become aware of the shape of her nose since college. Several years ago, she noticed the prominence of her nasal dorsum and the bulky mid dorsal area when she looks in the mirror. In addition, she complains of difficulty breathing through her right nostril. She reports to breathing better through the left nostril, and when she pulls her right cheek inferiorly and laterally, she experiences improved airflow through the right nostril (positive Cottle sign).

PMHX/PDHX/MEDICATIONS/ALLERGIES/SH/FH

The patient has no previous history of septoplasty, cosmetic rhinoplasty, or nasal trauma (previous nasal surgery is particularly important because the anatomy may be altered. If the septal cartilage has be previously harvested or adjusted and there is a need for cartilage grafting, the ear cartilage can be used). She denies any seasonal or drug allergies (important to note symptoms of allergic rhinitis or recent upper respiratory tract infections). There is no history of psychiatric disorders or treatment (patients with certain psychiatric disorders may not be candidates for elective cosmetic procedures). There is no history of smoking or cocaine or other drug use (cocaine-induced vasoconstriction will compromise wound healing and increase the risk of septal perforation). She also has no history of granulomatous or autoimmune disorders (such as Wegener granulomatosis, which can affect the nasal mucosa) or of epistaxis (prior history of unexplained epistaxis should be investigated for blood dyscrasias such as von Willebrand disease).

EXAMINATION

Examination of the nose for cosmetic surgery has to include both cosmetic and functional factors. Cosmetic evaluation should encompass the entire face, but for planning purposes, the nose can be examined in five regions:

1. Skin
2. Radix
3. Dorsum
4. Tip
5. Nostrils and alar base

Each region is evaluated in three dimensions. The functional aspects of the nose (mainly breathing) require a careful endonasal speculum examination. Correction of cosmetic parameters may cause or exacerbate nasal function (e.g., narrowing the nose may compromise breathing).

General. The patient is a well-developed and well-nourished woman with realistic expectations and knowledge of nasal cosmetic surgery.

Maxillofacial. There is no evidence of upper respiratory infection (no postnasal drip, discharge, or erythema of mucous membranes).

Examination of the Nose

- **Skin.** The skin meets the criteria of Fitzpatrick type II with no evidence of acne or excessive sebaceous secretions. Skin and soft tissue envelope have adequate thickness over the dorsum and tip (Figure 12-3).
- **Radix.** Soft tissue nasion is between the lash and crease line of the upper lid (within normal limits). The nasofacial angle is 34° (within normal limits).
- **Dorsum.** There is a prominent dorsal hump on the profile view (Figure 12-4). The mid dorsum is rectangular in shape on the frontal view. The nasal dorum is wide but symmetrical.
- **Tip.** The tip is slightly bulbous with prominent lower lateral cartilages. The nasolabial angle is 100° (normal is approximately 105°).
- **Nasal base.** There is adequate width (coincident with the medial canthus). The nostrils are symmetrical, with no significant nostril show or hanging columella.
- **Speculum exam.** Linear deviation of the quadrangular cartilage (nasal septum) to the right and partial blockage of the right internal nasal valve (the angle formed by the nasal septum and upper lateral cartilage). There is compensatory inferior turbinate hypertrophy on the left, with mild erythema of the nasal mucosa and turbinates.

IMAGING

Preoperative and serial postoperative photoimaging is mandatory for cosmetic procedures. Standard photography for cosmetic rhinoplasty includes frontal, right and left lateral, right and left oblique, and basal ("worm's eye") views. Photographs should be standardized to allow optimal preoperative and postoperative comparisons.

CEPHALIC   **DORSUM**

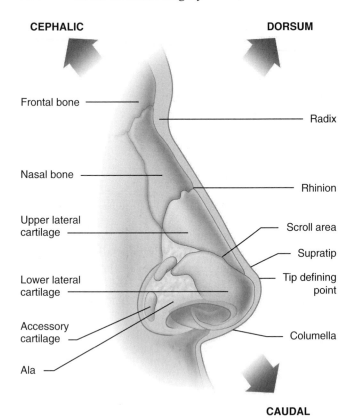

CAUDAL

Figure 12-3 Anatomy of nasal structures as seen from profile.

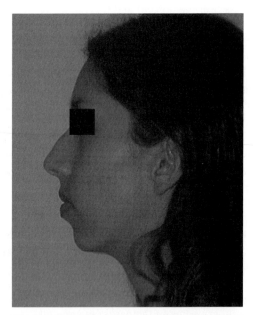

Figure 12-4 Preoperative facial profile before septorhinoplasty.

Computed tomography (CT) is not necessary for cosmetic rhinoplasty, but it can be used in selected cases to delineate the severity of septal deviation and identify sinus pathology.

LABS

No routine laboratory testing is indicated for cosmetic rhinoplasty unless dictated by the medical history.

ASSESSMENT

Patient desires cosmetic rhinoplasty: prominent dorsal hump on profile; wide nasal dorum on frontal view ("boxy dorsum"); bulbous tip as seen on the frontal view, with good projection; deviated septum with compromised right nasal valve function

It is important to assess both the cosmetic and the functional aspects of the diagnosis.

TREATMENT

Treatment is dependent not only on the physical findings (diagnosis) but, more important, also on the patient's desires and expectations. This is best achieved by establishing an open line of communication and exact identification of patient goals. This patient complains of a large nose and difficulty breathing through the right nostril. Treatment should address both the aesthetic and functional disturbances. Cosmetic alterations frequently exacerbate functional parameters. The surgical plan must be developed preoperatively, based on the patient's function and cosmetic desires and needs.

The surgical approach (endonasal versus open rhinoplasty) is dependent on the complexity of the case and the experience and preference of the surgeon. Incisions for endonasal rhinoplasty include (Figure 12-5):

- Intercartilaginous or limen vestibula incision (between the upper and lower lateral cartilages)
- Intracartilaginous or cartilage splitting incision (through the upper aspect of the lateral crura of the lower lateral cartilage)
- Infracartilaginous or marginal incision (on the inferior aspect of the lower lateral cartilage)

Standard incisions to approach the nasal septum include the transfixion incision (through the membranous septum) or the Killian incision (incision over the cartilaginous septum). Most simple rhinoplasties can be done via an endonasal approach. However, if complex tip work or spreader grafts are required, an open transcollumellar incision allows greater access and visibility than the cartilage delivery approach. The scar from this incision is usually not visible several months after the procedure.

For any rhinoplasty surgery, a treatment plan should be outlined to address patient desires within the confines of the surgeon's ability to achieve the outcome and without compromise of nasal function. The following surgical plan was made for this patient:

Open Septorhinoplasty

1. Septoplasty and harvest of septal cartilage
2. Submucus resection and turbinate outfracture
3. Transcolumellar incision for access to the dorsum, septum, and nasal valve
4. Reduction of the nasal dorsum (rasp or osteotome reduction)
5. Nasal tip refinement (resection and/or suture techniques can be used based on the surgeon's preference)

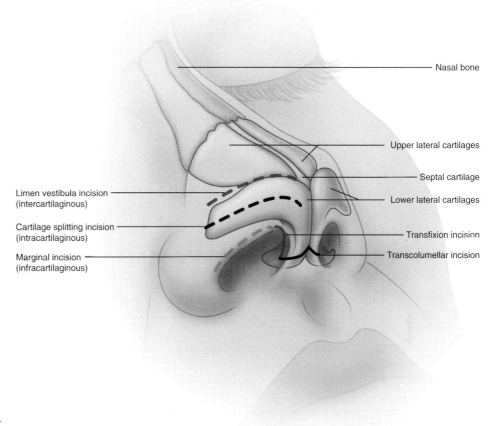

Nasal bone

Upper lateral cartilages

Septal cartilage

Lower lateral cartilages

Transfixion incision

Transcolumellar incision

Limen vestibula incision
(intercartilaginous)

Cartilage splitting incision
(intracartilaginous)

Marginal incision
(infracartilaginous)

Figure 12-5   Common sites of incisions for rhinoplasty.

6. Bilateral spreader grafts (from septum) for opening of the nasal valves
7. Bilateral low to high nasal osteotomies for narrowing of the dorsum and closure of the "open book" deformity

Under general anesthesia, lidocaine with epinephrine was injected along the nasal septum, columella, dorsum, and nostril areas, and adequate time was given for vasoconstriction (some surgeons limit the amount of subcutaneous local anesthetic injection to minimize tissue distortion for improved intraoperative assessment). A septoplasty and septal cartilage harvest were performed via a left hemitransfixion incision (a minimum of 1-cm strut of dorsal and caudal cartilage should be left intact for adequate support) followed by submucosal resection with lateral displacement of the right inferior turbinate. Careful attention was given to maintain adequate dorsal and columellar cartilage to avoid a saddle nose deformity. An open rhinoplasty (inverted V transcolumellar with infracartilaginous incisions) was performed with subsequent resection of 4 mm of the cephalic margin of the lower lateral cartilages (cephalic trim or volumetric reduction). Domal equalization and creation sutures were used to provide tip definition (some surgeons may elect to split the domes). Reduction of the bony dorsum was performed using a rasp, followed by excision of the cartilaginous dorsum using fine scissors. Strut and shield grafts were not used in this patient (although some authors suggest that strut and shield grafts be used in most patients). The nasal tip was supported by suturing the medial crura of the lower lateral cartilages to the nasal septum (a columellar strut can be used to achieve greater tip projection). The septum was disarticulated from the upper lateral cartilages bilaterally, and a spreader graft was placed (to increase the internal nasal valve). Finally, low-to-high lateral nasal osteotomies were performed, and the nasal complex was fractured in to close the open "book deformity" and address the width of the dorsum. Figure 12-6 demonstrates the postoperative patient profile.

COMPLICATIONS

Cosmetic rhinoplasty is a difficult procedure to master. It is imperative to recognize complications early and not ignore a potentially correctable finding. Management of a dissatisfied patient can be challenging, but foresight, honesty, and a caring approach frequently aid in resolving an unsatisfactory outcome. These unsatisfactory outcomes may include a polly beak, saddle-nose, open roof deformity, undercorrection, dorsal irregularities, nasal tip deformities, or asymmetrical dorsum/tip. An overall revision rhinoplasty rate of 5% to 15% has been reported. Other reported complications include hemorrhage (1% to 4%), infection (0% to 3%), septal perforation (0.1%), skin sloughing (rare), and nasal obstruction (1% to 10%).

Patients undergoing open rhinoplasty should be informed about the postoperative anesthesia or profound hypoesthesia

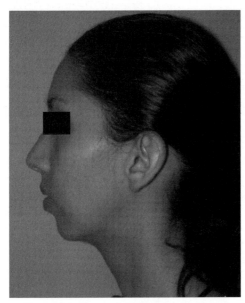

Figure 12-6 Postoperative facial profile after septorhinoplasty.

of the nasal tip. This is usually temporary but can take 6 months to 1 year to resolve.

DISCUSSION

The most important factor is a successful cosmetic rhinoplasty is patient selection. Equally important is the surgeon's ability to recognize his or her limitations in meeting the patient's cosmetic demands. The nose needs to be examined in conjunction with the rest of the face, and considerable attention needs to be given to the patient's ethnic background. Most normal anatomical nasal measurements in the literature are for Caucasians, and therefore treatment planning must be done with caution. A systematic approach to analyze the nose both as a component of the face and as an independent entity is essential. For example, a prominent nose may be accentuated by a hypoplastic mandible or chin, and the patient may benefit from an advancement genioplasty or alloplastic augmentation. Additionally, both cosmetic and functional aspects need to be addressed and anticipated. It is imperative for the surgeon to realize that an optimal cosmetic outcome may compromise nasal function. A good example is internal nasal valve compromise secondary to excessive nasal dorsum narrowing. Additional procedures such as spreader grafts (cartilaginous graft between nasal septum and upper lateral cartilage) to widen the nasal valve area may be considered.

Bibliography

Beekhuis GH: Nasal obstruction after rhinoplasty: etiology and techniques for correction, *Laryngoscope* 86:540, 1976.

Daniel RK: *Rhinoplasty: an atlas of surgical techniques,* New York, 2002, Springer.

Kamer FN, McQuown SA: Revision rhinoplasty, *Arch Otolaryngol Head Neck Surg* 114:257, 1988.

Maniglia AJ: Fatal and major complications secondary to nasal and sinus surgery, *Laryngoscope* 99:276, 1989.

Teichgraeber JF, Riley WB, Parks DH: Nasal surgery complications, *Plast Reconstr Surg* 85:527, 1990.

Teichgraeber JF, Russo RC: Treatment of nasal surgery complications, *Ann Plast Surg* 30:80, 1993.

Cervicofacial Rhytidectomy (Facelift)

Chris Jo, DMD, and Shahrokh C. Bagheri, DMD, MD

CC

A 52-year-old white woman presents to your office for evaluation for possible facial cosmetic surgery. She complains of excessive skin laxity and wrinkling in her face and neck.

Although the majority of patients seeking facial cosmetic surgery are females, there is an increasing trend of male patients. Given the elective nature of facial cosmetic surgery, the chief complaint should strongly influence the selection of surgical procedures. It is our belief that for successful cosmetic surgery, the surgeon should focus on facilitating patient desires, as opposed to "selling" any procedure that falls within the surgeon's armamentarium.

HPI

The patient has no history of prior facial cosmetic surgery. She had recently attended a cosmetic seminar at your office, which has sparked her interest in facial surgery (unlike other aspects of oral and maxillofacial surgery, a successful facial cosmetic practice requires adequate marketing and patient education). The patient specifically points to her jowls, cheeks, and submental regions, explaining that she has progressively noticed "sagging" of her face and neck over the past 3 years. She is constantly aware of her appearance to the point that it consistently bothers her, and she desires a more youthful appearance of her face. She reports using sunscreen and tries to avoid sunlight exposure because she does not tan and burns rather easily (Fitzpatrick type I skin).

The two most important factors related to the aging of skin are sunlight exposure and individual genetic characteristics. The latter cannot be altered, and therefore exposure to sunlight is the single most important factor in skin care. Many skin care products are available on the market, most of which work by either promoting hydration, protecting from ultraviolet light, or facilitating exfoliation of superficial epithelium and dead cells.

PMHX/PDHX/MEDICATIONS/ALLERGIES/SH/FH

The patient has hypertension, which is well controlled with Lopressor HCT (combination β-blocker with thiazide diuretic [metoprolol, hydrochlorothiazide]). The perioperative control of blood pressure is paramount for prevention of postoperative hematoma).

She is also taking aspirin 81 mg daily for cardioprotective effects (aspirin or other nonsteroidal antiinflammatory drugs that interfere with platelet function should be stopped before facelift procedures. Generally, it is recommended to discontinue aspirin 2 weeks before and for 1 week after the procedure, to reduce the risk of hematoma formation).

She denies smoking or illicit drug use (smoking is associated with an increased risk of flap necrosis. Ideally, all nicotine-containing products should be stopped 4 to 6 weeks before cervicofacial rhytidectomy. Patients unable to quit smoking may be candidates for less invasive procedures such as the "S-lift," or short flap rhytidectomy).

There is no prior history of fever blisters (prophylaxis is required when concomitant laser or chemical resurfacing is performed). Facelift procedures should be postponed in the presence of active herpes simplex virus blisters.

EXAMINATION

General. The patient is a well-developed and well-nourished, pleasant woman in no apparent distress.

Maxillofacial (divided into bony and soft tissue examination).

- **Bony structure.** The facial structures are symmetrical with good malar projection and symmetrical mandibular angles. There is no orbital dystopia (difference in position of the globe). The bony nasal pyramid and nasal tip are midline, with no dorsal hump. Examination of the nasal septum reveals no deviation. The hyoid bone is in good position (a low, anterior hyoid position compromises aesthetic results in the neck).
- The maxillary and mandibular dental midlines are coincident with the face. The occlusion is class I skeletal relationship. The chin is symmetrical with good anteroposterior and vertical dimensions (recognition and subsequent correction of microgenia can significantly improve the facial contour of the chin and neck).
- **Soft tissue.** The eyebrows are in good position (in the female patient, the apex of eyebrow should be approximately 8 to 10 mm above the superior orbital rim and between the lateral limbus and canthus).
- Upper eyelids show minimal dermatochalasis (excessive eyelid skin laxity).
- There is no lateral hooding (excess skin of the lateral portion of the upper eyelid descending past the eyelid margin and obstructing vision in the lateral gaze).
- There is no upper eyelid ptosis (upper lid margin should cover 2 to 3 mm of the superior iris). The lower eyelids show good contour with no fat herniation. The snap test is normal (lower lid should reapproximate the globe

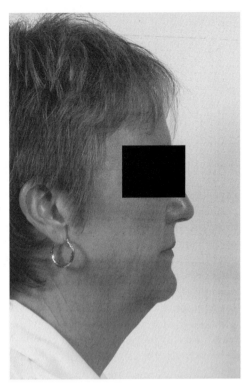

Figure 12-7 Preoperative profile view illustrating the extent of soft tissue descent and laxity with mandibular jowling and blunting of the cervicomental angle.

within 1 second when it is pulled inferiorly and released).
- The nasolabial groove is deepened (formed by insertions of the zygomaticus muscles) and the nasolabial fold is full (caused by descent of the malar fat pad).
- There is moderate jowling most pronounced at the lower facial third and neck, causing blunting of the inferior border of the mandible.
- Moderate submental lipomatosis and skin laxity are present with poorly defined cervicomental (cervical-submental) angle and visible platysmal bands (Figure 12-7). An aesthetically pleasing neck is defined as having a cervicosubmental angle of 115° ± 10°, distinct inferior border of the mandible, anterior border of the sternocleidomastoid muscle, a depression posterior and inferior to the angle of the mandible, gentle contours without bands or folds, smooth skin, proportionate length, and a slight prominence of the thyroid cartilage in men.
- **Dermatological.** The patient has fair skin (Fitzpatrick skin type I: ivory white fair skin that never tans and always burns).
- She is Glogau type II skin classification (early to moderate photoaging with wrinkles in motion, typically appearing in the fourth decade of life).
- There are fine dynamic cervicofacial rhytids in the periorbital (crow's feet) and perioral (marionette lines) regions.

IMAGING

Standard preoperative and postoperative photodocumentation is mandatory for the facelift patient and should include a full frontal view in repose and with a full smile, right and left three-quarter oblique views, and bilateral profile views.

LABS

In the absence of any significant medical problems, no routine laboratory testing is necessary for a cervicofacial rhytidectomy. Coagulation studies may be obtained if there is any suspicion of undiagnosed blood dyscrasias. An electrocardiogram is obtained based on patient age and risk factors for cardiovascular disease. A complete blood count and electrolyte panels can be obtained as needed.

ASSESSMENT

Patient desiring facelift procedure secondary to cutis laxis, designated as type III cervical facial laxity (defined as moderate redundancy and jowling, platysmal banding, accentuated nasolabial folds, and variable degrees of cervical facial lipomatosis)

Dedo's classification of facial profiles categorizes the lower facial third into six distinct groups:
- Class I (normal)
- Class II (cervical skin laxity)
- Class III (submental lipomatosis)
- Class IV (platysmal banding)
- Class V (retrognathia or microgenia)
- Class VI (low hyoid bone)

TREATMENT

Cervicofacial rhytidectomy and submental lipectomy with platysmaplasty (commonly known as a "full facelift") is the gold standard for treatment of type III cervical facial laxity. All modern facelift techniques involve modifications to the SMAS to achieve lasting cosmetic outcomes. The SMAS was first accurately described in 1976 by Mitz and Peyronie. Four basic approaches can be applied for correction of cervicofacial redundancy:
1. Meloplication (e.g., barbed suture)
2. An S-lift (described by Saylan, which now has several modifications for incision designs and SMAS suspension suturing techniques)
3. Superficial plane facelift
4. Deep plane facelift

Each technique has various modifications described in the literature. The two most commonly used rhytidoplasty techniques used are the S-lift and the superficial plane facelift with various incision designs for management of the SMAS, the platysma muscle, and suspension suturing techniques.

The superficial rhytidectomy with platysmaplasty is described here:

The incision design must be carefully planned and differs between surgeons based on preference and technique (needs modification for male patients to preserve sideburns). First, the preauricular region is marked along the preauricular skin crease. Some surgeons prefer an endaural for improved scar camouflage, but it is often criticized for causing tragal deformities. The retroauricular incision is carried onto the posterior surface of the conchal bowl (in the crease for men) up to the level of the external auditory canal. It then makes a right angle turn onto the mastoid skin and gently fades into the hairline. The temporal incision can extend superiorly from the preauricular incision as a temporal extension or can be made perpendicular to end at the anterior temporal tuft of hair (this incision should be beveled to allow regrowth of hair to hide the scar). A 3-cm curvilinear horizontal incision is marked in the submental region 3 mm posterior to the submental crease. This incision will be used for submental lipectomy and platysmaplasty.

Next, tumescent solution is injected into the submental and submandibular triangles and bilateral cheek areas in the superficial fat layer (tumescent has been shown to facilitate dissection and reduce postoperative complications). Local anesthetic with epinephrine can be injected into the incision sites.

Dissection begins in the submental region. A skin subcutaneous flap is elevated (leaving 3 to 5 mm of fat attached to the dermis). The boundaries of dissection should be the inferior border of the mandible, anterior border of the sternocleidomastoid, and 3 cm beyond the inferior border of the area of neck ptosis. Excessive fat is sharply removed and gentle open liposuction is performed. The central aponeurosis/fascia-platysma muscle complex and deep fat are sharply excised to identify the anterior borders of the platysma muscle. A suture platysmaplasty is performed to close this decussation (platysma suspension sutures and "Giampapa sutures" can be placed here to engage the anterior platysma border at the depth of the new cervicosubmental angle, which will be suspended later to the contralateral mastoid fascia).

Next, the preauricular and postauricular incisions are made along the previous markings. A superficial flap is developed using facelift scissors. This dissection joins the submental dissection that was previously carried out. Once the flap has been completely developed, the SMAS and platysma may be mobilized in a posterosuperior vector via a variety of techniques (imbrication, plication, lateral SMAS-ectomy, etc.).

We prefer the lateral SMAS-ectomy as described by Baker in 2000, in which a 1.5- to 2-cm strip of SMAS parallel to the nasolabial fold (from the malar eminence to angle of the mandible) is sharply excised and the margins reapproximated with 3-0 Vicryl sutures. This maneuver elevates the SMAS in a posterosuperior vector. Other surgeons prefer to fold the SMAS upon itself (plication) with sutures, whereas others prefer to incise the posterior aspect of SMAS and perform sub-SMAS dissection with imbrication of the SMAS. The posterior border of the platysma/SMAS is identified and suspended to the mastoid fascia (if platysma suspension sutures

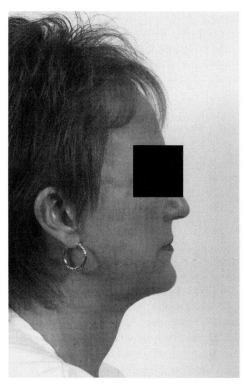

Figure 12-8 Postoperative profile view following a full face and neck lift using a superficial rhytidectomy technique. Note the creation of a distinct cervicomental angle and improvement of the mandibular jowl and nasolabial folds.

were placed earlier, they are also sutured to the mastoid fascia).

The skin-subcutaneous tissue flap is then allowed to passively redrape by sweeping the flap in a posterosuperior vector without excessive tension. The flap beds are checked for hemostasis (meticulous attention to hemostasis will reduce the incidence of postoperative hematoma). Platelet-rich plasma or fibrin glue can be sprayed beneath the flaps (shown to decrease incidence of seroma, edema, and ecchymoses). Key sutures are placed superiorly at the superior helix and at the lobule of the ear. Excess skin in the preauricular and postauricular region is excised with facelift scissors and closed in layers (5-0 PDS in subcutaneous and 6-0 Ethicon for skin) and removed in 7 days. The excess skin in the temporal (vertical or horizontal) and mastoid region is excised and carefully closed. Finally, the submental incision is inspected for hemostasis and closed in layers. A pressure dressing is applied (some surgeons still prefer to use drains instead of platelet-rich plasma or fibrin sealant) (Figure 12-8).

COMPLICATIONS

Hematoma is the most common postoperative complication (incidence of 0% to 9%) and can lead to prolonged facial edema and skin necrosis. Hematomas (most commonly occurring within the first 24 hours) can be classified as either large ("major" or "expanding") hematomas that require immediate surgical intervention (evacuation of hematoma and achieve hemostasis) or minor hematoma ("microhematoma") that can be treated with needle aspiration and/or massage therapy. Signs include increased facial pain (especially when unilateral), swelling, tightening of facial dressing, or ecchymosis of buccal mucosa, lips, and neck.

Jones and Grover in 2004 reviewed 678 consecutive superficial facelifts and found no significant difference in major hematoma rates between groups treated with pressure dressing, drains, fibrin glue, or tumescence (overall rate of 4.4%). When comparing tumescent with and without epinephrine, they found that the epinephrine-containing group had a 4.8% hematoma rate compared with 0% none in the control group. A separate study by the same authors showed that a tumescent technique significantly reduces the incidence of skin necrosis (14:1), alopecia (19:1), hypertrophic scarring (25:1), stretched scarring (21:1), and subsequent scar revision. Griffin and Jo in 2006 reviewed 178 consecutive facelifts and reported a 2.8% incidence of major hematoma and 1.7% incidence of minor hematoma after superficial rhytidectomy.

In 1976, Berner and associates found that postoperative hypertension to be an etiological factor in hematoma formation after rhytidectomy. Straith and colleagues in 1977 found that an admission blood pressure greater than 150/100 mm Hg had a 2.6 times greater incidence of hematoma formation. In the following year, Rees and Aston found that intraoperative hypotension increases the risk of hematoma, which was attributed to subsequent rebound hypertension. All three studies strongly suggest that blood pressure should be well controlled throughout the perioperative period. Kamer and Kushnick in 1995 found a twofold increase in expanding hematoma (2% versus 4.2%) when propofol was used for anesthesia, which caused a drop in systolic blood pressure by 26% versus a 16% drop in the control group not receiving propofol.

Fibrin glue has been used to reduce the incidence of seroma. Oliver and colleagues in 2001 prospectively showed that fibrin glue reduces the amount of serosanguinous output, which obviated the need for drains to prevent seromas (no effect on incidence of major hematoma). Marchac and Sandor in 1994 reported a significant reduction in major hematoma and ecchymoses when using fibrin sealant, without the need of drains or pressure dressings. However, in a later study, Jones and Grover did not find a difference in major hematoma rates when fibrin glue was used.

Platelet-rich plasma is used by some surgeons for its ability to enhance soft tissue healing and decrease the amount of edema and ecchymoses. Man and colleagues in 2000 and Powell and colleagues in 2001 reported the benefits of platelet-rich plasma when used in cervicofacial rhytidectomy. Neither fibrin glue, platelet-rich plasma, nor other adjunctive maneuvers is a good substitute to meticulous hemostasis for prevention of major postoperative hematomas (Palaia and colleagues in 2001 found that DDAVP [desmopressin] reduces the incidence of minor hematoma).

Seromas can also cause delayed wound healing and therefore should be aspirated. Perkins and associates in 1997 found

that placing suction drains significantly decreases the incidence of seroma (37% without drains versus 15% with drains). However, hematoma rates remained similar in the two groups. The differential diagnosis of a fluctuant swelling beneath the flap must also include a parotid pseudocyst (resulting from damage to the parotid gland parenchyma). McKinney and associates in 1996 found that placing a suction drain, rather than repeated aspirations and pressure dressings, allowed more rapid resolution of parotids pseudocysts (within 1 week).

Postsurgical auricular deformities (downward and forward auricular displacement and rotation, increased auriculocephalic angle, hidden or buried tragus, pixie ear deformity) can occur but can be minimized by attention to suture anchoring of the soft tissue flaps.

Direct injury to facial nerve branches is a rare complication. Almost all motor nerve injuries are temporary. One review of 7000 cases of superficial rhytidectomy from multiple surgeons reported 55 cases of motor nerve injury (temporal and marginal mandibular branches most commonly injured), seven of which were permanent. Hamra in 1992 found that deep plane dissection was most likely to encounter temporary paresis of the upper lip and cause injury to the frontal branch. He also found a higher incidence of pseudoparesis of the lower lip due to platysmal transaction.

The greater auricular nerve (C2-3) is the most common sensory nerve to be injured during a facelift. It crosses the posterior border of the sternocleidomastoid muscle at Erb's point (along with three other cutaneous branches of the cervical plexus: lesser occipital, transverse cervical, and supraclavicular nerves). It supplies the skin of the back of the ear, mastoid region, and angle of the mandible.

Daane and Owsley in 2003 reviewed 2002 cases and found 1.7% incidence of pseudoparalysis of the marginal mandibular nerve, in which the lower lip eversion was intact but an asymmetrical "full denture-type smile" was caused by injury to the cervical branch of the facial nerve or direct platysmal injury. All cases fully recovered within 3 weeks to 6 months.

The most feared of all complications is flap necrosis and slough (incidence of 0% to 3%). This is the result of vascular compromise (decreased arterial perfusion, venous congestion, small vessel disease seen with diabetes mellitus and smoking). Other causes include late hematoma evacuation and wide undermining with a wound closed under tension. Small areas of necrosis along the flap edge most commonly occur in the postauricular region (allow to heal by secondary intention). Smoking significantly increases the risk of skin slough because of its negative effect on wound healing and flap vascularity. Rees and colleagues in 1984 reported a 12 times greater risk for skin slough in smokers. Webster and associates in 1986 found that a conservative technique was safe in smokers and advocated using the S-lift for noncompliant patients. It is recommended that the patient stop smoking 4 to 6 weeks preoperatively and 2 to 4 weeks postoperatively. Wellbutrin is reported to be a good therapy for smoking cessation. Ice packs should be avoided because they may cause decreased flap perfusion.

DISCUSSION

Facial aging is the result of progressive gravitational descent of soft tissue that occurs in a predictable course based on anatomical and biologic certainties, which must be understood for facial rejuvenation surgery. The genetic differences between individuals will give each patient their own unique variations (timing and extent) of facial aging (skin laxity, soft tissue descent, fat atrophy and volume loss, orbital fat herniation, loss of facial volume, bony resorption of the anterior facial skeleton, and skin changes). Facial subcutaneous tissue, fascia, and overlying skin are supported or "anchored" by four true retaining ligaments (orbital, zygomatic, buccal-maxillary, and mandibular) and by three false retaining ligaments (platysma-auricular, buccal-maxillary, and masseteric-cutaneous). Areas of the face that have loosely adherent areolar tissue become preferentially ptotic. These loose areolar planes exist in the forehead and eyebrow region, the temporal region, the anterior and middle cheek, and in the lower face and neck, and they account for the characteristic pattern of facial aging in the upper face, mid-face, and lower face and neck.

The aging pattern of the upper face is characterized by horizontal forehead lines (frontalis muscle hypertrophy), oblique and transverse frown lines (corrugator and procerus muscles, respectively), soft tissue descent over the lower forehead (due to depressor muscle tone overwhelming frontalis muscle), and soft tissue descent of the unsupported temporal tissue overlying the temporalis fascia (causing eyebrow ptosis and contributing to an aged upper eyelid appearance). Rejuvenation of the upper face will be discussed in a separate section (see sections on Endoscopic Brow-Lift and Upper and Lower Eyelid Blepharoplasty later in this chapter).

The aging pattern of the mid-face is characterized by attenuation and lengthening of the soft tissues causing ptosis and pseudoherniation of the orbital fat pads and suborbicularis oculi fat pad. Also, loss of support from the retaining ligaments of the mid-face causes descent of the malar fat pad resulting in a deepened nasolabial groove, thickened nasolabial fold, and a hollowing of the upper mid-face.

The aging pattern of the lower face and neck is characterized by ptosis of midfacial soft tissue and fat (facial SMAS complex loses adherence and support from deep facial fascia and bone) that descends behind the mandibular retaining ligament and below the inferior border of the mandible (results in "jowling" and blunting of the inferior border of the mandible). The major plane of aging in the neck is the deep fat (areolar) layer (subfascia-platysma layer) due to the release of central adherence between the superficial cervical fascia and superficial layer of deep cervical fascia. This manifests as laxity in the submental region, blunting of the cervical-submental angle with lipomatosis or fat atrophy of the superficial fat layer, lipomatosis of the central deep fat layer, and platysma bands.

Most facial cosmetic surgeons prefer the superficial plane facelift due to its technical simplicity, decreased operating time, decreased recovery time, decreased morbidity, and good patient satisfaction. Many other surgeons advocate the deep plane facelift for its long-term stability and more natural rejuvenated appearance. Deep plane rhytidectomy was first introduced by Skoog in 1974 and has been popularized by the works of Owsley, Hamra, Barton and others. The philosophy behind deep place facelifts is that the skin, subcutaneous tissue, platysma muscle, and SMAS should be elevated as one unit off the underlying facial muscles and repositioned to restore a more youthful appearance. This composite rhytidectomy technique is beyond the scope of this section.

Recently, minimally invasive techniques (contour thread lifts) have been developed to rejuvenate the aging face. Although it is celebrated for its simplicity in technique, its short- and long-term stability is questionable.

Examination and treatment for facial cosmetic surgery should focus on the hard and soft tissues. Optimal cosmetic results are often obtained by combining surgical procedures that involve the underlying bony architecture, as well as the soft tissue envelope. Recent trends in maxillofacial aesthetics place greater emphasis on addressing the hard tissue deformities of the dentofacial region. Knowledge of orthognathic surgery, orthodontics, and dental aesthetics can be beneficial to the facial cosmetic surgeon, allowing oral and maxillofacial surgeons to better serve the cosmetic needs of many patients.

Bibliography

Baker D: Rhytidectomy with lateral SMASectomy, *Fac Plast Surg* 16:209-213, 2000.

Berner RE, Morain WD, Noe JM: Postoperative hypertension as an etiological factor in hematoma after rhytidectomy, *Plast Reconstr Surg* 57:314, 1976.

Brink RR: Auricular displacement with rhytidectomy, *Plast Reconstr Surg* 108(3):743-749, 2001.

Chisholm BB: Surgical facial rhytidectomy: the evolution of an esthetic concept, *Oral Maxillofac Surg Clin N Am* 12:719-728, 2000.

Daane SP, Owsley JQ: Incidence of cervical branch injury with "marginal mandibular nerve pseudo-paralysis" in patients undergoing face lift, *Plast Reconstr Surg* 111(7):2414-2418, 2003.

Evans TW, Stepanyan M: Isolated cervicoplasty, *Am J Cosmet Surg* 19:91-113, 2002.

Ghali GE, Smith BR: A case for superficial rhytidectomy, *J Oral Maxillofac Surg* 56:349-51, 1998.

Griffin JE, Epker BN: Correction of cervicofacial deformities, *Atlas Oral Maxillofacial Surg Clin N Am* 12:179-197, 2004.

Griffin JE, Jo C: Complications after superficial plane cervicofacial rhytidectomy: a retrospective analysis of 175 consecutive face-lifts and review of the literature, *J Oral Maxillofac Surg* Aug/Sept, 2007.

Hamra ST: Composite rhytidectomy, *Plast Reconstr Surg* 90:1-11, 1992.

Hamra ST: Prevention and correction of the "face-lifted" appearance, *Fac Plast Surg* 16:215-229, 2000.

Jones BM, Grover R: Reducing complications in cervicofacial rhytidectomy by tumescent infiltration: a comparative trial evaluating 678 consecutive face lifts, *Plast Reconstr Surg* 113(1): 398-403, 2004.

Jones BM, Grover R: Avoiding hematoma in cervicofacial rhytidectomy: a personal 8-year quest. Reviewing 910 patients, *Plast Reconstr Surg* 113(1):381-387, 2004.

Kamer F, Kushnick SD: The effect of propofol on hematoma formation in rhytidectomy, *Arch Otolaryngol Head Neck Surg* 121(6):658-661, 1995.

Man D, Plosker H, Wildland-Brown JE: The use of autologous platelet-rich plasma (platelet gel) and autologous platelet-poor plasma (fibrin glue) in cosmetic surgery, *Plast Reconstr Surg* 107(1):229-237, 2000.

Marchac D, Sandor G: Face lifts and sprayed fibrin glue: an outcome analysis of 200 patients, *Br J Plast Surg* 47(5):306-309, 1994.

McKinney P, et al: Management of parotid leakage following rhytidectomy, *Plast Reconstr Surg* 98(5):795-797, 1996.

Mitz V, Peyronie M: The superficial musculo-aponeurotic system (SMAS) in the parotid and cheek area, *Plast Reconstr Surg* 38:80-88, 1976.

Newman JP, et al: Distortion of the auriculocephalic angle following rhytidectomy: recognition and prevention, *Arch Otolaryngol Head Neck Surg* 123(8):818-820, 1997.

Obagi S, Bridenstine JB: Chemical skin resurfacing, *Oral Maxillofac Surg Clin N Am* 12:541-553, 2000.

Oliver DW, et al: A prospective, randomized, double-blind trial of the use of fibrin sealant for face lifts, *Plast Reconstr Surg* 108(7):2102-2105, 2001.

Palaia DA, Rosenberg MH, Bonanno PC: The use of DDAVP desmopressin reduces the incidence of microhematomas after facialplasty, *Ann Plast Surg* 46(5):163-166, 2001.

Perkins SW: Achieving the "natural look" in rhytidectomy, *Fac Plast Surg* 16:269-282, 2000.

Perkins SW, Williams JD, Macdonald K, et al: Prevention of seromas and hematomas after face-lift surgery with the use of postoperative vacuum drains, *Arch Otolaryngol Head Neck Surg* 123(7):743-745, 1997.

Powell DM, Chang E, Farrior EH: Recovery from deep-plane rhytidectomy following unilateral wound treatment with autologous platelet gel (a pilot study), *Arch Fac Plast Surg* 3:245-250, 2001.

Rees TD, Aston SJ: Complications of rhytidectomy, *Clin Plast Surg* 5:109-119, 1978.

Rees TD, Liverett DM, Guy CL: The effect of cigarette smoking on skin-flap survival in the face lift patient, *Plast Reconstr Surg* 73:911-915, 1984.

Rubin LR, Simpson RL: The new deep plane face lift dissections versus the old superficial techniques: a comparison of neurologic complications, *Plast Reconstr Surg* 97(7):1461-1465, 1996.

Saylan Z: The S-lift for facial rejuvenation, *Int J Cosmet Surg* 7:17-24, 1999.

Saylan Z: The S-lift: less is more, *Aesthetic Surg J* 19:406-409, 1999.

Straith RE, Raghava R, Hipps CJ: The study of hematomas in 500 consecutive face lifts, *Plast Reconstr Surg* 59:694-698, 1977.

Webster RC, Davidson TM, White MF, et al: Conservative face lift surgery, Arch Otolaryngol 102:657-662, 1976.

Webster RC, Kazda G, Hamden US: Cigarette smoking and face lift: conservative versus wide undermining, *Plast Reconstr Surg* 77:596-604, 1986.

Webster RC, Smith RC, Smith KF: Face lift, part i: extent of undermining of skin flaps, *Head and Neck Surgery* 5:525-534, 1983.

Webster RC, Smith RC, Smith KF: Face lift, part II: etiology of platysma cording and its relationship to treatment, *Head Neck Surg* 6:590-595, 1983.

Webster RC, Smith RC, Smith KF: Face lift, part III: plication of the superficial musculoaponeurotic system, *Head Neck Surg* 6:696-701, 1983.

Upper and Lower Eyelid Blepharoplasty

Chris Jo, DMD, and Shahrokh C. Bagheri, DMD, MD

CC

A 48-year-old woman presents for consultation regarding excess skin on her upper and lower eyelids (dermatochalasis). Her coworkers constantly tell her that she "looks tired all the time."

HPI

The patient was able to point out areas of excess skin over both upper and lower eyelids in front of a mirror. In addition, she complains about the "dark circles and bags" under her eyes. She does not complain about any visual field restrictions (can be caused by advanced dermatochalasis or lateral/temporal "hooding"). There is no history of dry eyes or other ocular problems and she has not had any previous facial cosmetic surgery.

PMHX/PDHX/MEDICATIONS/ALLERGIES/SH/FH

The patient has no history of thyroid disease (Graves ophthalmopathy may manifest as eyelid edema, lid retraction, or early proptosis and may mimic fat prolapse or aging). There is no history of coagulopathies or bleeding tendencies. The patient does not use aspirin, nonsteroidal antiinflammatory drugs, vitamin E, herbal medications, or anticoagulants (medications that affect platelet or coagulation function and potentially increase the risk of retrobulbar hemorrhage must be discontinued at least 10 to 14 days before the procedure).

EXAMINATION

General. The patient is a well-developed and well-nourished woman in no apparent distress.

Ocular. Examination of the pupillary reactions, visual fields, visual acuity, and extraocular muscles reveals no abnormalities. Schirmer's test is normal (measures baseline tear production and can be used as needed to document preoperative lacrimal gland function) (Figure 12-9).

Forehead–eyebrow–upper lid complex. This area is assessed first to evaluate for brow ptosis. The distance from the patient's upper lid margin to the lower edge of the brow during primary gaze measures at 10 mm (normal range). If this measurement is less than 10 mm, it is suggestive of brow ptosis, which can also contribute to the amount of temporal hooding (another reference is the distance from mid-pupil to the high point of the brow, which is about 25 mm). In cases of significant brow ptosis, added consideration to brow-lift procedures is warranted (the eyebrows can be elevated to the ideal position with the thumb and index finger, while examining the upper eyelid). There are no horizontal glabellar (caused by procerus muscle) or vertical (caused by corrugator supercilii) furrows at rest.

- **Upper eyelid.**
  - **Skin** (examined with eyebrows/forehead completely relaxed). Excessive skin is centered over the mid eyelid. The redundant eyelid skin is predominantly above the eyelid crease (smooth forceps can be used to pinch the excess tissue to demonstrate the amount of skin laxity). There is no ectropion (everted eyelid), entropion (inverted eyelid), or lagophthalmos (eyelid incompetence). Bell's phenomenon is intact (protective reflex to prevent corneal abrasion/erosion). Upper eyelid margin position is ideal (should cover 2 to 3 mm of superior iris).
  - **Herniated or prolapsed fat** (upper eyelid has two preaponeurotic fat pads). Areas of herniated/prolapsed orbital fat are noted nasally (most commonly noted in this area). Gentle pressure on the globe while the eye is closed accentuates nasal fat herniation.
  - **Eyelid crease.** The eyelid crease is identified at 9 mm above the lid margin (within normal limits) at the level of the pupil.
  - **Examination for blepharoptosis (eyelid ptosis).** The vertical interpalpebral fissure distance is measured at 10 mm (normal is 10 to 12 mm centrally). This is the distance from the mid upper to the mid lower eyelid margin during primary gaze. A smaller distance is suggestive of blepharoptosis and levator disinsertion/dysfunction, in which the upper eyelid has decreased excursion upon superior gaze. This distance is increased with upper eyelid retraction as seen in thyroid ophthalmopathy.
  - **Evaluation for prolapsed lacrimal gland.** No fullness in the temporal region is noted; fullness in this area would be suggestive of lacrimal gland prolapse or descent of the retro-orbicularis oculi fat.
- **Lower eyelid.** The lower eyelids should be examined in conjunction with upper eyelid examination even when the patient desires only upper eyelid surgery. The lower eyelid should be evaluated for excess skin, laxity, orbital fat herniation and retraction.
  - **Skin.** A moderate amount of excess skin is observed when the patient is looking up.
  - **Orbital fat.** The medial, central, and temporal areas (corresponding to the three lower orbital fat pads) are

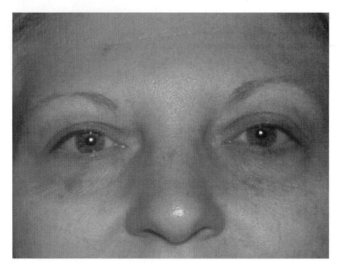

Figure 12-9   Preoperative frontal view of patient.

examined as the patient looks up. Gentle pressure over the closed upper eyelid demonstrates accentuation of orbital fat herniation.

○ **Lower eyelid retraction.** The lower eyelid is slightly above the level of the inferior limbus (no scleral show).

○ **Lower eyelid laxity.** The snap test is normal (lower lid reapproximates the globe within 1 second when it is pulled inferiorly and released).

IMAGING

Preoperative and serial postoperative photoimaging is mandatory for cosmetic procedures. Close-up views of the eyelids in closed and open eyelid positions are recommended.

LABS

No routine laboratory studies are indicated for cosmetic eyelid surgery unless dictated by the medical history.

ASSESSMENT

Patient desires bilateral upper and lower eyelid blepharoplasties secondary to dermatochalasis (excess eyelid skin laxity) and prolapse of preaponeurotic fat

TREATMENT

Bilateral upper eyelid blepharoplasty with resection of prolapsed fat is the treatment of choice to recreate an aesthetically pleasing upper eyelid shelf for this patient. Because no eyebrow ptosis is present, a forehead/brow-lift procedure would not be indicated. We emphasize that each patient presents with unique aesthetic needs mandating differences in the amount of skin, muscle, or fat that must be removed to achieve the optimal cosmetic result.

Blepharoplasties can be performed under local anesthesia in a cooperative patient, or general anesthesia can be used as

needed. Intravenous sedation is ideal for patient comfort. Before the administration of a sedative-hypnotic or local anesthetic, the eyelids should be reexamined and marked in the upright position (after administration of topical tetracaine).

The eyelids are marked in the upright or semireclined position before the administration of sedation. The upper eyelid is elevated and the inferior incision line is marked in the natural supra tarsal lid crease, approximately 1 cm above the lid margin (natural eyelid crease is 7 to 10 mm centrally in women and 6 to 8 mm centrally in men). Medially, the marking ends above the lacrimal punctum (extending the incision beyond the punctum will increase the risk of webbing), with a slight downward taper. Laterally, it is extended approximately 1 cm beyond the lateral canthus with a general upward slope (at the level of the lateral canthus, the incision should be approximately 5 mm above the level of the canthus). The superior incision line is marked as the excess skin is pinched with smooth forceps and the forehead/eyebrow is stabilized (a slight eversion of the upper eyelid margin with less than 1 mm of lagophthalmos will ensure an adequate but not overly aggressive skin resection). A minimum of 20 mm of skin must remain between the upper eyelid margin and the lower eyebrow margin to prevent postoperative lagophthalmos. The superior incision is marked with the skin held by the forceps, curving into the inferior incision medially and laterally in an elliptical fashion (modifications to the incision design can be made at the medial and lateral junctions depending on the clinical situation). The markings are again verified with smooth forceps to ensure symmetry and lid competence. (When simultaneous lower eyelid blepharoplasty with a skin incision is planned, a minimum of 5 mm between the two incisions must be maintained laterally.)

After injection of local anesthetic with epinephrine, the incision can be made with various techniques (blade, radiofrequency, or CO_2 laser). The authors prefer to use CO_2 laser (at 5-W continuous wave) to make the skin incision along the previously marked incision line. The skin is sharply excised from the underlying muscle with the laser by using forceps to grasp the lateral point of the ellipse with gentle upward traction. Upper eyelid skin is the thinnest skin in the body and very mobile tissue, especially in the elderly patient. For these reasons, the CO_2 laser is ideal due to its precision. Some surgeons prefer to resect skin and muscle (orbicularis oculi) as a single unit, whereas others address the two separately.

A 3-mm strip of orbicularis oculi muscle, along the superior aspect of the wound, is excised from the lateral pole to the medial pole with curved scissors (removal of redundant orbicularis muscle is necessary to obtain optimal results in most patients). After excision of the muscle, the orbital septum is exposed. The yellowish fat pads are visible through the septum. Gentle ballottement of the globe will accentuate the prolapsed fat (supine position can mask the excess fat that is usually prolapsed when the patient is upright).

The orbital septum is incised and the fat is allowed to herniate through, assisted by gentle traction (excessive traction can shear terminal branches of the ophthalmic artery and vein). The herniated fat can be clamped with a hemostat and then excised with electrocautery (which will achieve hemostasis simultaneously) or simply excised with the laser as the fat is passively draped over a cotton swab (to avoid overresection). Not all patients require fat excision.

Hemostasis must be achieved before closure. The skin is closed using 6-0 nylon suture in a running fashion (some surgeons prefer using absorbable sutures). An ophthalmic-grade antibiotic ointment is applied, and a cold compress (4 × 4-inch gauze soaked in ice water) is used to minimize edema (preoperative dose of steroids can also be used).

The lower eyelid blepharoplasty was conducted using a subcilliary incision with a lateral extension within a natural skin crease, allowing for a minimum of 5 mm between upper and lower eyelid incisions. A skin muscle flap was elevated, the orbital septum was incised, and any excess periorbital fat was gently removed in a similar fashion, with careful attention to hemostasis. A strip of skin and muscle was removed along the incision line to remove any excess skin and restore the lower eyelid to a more youthful appearance. Upon closure, attention is given to resuspension of the lateral aspect of the flap to the periosteum of the lateral orbital rim. Alternatively, lower eyelid blepharoplasties can be performed via a transconjunctival approach for removal of fat only, or it can be combined with a skin pinch technique to remove excess skin without disrupting the orbicularis oculi muscle. Some surgeons advocate redistributing the fat instead of excising it. The ideal technique will be determined by the surgeon's preference and the patient's clinical presentation.

Postoperative care includes local wound care and application of antibiotic ointment. Overexertion must be avoided (especially during the first 48 hours postoperatively), which can increase postoperative edema and increase the risk of hematoma formation (especially a retrobulbar hematoma, which is a surgical emergency). Control of nausea and vomiting with antiemetics and control of hypertension is essential. Sutures are removed in 5 to 7 days. Figure 12-10 is a postoperative photograph of the patient at 6 weeks after upper and lower eyelid blepharoplasties.

COMPLICATIONS

Retrobulbar hematoma/bleeding causing loss of vision. Retrobulbar hematoma after cosmetic blepharoplasty is the most feared but fortunately rare (0.04%) complication. It is more commonly reported in patients who failed to report the use of anticoagulation medications such as aspirin or herbal medications A hematoma may be caused by shearing of small vessels in the fat pads, located posteriorly, or by uncontrolled hemostasis after excision of the fat (the fat pads retract when released, making it difficult to control any small bleeders, so it is prudent to achieve hemostasis while the fat is being excised with electrocautery or laser). The other theorized source of retrobulbar hematoma is hemorrhage from the cut edges of the orbicularis oculi muscle that gains retrobulbar access through the opened septum. The earliest sign is unilateral eye pain. This will progress to proptosis, ophthalmoplegia, and decreased pupillary reflex with eventual visual disturbances (color discrimination is affected first, especially the color red). Sustained increased intraocular pressures result in central retinal artery occlusion and optic nerve ischemia, causing irreversible damage. Treatment includes immediate removal of skin sutures and decompression of the orbit (may require a lateral canthotomy and inferior cantholysis). Medical management includes high-dose steroids (dexamethasone 3 to 4 mg/kg, followed by a tapering dose), mannitol, acetazolamide, and papaverine (to decrease vascular spasm). Bed rest, elevation of the head, and avoidance of Valsalva maneuvers are important supportive measures.

Wound dehiscence. Due to the vascularity and quick healing time in the eyelids, wound dehiscence is uncommon. It can be seen after postoperative complications such as prolonged bleeding, hematoma, or infection. Patient noncompliance is another risk factor (early return to strenuous activity, eye rubbing). Management includes local wound care and allowing for healing by secondary intention, which generally occurs without scarring or cosmetic deformity.

Lagophthalmos and corneal abrasion. Transient lid incompetence is common following upper eyelid blepharoplasty. An intact Bell's phenomenon will protect the cornea from corneal abrasions and exposure keratitis, when tear production is normal. Lagophthalmos with decreased tear production and/or a poor Bell's phenomenon will increase the risk of exposure-related corneal complications. Lubrication ointment and an eye patch (plastic wrap placed over the eye works well) should be used during sleep until lagophthalmos resolves (as the lid skin stretches). Manual lid massage can be initiated 2 weeks after surgery to facilitate resolution. Full-thickness skin grafts (from contralateral eyelid, banked tissue, or periauricular skin) may be required in cases of overly aggressive skin resection.

Eyelid ptosis. Postoperative eyelid ptosis may be caused by surgical injury or from an undiagnosed preexisting condition. Acquired senile ptosis (caused by dehiscence or disin-

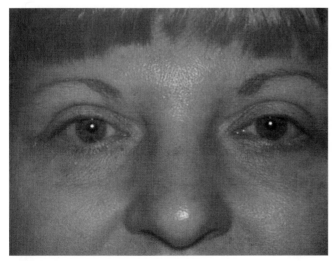

Figure 12-10 Frontal view of patient 6 weeks after bilateral upper and lower blepharoplasties.

sertion of the levator aponeurosis), accompanied by varying degrees of dermatochalasis of the upper eyelid, is common in the elderly population. Blepharoplasty performed in these patients without ptosis repair may result in postoperative exaggeration of the drooping eyelid. Therefore it is prudent to identify such patients by properly examining their levator function (normal excursion of 15 mm is considered excellent, greater than 8 mm is good, 5 to 7 mm is fair, and less than 4 mm is poor) and upper eyelid position at rest (normally covers 1 to 2 mm of the superior limbus). Periorbital edema and hematoma can cause transient ptosis. Otherwise, surgery for postoperative ptosis repair should be delayed 3 to 6 months to allow for resolution.

Keratoconjunctivitis sicca (dry eye syndrome). Tear production begins to decrease in the fifth decade of life. Blepharoplasty may produce subtle changes (increased width of palpebral fissure, lower eyelid retraction, lagophthalmos) unmasking the borderline dry eye patient. Preoperative Schirmer's testing (5×35-mm filter paper placed on the lower conjunctiva for 5 minutes; less than 10 mm of wetting is considered abnormal) is recommended by some. However, McKinney and Byun found that Schirmer's test was not a good predictor of postblepharoplasty complication of dry eye. Instead, the history (increased blinking, dryness, contact lens intolerance, grittiness, and pain) and anatomy (presence of scleral show, lagophthalmos, snap test, and negative vector) were found to be more important predictors of postoperative dry eye complications. Treatment options include topical ocular lubricants, wetting drops, ointments (nighttime), and punctal plugs.

Infection. Orbital cellulitis or abscess following blepharoplasty is extremely rare. Prevention includes identification and treatment of preexisting infectious diseases of the eyelid, conjunctiva, sinuses, and lacrimal sac. Appropriate surgical management may include opening a portion of the incision to allow drainage and systemic antibiotic coverage.

Cosmetic deformity (asymmetry, inappropriate fat resection, or lid malpositioning). Incomplete or overzealous resection of fat may cause residual fat bags or periorbital hollowing, respectively. Asymmetries of the lid arch, height and width of the palpebral fissure, residual fat, and lid crease are not uncommon. Photodocumentation of preexisting asymmetry and patient counseling are important. Using careful surgical technique and attention to detail will reduce the risk of asymmetry. Eyelid malpositioning (scleral show, ectropion, entropion, rounded eye) is mostly seen in lower eyelid blepharoplasty. Damage to the levator muscle, aponeurosis, or Mueller muscle can result in upper lid malpositioning.

DISCUSSION

Examination of the blepharoplasty patient should encompass the whole face and not be limited to the eyelids. Particular attention is given to the position of the upper lid (upper lid ptosis) and brow. Brow ptosis can cause excessive upper eyelid folds. This needs to be recognized and addressed in the treatment plan for possible brow-lift procedures.

Correct diagnosis is the first step to a successful outcome. The evaluation of the upper eyelid itself can be categorized into skin, muscle, and fat. Not all patients require surgical excision of all three components. Younger patients can demonstrate fat herniation/prolapse (especially the nasal/medial fat pad) without excess skin. A transconjunctival upper blepharoplasty (removal of excess medial upper eyelid fat) may be suitable for some patients. The aging patient may have excess eyelid skin and laxity (dermatochalasis), which will require skin excision only. However, most patients with varying degrees of dermatochalasis will require a small strip of orbicularis oculi muscle to be resected for a better-defined supratarsal crease and cosmetic outcome. Once the skin and muscle have been excised, the fat pads can be reevaluated under direct vision. Gentle ballottement of the globe will accentuate the fat pads (which are normally prolapsed in the upright position but are retracted in the supine position). If fat prolapses into the wound upon ballottement, the septum should be incised and the fat gently excised. It is important to keep in mind that the medial/nasal fat compartment is composed of two individual fat pads. It is also prudent to avoid excess traction on the fat pads, which can result in overresection of fat and sheering of the posterior vessels.

Management of the prolapsed lacrimal gland. A prolapsed lacrimal gland (superior lateral compartment of the orbit) should not be mistaken for a herniated fat pad. A prolapsed lacrimal gland can be repositioned using suture suspension techniques (suture leading edge of gland to the periosteum just posterior to the superior orbital rim) but should not be excised (increased risk of postoperative dry eye).

Adjunctive procedures during upper eyelid blepharoplasty. Corrugator supercilii muscle can be resected via the upper blepharoplasty incision, when indicated (to treat vertical glabellar rhytids). Some surgeons prefer to use this incision to facilitate subperiosteal dissection during endoscope-assisted forehead lift. If simultaneous forehead/eyebrow lifting is to be performed, the upper eyelid skin resection should be more conservative and marked with the eyebrow lifted to the ideal position (either procedure can be done first depending on the surgeon's preference). Simultaneous laser resurfacing can also be performed.

The male patient requesting upper eyelid blepharoplasty. There is an increasing number of male patients seeking facial cosmetic surgery—in particular, eyelid procedures. It is important to note the differences in anatomy and aesthetic norms between the two genders. The male eyebrow should rest on the superior orbital rim (in females the apex of the brow should be 8 to 10 mm above) and is more flattened compared with the "arched" female brow. However, males can experience eyebrow ptosis and should be appropriately managed. Men's eyelid crease is typically lower, flatter, and less defined. In addition, the inferior skin incision is typically 6 to 8 mm above the upper eyelid margin centrally (in women, it is 7 to 10 mm) and remains more flattened.

Special considerations for the Asian patient requesting blepharoplasty. The Asian patient requesting upper eyelid blepharoplasty deserves special attention. More than 50% of

East Asians do not have a superior palpebral fold or supratarsal crease ("single eyelid"), and most of these patients requesting blepharoplasty seek surgical creation of a palpebral furrow or supratarsal crease ("double eyelid"). In the Asian "single eyelid," the superficial lamina of the levator aponeurosis/ expansion does not penetrate the orbital septum and orbicularis oculi muscle to insert to the overlying dermis, as it does in the western "double eyelid." Instead, these fibers terminate on the tarsal plate (the height of the superior tarsal plate is between 5 to 6 mm in Asians and 10 to 12 mm in Caucasians), and no palpebral fold is formed upon eyelid opening. The goal of Asian blepharoplasty is to create a well-defined supratarsal crease (the size and shape are dictated by patient desires) via various surgical techniques using supratarsal fixation sutures to adjoin the levator aponeurosis to the pretarsal skin. Several techniques can be used to create the "double eyelid" and manage the epicanthal fold, depending on the individual patient anatomy and expectations.

Bibliography

Carraway JH: Surgical anatomy of the eyelids, *Clin Plast Surg* 14:693-701, 1987.

Cook BE, Lemke BN: Cosmetic blepharoplasty upper eyelid techniques, *Oral Maxillofacial Surg Clin N Am* 12(4):673-687, 2000.

Fagien S: Advanced rejuvenative upper blepharoplasty: enhancing aesthetics of the upper periorbita, *Plast Reconstr Surg* 110:278-289, 2002.

Fagien S: Discussion: The value of tear film breakup and Schirmer's tests in preoperative blepharoplasty evaluation, *Plast Reconstr Surg* 104:570-573, 1999.

Ghali GE, Lustig JH: Complications associated with facial cosmetic surgery, *Oral Maxillofac Surg Clin N Am* 15:265-283, 2003.

Holt JE, Holt GR: Blepharoplasty: indications and preoperative assessment, *Arch Otolaryngol* 111:394-397, 1985.

Hughes SM: Evaluation of the cosmetic blepharoplasty patient, *Oral Maxillofac Surg Clin N Am* 12(4):649-670, 2000.

Januszkiewicz JS, Nahai F: Transconjunctival upper blepharoplasty, *Plast Reconstr Surg* 103:1015-1019, 1999.

Lisman RD, Hyde K, Smith B: Complications of blepharoplasty, *Clin Plast Surg* 15:309-335, 1988.

McCurdy JA: Upper blepharoplasty in the Asian patient: the "double eyelid" operation, *Fac Plast Surg Clin N Am* 10:351-368, 2002.

McCurdy JA: Upper lid blepharoplasty: the double eyelid operation — external approach, *Fac Plast Surg Clin N Am* 4:7-23, 1996.

McKinney P, Byun M: The value of tear film breakup and Schirmer's tests in preoperative blepharoplasty evaluation, *Plast Reconstr Surg* 104:566-568, 1999.

Millay DJ, Larrabee WF: Ptosis and blepharoplasty surgery, *Arch Otolaryngol Head Neck Surg* 115:198-201, 1989.

Niamtu J: Cosmetic blepharoplasty, *Atlas Oral Maxillofac Surg Clin N Am* 12:91-130, 2004.

Seckel BR, et al: Laser blepharoplasty with transconjunctival orbicularis muscle/septum tightening and periocular skin resurfacing: a safe and advantageous technique, *Plast Reconstr Surg* 106:1127-1145, 2000.

Seiff SR: Anatomy of the Asian eyelid, *Fac Plast Surg Clin N Am* 4:1-5, 1996.

Ullmann Y, et al: The surgical anatomy of the fat in the upper eyelid medial compartment, *Plast Reconstr Surg* 99:658, 1997.

Zukowski ML: Endoscopic brow surgery, *Oral Maxillofac Surg Clin N Am* 12(4):701-708, 2000.

Genioplasty

Piyushkumar P. Patel, DDS, and Shahrokh Bagheri, DMD, MD

CC

A 25-year-old woman presents for consultation regarding chin augmentation. She explains, "I would like my chin to be bigger."

HPI

The patient states that she has been unhappy with the appearance of her lower face. In particular, she feels that her chin is small and that it influences her neck and facial profile. She has no prior history of facial cosmetic surgery or orthodontic treatment.

PMHX/PDHX/MEDICATIONS/ALLERGIES/SH/FH

Noncontributory.

EXAMINATION

General. The patient is a well-developed and well-nourished woman in no apparent distress.

Psychiatric evaluation. Mood and affect are appropriate. In the past, studies have demonstrated that over half of patients seeking facial aesthetic surgery can be assigned a formal psychiatric diagnosis, such as personality trait disorders, neurosis, and psychosis. However, trends and acceptance of aesthetic surgery have since matured, and recent studies demonstrate that individuals seeking aesthetic surgery are less likely to be psychologically distressed. Physical attractiveness may play a critical role in the development of self-concept or even career goals (such as modeling). Modern surgical interventions can safely enhance physical appearance, which in turn elevates self-confidence and personal well-being.

Maxillofacial. Chin deformities can manifest in any of the three dimensions (vertical, horizontal, and transverse) in isolation or in combination. The vast majority, however, are in the horizontal plane only. Careful scrutiny of the skeletal, dental, and soft tissue structures is required to obtain a good result.

On frontal view, the patient exhibits good symmetry. The maxillary midline is coincident with the facial midline. The patient shows 2 to 3 mm of maxillary anteriors at rest (vertical maxillary excess can result in a clockwise rotation of the mandible and thus cause a retrognathic/microgenic appearance). The chin is symmetrical with soft tissue menton lying on the facial midline. Chin pad tissue thickness is approximately 10 mm (normal, 8 to 11 mm). On smiling, the lower lip is symmetrical. On elevation of her lower lip, no mentalis muscle hyperactivity or chin pad fasciculations were seen (if alloplastic augmentation is to be used, muscle hyperactivity may place excessive force on the implant, leading to increased bone resorption or displacement of the implant).

On profile examination (Figure 12-11), the patient exhibits a good nasal projection with a mild dorsal hump (a large nose will make the chin look small, and vice versa). The labiomental angle is obtuse at 160° (ideally, the depth of the fold/sulcus should lie 4 mm posterior to a line drawn from the lower vermilion border to the pogonion. If the sulcus is shallow or high, augmentation results in enlargement of the lower face [chin and lip]; however, if the fold is deep and more inferiorly positioned, augmentation will predominantly accentuate the chin). The patient demonstrates a convex facial profile with a retrognathic appearance. The cervicomental angle is obtuse at 150° (normal, 110° to 120°). On posturing the mandible forward, there is significant improvement in the neck aesthetics (patients with microgenia can have altered neck aesthetics). There is a lack of the visible separation of the mandible and neck, giving the appearance that the face "flows" into the neck. To the untrained eye, this may appear to be secondary to tissue laxity or lipomatosis. Microgenia can further aggravate this condition. In such a case, the soft tissues of the neck should be examined with forward posturing of the mandible; if this produces less-than-optimal improvement in neck aesthetics, cosmetic neck surgery may be indicated.

Intraoral. Oral hygiene is excellent (some clinicians will not place an alloplastic implant in patients with active periodontal disease. Also, this may be an indicator of the patient's ability to keep the wound clean if an intraoral approach is to be used). The patient has a Class I molar and canine relationship (a Class II malocclusion indicates that a skeletal abnormality exists—the patient should be informed of the option of orthodontic realignment and orthognathic surgery). The mandibular anterior teeth are in good position, neither retroclined nor proclined. Eversion of the lower lip results in deepening of the labiomental sulcus (this occurs with excess proclination of the anterior teeth).

IMAGING

Standard photographs of the frontal and profile views, both in repose and on smiling, are recommended. A panoramic radiograph and a lateral cephalogram are recommended for the work-up of patients requiring a genioplasty.

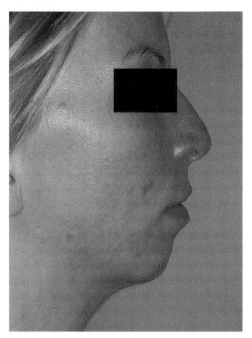

Figure 12-11 Preoperative profile view of the patient demonstrates a deficient chin in the horizontal plane.

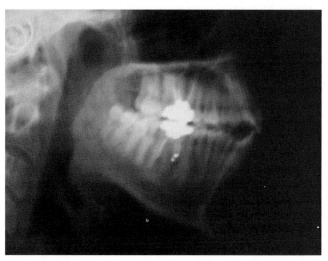

Figure 12-12 Preoperative lateral cephalogram showing the deficiency of the chin in the anteroposterior dimension and a Class I molar relationship.

The panoramic radiograph is used to delineate the proximity of the mandibular canal/mental foramen, and the apices of the mandibular anterior dentition, in anticipation for a genial osteotomy. In addition, it provides a general overview of any mandibular osseous pathology.

Lateral cephalometric evaluations have been used to help determine the desired horizontal and vertical dimensions of the chin. Information gained from the cephalometric tracings includes the relationship of the maxilla and mandible to the skull base and to each other. It is important to identify any skeletal or occlusal disparities that can be corrected before or concomitant with a genioplasty procedure. Ideally, the chin should rest slightly posterior to the lower lip, and the lower lip should be posterior to the upper lip. Increasing sagittal projection beyond these relations may risk an unaesthetic result.

The lateral cephalogram for this patient shows the deficiency of the chin in the anteroposterior dimension and a Class I molar relationship (Figure 12-12).

LABS

No routine laboratory testing is indicated for genioplasty procedures unless dictated by the medical history.

ASSESSMENT

Horizontal microgenia, in a patient who desires chin augmentation

TREATMENT

Genioplasty refers to a horizontal osteotomy of the anterior mandible. Chin implant refers to either an alloplastic implant or an autogenous implant. Alloplastic chin implants and sliding genioplasty represent the two currently accepted methods for chin augmentation. The anticipated soft tissue changes in response to hard tissue movements are shown in Table 12-1.

Careful treatment planning, meticulous surgical technique, and the surgeon's artistic sense are three important factors for successful and predictable chin surgery. For intraoral access, it is important to plan an incision that will achieve the following goals:

- Ease of wound closure, ensuring that movable mucosa rather than attached gingiva forms the wound margin
- Avoidance of periodontal problems following wound contraction and scar formation
- Prevention of mental or inferior alveolar nerve severance
- Ability to resuspend the mentalis muscle to prevent chin (mentalis) droop

An incision in the depth of the vestibule will result in excess scar formation and should be avoided. A U-shaped incision extending from canine to canine that leaves 10 to 15 mm of mucosa anterior to the depth of the vestibule is ideal. The mentalis muscle is incised in an oblique fashion, leaving an ample amount superiorly to allow for closure. The mentalis muscle is stripped in a subperiosteal plane, exposing the symphysis. The mental nerves are identified bilaterally, and the periosteum is freed circumferentially around the foramen. Careful dissection in this area will allow the surgeon to preserve all branches of this nerve. The planned osteotomy should lie a minimum of 5 mm below the longest tooth root (usually the canine) as well as a minimum of 10 to 15 mm superior to the inferior border. The osteotomy should also extend 4 to 5 mm below the lowest point of the mental foramen. It should be remembered that the angle of the osteotomy can influence vertical and horizontal changes. An osteotomy that is more parallel with the occlusal plane will allow a greater vector of advancement in the horizontal dimension

Table 12-1.   Soft Tissue Response to Hard Tissue Movements

Procedure	Soft Tissue Response (% of hard tissue movement)	Comment
1. Advancement		
Osteotomy (genioplasty)	90-100% horizontal	Labiomental fold deepens
Alloplast onlay	80-90% horizontal	Labiomental fold deepens
Bone onlay graft	60-70% horizontal	
2. Vertical augmentation		
With interpositional graft	80-90% of vertical augmentation	Labiomental fold flattens
3. Reduction Genioplasty		
Vertical reduction with wedge removal	90% of vertical reduction	
Vertical reduction with osteotomy of inferior border	25%	Highly unpredictable
Horizontal reduction (sliding)	90-100%	Labiomental fold flattens
Horizontal reduction (degloving with bur reduction)	25-30%	Overall flattening of chin

Modified from Peterson L, Indresano AT, Marciani RD, Roser SM: *Principles of oral and maxillofacial surgery, vol III,* Philadelphia, 1992, JB Lippincott.

movement. If vertical shortening is desired, the angle should be more acute. The midline should be marked with a burr (fissure type) to prevent postoperative iatrogenic asymmetries. The osteotomy is completed with a reciprocating saw. The orientation of this saw should remain constant to ensure a symmetrical cut through the buccal and lingual cortices, to prevent interferences that may hamper the proposed movement. Once the osteotomy is completed and the fragment is repositioned, it can be secured through a variety of methods, including the use of wires, prebent chin plates, or lag screws. The wound should be closed in layers, and it is essential that the mentalis muscle is accurately repositioned. A dressing is applied to facilitate soft tissue reattachment and prevent hematoma formation.

Alloplastic augmentation can also be considered for the treatment of a genial deficiency. A wide range of materials can be used. The materials most commonly used include high-density polyethylene (Medpor; Porex Surgical Products Group, Newman, GA), hard tissue replacement polymer, polyamide mesh (Supramid, S. Jackson Inc., Alexandria, VA), solid medical-grade silicone rubber (Silastic), hydroxyapatite, and Gore-Tex (W.L. Gore and Associates, Flagstaff, AZ). Prior to it's removal from the American market various forms of Proplast (Vitek, Houston. TX) was used for genial augmenatation, such as Proplast I (PTFE and graphite), Proplast II (PTFE and alumina) and Proplast hydroxyapatite. Many surgeons believe that Silastic meets most of the criteria for an ideal alloplastic implant. The ideal characteristics of an alloplastic implant include the following:
- Anatomical configuration that has a posterior surface that contours to the external surface of the mandible and an external implant shape that imitates the desired outcome
- Readily implantable and nonpalpable
- Margins of the implant blend onto the bony surfaces
- Easily removable
- Malleable, comfortable, and inert
- Easily modifiable by the surgeon during the procedure

Placement of alloplastic implants via an extraoral submental incision can be combined with other procedures such as submental liposuction or platysmal placation. The surgeon's experience is usually the deciding factor on whether an implant or an osteotomy is performed. It is generally accepted that mild to moderate abnormalities can be corrected with either alloplastic implantation or genioplasty, whereas with severe abnormalities, sliding genioplasty should be performed. Genioplasty is a more versatile procedure as it can address abnormalities in any of the three dimensions. There is some debate on the superiority of either procedure for augmentation.

This patient underwent advancement of 7 mm with use of a prebent chin plate that was secured with six monocortical screws (Figure 12-13, *A*). Figure 12-13, *B* demonstrates the preservation of the branches of the mental nerve, after careful dissection and plate stabilization. Figure 12-14 shows the postoperative lateral cephalogram and profile view at 4 weeks.

COMPLICATIONS

The most common complication after genioplasty surgery is a neurosensory disturbance, followed by hematoma and infection. Soft tissue changes such as chin ptosis, excessive lower tooth display, devitalization of teeth, creation of mucogingival problems, asymmetry, and unaesthetic results are also known complications. Mandibular fracture, hemorrhage causing lingual hematoma and possible airway compromise, and avascular necrosis of the mobilized segment are possible but rare complications of this procedure.

Injury rates to the mental nerve have been reported to range from 0% to 20% at 1 year postoperatively. Etiologies of nerve injury include inadequate exposure, poorly designed flaps, inadequate protection during osteotomy, excessive stretching, or compression. The majority of patients undergoing genioplasty experience a transient neurosensory deficit probably secondary to neuropraxia. However, most studies

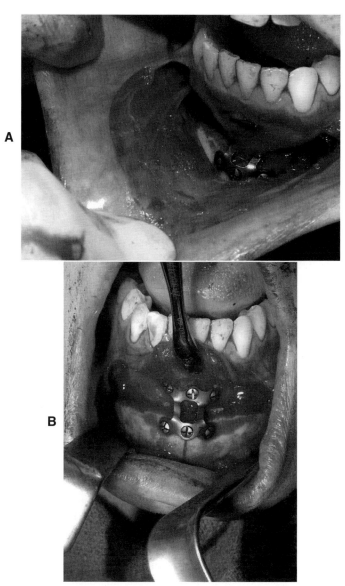

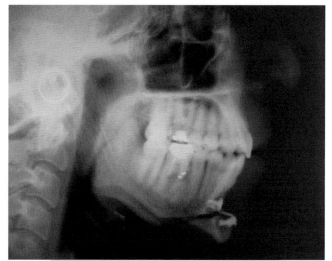

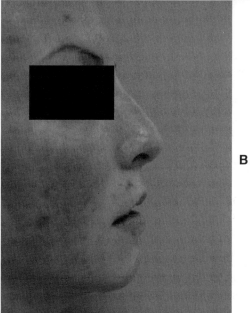

Figure 12-13 **A,** Intraoperative view showing the placement of a 7-mm prebent chin advancement plate. **B,** Intraoperative view showing the preservation of all branches of the mental nerve.

Figure 12-14 **A,** Postoperative lateral cephalogram showing the position of the chin after 7-mm advancement. **B,** Postoperative lateral view at 4 weeks after 7-mm advancement genioplasty.

show resolution of any neurosensory deficit after several months. Reduction in response to light touch (a sensitive marker for neurosensory deficit) has an incidence of 3.4%. This complication is associated with no adverse effect on the quality of life.

The inferior alveolar nerve travels inferiorly and anteriorly past the mental foramen before looping back and exiting the mental foramen (Figure 12-15). It is recommend that the osteotomy line remain 5 mm (4.5 mm minimum) below the mental foramen to avoid injury to the inferior alveolar nerve.

Guyot and associates have proposed a new pattern of sensory innervation of the chin with three territories—labial territory (mental nerve supplies this area), mental territory (cutaneous branch of the mylohyoid nerve), and submental territory (cervical branches of the cervical plexus). They pos-

tulate that when a horizontal osteotomy is performed using a reciprocating saw, sectioning involves not only bone but also some soft tissue of the floor of the mouth. In this area, the potential for injury to the mylohyoid muscle exists along with injury to the mylohyoid nerve. This can result in neurosensory deficits of the skin overlying the chin without involvement of the mental nerve. Other anatomical structures at risk include the submental and sublingual arteries. It should be noted that some authors believe the cutaneous branch of the mylohyoid nerve innervates an inconsistent area of the submental region.

Relapse in the immediate postoperative period is uncommon except in the case of fixation failure. There is generally good stability of the segment following genioplasty.

"Witch's chin deformity" is a term originally coined by Gonzales-Ulloa in 1971 to describe chin ptosis. Loss of

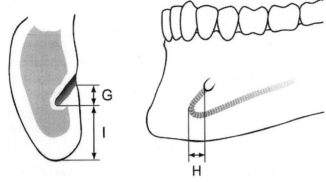

Figure 12-15 Terminal mandibular canal in relationship to the mental foramen, demonstrating the looping of the nerve before exiting at the foramen. Looping terminal mandibular canal and mental foremen. G, distance from terminal mandibular canal to mental foramen; H, advanced anterior distance from terminal mandibular canal to mental foramen; I, distance from terminal mandibular canal to inferior border of body near the mental foramen. The average distances of G, H, and I were 4.5 ± 1.9 mm, 5.0 ± 1.8 mm, and 9.2 ± 2.7 mm, respectively. *(From Hwang K: Vulnerability of the inferior alveolar nerve and mental nerve during genioplasty: an anatomic study,* J Craniofac Surg *16:10-14. 2004.)*

mentalis muscle origination plays an important role in the pathogenesis of this problem. The mentalis muscle is the only muscle of significance when performing a genioplasty. It is the sole elevator of the lower lip, providing the majority of the lip's vertical support. If the muscle is not precisely reattached at the end of the surgery, chin ptosis and increased exposure of the lower incisors can occur. Advocates of alloplastic augmentation report that if the implant is placed through a submental approach, the mentalis muscle can be left attached.

The most common complications of alloplastic augmentation are infection, bone resorption under the implant (although this has been shown to have no clinical consequences), extrusion, malpositioning or displacement of the implant, and improper sizing of the implant.

DISCUSSION

Horizontal sectioning of the anterior mandible (genioplasty) was first described by Hofer in the German literature. This initial operation was performed on a cadaver, with preoperative and postoperative photographs demonstrating the results. Trauner and Obwegeser introduced the intraoral approach in 1957. Since then a number of technical variations have been described. Despite the versatility of the horizontal mandibular osteotomy, the biologic basis was not studied until the mid 1980s. Ellis and colleagues demonstrated that maintaining the soft tissue pedicle (the digastric musculature and the periosteum on the inferior and lingual border) is associated with less osseous resorption in the postoperative period. Storum and associates demonstrated that close apposition of the margins of the osteotomy is important for vascular bridging and early osteogenesis.

In patients with skeletal discrepancies who would benefit from conventional orthognathic surgery, Proffit and colleagues suggested three specific indications for an isolated genioplasty as a camouflage procedure:
1. The borderline extraction patient with a good nasolabial angle, protruding mandibular incisors, and a deficient chin
2. A patient with a short mandibular ramus in whom advancement may lead to an unstable result
3. A patient with asymmetry that does not involve a significant malocclusion

Macrogenia can be seen in isolation or associated with mandibular hyperplasia. Some patients who are under the care of an orthodontist and would benefit from a mandibular setback are never referred to a surgeon, for a variety of reasons. In these cases, the orthodontist extracts lower premolars, followed by retroclining of the mandibular incisors. This results in a normal occlusal relationship; however, the patients usually exhibit macrogenia. Macrogenia can be classified into three subgroups depending on the vectors of growth—anterior, vertical, or a combination. This can be corrected using either reduction of the mental protuberance with a bur or a horizontal sliding osteotomy. Removal of excess bone with a bur will not result in appreciable improvement of the soft tissue contour. The soft tissues drape poorly over the newly contoured bone, resulting in a double chin appearance. Lower lip ptosis can also be seen if the periosteum does not attach to the newly contoured bone. Lip incompetence and a lack of cervicomandibular definition can also be associated with this technique. Submental ostectomy (burring down) of the prominence is acceptable when only a small amount of reduction is needed. Posterior repositioning with an osteotomy has been shown to produce a better result. However, this technique has the potential for mental nerve injury not only from the procedure but also from the need to dissect around the inferior border to reduce the projecting wings. Submental ostectomy with soft tissue excision via an extraoral approach has been shown to avoid the negative sequelae of excessive submental tissue and chin ptosis.

Alantar and colleagues have shown that the mean number of branches of the mental nerve as it exits the foramen is two. However, the number of branches can range from one to four. The branches of the mental nerve are known to run in an oblique direction; the mean angle between the most medial branch and the long axis of the orbicularis oris muscle is 36°. Based on this, it is recommended that an incision should not be made parallel to the fibers of the orbicularis oris muscle. Damage can be avoided if the incision is made with an angle of 36° to the long axis of the lip. Labial incisions should thus have a U shape. The two sides of the U should be as parallel as possible to the lower labial branches (36°). Limiting the proximal extension of the incision to the canine region also reduces the incidence of neuronal injury.

Bibliography

Alantar A, et al: The lower labial branches of the mental nerve: anatomic variation and surgical relevance, *J Oral Maxillofac Surg* 58:415-418, 2000.

Chang EW, et al: Sliding genioplasty for correction of chin abnormalities, *Arch Fac Plast Surg* 3:8-14, 2001.

Chaushu G, et al: The effect of precise reattachment of the mentalis muscle on the soft tissue response to genioplasty, *J Oral Maxillofac Surg* 59:510-516, 2001.

Ellis E, et al: Advancement genioplasty with and without soft tissue pedicle, *J Oral Maxillofac Surg* 42:637-645, 1984.

Frodel JL, et al: Evaluation of vertical microgenia, *Arch Fac Plast Surg* 6:111-119, 2004.

Guyot L, et al: Alteration of chin sensibility due to damage of the cutaneous branch of the mylohyoid nerve during genioplasty, *J Oral Maxillofac Surg* 60:1371-1373, 2002.

Hofer O: Die osteoplastiche verlaengerung des unterkiefers nach voneiselber bei mikrogenia, *Dtsh Zahn Mund Kieferheilkd* 27:81, 1957.

Hoffman GR, Moloney FB: The stability of facial osteotomies. Part 6. Chin setback, *Aust Dent J* 41:178-183, 1996.

Hoffman GR, Moloney FB: The stability of facial osteotomies. Part 3. Chin advancement, *Aust Dent J* 40:289-295, 1995.

Hwang K: Vulnerability of the inferior alveolar nerve and mental nerve during genioplasty: an anatomic study, *J Craniofac Surg* 16:10-14. 2004.

Hwang K, et al: Anatomic studies. Cutaneous sensory branch of the mylohyoid nerve, *J Craniofac Surg* 16:343-345, 2005.

Kim SG, et al: Unusual complication after genioplasty, *Plast Reconstr Surg* 109:2612-2613, 2002.

Lesavoy M, et al: A technique for correcting witch's chin deformity, *Plast Reconstr Surg* 97:842-846, 1999.

Nishioka GJ, et al: Neurosensory disturbances associated with the anterior mandibular horizontal osteotomy, *J Oral Maxillofac Surg* 46:107-110, 1988.

Proffit WR, Turvey TA, Mariarty JD: Augmentation genioplasty as an adjunct to conservative orthodontic treatment, *Am J Orthod* 79:473-491, 1981.

Reed EH, Smith RG: Genioplasty: a case for alloplastic chin augmentation, *J Oral Maxillofac Surg* 58:788-793, 2000.

Storum KA: Microangiographic and histologic evaluation of revascularization and healing after genioplasty by osteotomy of the inferior border of the mandible, *J Oral Maxillofac Surg* 48:210-216, 1988.

Strauss RA, Abubaker AO: Genioplasty: a case for advancement osteotomy, *J Oral Maxillofac Surg* 58:783-787, 2000.

Trauner R, Obwegeser H: Surgical correction of mandibular prognathism and retrognathism with consideration of genioplasty, *Oral Surg* 10:677, 1957.

Zide BM, et al: Chin surgery I. Augmentation—the allures and the alerts, *Plast Reconstr Surg* 104:1843-1853, 1999.

Zide BM, Longaker MT: Chin surgery II. Submental ostectomy and soft tissue excision, *Plast Reconstr Surg* 104:1854-1860, 1999.

Endoscopic Brow-Lift

Chris Jo, DMD, and Shahrokh C. Bagheri, DMD, MD

CC

A 52-year-old woman presents to your office with a chief complaint of "My eyebrows have been drooping down slowly year after year, and I want them lifted back up."

HPI

The patient points to one eyebrow and lifts it superiorly with her fingers in front of a mirror, stating "This is where my eyebrows used to be and should be, but now look how flat they are" (this maneuver may unmask pseudo upper eyelid dermatochalasis caused by the descended brow). She also brings a picture of when she was in her 30s to illustrate her desired surgical outcome. She denies any previous facial cosmetic surgery and appears to have reasonable expectations (surgeons should be cautious about patients with unreasonable expectations of cosmetic surgery).

PMHX/PDHX/MEDICATIONS/ALLERGIES/SH/FH

Noncontributory. The patient is not on any medications that would affect platelet function (e.g., aspirin) or the coagulation cascade.

EXAMINATION

Forehead–eyebrow–upper lid complex. The forehead exhibits minimal horizontal rhytids (wrinkles) at rest and moderate dynamic horizontal furrows (caused by frontalis muscle hypertrophy/hyperactivity compensation for brow ptosis). Hairline (trichion) is 5 cm from the orbital ridge (within normal limits). There are mild horizontal radix and vertical glabellar furrows at rest (caused by the procerus and corrugator supercilii muscles respectively). The eyebrow (examined with the patient completely relaxed and in a neutral position) is relatively flat in shape (attractive female eyebrows are arched, as opposed to flattened eyebrows in males). The positions of the eyebrows are recorded (the inferior border of the eyebrow is measured from the superior orbital rim). Figure 12-16 shows the ideal eyebrow position in a Caucasian female.

- **Medial brow region.** This is 1 mm below the superior orbital rim (ideally, the medial brow is 1 to 2 mm above the rim in females and males).
- **Brow apex** (halfway between the lateral limbus and lateral canthus): This is 3 mm above the superior orbital rim (ideally, the apex is 8 to 10 mm above the rim, or 25 mm diagonally from mid-pupil in females and 1 to 2 mm above the rim in males).
- **Tail of brow (lateral).** This is 2 mm above the superolateral orbital rim (ideally, the tail is located 10 to 15 mm above the superolateral orbital rim in females and 1 to 2 mm above the rim in males) and ends just lateral to the line connecting the lateral canthus and nasal ala (within normal limits).
- **Upper eyelid** (see also earlier information upper eyelid blepharoplasty for further details). This exhibits pseudodermatochalasis, or hooding, secondary to brow fat pad and eyebrow ptosis (descent of the forehead-eyebrow-brow complex), which resolves when the forehead-eyebrow complex is manually raised into an ideal position by the surgeon's thumb.

IMAGING

Preoperative and serial postoperative photoimaging is mandatory for cosmetic procedures. Close-up views of the forehead-eyebrow-upper eyelid complex in frontal, three-quarters, and profile positions are recommended.

LABS

Routine preoperative laboratory testing for outpatient brow-lift procedures is not indicated unless dictated by the medical history.

ASSESSMENT

Patient desires browlift procedure secondary to bilateral eyebrow ptosis caused by gravitational descent of the soft tissues of the upper facial third with age

TREATMENT

Upper facial rejuvenation with an endoscopic brow (forehead) lift is the treatment of choice to restore a youthful or aesthetically pleasing eyebrow position for this patient. The authors' preferred technique is described here.

Incisions. Three 2-cm vertical incisions (one in the midline and two parasagittal incision coincident with the lateral limbus) are made just behind the hairline down to bone, and two bilateral 3-cm vertical temporal incisions are made at 2 to 3 cm posterior to the hairline down to the deep temporal fascia (alternatively, some surgeons recommend two incisions coincident with the medial brow instead

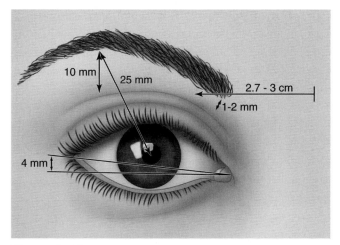

Figure 12-16 The ideal position of an aesthetically pleasing, youthful eyebrow for a Caucasian female.

of one midline incision when more medial elevation is required).

Dissection. Subperiosteal dissection is initially carried out blindly, using the three frontal incisions, posteriorly toward the lambdoid suture, anteriorly to approximately 2 to 3 cm above the superior orbital rim, and laterally to the temporal crest. The endoscope is introduced into the midline incision and used to assist the subperiosteal dissection toward the superior orbital rim (strong periosteal adherence to bone in this region), to avoid injury to the supraorbital and supratrochlear neurovascular bundles. It is important to release the periosteum down to the radix medially and past the orbital rims laterally.

The temporal incisions are then used to blindly dissect the initial 2 cm toward the lateral orbital rims. The endoscope is then used to assist the remainder of the dissection. The temporal dissection should remain 1 cm above the zygomatic arch to prevent injury to the frontal branch of the facial nerve. The anterior extent of dissection is sufficient once the sentinel vein (zygomaticotemporal vein) is encountered. The temporal zone of fixation (cojoined tendon) is penetrated and released with a periosteal elevator, connecting the subperiosteal dissection in the forehead region and the subtemporoparietal dissection in the temporal region (connecting all three optical cavities). Some surgeons recommend removing a strip of deep temporal fascia to enhance scar formation and to improve long-term stability.

Before elevating the forehead and eyebrow, it is important to incise and release the periosteum just superior to the arcus marginalis from the lateral orbital rim, along the superior orbital rim, and across the radix of the nose. Several techniques can be used to release the periosteum. The authors prefer to use technique described by Griffin and associates using the 50-W CO_2 laser (alternatively, other surgeons prefer to use a long Colorado needle). Corrugator supercilii or procerus muscles, or both, can be disrupted if needed.

Elevation and fixation. Various methods can be used to elevate and fixate the forehead-eyebrow complex. Evans describes a very precise technique using two-hole miniplates,

securing the forehead-eyebrow complex to the miniplate with 2-0 Vicryl suture. Griffin and associates describe a flap suspension suturing technique that secures the flap to the posterior scalp. It is important that the suture engages subcutaneous tissue, galea, frontalis muscle, subgaleal areolar fascia, and periosteum (most important) at the anterior aspect of the incision. Resorbable endotines have been recently introduced, which are drilled into the frontal bone, and then the spikes engage, holding the periosteum in place. The temporal tissues (superficial temporal fascia anteriorly to temporal fascia posteriorly) are suspended posteriorly by 2-0 Vicryl sutures through the temporal incision. The incisions are closed and a head dressing is placed.

COMPLICATIONS

Endoscopic brow-lift has minimal complications (infection, hematoma, nerve injury, alopecia, scarring, and brow malposition). As with all facial cosmetic procedures, relapse is the greatest concern for the surgeon, and long-term stability is one of the main goals of cosmetic surgery. Transient forehead paresthesia (anesthesia, hypoesthesia) is a consequence of surgery and is not considered a complication. Permanent nerve injury, although uncommon, may occur if the supraorbital or supratrochlear nerve is injured beyond a stretch injury (neuropraxia), and it is usually avoided by careful dissection assisted by an endoscope. Despite correct technique and thorough knowledge of the regional anatomy, nerve injuries can occur.

We emphasize that the evaluation of the brows should be done with particular attention to the upper eyelids. It is important to avoid performing an upper eyelid blepharoplasty on a patient who really requires a brow-lift procedure. Lifting the brow to an ideal position may subsequently cause lagophthalmos, due to excess upper eyelid skin excision.

DISCUSSION

Youthful or ideal appearance of the upper facial third. A youthful appearance of the upper third of the face includes a smooth forehead skin without rhytids or furrows, arched tapering eyebrows (for females), and a distinct supratarsal fold without excess skin or prolapsed fat. Males tend to have thicker and more horizontal eyebrows that are ideally 1 to 2 mm above and along the superior orbital rim. The goal of rejuvenation of the upper face is to not only restore the eyebrow to an aesthetically pleasing form with a brow-lift procedure but also restore the upper eyelid with a blepharoplasty as needed (see earlier section on upper eyelid blepharoplasty) and smooth the forehead and glabellar rhytids or furrows with adjunctive procedures (see later). Figure 12-16 shows an aesthetically pleasing eyebrow position. It is important to note that there are variations in what is considered a "normal" or "aesthetically pleasing" eyebrow among different ethnic and racial groups.

Anatomy of aging of the upper facial third. The major plane of aging of the upper face is between the superficial fascia and deep fascia (gliding plane). This plane is called the subtemporoparietal areolar fascia (in the temporal region) and the subgaleal areolar fascia (in the frontal region). The frontalis muscle inserts into the dermis of the medial two thirds of the eyebrow only, medial to the temporal fusion line. The lateral third of the eyebrow is unsupported by the frontalis muscle and begins to descend as the lateral support mechanism attenuates (temporal zone of fixation and orbital osteocutaneous ligament). The forehead-eyebrow-temporal soft tissues slide over the deep fascia-pericranium and, due to its loose adherence, causes ptosis of the eyebrows with a relatively greater effect on the lateral brow. Depressor action of the orbicularis oculi, depressor supercilii, corrugator supercilii, and procerus muscles and descent of the brow fat pad contribute to this aging process. Even though the changes in the sub-SMAS plane are considered to be a main contributor to aging of the upper face, long-term stability of forehead/eyebrow lift procedures depends on scarification of the periosteum to bone.

Alternative surgical procedures for forehead-eyebrow rejuvenation. Traditional approaches to the forehead and brow-lift include a direct brow-lift (incision/excision directly above the eyebrow), a mid-forehead lift (incision/excision along a horizontal forehead furrow), and the coronal lift (incision/excision along and/or within the hairline). The coronal lift (either coronal or pretrichial incisions) is still commonly used by some surgeons and has indications. More recently, minimally invasive barbed sutures (contour threads) have been introduced, but their long-term stability has come into question.

Adjunctive procedures. The endoscopic brow-lift can be an isolated procedure or combined with other facial cosmetic procedures (facelift, upper or lower blepharoplasty, Botox injections, etc.) depending on the patient needs and desires. It is important to realize that the upper eyelid and eyebrow positions have a close relationship and must be examined together (refer to upper and lower eyelid blepharoplasty section). Botox is commonly used to treat vertical glabellar rhytids (corrugator supercilii muscle), horizontal forehead rhytids (frontalis muscle), and horizontal rhytids at the radix (procerus muscle). It can be used to achieve some elevation of the brow by reducing the downward force caused by the orbicularis oculi muscle.

Bibliography

Adamson PA, Johnson CM, Anderson JR, et al: The forehead lift, *Arch Otolaryngol* 111:325-329, 1985.

Beeson WH, McCollough EG: Complications of the forehead lift, *Ear Nose Throat J* 64:28-42, 1985.

Cook TA, Brownrigg PJ, Wang TD, et al: The versatile midforehead browlift, *Arch Otolaryngol Head Neck Surg* 115:163-168, 1989.

Evans TW: Endoscopic facial aesthetic surgery. In Fonseca RJ, editor: *Oral and Maxillofacial Surgery,* Philadelphia, 2000, WB Saunders, pp 457-490.

Griffin JE, Frey BS, Max DP, et al: Laser-assisted endoscopic forehead lift, *J Oral Maxillofac Surg* 56:1040-1048, 1998.

Griffin JE, Owsley TG: Management of forehead and brow deformities, *Atlas Oral Maxillofac Surg Clin N Am* 12:235-251, 2004.

Knize DM: An anatomically base study of the mechanism of eyebrow ptosis, *Plast Reconstr Surg* 97:1321-1333, 1996.

Liebman EP, Webster RC, Berger AS, et al: The frontalis nerve in the temporal brow lift, *Arch Otolaryngol* 108:232-235, 1982.

Ramirez OM, Robertson KM: Update in endoscopic forehead rejuvenation, *Fac Plast Surg Clin N Am* 10:37-51, 2002.

Zukowski ML: Endoscopic brow surgery, *Oral Maxillofac Surg Clin N Am* 12(4):701-708, 2000.

Botulinum Toxin A (Botox) Injection for Facial Rejuvenation

Eric P. Holmgren, MS, DMD, MD, and Shahrokh C. Bagheri, DMD, MD

CC

A 44-year-old Caucasian woman presents to your office for consultation regarding the wrinkles on her forehead. (The majority of the patients seeking facial rejuvenation are female, but there is growing interest in the male population.)

HPI

During an orthognathic surgery consultation for her daughter several months earlier, the patient noticed the Botox pamphlets in the waiting room at your office (unlike other branches of oral and maxillofacial surgery, a busy cosmetic surgery practice is usually heavily dependent on marketing and advertisement). The patient states that "these lines" have recently appeared on her forehead and that she is tired of looking like she is "scowling" or "frowning." Her husband has mentioned to her that the wrinkles make her appear "angry." Several of her friends have had satisfactory results with Botox injections for glabellar and periorbital lines. She has many questions regarding the safety and outcome of Botox injections for elimination of wrinkles.

PMHX/PDHX/MEDICATIONS/ALLERGIES/SH/FH

The patient does not have any known medical conditions. Specifically, she has no known history of neuromuscular diseases, including myasthenia gravis, amyotrophic lateral sclerosis, multiple sclerosis, Eaton-Lambert syndrome, or other motor neuron–related disorders (despite the absence of specific studies, Botox should be used cautiously in individuals with neuromuscular disorders due to potential exacerbation of any preexisting conditions). There is no significant family history of neuromuscular disorders.

She is not taking any aminoglycoside antibiotic or other medications that could interfere with neuromuscular transmission (it is recommended that Botox injections be delayed or avoided in patients taking aminoglycosides). She is not taking aspirin or a nonsteroidal antiinflammatory drug or other medications that can interfere with coagulation or platelet function (increases the risk for hematoma formation and bruising). She smokes one-half pack of cigarettes per day (smoking is not a contraindication for Botox injection).

There is no history of allergies to human albumin or any previous adverse reactions to Botox. (Botox that was manufactured after 1997 has a lower albumin concentration, and therefore presumably a lower risk of clinical antigenicity.) She is not pregnant or lactating (Botox is contraindicated during nursing or pregnancy and is classified by the FDA as Pregnancy Category C, meaning that its safety profile during pregnancy has not been studied. It is unknown whether the toxin can cross the placenta or if it is excreted during lactation. However, the localized application of the drug would suggest the safety of application during pregnancy or nursing).

EXAMINATION

General. The patient is a thin, athletic, well-dressed woman. She has extensive amounts of makeup that mask some of her facial features of aging. She is wearing her hair in a fashion to reduce the visibility of the forehead lines (subtle observations about appearance may be the key to successful patient rapport).

Maxillofacial. There are no pustules or signs of active dermatological infections or pathology in the facial region (injections are contraindicated if an active infection exists at the injection site). There is no marked facial asymmetry or hypertrophic facial scarring (thick skin or a susceptibility to hypertrophic scars may be a relative contraindication to injections). There is no significant eyebrow ptosis (this is important for injection around the eyes or the forehead. Impairment of functioning of the frontalis can also lower the brow position from unopposed muscle action, resulting in an unappealing outcome. Similarly, large amounts of Botox injected around the eye can diffuse toward the levator palpebrae muscle, causing impaired eyelid closure. The degree of preoperative ptosis can be documented for postoperative comparison).

Several prominent horizontal forehead wrinkles (due to frontalis muscle action) are present at rest (Figure 12-17, *A*), which are accentuated with animation (Figure 12-17, *B*), and multiple hyperdynamic rhytids (lines on face) are seen lateral to the eye that are most pronounced on animation (the obicularis oculi region is also known as "crow's feet") (Figure 12-17, *C*). At rest, fine vertical glabellar furrows are present, and on animation and frowning, the glabella muscle bulge becomes significantly prominent (the corrugator muscle is responsible for the vertical glabellar furrows and the procerus muscle is responsible for the horizontal glabellar furrows). A glabellar-spread test was performed, revealing that the glabellar lines are substantially decreased when physically manipulated or spread apart (a good indication that the muscle and its overlying soft tissue are the etiology of the lines). During physical examination, it is important to distinguish between dynamic and static wrinkles. Botox will decrease dynamic

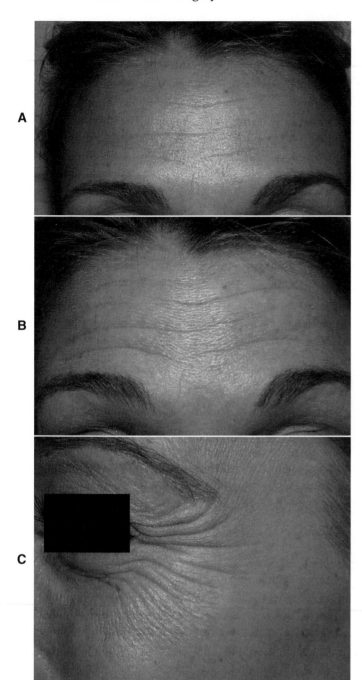

Figure 12-17 A, Forehead wrinkles secondary to the frontalis muscle functioning. **B,** Forehead lines accentuated during frontalis function. **C,** Hyperdynamic periorbital lines (crow's feet) accentuated with animation.

wrinkles because of its effect on muscles. Static wrinkles may be treated using soft tissue fillers to decrease skin laxity at rest.

No significant horizontal lines were present at the nasal root ("bunny lines"), and no prominent perioral vertical ("lipstick") rhytids are visible.

Intraoral. No abnormalities or lesions are noted (important to conduct an oral cancer screening examination, especially in a patient with a history of smoking).

Neck. There is no cervicomental lymphadenopathy (enlarged lymph nodes are indicative of ongoing pathological, inflammatory, or infectious processes).

IMAGING

Standard facial photodocumentation of the areas to be treated is recommended (but not essential) for Botox injection. Comparisons of preinjection and postinjection photographs may be important for future dosing and for surgeon education toward optimal results.

LABS

No routine laboratory tests are indicated. Patients on large doses of anticoagulation are at risk for small hematoma formation at the injection site. The treating surgeon should inquire about any coagulation studies to assess the risk and educate the patient about this potential temporary, yet undesired, effect.

ASSESSMENT

Multiple areas of hyperfunctioning facial muscles, and signs of aging involving the periorbital, glabellar, and horizontal forehead regions

The patient desires injection of Botox for effacement of the wrinkles associated with her periorbital and forehead regions (while there may be many findings amendable to cosmetic surgery, the assessment and treatment are dictated by patient desires).

TREATMENT

After a complete discussion of the procedure, risks, and alternatives, the patient signed the informed consent (which addressed all of the complications listed later). One hundred units of botulinum toxin A was reconstituted with 3.3 ml of unpreserved normal saline (according to a study by Alam and associates in 2002, the use of preservative-containing normal saline is less painful than the use of preservative-free saline. However, this is not in accordance with the manufacturer's recommendations). Botox is available in a sealed vacuum container that allows for easy reconstitution with saline. The resulting solution provides 3 units/0.1 ml, or 15 units/0.5 ml. Botox should be reconstituted gently (shaking and trauma to the toxin can diminish its potency) with a 21-gauge needle and then gently drawn into a tuberculin syringe. The syringe can be used with a short 30-gauge needle.

The patient was seated upright, close to a 60° position. After the injection sites were prepared with alcohol, the patient was asked to frown (or to lower eyebrows) to highlight the regions of maximum muscular contraction. Six injection sites were identified to inject the frontalis muscle. To minimize the chance for blepharoptosis, the injections were performed at least 1 cm above both the central eyebrow and the supraorbital ridge. To prevent inhibiting temporalis function, it is important to avoid injections on the forehead lateral to the lateral canthus. The goal of forehead injections is not to completely eliminate the frontalis muscle action, as this can cause undesirable brow ptosis. Ice packs were applied immediately before injection to blunt the pain response from needle injection. The needle was inserted into the belly of the muscle, aspiration was performed, and then Botox was slowly injected. After the injections, no manipulation was performed, and an ice pack was placed on the area (manipulation can enhance diffusion into other muscles, affecting the levator palpebrae superior and causing blepharoptosis, especially with injections near the eyelid). Attention was then turned to the obicularis oculi region. After preparing the area with alcohol, a total of 9 units was injected into three sites bilaterally just below the skin (to minimize diffusion in this area). A total of 36 units was used for the forehead and crow's feet regions (18 units for the forehead and a total of 18 units for the two eyes).

Ice was placed on the injection sites for as long as the patient could tolerate it. The patient was instructed to remain upright for at least 4 hours and was allowed to apply makeup 4 hours after injection (the delay is to minimize manipulation and thus diffusion of the toxin). She can resume exercise the next day. She was instructed to expect a noticeable effect in 3 to 4 days with maximum benefit in 30 days (Figure 12-18). Follow-up was made in 1 week. The areas can be reinjected after a minimum of 3 months has elapsed (earlier injections can increase the chance of the development of antibodies).

COMPLICATIONS

Since its introduction, many patients have been safely treated with Botox. The complications of treatment using Botox include the following:

- Undesired effect (can be related to patient expectations, rate of metabolism, dosing, anatomical variations, or inadequate site of injection)
- Short duration of the desired effect
- Postinjection bruising (this can be minimized by avoiding aspirin or nonsteroidal antiinflammatory drugs 7 to 14 days before injection and is most common in the periorbital region)
- Blepharoptosis—reported occurrences in 1% to 2% of periorbital injections (this can be treated with an α_2-adrenergic agonist [aproclonidine 0.5% eye drops to be used 30 minutes before social situations]; this stimulates Mueller's muscle, causing hours of transient lid opening)
- Transient headaches, pain, edema, and erythema at the injection site
- Formation of neutralizing antibodies (this has been reported to occur with repeat injections within 1 month of the previous and was reported with doses greater than 100 units per treatment session; this has not been reported for the cosmetic use of Botox, but it is recommended to wait at least 3 months between injections)
- Hematoma formation at the injection site

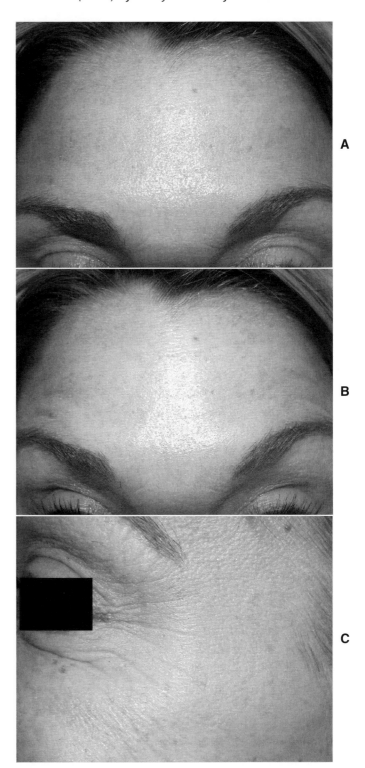

Figure 12-18 **A,** One-month postoperative view at rest showing significant reduction of horizontal forehead lines. **B,** One-month postoperative view upon brow elevation and, showing significant reduction of horizontal forehead lines with animation. **C,** One-month postoperative view of the lateral periorbital lines (crow's feet) seen during animation.

DISCUSSION

Botox is a formulation of botulinum toxin A purified neurotoxin complex produced from fermentation of the gram-positive spore-forming bacteria *Clostridium botulinum* type A. When injected into striated muscle, it produces a dose-dependent local muscle weakness by preventing the release of acetylcholine from nerve terminal at the neuromuscular junction (chemical deinnervation). The action involves a four-step process that culminates with the cleavage of the 25-kDa synaptosome-associated protein (SNAP), which is essential for the exocytosis of acetylcholine. The paralytic effect is temporary, because there is a gradual recovery of the activity of the nerve terminal over a 3- to 6-month time-frame. The unit of measurement for Botox is derived from research with mice. One unit of Botox is the lethal dose in 50% of mice (LD_{50}). The LD_{50} is 2500 to 3000 units in humans (40 units/ kg). Dosing for the clinical effects of Botox can vary among individuals; those with thicker muscles and male patients often require more Botox units to achieve the desired effect.

Unopened vials of Botox can be stored for 24 months in a refrigerator (2° to 8°C) and, once reconstituted, varying opinions exist regarding its shelf-life beyond the manufacturer's recommendation of only 4 hours. Studies have suggested no clinical difference for up to 6 weeks after reconstitution, but others have noticed diminished potency beyond 48 hours. To the date of this publication, the FDA-approved use of Botox includes treatment for dystonia, torticollis, blepharospasm, strabismus, wrinkles caused by the procerus and corrugator muscles (glabellar region), and severe primary axillary hyperhidrosis on patients younger than 65 years. However, common off-label uses are numerous and include hyperhydrosis for palms, Frey syndrome, migraine headaches, myofascial pain, bruxism, masseter hypertrophy, chronic temporomandibular joint dislocation, limb spasticity, platysmal banding, and others.

In the oral and maxillofacial surgery office, injections are commonly made into the upper face region, such as the glabella, lateral canthal lines (crow's feet), and forehead (frontalis). Selective brow-raising techniques can be used. By injecting the lateral obicularis muscle without injecting the frontalis in select areas, the brow peak can rise as a result of unopposed frontalis muscle action. Noncosmetic injections for trigger pain regions of the temporalis and masseter muscle can be performed as well with Botox. Lower face injections to treat "lipstick lines" should be reserved for experienced surgeons and may cause oral incompetence. Also, the concomitant use of fillers such as a non–animal-source hyaluronic acid (Restylane) can be used to augment static wrinkles. Patient satisfaction has been shown to be increased with the use of these two techniques.

Bibliography

Alam M, Dover JS, Arndt KA: Pain associated with injection of botulinum A exotoxin reconstituted using isotonic sodium chloride with and without preservative: a double-blind, randomized controlled trial, *Arch Dermatol* 138(4):510-514, 2002.

Carruthers J, Carruthers A: A prospective, randomized, parallel group study analyzing the effect of BTX-A (Botox) and non-animal sourced hyaluronic acid (NASHA, Restylane) in combination compared with NASHA (Restylane) alone in severe glabellar rhytides in adult female subjects: treatment of severe glabellar rhytides with a hyaluronic acid derivative compared with the derivative and BTX-A, *Dermatol Surg* 29:802-809, 2003.

Castro WH, Gomez RS, da Silva Oliveira J, et al: Botulinum toxin type A in the management of masseter muscle hypertrophy, *J Oral Maxillofac Surg* 63(1):20-24, 2005.

Connor MS, Karlis V, Ghali GE: Management of the aging forehead: a review, *Oral Surg Oral Med Oral Pathol Oral Radiol Endod* 95(6):642-648, 2003.

Frampton J, Easthope S: Botulinum toxin A (Botox cosmetic): a review of its use in the treatment of glabellar frown lines, *Am J Clin Dermatol* 4(10):709-725, 2003.

Freund B, Schwarz M, Symington JM: Botulinum toxin: new treatment for temporomandibular disorders, *Br J Oral Maxillofac Surg* 38:466-471, 2000.

Hexsel DM, De Almeida AT, Rutowitsch M, et al: Multicenter, double-blind study of the efficacy of injections with botulinum toxin type A reconstituted up to six consecutive weeks before application, *Dermatol Surg* 29(5):523-529, 2003.

Kane M: Botox injections for lower facial rejuvenation, *Oral Maxillofac Surg Clin N Am* 17(1):41-49, 2005.

Niamtu J 3rd: Botulinum toxin A: a review of 1,085 oral and maxillofacial patient treatments, *J Oral Maxillofac Surg* 61(3):317-324, 2003.

Rohrich R, Janis J: Botox for the treatment of dynamic and hyperkinetic facial lines and furrows: adjunctive use in facial aesthetic surgery, *Plast Reconstr Surg* (5 suppl):112, 2003.

Solish N, Benohanian A, Kowalski JW; Canadian Dermatology Study Group on Health-Related Quality of Life in Primary Axillary Hyperhidrosis: Prospective open-label study of botulinum toxin type A in patients with axillary hyperhidrosis: effects on functional impairment and quality of life, *Dermatol Surg* 31(4):405-413, 2005.

Trindade De Almeida AR, Kadunc BV, et al: Foam during reconstitution does not affect the potency of botulinum toxin type A, *Dermatol Surg* 29(5):530-531, 2003.

Vartanian AJ, Dayan SH: Facial rejuvenation using botulinum toxin A: review and updates, *Fac Plast Surg* 20(1):11-19, 2004.

13 Syndromes of the Head and Neck

Chris Jo, DMD

This chapter addresses:
- Cleft Lip and Palate
- Nonsyndromic Craniosynostosis
- Apert Syndrome
- Crouzon Syndrome
- Hemifacial Microsomia
- Obstructive Sleep Apnea Syndrome

A multitude of anomalies and syndromes occur in the head and neck, most of which are beyond the scope of this book. This chapter covers some of the most common anomalies or syndromes associated with the craniomaxillofacial region. Congenital anomalies include nonsyndromic craniosynostosis, hemifacial microsomia, and cleft lip and palate (CLP). Congenital syndromes include Apert and Crouzon syndromes. Unlike the other syndromes in this section, which are congenital, obstructive sleep apnea syndrome (OSAS) is included here because the pathogenesis and manifestation of this syndrome are based on anatomical anomalies of the head and neck. Oral and maxillofacial surgeons are uniquely trained and play an integral role in the surgical management of these patients, whether or not syndromic.

The intent of this chapter is to familiarize readers with the pathogenesis, presentation, and management strategies of such anomalies. The chapter is structured so that key features of each syndrome or anomaly are emphasized. The reconstructive strategies and rationale for treatment are discussed. Because of the complexity of craniofacial deformities involved in the growing child, the reconstructive efforts are generally staged. There is no consensus on the best timing of each stage, but the general guidelines are presented. Various surgical strategies, depending on the surgeons' preference and clinical situation, can be used. These are presented in the chapter along with their rationale of treatment. Table 13-1 outlines the characteristics of some craniofacial syndromes.

Table 13-1. Characteristics of Some Craniofacial Syndromes

Syndrome	Prevalence/ Inheritance	Genetic	Synostosis/Orbit	Limbs	Central Nervous System
Apert syndrome	15.5:1 million, AD or sporadic or new mutation Males = females	Ser253Trp or Pro253 Arg on Ig II or III of *FGFR2*	Early fusion of coronal suture, widely patent midline calverial defect	Fusion of digits 2, 3, and 4 Less common is fusion of digits 2, 3, 4, and 5, with digit 1 free	Patent sutures (except coronal) and open synchondroses, agenesis of septum pellucidum, agenesis of corpus callosum, cavum septum pellucidum, developmental delay
Crouzon syndrome	15-16:1 million, AD	15 mutations of Ig III domain of *FGFR2*	Variable sutures involvement and skull shape, extropia, exposed conjunctiva, and keratitis	None	Cerebellar tonsil herniation, jugular foramen stenosis, venous obstruction, and increased intracranial pressure Headache (29%), seizure (10%), mental retardation (3%)
Pfeiffer syndrome	16-40/million, AD	*FGFR1, FGFR2*	Pronounced extrobism	Broad thumbs	Three types: type 1, normal life expectancy and intelligence; type 2, cloverleaf skull, exorbitism, elbow ankylosis, broad thumb and great toes; type 3, same as type 2 without cloverleaf. Types 2 and 3 with ventriculomegaly, progressive hydrocephalus, and cerebellar herniation

AD, Autosomal dominant.

Cleft Lip and Palate

John M. Allen, DMD, and Chris Jo, DMD

CC

As a member of the craniofacial multidisciplinary team, you are asked to evaluate a 4-week-old male infant born with a left complete CLP.

There are both ethnic and racial variations in the incidence of CLP. CLP is most common in Asians (3.2:1000), followed by whites (1.4:1000), and, least common, individuals of African descent (0.43:1000). CLP occurs more commonly in males, and on the left side. Isolated cleft palate (CP) is a different genetic entity with no racial predilection, and it is more common in females.

HPI

The infant was born at a community hospital with no obstetric complications. He was subsequently diagnosed with a nonsyndromic CLP and was referred to the cleft team at your institution for further evaluation and treatment. The pregnancy was uncomplicated with no known environmental exposures.

Modern high-resolution ultrasonographic studies are able to diagnose complete CLP as early as 16 weeks in utero, and therefore the prenatal diagnosis of CLP has become more common.

PMHX/PDHX/MEDICATIONS/ALLERGIES/SH/FH

Except for the CLP, the child has no other medical problems. He was born with Apgar scores of 8 and 9, at 1 and 5 minutes, respectively. There are no facial or systemic anomalies characteristic of any known syndromes (see Discussion), including any associated cardiac, respiratory, ophthamological, or musculoskeletal abnormalities. There is no family history of CLP or CP.

Pedigree analysis has demonstrated an increase incidence when a family member has CLP. In addition, if a couple has a child with CLP, the risk of having an affected second child is significantly (fortyfold) increased.

EXAMINATION

General. The 4-week-old Caucasian male infant is in the 25th percentile for weight and height (likely due to difficulty with feeding).

Maxillofacial. The cleft lip (CL) is complete, penetrating the entire thickness of the lip, alveolus, nasal tip cartilages, and floor of the nose. The cleft is unilateral, left of midline (left side prevalence), and continuous with the palate (CLP is most commonly expressed unilaterally, with a 2:1 predilection for the left side).

Intraoral. The cleft continues through the hard palate and soft palate (structures anterior to the incisive foramen form the primary palate and posterior to the incisive foramen form the secondary palate). Throughout the cleft, the nasal cavity, nasal conchae, and posterior pharyngeal wall are readily visible. The nasal mucosa appears inflamed and ulcerated (due to irritation of the fragile tissue from feeding). Bidigital palpation identifies solid supportive bone along the palatal shelves bordering the cleft site (it is important to palpate the hard palate of any infant in order to detect the presence of a notch in the posterior border of the hard palate, suggesting the presence of a submucous cleft).

IMAGING

No imaging studies are indicated for the diagnosis and management of isolated CLP. When craniosynostosis or syndromic anomalies are suspected, craniofacial and head computed tomography (CT) scans are indicated.

LABS

Baseline hemoglobin and hematocrit are indicated before surgical correction of any cleft. In general, a hemoglobin level of 10 mg/dl is deemed necessary before surgical intervention for lip repair (although there is no scientific rationale for this determination).

ASSESSMENT

Four-week-old Caucasian male infant with an isolated, complete, nonsyndromic CLP

Although there are several classification systems for facial clefting, including one by Tessier, they are not routinely used at most centers.

CL is a unilateral or bilateral gap in the upper lip and jaw that forms during the third through seventh weeks of embryonic development. It develops from failure of fusion of the medial nasal process and the maxillary process. CLs are described as either complete or incomplete. A complete CL is a cleft of the entire lip and alveolar arch or premaxilla; an incomplete CL involves only the lip. A CP is a gap in the hard and/or soft palate that forms during the fifth through twelfth weeks of development. CP forms as a result of failure of attachment and alignment of the levator veli, tensor veli palatini, uvular, palatopharyngeus, and palatoglossus muscles. The primary palate is formed by the lip, alveolar arch, and palate anterior to the incisive foramen (known as the premaxilla). The secondary palate is formed by the soft and hard palates posterior to the incisive foramen.

TREATMENT

There is no general consensus regarding the timing and techniques used for CLP surgery. Individual craniofacial centers and craniofacial surgeons follow various protocols according to their own experience, rationale, and preferences. The functional needs, aesthetic concerns, and ongoing growth of affected individuals all create specific concerns that complicate the treatment process. Presurgical dentofacial orthopedics is increasingly used to optimize primary CL repair.

Table 13-2 outlines the sequence of management of patients with CLP. CL repair is usually addressed at 10 to 14 weeks of age. One advantage of waiting until this age is that it allows time for a thorough medical evaluation to determination of any congenital defects. The surgical procedure is generally easier to perform when the child is slightly larger, with anatomical landmarks being more prominent and well defined. In addition, it has historically been accepted that the safest anesthesia time period for infants occurs when one follows the "rule of tens"—surgery can be performed when the child is at least 10 weeks of age, weighs at least 10 lb, and has a minimum hemoglobin value of 10 mg/dl (however, there is no current scientific rationale to support this rule). With modern intraoperative pediatric monitoring techniques, general anesthesia

can be performed safely at an earlier age as needed, although there is no documented benefit to perform lip repair before 3 months of age. Excessive scarring and inferior aesthetic results have been found to occur when surgery is performed earlier than age 3 months. CP repair is usually performed between 9 to 18 months of age. CP repair is intended to coincide with the progression of natural speech development and growth. In deciding upon the timing of repair, the surgeon must consider the delicate balance between facial growth restriction after early surgery, and early speech development that requires an intact palate. Most children require an intact palate to produce certain sounds by 18 months of age. If developmental delay is present and speech is not anticipated to develop until later, then CP repair can be delayed.

There is very little evidence to support palate repair before 9 months of age. Surgical repairs before this time are associated with a higher incidence of maxillary hypoplasia later in life and show no improvement in speech. After initial CP repair, 20% of the children develop inadequate closure of the velopharyngeal mechanism (velopharyngeal insufficiency). This is usually diagnosed at 3 to 5 years of age, when a detailed speech examination can be performed. Surgery is performed to correct the anatomical defect, with the goal of improving closure between the oral and nasal cavities and reducing nasal air escape during the production of certain sounds. Approximately 75% of patients with any type of cleft will present with clefting of the maxilla and alveolus. Bone graft reconstruction of the alveolus is performed during the mixed dentition period before eruption of the permanent canine and/or permanent lateral incisor. The timing of this

Table 13-2.   Sequence of Management of the Cleft Patient

Procedure	Age or Timing	Comments
Dentofacial orthopedics	First few weeks of life	Improves tension-free lip closure
Lip adhesion (two-stage repair)	After dentofacial orthopedics and before definitive nasolabial repair	Some centers prefer one-stage closure and do not perform lip adhesions
Definitive nasolabial repair	Traditionally done at 10 weeks (no scientific basis) Centers now advocate lip closure at 3 to 6 months	Timing may vary based on cleft type
Cleft palate repair	Before 1 to 2 years Some centers advocate closure at 8 to 10 months Some centers advocate two-staged repair, using an obturator to delay palate closure	Earlier repair (before 1 year) is advocated to improve speech development Maxillary growth should be monitored with earlier repairs
Correction of velopharyngeal insufficiency (pharyngeal flap or sphincter pharyngoplasty)	Speech assessment begins at $1^1/_2$ to 2 years	Velopharyngeal insufficiency may occur after maxillary advancement as well, and can be corrected 6 to 12 months later
Nasolabial revisions	Before 3 years	
Phase I orthodontics	Before alveolar cleft bone grafting	Differentially expanding the anterior maxilla
Alveolar bone grafting	At 8 to 12 years (when maxillary canine root is $^1/_2$ to $^2/_3$ formed)	Bone graft from anterior ilium is usually preferred
Phase II orthodontics	Permanent dentition phase	
Correction of maxillary hypoplasia (orthognathic surgery and/or distraction osteogenesis)	After completion of growth	Distraction osteogenesis should be considered when maxillary advancement is greater than 10 mm
Rhinoplasty	At 6 to 12 months after maxillary advancement	

Modified from Kaban LB, Troulis MJ, editors: *Pediatric oral and maxillofacial surgery,* Philadelphia, 2004, Elsevier.

procedure is based on dental development and not chronological age. Reconstruction of the alveolus before the mixed dentition stage has been associated with a high degree of maxillary growth restriction, requiring orthognathic correction later in life. Autogenous bone grafted from the iliac crest has provided the best results for reconstruction of alveolar cleft defects.

Orthognathic reconstruction of maxillary and mandibular discrepancies is generally performed from 14 to 18 years of age based on individual growth characteristics. This is performed in conjunction with orthodontics before and after surgery. Orthognathic surgery before this time-frame is performed only for severe cases of dysmorphology.

Lip and nasal revision is best treated once the majority of growth is complete, which generally occurs after 5 years of age but is usually performed only for severe deformities. Nasal revision is generally performed after age 5, when most of the nasal growth is complete. When orthognathic reconstruction is planned, rhinoplasty is best performed after orthognathic surgery as maxillary advancement improves many characteristics of nasal form.

Treatment techniques for CL. Unilateral CL repair, as previously mentioned, is usually performed after 10 weeks of age. The technique most commonly used is the "Millard rotation-advancement" technique. The basic intent of the repair is to create a three-layer closure of skin, muscle, and mucosa that approximates the normal tissue and excises hypoplastic tissue at the cleft margins. The orbicularis oris muscle is adapted to form a continuous sphincter. The incision lines of the Millard technique also fall within the natural contours of the lip and nose on closure, which helps promote a natural form of symmetry. The "C-flap" can be used to lengthen the columella, create a nasal sill, or can be banked for later use.

The Randall-Tennison technique represents a Z-plasty technique that is used by some surgeons for unilateral CL repair. This technique, however, does not achieve the same semblance of symmetry as that obtained using the Millard technique.

Primary nasal reconstruction may be performed at the time of lip repair to reposition the displaced lower lateral cartilages and alar tissues. Various techniques have been advocated, each with considerable variation. The repair essentially involves releasing the alar base, augmenting the area with allogenic subdermal grafts, or proceeding with open rhinoplasty with minimal dissection to avoid scar formation.

Bilateral lip repair is a very challenging technical procedure, primarily due to the lack of quality tissue present and the manner of separation of the tissues caused by the clefting. The typically shortened columella and rotation of the premaxilllary segment make achieving acceptable aesthetic results difficult. Variations to surgical approaches range from aggressive lengthening of the columella with preservation of hypoplastic tissue to conservative primary nasal reconstruction as performed with McComb's unilateral CL technique. McComb's technique involves release and repositioning of the lower lateral cartilages and alar base on both sides without aggressive degloving of the entire nasal complex. Aggressive

corrective techniques often produce initial results that are very good. Long-term results, however, are not so favorable due to the progression of natural growth processes. Excessive angulations and lengthened structures provide a less-than-optimal aesthetic effect. Revision of these deformities is usually very difficult, and sometimes impossible. In general, if hypoplastic tissue is excised and incisions within the medial nasal base and columella are avoided, long-term aesthetic results are excellent.

Treatment techniques for CP. Successful CP repair during infancy depends on two objectives. The first involves water-tight closure of the entire oronasal communication involving the hard and soft palate. The second involves the anatomical repair of the musculature within the soft palate, which is critical for the creation of normal speech. The soft palate functions in coupling and decoupling of the oral and nasal cavities in the production of speech. The tensor and levator palatini and uvularis muscles, which usually join at the midline, forming a continuous sling, are separated and insert along the posterior edge of the hard palate. Surgical treatment of a CP is concerned with closing the palatal defect and release of the abnormal muscle insertions. The timing for CP repair is correlated with the development of speech, which usually occurs around 18 months for a normally developing child. The velum or soft palate must be closed before the development of speech. If repair occurs after this time, compensatory speech articulations may result. The timing of surgery must also be balanced with the known biologic consequences of performing surgery during infancy, specifically during the growth phase, which could result in maxillary growth restriction. When repair of the palate is performed between 9 and 18 months of age, the incidence of maxillary restriction is approximately 25%. If repair is carried out earlier than 9 months of age, the incidence of severe growth restriction requiring future orthognathic surgery is greater. In addition, CP repair before 9 months of age is not associated with any increased benefit in terms of speech development. Performing CP repair between 9 and 18 months of age seems to best address the functional concerns of speech development and the potential negative impact surgery has on growth.

An approach used to address the speech issues with growth-related concerns involves staging the closure of the secondary palate with two procedures. This involves repair of the soft palate early in life, followed by closure of the hard palate later during infancy. The intent of this approach is that timely repair of the soft palate, which is critical for speech, is accomplished with hard palate repair being delayed until further growth has occurred. This technique offers the advantage of less growth restriction, easier repair of larger clefts, and less chance for fistula formation.

The basic premise for CP repair involves mobilization of multilayered flaps to close the defect created due to the failed fusion of the palatal shelves. The nasal mucosa is first closed, followed by reconstruction of the levator and tensor palatini muscles. The abnormal insertion of the levator and tensor palatini muscles on the hard palate must be removed and reconstructed to join in the midline. The musculature making up the velopharyngeal mechanisms are also reconstructed to allow the soft palate to close the space between the nasopharynx and oropharynx in order to create certain speech sounds. Closure of the oral mucosa completes the repair.

Many techniques have been devised for CP repair. The Bardach technique involves creation of two large full-thickness flaps on each palatal shelf, which are layered and brought to the midline for closure (Figure 13-1, *A, B*). This

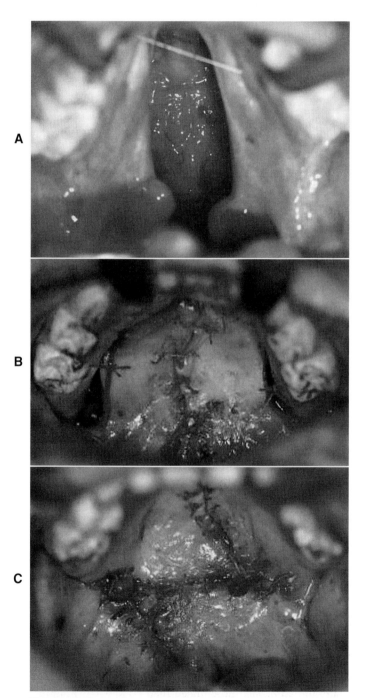

Figure 13-1 **A,** Complete cleft palate. **B,** Immediate postoperative photograph demonstrating cleft palate closure using the Bardach technique. **C,** Immediate postoperative photograph demonstrating cleft palate closure using the Furlow double-opposing Z-plasty technique.

technique allows for preservation of the palatal neurovascular bundle, which is contained within the pedicle of each flap. The Von Lagenbeck technique is similar to the Bardach technique but it preserves an anterior pedicle for increased blood supply to the flaps. It also involves elevation of large muco-periosteal flaps from the palate with midline approximation of the cleft margins. Long lateral releasing incisions are made at the border of the palatal and alveolar bone to allow mobilization. The levator muscles are detached from their abnormal insertion along the hard palate. The Furlow double-opposing Z-plasty technique involves two Z-plasties—one on the oral mucosa and one in the reverse orientation on the nasal mucosa (Figure 13-1, *C*). The levator muscle on one side is included in the posteriorly based oral mucosa Z-plasty, whereas the levator muscle from the opposite side is included within the posteriorly based nasal mucosal Z-plasty flap. This procedure produces palatal lengthening, reorients, and provides overlap of the malpositioned levator muscles. The Furlow Z-plasty has been reported to be associated with a higher rate of fistula formation at the junction of the soft and hard palates.

The Wardill-Kilmer-Veau technique represents a V-Y advancement of the mucoperiosteum of the hard palate and is intended to lengthen the palate in the anteroposterior plane at the time of palatoplasty. Bone is left exposed in the area where the flaps were advanced. These areas granulate and epithelialize within 2 to 3 weeks but form excessive scar tissue that may contribute to maxillary growth disturbances. The Vomer flap is used to achieve closure of the hard palate. A wide superiorly based flap of nasal mucosa is elevated from the vomer and attached to the palatal shelf to close the defect. The vomer flap avoids the need for elevating large mucoperiosteal flaps from the hard palate thus avoiding possible maxillary growth disturbances. For very wide clefts, a pharyngeal flap may be used. This technique allows the central portion of the cleft to be filled with posterior pharyngeal wall tissue, making the closure of the nasal and palatal mucosa easier. Patients with Pierre Robin sequence (malformation) or Treacher Collins syndrome have exceptionally wide clefts that are difficult to close without tension. The pharyngeal flap seems to address the concerns for CP repair with these patients. Pharyngeal flaps, however, are involved with an increased risk of bleeding, snoring, obstructive sleep apnea, and hyponasality.

COMPLICATIONS

The complications associated with cleft repair are essentially related to the technique used for treatment. The overall goals include nasal lining closure, adequate exposure, and release of soft tissue attachment along the bony borders of the cleft from the alveolar crest to the pyriform rim and closure of the oral mucosa with well-vascularized tissue that contains attached mucosa at the alveolar crest. Failure to address these concerns during treatment will ultimately lead to complications that include wound infection with fistula formation, mucosal dehiscence, hypertrophic scar formation, and hemorrhage.

It is also important to note that many patients with CLP have coexisting systemic abnormalities that may negatively affect the outcome of the treatment provided. Patients who present with systemic abnormalities in general are expected to have a higher incidence of complications compared with healthy patients. For the surgical correction of CLP, Lees and Piggott observed a high incidence of intraoperative and postoperative complications related to the respiratory system.

The most significant complication or unfavorable result of palate closure is the development of velopharyngeal insufficiency. This is manifested as a resonance problem with creation of hypernasal or hyponasal speech. Velopharyngeal insufficiency can be secondary to maxillary orthognathic (advancement) surgery or the use of pharyngeal flaps. The resonance occurs from the modification of oronasal portals that are either too large or too narrow. Correction of this problem involves reconstructive surgery with revision or creation of a new pharyngeal flap, accompanied by aggressive speech therapy.

A common complication of lip repair is the "whistle" deformity, which occurs due to vertical retraction of the scar or from inadequate advancement and rotation of the skin flap. Various lip-lengthening procedures can be performed secondarily, such as the V-Y advancement, which will correct the deformity and create a normal lip seal.

In cases of complete bilateral CLP, collapse of the alveolar segments posterior to the premaxilla is a common occurrence when orthodontic or palatal retention devices are not utilized. Correction of segment collapse is very complex, involving multiple surgeries over an extended period of time.

DISCUSSION

CL and/or CP malformations are the most common congenital abnormalities in the facial region. Worldwide, the incidence of CL is approximately 1:700 live births. The incidence of CP is approximately 1:2000 live births. CLP patients routinely have impaired facial growth, dental anomalies, speech disorders, poor hearing, psychological difficulties, and poor social relationships. Due to the multiple factors associated with CLP, specialty multidisciplinary teams are involved with the overall care of these patients. The involvement of the team starts during the immediate neonatal period and continues through completion of growth and adolescence. The multidisciplinary team is composed of a craniofacial surgeon, an oral and maxillofacial surgeon, a pediatrician, an otolaryngologist, a pediatric dentist, an orthodontist, an audiologist, a speech and language therapist, a geneticist, a psychologist, and a social worker.

CP deficiencies commonly go undetected during infancy, only to be identified later during childhood when the resultant anomaly becomes very apparent with the emergence of speech, feeding, and growth complications. It is therefore very important to accurately assess the palatal anatomy of any infant before such deficiencies create significant problems. During the initial inspection/examination of the palatal anatomy of infants, the presence of a submucous cleft is quite frequently missed. With submucous clefts, on visual inspection the palate appears intact; however, the overlying oral and nasal mucous membranes are expanded against the cleft area, giving the illusion of an intact palate. Digital palpation identifies a notch or discontinuity along the posterior aspect of the bony hard palate. The submucous cleft represents a deficiency in the musculature of the palate due to failed midline fusion of the palatal muscles, namely, the levator veli palatini, tensor veli palatini, uvulus, palatoglossus, and palatopharyngeus muscles. A bluish midline streak is often present over the soft palate, which indicates the splitting of the muscle layers.

Concerns that are associated with CLP include the following:

Feeding. Approximately 25% of CLP infants have early feeding difficulties with poor weight gain for the first 2 to 3 months. Feeding sessions are prolonged due in part to ulceration of the nasal mucosa. Some infants also have increased metabolic needs due to congenital heart disease or airway obstruction. Initial poor weight gain usually resolves following cleft closure, and any deficiency in growth is corrected by 6 months of age. Height and weight progressions are routinely monitored.

Speech and language development. Even when the palate is repaired, children are still at risk for subsequent speech disorders. It is reported that 25% of children with CLP develop normal speech after primary surgery, while the other 75% require many surgical interventions throughout childhood and adolescence. Speech problems arise from velopalatal insufficiency, dental and occlusal problems, oronasal fistulas, and hearing problems. Approximately 15% to 20% of patients who have CP repair within the first 12 to 15 months of life have velopharyngeal insufficiency. As mentioned earlier, surgical intervention must be coordinated with the development of speech. Speech and language therapy must also be provided during this time. The monitoring of speech continues into adolescence and adulthood in conjunction with active orthodontic and surgical management.

Hearing. Patients with CP are at increased risk of middle ear effusions and subsequent infections. The attachment of the levator veli palatini muscle around the eustachian tube is abnormal and leads to poor aeration and drainage of the middle ear. Regular assessment by the ENT surgeon and audiologist is recommended so that poor hearing is not a contributing factor to compromised speech.

General dental welfare. Children with CLP are at great risk for developing malocclusion. When the cleft involves the alveolar process, odontogenic structures within this region are routinely absent or malformed. Orthodontic intervention is generally initiated during the preschool years. Active occlusal manipulation and correction should not be instituted until the permanent dentition has erupted.

Genetics. There are three types of genetic risk groups for CLP: the *syndromic* group, identified by physical examination; the *familial* group, identified by history; and *isolated defects,* identified by exclusion of the first two groups. As earlier mentioned, the incidence of CL is approximately 1:700 live births, and the incidence of CP is approximately

1:2000 live births. With one parent and one child affected, the chance of a second child having a cleft is 10%. When both parents are without clefts and two children have clefts, the chance of a third child having a cleft is 19%. When one parent has a cleft and two offspring are normal, the chance of the third child being born with a cleft is 2.5%.

Environment. Epidemiological studies have demonstrated a relation between exposure of environmental factors or teratogens during pregnancy and the development of CLP. These factors or teratogens include alcohol consumption, cigarette smoking, folic acid deficiency, corticosteroids, benzodiazepines, and anticonvulsants.

Bibliography

Bryne PJ, Sands NR: Secondary bone grafting of residual alveolar and palatal clefts, *J Oral Surg* 30:87-92, 1972.

Carici F: Recent developments in orofacial cleft genetics, *J Craniofac Surg* 142(2):130-143, 2003.

Chung K, Kowalski C, Kim HM, et al: Maternal cigarette smoking during pregnancy and the risk of having a child with cleft lip/palate, *Plast Reconstr Surg* 105(2):485-491, 2000.

Copeland M: The effect of very early palatal repair on speech, *Br J Surg* 43:676, 1990.

Costello BJ, Ruiz RL, Turvey T: Surgical management of velopharyngeal insufficiency in the cleft patient, *Oral Maxillofac Surg Clin N Am* 539-551, 2002.

Costello BJ, Shand J, Ruiz RL: Craniofacial and orthognathic surgery in the growing patient, *Select Readings Oral Maxilllofac Surg* 11(5):1-20, 2003.

Dorf DS, Curtin JW: Early cleft repair and speech outcome: a ten year experience. In Bardach J, Morris HL, editors: *Multidisciplinary management of cleft lip and palate,* Philadelphia, 1990, WB Saunders, pp 341-348.

Glenny AM, Hooper L, Shaw WC, et al: Feeding interventions for growth and development in infants with cleft lip, cleft palate or cleft lip and palate, *Cochrane Database Syst Rev 2,* 2005.

Habel A, Sell D, Mars M: Management of cleft lip and palate, *Arch Dis Child* 74(4):360-366, 1996.

Lees VC, Pigott RW: Early postoperative complications in primary cleft lip and palate surgery: how soon may we discharge patients from hospital? *Br J Plast Surg* 45:232-234, 1992.

Marsh JL: Craniofacial surgery: the experiment on the experiment of nature, *Cleft Palate Craniofac J* 33:1, 1996.

McComb H: Primary correction of unilateral cleft lip nasal deformity: a ten year review, *Plast Reconstr Surg* 75:791-799, 1985.

Murray JC: Gene/environment causes of cleft lip and/or palate, *Clin Genet* 248-256, 2002.

Padwa BL, Sonis A, Bagheri SC, et al: Children with repaired bilateral cleft lip/palate: effect of age at premaxillary osteotomy on facial growth, *Plast Reconstr Surg* 105:1261, 1999.

Posnick JC: The staging of cleft lip and palate reconstruction: infancy adolescence. In Posnick JC, editor: *Craniofacial and maxillofacial surgery in children and young adults,* Philadelphia, 2000, WB Saunders, pp 785-826.

Posnick JC: Cleft orthognathic surgery: The unilateral cleft lip and palate deformity. In Posnick JC, editor: *Craniofacial and maxillofacial surgery in children and young adults.* Philadelphia, 2000, WB Saunders, pp 860-907.

Ruiz RL, Costello BJ, Turvey T: Orthognathic surgery in the cleft patient. In Ogle O, editor: Secondary cleft surgery, *Oral Maxillofac Surg Clin N Am* 491-507, 2002.

Spritz RA: The genetics and epigenetics of orofacial clefts, *Curr Opin Pediatr* 13(6):556-600, 2001.

Takato T, Yonohara Y, Mori Y: Early correction of the nose in unilateral cleft lip patients using an open method: a ten year review, *J Oral Maxillofac Surg* 53A:28-33, 1995.

Nonsyndromic Craniosynostosis

Chris Jo, DMD, and Shahrokh C. Bagheri, DMD, MD

CC

A 7-month-old male infant is referred by his pediatrician for evaluation of a craniofacial dysmorphology.

HPI

The mother of this 7-month-old, otherwise healthy, male (craniosynostosis has a male predilection) has been concerned about the abnormal shape of his head, which was noticed immediately after birth (craniosynostosis is the premature fusion of the cranial sutures occurring during intrauterine life. The deformity is often noticeable early). The pediatrician has been closely observing this skull deformity for changes and resolution. It was initially assumed to be deformational plagiocephaly (skull deformity caused by vaginal delivery or early fetal decent into the pelvis) and later was thought to be secondary to a positional plagiocephaly, an acquired skull deformity caused by a repetitive head position during sleep (nonsynostotic posterior plagiocephaly has increased since the American Academy of Pediatrics issued a recommendation to place infants on their back during sleep to reduce the risk of sudden infant death syndrome [SIDS]). Despite conservative management, the child continued to exhibit the cranial deformity, which appeared to slightly worsen over time. He is otherwise in good health, and the mother denies any behavioral abnormalities. He is referred for craniofacial evaluation (the rate of detectable cranial abnormalities secondary to craniosynostosis has been reported as high as 1:1700 to 1:1900 births).

PMHX/PDHX/MEDICATIONS/ALLERGIES/SH/FH

Noncontributory. The patient is up to date with all childhood immunizations, and there is no previous surgical history. The patient had an otherwise uneventful vaginal delivery.

There is no significant family history (Mendelian inheritance patterns are rare for nonsyndromic craniosynostosis, and are usually associated with other abnormalities, except for metopic suture craniosynostosis, which reveals a 5% positive family history).

With the exception of metopic craniosynostosis (which has a 43% incidence of associated malformations with no clear syndromic diagnosis), patients with nonsyndromic craniosynostosis are typically healthy and do not exhibit other malformations that are commonly present in syndromic craniosynostosis.

EXAMINATION

General. The patient is a well-developed and well-nourished, pleasant child in no apparent distress.

Maxillofacial. Examination of the skull reveals a mild dysmorphology (the exact dysmorphology varies greatly and depends on which portion or portions of the sagittal suture are involved) in which the cranial vault is narrow in the bitemporal and biparietal dimensions and abnormally elongated in the anteroposterior dimension (this is called scaphocephaly, meaning "long and narrow"). Frontal and occipital bossing is apparent (described as "keel-like" appearance).

There is no midfacial or mandibular hypoplasia or asymmetry and no orbital dystopia (a relative discrepancy in globe position in the vertical and/or horizontal planes) or exophthalmos (anterior position of the globe relative to the orbital rims).

The fundoscopic examination is normal with no evidence of papilledema (edema of the optic disc, which is indicative of elevated intracranial pressure).

Intraoral. The results of the examination are within normal limits (nonsyndromic craniosynostosis is not associated with increased incidence of CLP).

Extremities. There are no deformities (nonsyndromic craniosynostosis does not have any associated abnormalities of the extremities).

IMAGING

Plain film complete skull series comprise the initial diagnostic radiographs of choice (the clinical diagnosis of craniosynostosis must be confirmed radiographically), and in this case, the radiographs reveal the absence of the entire sagittal suture (sagittal suture synostosis can involve the entire suture, anterior portion only, or posterior portion only). If sutures appear patent on a radiographic study that is of diagnostic quality, then craniosynostosis can be ruled out.

Craniofacial axial and coronal (or reformatted) cut CT scans and three-dimensional reconstructions provide more detailed morphological information, which is very useful during surgical planning (CT scans are also indicated when plain films are nondiagnostic). CT scans show a scaphocephalic skull deformity, which is consistent with synostosis of the sagittal suture.

Head CT showed no masses (possibility of intracranial mass should be included in the differential diagnosis of cranial vault abnormalities) and no hydrocephalus (usually not encountered in single-suture craniosynostosis but may occur independently), which can be seen in approximately 10% of cases where multiple sutures are involved.

LABS

In an otherwise healthy 7-month-old patient, preoperative laboratory evaluation should include hemoglobin and hematocrit levels.

ASSESSMENT

Nonsyndromic craniosynostosis involving the entire sagittal suture

TREATMENT

There are two primary goals in the surgical management of nonsyndromic craniosynostosis: (1) release of the fused suture(s) to allow unrestricted growth of the brain and (2) reconstruction of all dysmorphic skeletal components to correct the anatomic form. The surgical team should be composed of a pediatric craniofacial surgeon and a pediatric neurosurgeon for optimal results ("strip craniectomy" previously performed by neurosurgeons working independently did not address the dysmorphology of the craniofacial skeleton and resulted in residual deformities). Modern craniofacial management includes a formal craniotomy performed by a neurosurgeon and simultaneous skeletal reconstruction by the craniofacial surgeon. Reconstruction and reshaping includes the removal, dismantling, and reassembly of all dysmorphic skeletal components into an anatomically desirable shape. The extent of the surgery depends on the suture(s) involved and the resultant skeletal deformity.

Although craniosynostosis is surgically addressed during the first year of life, the exact timing of craniosynostosis repair is controversial. Some surgeons prefer early surgical correction when the child is 3 to 6 months of age. In theory, early release of the suture or sutures allows the expanding brain to naturally reshape the cranial vault, minimizing the later-staged reconstructive efforts. Other surgeons prefer delaying the surgical correction until 9 to 11 months of age, permitting more growth of the cranial vault before reconstruction. The more stable cranial skeleton will potentially result in fewer postsurgical deformities. Also, increased bony calcification allows for easier rigid fixation of the bony segments.

The surgical correction of nonsyndromic sagittal suture craniosynostosis involves a biparietal craniotomy for release of the fused suture and reshaping of the posterior and anterior cranial vault. The abnormal cranial components are dismantled and osteotomized into strips for reshaping of the cranial vault. The objectives are to increase the bitemporal and biparietal width and to decrease the anteroposterior length of the cranial vault (reduce frontal and occipital bossing). The bony segments are placed into the correct anatomic position and secured with rigid miniplates with monocortical screws. Most bony gaps, including full-thickness defects will com-

pletely fill with bone when the surgery is performed by age 2, because of the osteogenic potential of the periosteum and dura mater. Complete healing of these defects is less predictable when surgery is performed between ages 2 and 4. After the age of 4, these defects may not heal without immediate reconstruction (with bone grafting or other alloplastic material).

If the entire sagittal suture is involved, reconstruction can be done in a single-stage (associated with increased difficulty, surgical time, blood loss, and morbidity) or two-staged operation. The staged reconstruction involves addressing and reshaping the posterior two thirds of the cranial vault, which will correct the bitemporal and biparietal width and improve the anteroposterior cranial dimension. This will not correct the frontal bossing, which will need to be addressed during the second surgical phase 6 to 12 weeks later. Others in the past have advocated strip craniectomy (at least 3 cm wide) from anterior fontanelle to just beyond the lambdoidal suture as adequate treatment when the child is between 3 months and 1 year of age. This technique (along with its endoscopically assisted variation) has been criticized for its less-than-ideal cosmetic results.

When only the posterior portion of the sagittal suture is fused, surgical reshaping of the posterior two thirds of the cranial vault can be accomplished via a postauricular coronal scalp incision, with the patient in a prone position. Formal biparietal and occipital craniotomy is performed by the neurosurgeon. The bone flaps are removed, osteotomized, placed into correct anatomical position, and secured with bone plates using monocortical screws. If only the anterior portion of the sagittal suture is involved, the resulting deformity is primarily frontal bossing. A coronal flap is elevated and a bifrontal craniotomy is performed, with the patient supine. The anterior cranial vault is reshaped and fixated, as was previously described.

COMPLICATIONS

Despite having very low complication rates associated with craniofacial surgery, both intraoperative and postoperative complications can occur. Massive blood loss and postoperative infection are the most common and most feared complications (Box 13-1).

Other minor complications include ocular complications (diplopia, temporary ptosis, strabismus, corneal abrasion, and, very rarely, visual loss), seizures (rare), cerebrospinal fluid leak, elevated intracranial pressure, electrolyte disturbances (syndrome of inappropriate antidiuretic hormone secretion or cerebral salt-wasting syndrome resulting in hyponatremia), airway embarrassment, fixation failure or translocation/migration, damage to the lacrimal drainage apparatus, and residual deformity requiring secondary procedures.

DISCUSSION

Virchow first coined the term *craniostenosis* in 1851. The word *craniosynostosis* describes the process of premature

Box 13-1.   Intraoperative and Postoperative Complications in Craniofacial Surgery

Intraoperative Complications

- **Venous air embolism.** Neonatal and pediatric calvaria have a large number of diploic and emissary channels that become exposed during a craniotomy procedure. Because the operative field is typically above the level of the heart, air could enter into these exposed vascular channels and travel to the right atrium. A symptomatic air embolus could lead to profound hypotension and cardiovascular collapse. If venous air embolism is suspected, surgery should be stopped, the head of bed lowered, the surgical field irrigated and covered with a wet sponge, and bone wax can be applied to the osteotomized bony edges. Nitrous oxide should be discontinued. A closed cardiac massage may be indicated in a severely compromised patient to force the air into pulmonary circulation. A thoracotomy and direct massage with aspiration of intracardiac air is the last resort for failed attempts.
- **Oculocardiac reflex.** Transcranial and fronto-orbital surgery can trigger the oculocardiac reflex in response to orbital manipulation and pressure, leading to bradycardia and hypotension. Care must be taken to prevent excessive orbital pressure and flap retraction. The anesthesia team should be notified during such maneuvers. Severe bradycardia and hypotension will require the administration of atropine.
- **Dural lacerations.** David and Cooter reported a 31% incidence of iatrogenic dural tears in a series of 53 patients. Others have reported an incidence of 5% to 60%. Direct repair usually has no detrimental sequelae.
- **Major blood loss.** The continual ooze of blood from the vascular osteotomy sites over several hours of surgical time can accumulate to loss of a large portion of the patient's blood volume. The incidence of perioperative blood transfusions is variable and has been reported to be as high

as 80% to 100% of patients undergoing cranial vault reconstruction. However, this is not universally accepted by all craniofacial surgeons. Major blood loss resulting in hypovolemic shock has a reported incidence of 0.3% to 4.6%. Appropriate fluid resuscitation with crystalloid, colloid, blood, and replacement of coagulation factors (fresh frozen plasma) should be anticipated.
- **Death.** Reported mortality rates from craniofacial surgery ranges from 0% to 4.3%. Massive intraoperative bleeding, postoperative bleeding, intracranial bleeding, cerebral edema, infection, inadequate volume replacement, respiratory obstruction, and anesthetic complications are the most common causes.

Postoperative Complications

- **Infection.** Infection can be in the form of osteitis/osteomyelitis, meningitis, or intracranial abscess and is the most common postoperative complication (infection rates range from 1% to 14%). Separation of nasal and paranasal sinuses from intracranial cavity is paramount in reducing the incidence of infection. The use of appropriate perioperative antibiotics, intraoperative antibiotic irrigation (or saline with dilute iodine), and reduction of surgical time also reduces infection rates. Monobloc advancement procedures have a higher rate of infection compared with other intracranial procedures.
- **Extradural and subdural hematomas.** These are a relatively rare occurrence. Poole reported less than a 1% incidence of hematoma. Suction drainage is not advocated because of concern that it can cause bleeding, cerebrospinal fluid leakage, infection, or draw nasal/sinus contamination intracranially. Close neurological observation is needed to look for signs of an evolving intracranial hemorrhage.

---

fusion of cranial sutures (six major suture areas and seven minor sutures), which results in craniostenosis (outdated terminology). The craniofacial deformity is directly proportional to the area of sutures fused. Many classification systems have been developed to describe various subtypes of craniosynostosis. Three broad categories of craniosynostosis have been identified: simple (single suture) or compound (two or more sutures), primary or secondary (related to other disorder), and isolated (nonsyndromic) versus syndromic (Crouzon, Apert, Carpenter, Pfeiffer, Saethre-Chotzen, and other syndromes).

There are several different types of craniosynostosis. Sagittal suture craniosynostosis is the most common form of nonsyndromic single-suture synostosis, with a prevalence of approximately 1:5000 live births and 3:1 male predilection. It is characterized by a scaphocephalic deformity (long and narrow cranial vault) due to the premature fusion of the entire or part of the sagittal suture. Absence or premature fusion of the sagittal suture results in no growth perpendicular to the suture and arrested development of the two parietal bone plates, causing bitemporal and biparietal narrowing. There is compensatory growth at the major sutures that remain patent (i.e., coronal, lambdoid, and metopic sutures) as the brain

continues to expand, causing an abnormal anteroposterior elongation of the cranial vault. This results in frontal and occipital bossing, often described as "keel-like." Portions of the sagittal suture (anterior or posterior portions) or the entire suture can be fused and determine the extent of the cranial deformity. Several theories have been proposed for the etiology of craniosynostosis. Virchow believed that the primary event was craniosynostosis and the associated cranial base deformity was secondary to that event. Moss theorized that the cranial base deformity was the primary malformation resulting in premature fusion of the cranial sutures. Others theorized that mesenchymal defects result in both craniosynostosis and an abnormal cranial base. Growth of the midfacial skeleton will also be restricted if sutures along the anterior cranial base are prematurely fused. Regardless of the pathogenesis, the prematurely fused suture or sutures inhibits growth of the neurocranium perpendicular to the fused suture or sutures. There is compensatory overgrowth at the normal (open) sutures to accommodate the growing brain (brain volume triples during the first year of life). Thus a unilateral synostosis will result in a bilateral deformity. This phenomenon is known as Virchow's law. Despite this compensatory

Table 13-3. Types of Nonsyndromic Craniosynostosis

Suture(s) Affected	Head Shape	Name	Incidence	Elevated Intracranial Pressure	Central Nervous System (Mental Retardation)
Sagittal	Long and narrow	Scaphocephaly	1:5000	Absent	Slight
Coronal	One hemicranium smaller than other	Anterior plagiocephaly	1:10,000	Infrequent	Slight to moderate
Metopic	Triangular forehead	Trigonocephaly	1:15,000	Usually absent	Slight to moderate
Lambdoidal	One hemicranium smaller than other	Posterior plagiocephaly	1:150,000	Infrequent	Slight to moderate
Bilateral coronal	Short, broad, and tall	Brachycephaly (acrobrachycephaly)	Rare	Infrequent	Slight to moderate
Sagittal and coronal	Short and narrow	Oxycephaly	Rare	Usually present	High

Modified from Dufresne CR: Classifications of craniofacial anomalies. In Dufresne CR, Carson BS, Zinreich SJ, editors: *Complex craniofacial problems,* New York, 1992, Churchill Livingstone, pp 63-71.

growth, an increase in intracranial pressure (greater than 15 mm Hg) may still be seen.

Neurological impairment is a rare event in single-suture craniosynostosis (single-suture is most common, with the sagittal suture being most affected), especially when treated before the age of one (elevated intracranial pressure is seen in approximately 14% of children with untreated single-suture craniosynostosis and in 42% when two or more sutures are involved). However, if elevated intracranial pressure is left untreated, it may lead to irreversible neurological and cognitive damage.

The major cranial sutures are the sagittal, metopic, coronal (right and left), and lambdoidal (right and left). The minor sutures are the temporosquamosal, frontonasal, and frontosphenoidal. In the majority of nonsyndromic craniosynostosis, only one suture is involved. Involvement of the sagittal suture is the most common type. Table 13-3 lists the major nonsyndromic craniosynostosis, along with their characteristic features and incidence of occurrence.

Coronal suture craniosynostosis is the second most common type of nonsyndromic synostosis. Mutation of the fibroblast growth factor receptor 3 gene *(FGFR3)* has been implicated in its pathogenesis. Due to early fusion of the coronal suture (either right or left), there is hypoplasia of the frontal and parietal bones on the affected side resulting in flattening of the forehead (anterior plagiocephaly). Compensatory overgrowth of the unaffected sutures, including the contralateral coronal suture, results in frontal bossing of the unaffected side. Also, orbital dystopia (superior, posterior position of affected orbit), ipsilateral zygomatic hypoplasia, and nasal asymmetry commonly occur. Midfacial hypoplasia and orbital dystopia are seen because of the involvement of the anterior cranial base along the frontoethmoidal, frontosphenoidal, and sphenoethmoidal sutures. This results in "Harlequin eye" deformity on an anteroposterior skull film. Surgical correction involves a bifrontal craniotomy, orbital osteotomies, fronto-orbital advancement, and anterior cranial vault reshaping.

Bibliography

AAP Task Force on Infant Positioning and SIDS: Positioning and SIDS, *Pediatrics* 89:1120, 1992.

Carson BS, Dufresne CR: Craniosynostosis and neurocranial asymmetry. In Dufresne CR, Carson BS, Zinreich SJ, editors: *Complex craniofacial problems,* New York, 1992, Churchill Livingstone, pp 167-194.

David DJ, Cooter RD: Craniofacial infection in 10 years of transcranial surgery, *Plast Reconstr Surg* 80:213-223, 1987.

Dufresne CR: Classifications of craniofacial anomalies. In Dufresne CR, Carson BS, Zinreich SJ, editors: *Complex craniofacial problems,* New York, 1992, Churchill Livingstone, pp 63-71.

Eaton AC, Marsh JL, Pilgram TK: Transfusion requirements for craniosynostosis surgery in infants, *Plast Reconstr Surg* 95:277-283, 1995.

Faberowski LW, Black S, Mickle JP: Incidence of venous air embolism during craniectomy for craniosynostosis repair, *Anesthesiology* 92:20-23, 2000.

Fishman MA, Hogan GR, Dodge PR: The concurrence of hydrocephalus and craniosynostosis, *J Neurosurg* 36:621-629, 1971.

Gault DT, Renier D, Marchac D, Jones BM: Intracranial pressure and intracranial volume in children with craniosynostosis, *Plast Reconstr Surg* 90:230-271, 1992.

Golabi M, Edwards MSB, Ousterhout DK: Craniosynostosis and hydrocephalus, *Neurosurgery* 21:63, 1987.

Greensmith AL, Meara JG, Holmes AD, et al: Complications related to cranial vault surgery, *Oral Maxillofac Surg Clin N Am* 16:465-473, 2004.

Jones BM, Jani P, Bingham RM, Mackersie AM, et al: Complications in paediatric craniofacial surgery: an initial four year experience, *Br J Plast Surg* 45:225-231, 1992.

Meyer P, Renier D, Arnaud E, et al: Blood loss during repair of craniosynostosis, *Br J Anaesth* 71:854-857, 1993.

Phillips RJL, Mulliken JB: Venous air embolism during a craniofacial procedure, *Plast Reconstr Surg* 82:155-159, 1988.

Poole MD: Complications of craniofacial surgery, *Br J Plast Surg* 41:608-613, 1988.

Renier D, Sainte-Rose C, Marchac D, et al: Intracranial pressure in craniosynostosis, *J Neurosurg* 57:370, 1982.

Ruiz RL, Ritter AM, Turvey TA, et al: Nonsyndromic craniosynostosis: diagnosis and contemporary surgical management, *Oral Maxillofac Surg Clin N Am* 16:447-463, 2004.

Apert Syndrome

Mehran Mehrabi, DMD, MD, and Shahrokh C. Bagheri, DMD, MD

CC

A 14-year-old boy previously diagnosed with Apert syndrome presents to the craniofacial clinic for evaluation of his anterior open bite (apertognathia) with a chief complaint of "difficulty with chewing."

HPI

The patient was diagnosed with craniosynostosis (premature fusion of the cranial sutures) shortly after birth. Subsequently, he had fronto-orbital advancement at age 7 months. At age 2 years, he had a craniofacial advancement to address the midface hypoplasia. Currently, the parents are unhappy with the child's appearance because children at his school continually mock him regarding his appearance and, in particular, his open bite. They believe that it has affected his self-confidence and performance. The mother indicates that the child has difficulty biting hard foods such as steak or pizza and has to use his posterior teeth for mastication. He is currently undergoing presurgical orthodontic treatment in preparation for combined surgical-orthodontic correction of his skeletal malocclusion. The parents are also concerned about his continued "sunken" face appearance (midface hypoplasia) despite his corrective surgery at age 2 years (the midface hypoplasia frequently persists despite early surgical advancement and often needs to be reoperated after completion of midface growth).

PMHX/PDHX/MEDICATIONS/ALLERGIES/SH/FH

He was also diagnosed with a heart murmur at birth and subsequent corrective surgery without complications (cardiovascular and valvular abnormalities such as patent ductus arteriosus is seen in 10% of patients with Apert syndrome). He also had a history of hydronephrosis at birth that resolved without surgery (genitourinary abnormalities are seen in about 10% of patients). At age 4 weeks, he was diagnosed with pyloric stenosis, thickening of pyloric valve that results in gastric obstruction (gastrointestinal abnormalities are seen in 1.5% of patients) and successfully underwent a laparoscopic pyloroplasty. The family history reveals his two brothers and one sister are healthy (the majority of cases are sporadic in nature, although autosomal dominance inheritance has been reported). Cognitive assessments at school have revealed that he is slightly developmentally delayed for his age (65% of patients have an intelligence quotient of less than 70, which is defined as mental retardation).

EXAMINATION

General. The patient is moderately cooperative with poor attention span (secondary to developmental delay) but is able to follow simple commands. He has a short stature for his age and compared to his parents (megalocephaly [large head] results in the weight and height being above the 50th percentile early, but this decreases with age).

Maxillofacial. Examination of the skull reveals a steep frontal bone (Figure 13-2, *A*), flat occipital region, and bulging temporal region. He exhibits mild ocular esotropia (cross-eyed) as well as hypertelorism (diverging and widely spaced pupils, respectively). There is underdevelopment of his maxilla and zygomas bilaterally (midface hypoplasia) (Figure 13-2, *B*). Fundoscopic examination is normal with no evidence of papilledema (swelling of optic disc commonly seen in infants with Apert syndrome due to elevation in intracranial pressure).

Intraoral. The patient has anterior open bite (apertognathia) with a narrow high (V-shaped) maxillary arch (Figure 13-2, *C*). Class III molar relationship (Class III malocclusion with an anterior open bite is almost universal for Apert syndrome). Only two posterior molars are in contact on either side. There is no apparent hard or soft tissue clefting of the palate (seen in 30% of patients with Apert syndrome).

Extremities. The index, middle, and ring fingers are fused, and there is a common nail in both hands (symmetrical syndactyly) (Figure 13-2, *D*). The thumb and small fingers are not affected in either hand and show normal strength and mobility. The feet are normal and are not affected (lower extremities may be involved).

Skin. The child has yellow raised papules on the dorsum of the hands (acne vulgaris involving hands are seen in 70% of Apert syndrome).

IMAGING

A panoramic radiograph and periapical radiographs are required to evaluate for supernumerary teeth, root crowding, and morphology and to detect caries. When impacted teeth are present (excluding third molars), periapical films from various angles can be obtained to evaluate the buccolingual position of the tooth (Clark's rule). A lateral cephalometric radiograph, along with cephalometric analysis, is used for evaluation and treatment of the dentofacial deformity. A CT scan is not required but can be used for evaluation of opacified sinuses (which are not uncommon in maxillary hypoplasia) and for visualization of the three-dimensional anatomy as an

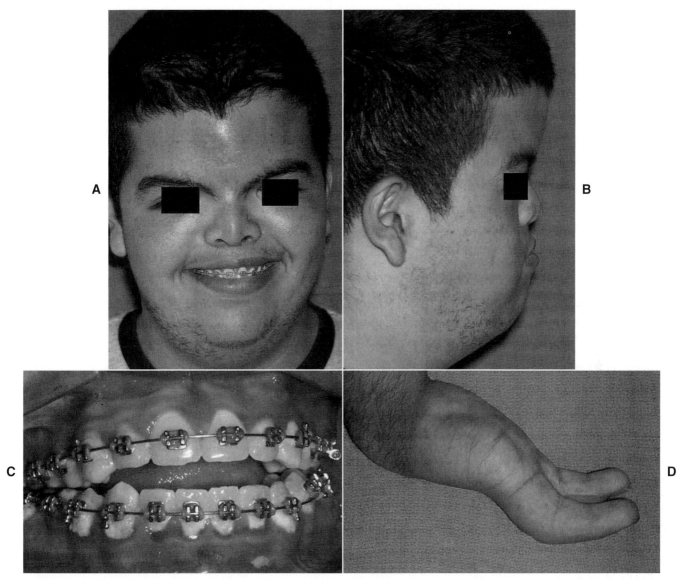

Figure 13-2 **A,** Frontal view demonstrating general appearance of the patient. **B,** Profile view demonstrating severe midfacial hypoplasia and frontal bossing. **C,** Intraoral view demonstrating apertognathia. **D,** Syndactyly (seen in both hands).

aid in treatment planning. Magnetic resonance imaging (MRI) is also not required but can be useful in select cases for evaluation of soft tissue anatomy such as brain parenchyma, orbital tissue, or pharyngeal structures. Obstructive sleep apnea (OSA) is commonly seen in patients with Apert syndrome, and the mentioned imaging modalities may be used to assess posterior airway anatomy.

In this patient, a panoramic radiograph and lateral cephalometric radiographs were obtained and used in treatment and cephalometric analysis. There were no teeth crowding, impactions, or supernumerary teeth; therefore, no periapical radiographs were obtained.

LABS

Preoperative laboratory testing includes a complete blood count (CBC) and basic metabolic panel, both of which demonstrated no abnormalities.

ASSESSMENT

Apert syndrome with maxillary hypoplasia and apertognathia requiring combined surgical orthognathic and orthodontic treatment

TREATMENT

The initial evaluation of patients with Apert syndrome at birth is focused on airway, central nervous system malformations, and feeding assessment. A retruded maxilla and limited nasopharyngeal airway would increase the work of breathing and may need advanced airway interventions. The inability to pass a nasogastric tube may indicate nasopharynx obstruction. Most often, these infants compensate with obligate mouth breathing and hence have an "open mouth" appearance. The central nervous system symptoms may manifest as seizures, hypotonia or hypertonia, and apnea. The high arched palate, possible clefting, and obligate mouth breathing make feeding challenging. These patients may need a nasogastric or orogastric feeding tube or placement of a percutaneous endoscopic gastrostomy tube.

Treatment of craniosynostosis is also dependent on age. Strip craniectomy, which allows for cranial decompression, has been performed in children younger than 3 months. However, due to unsatisfactory results, this procedure has been largely abandoned except for isolated sagittal synostosis. Fronto-orbital advancement is performed at age 6 to 9 months. In this procedure, the osteotomy is made across the nasofrontal junction, lateral orbital walls, and roof of the orbit. This increases the volume of the orbit along with the anteroposterior cranial dimension and decreases the bitemporal prominence. The fronto-orbital bar may be advanced up to 20 mm. Generally, there is no need for bone grafting (some surgeons use bone substitutes such as demineralized bone to fill in the defects), and the segments are commonly fixated using resorbable plating systems. A monobloc or craniofacial advancement is performed at age 9 months to 3 years. This procedure advances the cranium and midface simultaneously. This osteotomy consists of advancement of the frontal bone in two segments and a Le Fort III advancement. The retrofrontal (the space created behind the frontal bone) dead space makes this procedure dangerous and should be done only in patients with respiratory compromise. If a midface distraction or advancement is used, it is best done between ages 3 and 5 years with a subcranial (extracranial) Le Fort III advancement.

This patient was treated with a Le Fort III advancement. Mounted models with lateral cephalometric analysis were used to evaluated the extent of surgical movement. A custom-made prefabricated occlusal splint was used to guide the position of the maxilla intraoperatively. With a bicoronal, transconjunctival (or a subtarsal), and circumvestibular maxillary incision, osteotomies were made along the roof on the orbit, lateral orbital wall extended laterally and inferiorly to pterygomaxillary fissure. The medial orbital wall osteotomy was connected to inferior orbital fissure. This requires lifting the lacrimal sac without interruption of the medial canthal ligament. The nasofrontal osteotomy was extended laterally and inferiorly (behind the lacrimal groove) to meet the inferior cut. Then, a Rowe disimpaction forceps was used to mobilize and advance the midface. The position of the maxillary unit is dictated by the prefabricated splint. Bone grafts and/or distraction osteogenesis may be used in select patients. In patients with a normal occlusion, a Le Fort III with concurrent Le Fort I can be used. If the bizygomatic prominence is appropriate, Le Fort II osteotomy may be sufficient.

COMPLICATIONS

There are few reports in the literature on complications of Le Fort II and III orthognathic procedures. Complications of Le Fort I osteotomy have been extensively studied in the orthognathic surgery population and reported at a rate of about 6% to 9%. Most severe complications of Le Fort (I, II, or III) osteotomy result from an unwanted pterygomaxillary separa-

tion with fractures extending to skull base, the orbital wall, and pterygoid plates. This is seen with a higher frequency in patients with craniosynostosis. Skull base fractures can result in a subarachnoid hemorrhage; there have been seven reported cases of skull base fracture in patients with craniosynostosis. It is prudent to discuss this complication preoperatively. Other complications include the increased frequency of intracranial aneurysms seen in patients with Crouzon syndrome. Sporadic cases of blindness also have been reported following Le Fort I osteotomy.

There are various modifications of maxillary osteotomies at the pterygomaxillary junction that can be done to prevent an unfavorable fracture. A straight osteotome can be used at the tuberosity rather than the pterygomaxillary fissure. Swann shape osteotomes that are designed to direct force anteriorly or the use of an oscillating saw and endoscopic techniques have also been discussed. However, most surgeons use a curved osteotome directed anteriorly, medially, and inferiorly as a measure to prevent an unwanted fracture and to avoid the internal maxillary artery.

Relapse of the surgical move and development of an anterior open bite are more frequently seen with larger moves. Overcorrection may be appropriate, especially in younger patients. Another strategy to address this complication is to plan the surgical procedure in two stages, with an initial monobloc advancement followed by a Le Fort I osteotomy to close the anterior open bite.

DISCUSSION

Craniosynostosis, or abnormal premature closure of cranial sutures, was first described by Hippocrates in 100 BC. This may present as an isolated finding or in combination with other physical findings, designating it a "syndromic craniosynostosis." Apert, Crouzon, Pfeiffer, and Saether-Chotzen syndromes are the most commonly diagnosed syndromes that include craniosynostosis with midface hypoplasia. With involvement of the skull base with a hypoplastic midface, these are generally referred to as dysostosis syndromes.

Apert syndrome was first described in 1984 by S.W. Wheaton and later by Eugene Apert in 1906. This acrocephalosyndactyly (deformity of skull, face, and extremity) presents with a distinctive cranial vault shape, midface hypoplasia, and limb abnormalities such as symmetrical syndactyly, acne vulgaris, and nail abnormalities. There have been over 300 cases reported. The majority of cases are sporadic, but an autosomal dominance inheritance has also been observed. Advanced paternal age and parental consanguinity (seen in two patients) have been associated with increased risk.

Early fusion of the coronal sutures, along with a widely patent sagittal suture (extending from the glabella to the posterior fontanelle), produces a short anterior cranial fossa, a steep, wide, and flat forehead. This results in a bulging pterion and an obliquely contoured temporal bone. The occiput is also flat, which makes for a shorter anteroposterior dimension while increasing the vertical dimension. The resulting skeletal deformity of craniosynostosis is caused by poor skeletal development perpendicular to the prematurely fused suture. The remaining sutures widen excessively, producing the final cranial form. This is referred to as Virchow's law.

The midface hypoplasia consists of an underdeveloped maxilla in all dimensions with a reduction in the nasopharyngeal airway space. Oral examination may show a high arched palate, CP, dental crowding, and an anterior open bite. Ocular abnormalities present as orbital hypertelorism and exorbitism, which are generally not as severe as in Crouzon syndrome. Syndactyly consists of soft tissue fusion of the second, third, and fourth fingers or toes. This is seen with a variable extent of bony and fingernail fusion of the involved digits.

The effects of an abnormal skull shape on the brain include the development of progressive hydrocephalus (rare), distorted ventricle shape, agenesis of the septum pellucidum, corpus callosum, cavum septum pellucidum, and possible developmental delay. Two cranial nerves can be affected independent of cranial vault shape: I (9%), resulting in anosmia, and VIII, causing hearing impairment (10%).

Bibliography

Cohen MM, Kreiborg S: An updated pediatric perspective on the Apert syndrome, *Am J Dis Child* 147:989, 1993.

Ferraro NF: Dental, orthodontic, and oral/maxillofacial evaluation and treatment in Apert syndrome, *Clin Plast Surg* 18:291-307, 1991.

Girotto JA, Davidson J, Wheatly M, et al: Blindness as a complication of Le Fort osteotomies: role of atypical fracture patterns and distortion of the optic canal, *Plast Reconstr Surg* 102:1409-1421, 1998.

Juniper RP, Stajcic Z: Pterygoid plate separation using an oscillating saw in Le Fort I osteotomy. Technical note, *J Craniomaxillofac Surg* 19:153-154, 1991.

Katzen JT, McCarthy JG: Syndromes involving craniosysnostosis and midface hypoplasia, *Otolaryngol Clin North Am* 33:1257-1284, 2000.

Lanigan DT, Guest P: Alternative approaches to pterygomaxillary separation, *Int J Oral Maxillofac Surg* 22:131-138, 1993.

Lanigan DT, Romanchuk K, Olson CK: Ophthalmic complications associated with orthognathic surgery, *J Oral Maxillofac Surg* 51:480-494, 1993.

Lanigan DT, Tubman DE: Carotid-cavernous sinus fistula following Le Fort I osteotomy, *J Oral Maxillofac Surg* 45:969-975, 1987.

Lo LJ, Hung KF, Chen YR: Blindness as a complication of Le Fort I osteotomy for maxillary distraction, *Plast Reconstr Surg* 109:688-698, 2002.

Marsh J, Galic M, Vannier MW: The craniofacial anatomy of Apert syndrome, *Clin Plast Surg* 18:237-249, 1991.

Matsumoto K, Nakanishi H, Seike T, et al: Intracranial hemorrhage resulting from skull base fracture as a complication of Le Fort III osteotomy, *J Craniofac Surg* 14:545-548, 2003.

Newhouse RF, Schow SR, Kraut RA, et al: Life-threatening hemorrhage from a Le Fort I osteotomy, *J Oral Maxillofac Surg* 40:117-119, 1982.

Renier D, Arnaud E, Cinalli G, et al: Prognosis for mental function in Apert's syndrome, *J Neurosurg* 85:66-72, 1996.

Robinson PP, Hendy CW: Pterygoid plate fractures caused by the Le Fort I osteotomy, *Br J Oral Maxillofac Surg* 24:198-202, 1986.

Sakai Y, Kobayashi S, Sekiguchi J, et al: New method of endoscopic pterygomaxillary disjunction for a Le Fort I osteotomy, *J Craniofac Surg* 7:111-116, 1996.

Crouzon Syndrome

Deepak Krishnan, BDS, and Chris Jo, DMD

CC

A 16-year-old boy with a previous diagnosis of Crouzon syndrome presents to the craniofacial clinic for evaluation of his malocclusion with a chief complaint of "I am unable to chew with my front teeth, I do not like my face, and my upper jaw is smaller than my lower."

HPI

Shortly after birth, the patient was diagnosed with a familial craniofacial dysostosis syndrome that was characterized as Crouzon syndrome (most commonly caused by premature fusion of the coronal sutures resulting in brachycephaly; seen with an incidence of 1:25,000 live births). The initial craniofacial morphology was consistent with that of bilateral coronosynostosis. The skull showed significant brachycephaly (defined as a short and wide head with a cephalic index of over 80. The cephalic index is the maximum head width multiplied by 100, divided by maximum head length). The patient also demonstrated flat frontal and occipital bones with a bulging temporal region (temporal bossing).

Within several months of birth, the patient progressively showed signs of deficient growth of his maxilla and zygoma (midface hypoplasia), with moderately severe exophthalmos (due to hypoplasia of the midface causing shortened anteroposterior dimension of the orbital floor), resulting in mild exposure keratitis. The eyes showed mild exotropia (divergent strabismus) and hypertelorism (widened interpupillary distance). There were no signs of elevated intracranial pressures. At the age of 10 months, he underwent fronto-orbital advancement without any complications (primary cranio-orbital decompression and reshaping are performed at 10 to 12 months, unless there is elevated intracranial pressure requiring earlier intervention). Subsequently, at age 6 years, he had a midfacial advancement by craniofacial distraction to address the midface hypoplasia (final cranial vault and orbital reconstruction is performed between the ages of 5 and 7 years). At present, the parents complain of functional impairment due to his malocclusion and express generalized unhappiness with his appearance. They explain that he is the center of constant harassment by the other kids at school and that it has affected his self-confidence and academic performance. He is currently undergoing presurgical orthodontic treatment in preparation for combined surgical-orthodontic correction of his skeletal Class III malocclusion and apertognathia (orthognathic surgery is performed between the ages of 14 to 16 in females and 16 to 18 in males).

PMHX/PDHX/MEDICATIONS/ALLERGIES/SH/FH

The patient has a history of seizures (seizure disorder is seen in 10% of patients with Crouzon syndrome). He also has a conductive hearing loss and atresia of the internal auditory meatus (seen in approximately 55% of patients).

Family history reveals a sibling and a cousin with the diagnosis of Crouzon syndrome (both autosomal dominance inheritance with variability of expression and sporadic cases have been reported). Cognitive assessments at school have revealed slight developmental delay for his age (3% to 65% of patients have an intelligence quotient of less than 70, defined as mental retardation, emphasizing the variability in expression).

EXAMINATION

General. The patient is a well-developed and well-nourished boy in no apparent distress.

Maxillofacial. The head form is mildly brachycephalic. The supraorbital rims appear in good anteroposterior position. Examination of the face shows a flat forehead, moderate residual midfacial hypoplasia, and exophthalmos. Fundoscopic examination is normal with no evidence of papilledema or swelling of the optic disc (would be indicative of increased intracranial pressure).

Intraoral. There is an anterior open bite (apertognathia) with only molar occlusion, a narrow high (V shape) maxillary arch, and a high arched palate. The maxillary dental arch is constricted in the anteroposterior dimension. The patient is in Class III molar relationship with a negative overjet of 6 mm (Angle Class III malocclusion with an anterior open bite and narrow maxilla are almost universal for Crouzon syndrome). Bilateral posterior crossbites are evident (transverse maxillary deficiency is seen in up to two thirds of patients with Crouzon syndrome).

There is no hard or soft tissue clefting of the palate (low incidence of clefting, only seen in 2% to 3% of patients with Crouzon syndrome) or uvula (seen in 9% of patients with Crouzon syndrome). Two large lateral palatal swellings are present bilaterally, giving the appearance of a pseudo cleft (common in up to 50% of patients with Crouzon syndrome).

Extremities. No limb deformities are identified (Crouzon syndrome is not characterized by extremity abnormalities, in contrast to Apert or Pfeiffer syndrome).

IMAGING

A panoramic radiograph and lateral cephalogram are necessary plain radiographic studies before any orthognathic/craniofacial surgery. A posteroanterior cephalogram is also obtained for evaluation of suspected asymmetry. Periapical radiographs can be obtained for detailed evaluation of the dentition. Preoperative and postoperative photodocumentation (extraoral and intraoral) is required.

CT scans with three-dimensional reconstructions and stereolithographic models are adjunctive studies that are useful in treatment planning difficult cases or in the initial diagnosis of craniosynostosis.

For this patient, panoramic and lateral cephalometric radiographs were obtained for evaluation and cephalometric analysis. There was no dental crowding, impactions, or supernumerary teeth.

LABS

The baseline hemoglobin and hematocrit levels are the minimal preoperative laboratory testing necessary for craniofacial surgery in anticipation for potential blood loss. This patient had a hemoglobin level of 13 mg/dl and a hematocrit of 40%.

ASSESSMENT

Crouzon syndrome presenting with maxillary hypoplasia in the transverse and anteroposterior dimensions, and apertognathia requiring combined surgical orthognathic and orthodontic treatment

Craniosynostosis can be broadly categorized as syndromic craniosynostosis (craniofacial dysotosis) or nonsyndromic craniosynostosis. The reconstructive efforts are staged in multiple procedures (see HPI). This patient presents in the later stages of reconstruction for correction of the residual jaw deformities and malocclusion.

TREATMENT

On diagnosis of Crouzon syndrome, the initial assessment focuses on central nervous system malformations and feeding abnormalities. Maxillary hypoplasia and retrusion in combination with a narrow nasopharyngeal airway increase the work of breathing and may require advanced airway interventions. The central nervous system manifestations are usually the result of premature closure of cranial sutures leading to decreased cranial volume and increased risk for elevated intracranial pressure (risk of elevated intracranial pressure increases with the number of sutures involved).

The high arched palate, possible clefting, and obligate mouth breathing make feeding challenging. The inability to pass a nasogastric tube is suggestive of nasopharyngeal obstruction. Most often, these infants compensate by obligate mouth breathing. Feeding difficulties may require a nasogas-

---

> ### Box 13-2. Stages of Surgical Management of the Dysmorphologies Associated With Crouzon Syndrome
>
> **Stage 1.** Primary cranio-orbital decompression with reshaping and advancement is typically undertaken at 10 to 12 months of age. Some surgeons advocate earlier intervention at 6 to 9 months. Elevation of intracranial pressures warrant earlier intervention. During this stage, the coronal sutures are released bilaterally and osteotomies are performed on the anterior cranial vault and upper orbits (across the nasofrontal junction, lateral orbital walls, and roof of the orbit), thereby advancing and decompressing both compartments. This increases the volume of the orbits along with the anteroposterior cranial dimension and decreases the bitemporal prominence. Repeat craniotomy may be required in later childhood in the presence of increased intracranial pressure.
>
> **Stage 2.** Correction of midfacial deficiency and deformity with osteotomy and advancement can be performed as early as 5 to 7 years of age (cranial vault and orbits are 85% to 90% of adult size at this age). The presenting deformity (in the vertical, horizontal, and transverse planes) will dictate the type of osteotomy technique to be used. Monobloc, facial bipartition, or Le Fort III osteotomies can be used. An extracranial Le Fort III osteotomy is indicated when the supraorbital ridge is in good position and there is minimal ocular hypertelorism. If there is a residual deficiency in the supraorbital ridge and anterior cranial vault, along with midfacial deficiency, then a monobloc osteotomy is indicated to advance the entire orbit and midface. If there is significant hypertelorism, then a facial bipartition osteotomy (monobloc osteotomy with a vertical midline split and removal of a intraorbital wedge of bone) is indicated for orbital repositioning (this will also widen the maxillary arch).
>
> **Stage 3.** Orthognathic surgery to correct residual jaw deformities and malocclusion should be performed after completion of facial growth in conjunction with other cosmetic procedures such as malar or chin surgery.

---

tric or orogastric feeding tube or placement of a percutaneous endoscopic gastrostomy tube.

The surgical management of the dysmorphologies associated with Crouzon syndrome involves a staged reconstructive strategy. There is no clear consensus on the most appropriate timing and technique of each reconstructive stage; typically, there are three stages (Box 13-2):
- **Stage 1.** Primary cranio-orbital decompression with reshaping and advancement
- **Stage 2.** Correction of midfacial deficiency and deformity with osteotomy and advancement (monobloc, facial bipartition, or extracranial Le Fort III osteotomies)
- **Stage 3.** Orthognathic surgery

This patient was treated with a high Le Fort I osteotomy and bilateral sagittal split osteotomies for correction of his skeletal Class III deformity and apertognathia (see Chapter 7, the sections on Mandibular and Maxillary Orthognostic Surgery). He was also treated with an advancement genioplasty and malar implants for improved facial contours.

COMPLICATIONS

Complications of Le Fort II and III level maxillary osteotomies are discussed in the section on Apert Syndrome.

DISCUSSION

Crouzon syndrome was first described in 1912 by O. Crouzon and later in a series of 86 cases published by Atkinson in 1937. The reported prevalence in the literature is 15 to 16 per 1 million births, accounting for 4.5% of all cases of craniosynostosis. The syndrome follows an autosomal dominant mode of distribution, although reports of sporadic cases from new mutations occur. Variability of expression characterizes this syndrome.

Abnormalities of the central nervous system may include progressive hydrocephalus, chronic cerebellar herniation, and stenosis of the jugular foramen with venous obstruction. An increased frequency of cerebellar herniation has been attributed to earlier patterns of suture closure in Crouzon syndrome compared with Apert syndrome. Differences in skull development between Apert and Crouzon syndromes have been suggested, including earlier closure of sutures, fontanelles, and synchondroses in Crouzon syndrome. This leads to marked differences in shapes and the cranial volume of the skull in patients with Crouzon syndrome. Cranial malformation depends on the order and rate of progression of sutural synostosis. Brachycephaly is most common, but scaphocephaly, trigonocephaly, and cloverleaf skull may be observed.

Shallow orbits with ocular proptosis are an important diagnostic feature of Crouzon syndrome. Concomitant ocular findings include exotropia, poor vision or blindness, optic atrophy, nystagmus, exposure conjunctivitis, and keratitis, among others. Approximately 50% of patients with Crouzon syndrome have lateral palatal swellings that resemble a pseudocleft. CLP and a bifid uvula occur in lower frequencies.

Maxillary hypoplasia manifests as transverse and anteroposterior dental arch shortening. A high arched palate and a unilateral or bilateral crossbite are seen. Crowding, ectopic eruption, and missing teeth are not uncommon. Conductive hearing loss deficit is found in 55%, and atresia of the external auditory canals occurs in 13%. Crouzon syndrome should be distinguished from simple bilateral coronal synostosis and crouzonodermoskeletal syndrome.

Bibliography

Cohen MM Jr, MacLean RE: *Craniosynostosis diagnosis, evaluation and management,* ed 2, New York, 2000, Oxford University Press.

Fearon JA: The Le Fort III osteotomy: to distract or not to distract? *Plast Reconstr Surg* 107(5):1091-1103; discussion 1104-1106, 2001.

Flores-Sarnat L: New insights into craniosynostosis, *Semin Pediatr Neurol* 9(4):274-291, 2002 [erratum: *Semin Pediatr Neurol* 10(2):159, 2003].

Iannetti G, Fadda T, Agrillo A, et al: LeFort III advancement with and without osteogenesis distraction, *J Craniofac Surg* 17(3):536-543, 2006.

Posnick JC: Craniofacial dysostosis, *Oral Maxillofac Surg Knowledge Update* 2, 1998.

Ruiz RL: Update in craniofacial surgery, *Oral Maxillofac Surg Clin N Am* 16(4), 2004.

Hemifacial Microsomia

Chris Jo, DMD, and Shahrokh C. Bagheri DMD, MD

CC

A 12-year-old boy is referred by his orthodontist for evaluation of persisting facial asymmetry, explaining that, "My face and jaw are crooked" (possible male predilection, but some studies have shown an equal gender distribution).

HPI

The facial asymmetry was first noticed in early childhood and has progressively exacerbated (asymmetry in hemifacial microsomia usually progresses with age). The patient has been in a functional orthopedic and orthodontic appliance for several years, with no improvement. He presents with an obvious facial asymmetry and deviation of the face and mandible to the left side. The occlusal plane is canted toward the affected side. The patient denies any previous history of facial trauma (facial fractures in a growing child, especially to the mandibular condyle, can contribute to growth disturbances). He was born with an absent auricle with only some remnants of the lobule (E_3, Table 13-4). His left ear was reconstructed at age 6 (in a normal child, the ear is 90% of adult size at this age).

PMHX/PDHX/MEDICATIONS/ALLERGIES/SH/FH

Noncontributory. He is in the seventh grade and in good academic standing (mental and developmental retardation is not usually seen in patients with hemifacial microsomia).

EXAMINATION

General. The patient is a well-developed and well-nourished boy in no apparent distress.

Neurological. The patient is awake, alert, and oriented. Cranial nerves, other than the left vestibulocochlear (VIII) nerve, are intact (muscular impairments may be present, but this is not due to central or peripheral cranial nerve dysfunction. The facial nerve is intact bilaterally [N_0, or no facial nerve involvement]).

Maxillofacial. The examination results are consistent with hemifacial microsomia with obvious facial asymmetry. The left face appears hypoplastic (S_1, or minimal subcutaneous and muscle deficiency), and the facial midline is deviated to the left (the affected side). There is discrete vertical orbital dystopia (O_2, or abnormal orbital position). The left auricular reconstruction appears excellent but slightly anterior and inferior in position (E_3, or malpositioned remnant of lobule with absent auricle, usually in the anterior and inferior position).

The nasal tip is deviated 2 mm to the left of the facial midline, with slight shortening of the left ala. The left zygoma is moderately hypoplastic. The maxillary dental midline and chin are 2 and 6 mm to the left of the facial midline, respectively, but the maxillary and mandibular dental midlines are coincident. The right gonial angle is 4 mm lower than the left side (indicative of a vertical deficiency on the left ramus–condyle unit). The left condylar head is difficult to palpate (M_2, or short and abnormally shaped mandibular ramus with a severely hypoplastic condyle; confirmed radiographically).

The maxillary and mandibular occlusal planes are canted 3 mm downward on the right. The occlusion demonstrates a slight posterior crossbite and crowding of the anterior mandibular teeth on the left side. The molar relationship is Class I on the right side and Class II on the left side (malocclusion is prevalent in hemifacial microsomia, and the degree of malocclusion is proportional to the skeletal deformity. Dental crowding, inclination of the anterior teeth and unilateral crossbite on the affected side are characteristic findings).

The dentition is in the mixed stage and without any caries or soft tissue pathology (patients with hemifacial microsomia are five times more likely to have missing teeth than is the general population and frequently have delayed tooth development on the affected side. Dental agenesis and enamel hypoplasia are more likely to occur in persons with severe skeletal deformities. Enamel hypoplasia of the primary incisors on the affected side is thought to be an additional early developmental marker for hemifacial microsomia).

Lips and oral commissure are normal (macrostomia is seen in 35% of hemifacial microsomia). The soft palate, hard palate, and alveolar processes appear normal (approximately 7% to 15% of patients with hemifacial microsomia present with CLP).

IMAGING

A panoramic radiograph is the initial diagnostic radiographic study of choice, providing an excellent overview of the mandible and maxilla and demonstrating the degree of deformity of the mandibular ramus–condyle unit. Lateral and posteroanterior cephalometric radiographs are used to evaluate the degree of deformation, hypoplasia, and asymmetry of the maxilla and mandible in relation to the cranial base. CT scans with three-dimensional reconstructions provide the most detailed information. Stereolithographic models can be fabricated to assist in surgical planning, especially when severe asymmetries exist or when distraction osteogenesis is planned (models provide an excellent platform to contour custom-made prefabricated facial implants and vector planning for distraction osteogenesis). Standard preoperative and postoperative photodocumentation is required.

Table 13-4.	OMENS Classification of Hemifacial Microsomia

O	**Orbital distortion**
O_0	Normal orbital size and position
O_1	Abnormal orbital size
O_2	Abnormal orbital position
O_3	Abnormal orbital size and position
M	**Mandibular hypoplasia**
M_0	Normal mandible
M_1	Small mandible and glenoid fossa with a short ramus
M_2	Short and abnormal shaped ramus
M_3	Complete absence of ramus, glenoid fossa, and temporomandibular joint
E	**Ear anomaly**
E_0	Normal ear
E_1	Mild ear hypoplasia and cupping with all the structures present
E_2	Absence of external auditory canal with variable hypoplasia of the concha
E_3	Malpositioned lobule with absent auricle
N	**Nerve involvement**
N_0	Normal facial nerve
N_1	Upper facial nerve involvement (temporal and zygomatic branches)
N_2	Lower facial nerve involvement (buccal, mandibular, and cervical branches)
N_3	All branches of the facial nerve affected
S	**Soft tissue deficiency**
S_0	No apparent soft tissue and muscles deficiency
S_1	Minimal muscle and subcutaneous deficiency
S_2	Moderate deficiency
S_3	Severe deficiency with muscles and subcutaneous tissue hypoplasia

Modified from Horgan JE, Padwa BL, LaBrie RA, et al: OMENS-Plus: analysis of craniofacial and extracraniofacial anomalies in hemifacial microsomia, *Cleft Palate Craniofac J* 32(5):405-412, 1995.

For this patient, the panoramic radiograph demonstrates severe hypoplasia of the mandibular ramus–condyle unit (Figure 13-3). The auricular reconstruction is visible on the radiograph and is anterior and inferior in position compared with the normal side.

Figure 13-4 shows a stereolithographic model constructed from the CT scan illustrating the asymmetry, hypoplastic left zygoma, missing left zygomatic arch, occlusal canting, twisted maxilla, and severity of the condylar and ramus hypoplasia and deformity (although severely deformed, a small condyle is present: OMENS [see Table 13-4] M_2 or Kaban type IIB). The glenoid fossa is present (an absent fossa is classified as OMENS M_3 or Kaban type III).

LABS

Baseline preoperative hemoglobin and hematocrit levels are required for patients undergoing orthognathic or reconstructive surgery secondary to the potential for severe intraoperative blood loss. The hemoglobin and hematocrit for this patient were 15.5 g/dl and 42.1%, respectively.

ASSESSMENT

A 12-year-old boy with left-sided hemifacial microsomia

According to OMENS classification, the patient is classified as $O_2M_2E_3N_0S_1$ (see Table 13-4) or Kaban type IIB hemifacial microsomia.

TREATMENT

The goals of treatment for hemifacial microsomia are to:
- Increase the size of the underdeveloped/hypoplastic mandible and soft tissues on the affected side
- Establish a new articulation between mandible and temporal bone
- Correct the associated maxillary deformity
- Establish a functional occlusion
- Restore facial symmetry and establish an aesthetic appearance (residual deformities/asymmetries can be addressed with facial alloplastic implants or cranial bone grafts)

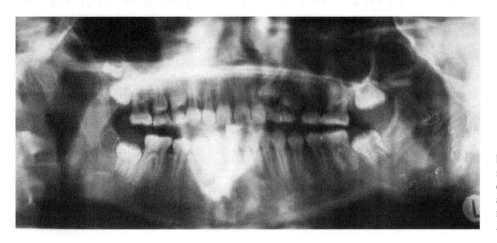

Figure 13-3 Panoramic radiograph showing the extent of the left mandibular ramus–condyle unit deformity and hypoplasia. Note the outline of the reconstructed left auricle. *(Courtesy Dr. Vincent J. Perciaccante.)*

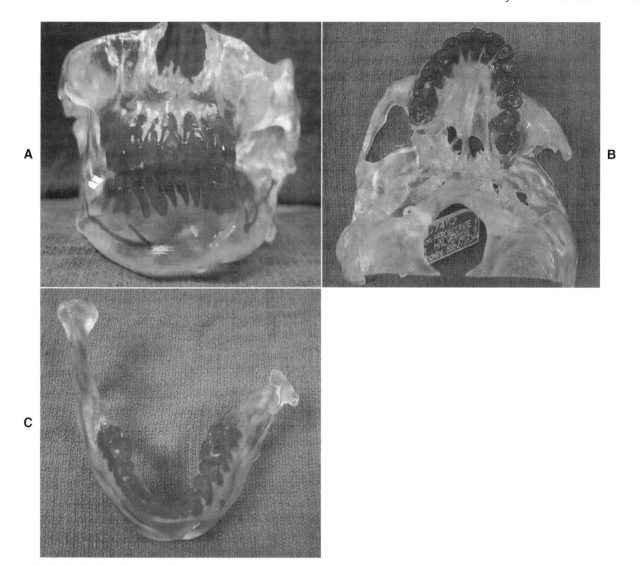

Figure 13-4   A-C, Stereolithographic model showing the extent of facial and mandibular asymmetry. Note the occlusal cant, deviation of the mandible to the affected side, twisting of the maxilla toward the affected side, hypoplasia of the midface and zygoma, agenesis of the left zygomatic arch, and, most important, the deformity of the hypoplastic ramus and condyle (glenoid fossa is deformed but present).   *(Courtesy Dr. Vincent J. Perciaccante.)*

Auricular reconstruction is ideally done at age 5 to 6 when the auricle is 85% to 90% of adult size and before the child enters grade school. This procedure is often accomplished using a contralateral costochondral graft from the sixth or seventh rib, which is shaped and placed under a skin flap anterior to the mastoid process. It is later elevated to provide projection to the ear. The lobular remnant can be rotated and incorporated into this framework.

Attempts at orthopedic/orthodontic appliances should be initiated early (may obviate the need for surgery in type I hemifacial microsomia and may optimize type II and III hemifacial microsomia for surgery). Surgical correction of the mandibular deformity (earliest skeletal manifestation of hemifacial microsomia) is the primary objective (usually in the mixed dentition phase). Lengthening the ramus–condyle unit and rotating the mandible to the facial midline (or slightly overcompensating) will cause an ipsilateral open bite and a contralateral crossbite (ideally done in a period of mixed dentition between the ages of 6 and 12). This will unlock the vertical growth potential of the maxilla in a growing child, improving the maxillary asymmetry and occlusal cant.

Several techniques for restoration of mandibular dimensions are available based on patient needs and surgeon preference. Costochondral or cranial bone grafts, vertical ramus osteotomy, or mandibular distraction osteogenesis can be used to lengthen and rotate the mandible by reconstructing the ramus–condyle unit (the glenoid fossa is reconstructed as needed).

Orthognathic surgery can be used in the final surgical stage. A Le Fort I osteotomy is performed once the patient's facial growth is complete, to correct any residual maxillary deformities (may require concurrent mandibular osteotomies and/or genioplasty if residual deformities exist in the mandible). Alloplastic facial implants or onlay cranial bone grafts can be used to restore midfacial (zygoma) and mandibular (gonial angle and antegonial notch) symmetry. Presurgical and postsurgical orthodontic treatment is essential for optimal results.

Due to the absent growth potential of the facial skeleton in the adult patient, correcting the mandibular defect (reconstruction of the mandibular ramus–condyle unit) will not "unlock" the maxilla's growth potential. Standard orthognathic surgery may be indicated for types I and IIA hemifacial microsomia patients (typically Le Fort I osteotomy and sagittal split or inverted-L osteotomies with bone grafting of the affected side). Combined Le Fort I osteotomy and reconstruction of the ramus–condyle unit (various methods discussed earlier) with or without contralateral mandibular osteotomy will be required for types IIB and III hemifacial microsomia patients. Bone grafts and alloplastic facial implants can be used adjunctively to restore facial symmetry.

This patient was treated with an intraoral mandibular osteotomy and distraction osteogenesis (advantageous due to the simultaneous expansion of the soft tissue matrix) using an intraoral double-vector device (Figure 13-5). Once growth is complete (typically by age 18 in males and age 16 in females), he can be reevaluated for orthognathic surgery and cosmetic maxillofacial recontouring with alloplastic implants.

COMPLICATIONS

A variety of complications can follow reconstruction (infection, nonunion, sensory and motor nerve injury, unfavorable scarring, relapse, and residual deformities), depending on the surgical modality. Many of the complications are dependent on the treatment and are synonymous to those observed in orthognathic surgery and distraction osteogenesis for the patient without hemifacial microsomia. These are discussed elsewhere in this book.

DISCUSSION

Hemifacial microsomia is a congenital craniofacial malformation of the first and second branchial arches, affecting the development of the mandible, temporomandibular joint, orbit, midface, ear, cranial nerves, and associated soft tissues. It has a reported incidence of 1:5000 to 1:5600 live births (second most common facial birth defect after CLP). Males and females are equally affected (some report 3:2 male predilection). The left and right sides are equally affected (16% reported to be bilateral). The mechanism of hemifacial microsomia is not completely understood. Some have postulated an intrauterine vascular insult to the stapedial artery (supplies the first and second branchial arches). Others speculate exposure to thalidomide and retinoic acid as an etiological factor. Although a 2% to 3% occurrence of hemifacial microsomia is reported in first-degree relatives, concordance is rarely seen in twins.

Several classification systems have been developed over the years. The Kaban classification is an adaptation of the Pruzansky system, which emphasizes the extent of mandibu-

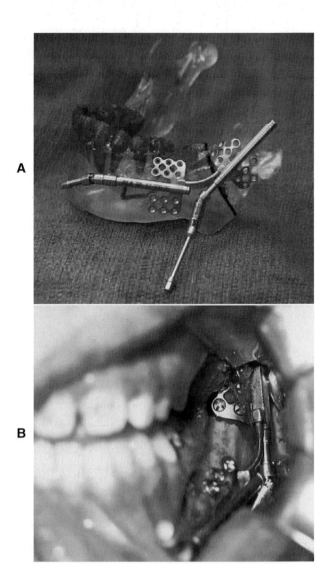

Figure 13-5   A, The stereolithographic model used for treatment planning the osteotomy and vector of distraction osteogenesis (also allowing prebending of the mesh plates for accurate adaptation). The double vector of the distraction device allows vertical elongation of the ramus–condyle unit, as well as horizontal elongation, and rotation of the mandible toward the unaffected side. Note the very high and posterior position of the mandibular foramen, which would make a vertical ramus osteotomy much more difficult. **B,** Intraoperative view showing the osteotomy and distraction device in place via a transoral approach.   *(Courtesy Dr. Vincent J. Perciaccante.)*

lar (ramus–condyle unit) and temporomandibular joint abnormalities. Kaban type I exhibits a mild hypoplasia of the mandibular ramus–condyle unit and its associated soft tissue structures but has a functional temporomandibular joint. Kaban type IIA exhibits a moderately hypoplastic and deformed mandibular ramus–condyle unit, but an articulation is present. Kaban type IIB exhibits a moderate to severe hypoplasia and deformity of the mandibular ramus–condyle unit and glenoid fossa with no articulation between the condyle and fossa (however, a posterior stop is present upon manipulation). Kaban type III exhibits complete aplasia of the mandibular ramus–condyle unit and therefore no functional articulation (no functional stop upon manipulation).

Table 13-5. Principal Maxillofacial Defects in Hemifacial Microsomia

Location	Principal Defects
Mandibular	Mandibular hypoplasia (89-100%)
	Malformed glenoid fossa (24-27%)
Ear	Microtia (66-99%)
	Preauricular tags (34-61%)
	Conductive hearing loss (50-66%)
Midfacial	Maxillary hypoplasia
	Zygomatic hypoplasia
	Occlusal canting
Soft tissue	Masticatory muscle hypoplasia (85-95%)
	Macrostomia (17-62%)
	Cranial VII nerve palsy (10-45%)

Table 13-6. Associated Defects in Hemifacial Microsomia

Craniofacial	General
Velopharyngeal insufficiency (35-55%)	Vertebral/rib defects (16-60%)
Palatal deviation (39-50%)	Cervical spine anomalies (24-42%)
Orbital dystopia (15-43%)	Scoliosis (11-26%)
Ocular motility disorders (19-22%)	Cardiac anomalies (4-33%)
Epibulbar dermoids (4-35%)	Pigmentation change (13-14%)
Cranial base anomalies (9-30%)	Extremity defects (3-21%)
Eyelid defects (12-25%)	Central nervous system defects (5-18%)
Hypodontia/dental hypoplasia (8-25%)	Genitourinary defects (4-15%)
Lacrimal drainage anomalies (11-14%)	Pulmonary anomalies (1-15%)
Frontal plagiocephaly (10-12%)	Gastrointestinal defects (2-12%)
Sensorineural hearing loss (6-16%)	
Preauricular sinus (6-9%)	
Parotid gland hypoplasia	
Other cranial nerve defects (e.g., V, VII, IX, XII)	

The OMENS classification system evaluates five major anatomic areas of abnormalities in hemifacial microsomia (Obit, Mandible, Ear, cranial Nerves, and Soft tissues). A score is given for each category based on the degree of abnormality (see Table 13-4), and the summation correlates with the severity of mandibular deformity. Several associated anomalies can exist in association with hemifacial microsomia (Tables 13-5 and 13-6). One study reported that over half of patients with hemifacial microsomia had at least one extracranial anomaly.

Goldenhar syndrome (oculoauriculovertebral spectrum) has been described as a variant of hemifacial microsomia. However, it appears that hemifacial microsomia is within the broad range of expression of the oculoauriculovertebral spectrum, which is synonymous with Goldenhar syndrome.

Bibliography

Berry G: Note on congenital defect (coloboma) of the lower lid, *Lond Ophthalmol Hosp Rep* 12:255, 1989.

David DJ, Mahatumarat C, Cooter RD: Hemifacial microsomia: a multisystem classification, *Plast Reconstr Surg* 80:525-335, 1987.

Enlow DH, Poston WR II: *Facial growth*, ed 3, Philadelphia, 1990, WB Saunders, p 81.

Fan WS, Mulliken JB, Padwa BL: An association between hemifacial microssomia and facial clefting, *J Oral Maxillofac Surg* 63:330-334, 2005.

Horgan JE, Padwa BL, LaBrie RA, et al: OMENS-plus: analysis of craniofacial and extracraniofacial anomalies in hemifacial microsomia, *Cleft Palate Craniofac J* 32:405-412, 1995.

Johnsen DC, Weissman BM, Murray GS, et al: Enamel defects: a developmental marker for hemifacial microsomia, *Am J Med Genet* 36:444-448, 1990.

Kaban LB, Moses MH, Mulliken JB: Surgical correction of hemifacial microsomia, *Plast Reconstr Surg* 82:9-19, 1988.

Kaye CI, Martin AO, Rollnick BR, et al: Oculoauriculovertebral anomaly: segregation analysis, *Am J Med Genet* 43:913-917, 1992.

Padwa BL, Kaban LB: Hemifacial microsomia, *Oral Maxillofac Surg Knowledge Updates* 2:145-157, 1998.

Obstructive Sleep Apnea Syndrome

Chris Jo, DMD, and Shahrokh C. Bagheri, DMD, MD

CC

A 46-year-old Caucasian man (2:1 to 3:1 male predilection, affecting up to 4% of men and 2% of women) is referred to your office by his primary care physician for the evaluation and management of OSAS.

HPI

The patient presents complaining of a long history of snoring and restless sleeping (sleep-disordered breathing includes hypopnea, apnea, and respiratory effort–related arousals). His wife of 20 years reports that he snores loudly, frequently stops breathing (apnea), making grunting, gasping, and choking sounds (bedroom partners are often the first to recognize the problem). The patient has noticed difficulty concentrating at work (OSAS decreases cognitive function) and difficulty staying awake during the day (daytime somnolence is a hallmark sign of OSAS). He scored over 10 on the Epworth Sleepiness Scale (a questionnaire to subjectively rate the level of daytime somnolence). He also complains of morning dry mouth, morning headaches, nocturia, and night sweats (common symptoms associated with OSAS). His primary care physician referred him to a sleep center for a polysomnogram (PSG), which found that his respiratory disturbance index (RDI) score was 51 (see Discussion).

PMHX/PDHX/MEDICATIONS/ALLERGIES/SH/FH

His past medical history is significant for hypertension (there is a direct relationship between OSAS and hypertension, resulting in cardiovascular morbidity), which is controlled with a β-blocker and a diuretic. His past surgical history is significant for tonsillectomy and adenoidectomy as a child (hypertrophic tonsils and adenoids increase the risk of OSAS in children, but this is more uncommon in adults).

He admits to drinking two or three beers a day (alcohol consumption can blunt the ventilatory response to hypercarbia and thereby worsen OSA) and occasional smoking (smoking can cause inflammation and edema of the upper airway mucosa, which increases airway resistance).

He is a sales manager working over 8 hours a day (overworking may contribute to lack of sleep, sleep-disordered breathing, and daytime somnolence). More recently, his coworkers have noticed that he is falling asleep at this desk (daytime somnolence also contributes to decreased productivity and can be particularly dangerous for individuals operating machinery or driving motor vehicles).

His father had similar signs and symptoms of OSAS that were untreated (a positive family history is commonly seen due to various genetic and environmental factors). He died at the age of 60 of a myocardial infarction (untreated OSAS significantly increases the risk of cardiovascular disease and cerebrovascular accident resulting in death).

EXAMINATION

Vital signs. His blood pressure is 150/95 mm Hg (stage I hypertension), heart rate 75 bpm, respirations 16, and temperature 37.6°C.

General. The patient is a moderately obese man in no apparent distress (obesity is an important risk factor for OSAS). His weight is 225 lbs, his body mass index is 32 kg/m^2 (class 1 obesity), and his waist-to-hip ratio is 1.2 (normal is 0.9 in males and 0.8 in females).

Maxillofacial. He displays mild retrognathia (retrognathia is a risk factor for OSAS). His neck measures 18 inches (neck circumference of 17 inches or greater in men increases the risk of OSAS and may be the best predictor of RDI in males).

Endonasal. The nares are equally patent bilaterally. There is no evidence of internal nasal valve collapse. A Cottle test is negative (a positive Cottle test may indicate internal nasal valve collapse). The nasal septum appears midline, and the inferior turbinates appear normal (deviated nasal septum and/or turbinate hypertrophy may cause nasal obstruction). There are no nasal polyps.

Intraoral. His occlusion is Class II division II. The oral tongue is normal in size. The soft palate and uvula are long and not completely visible. The tonsillar pillars are partially visible, and the tonsils are not present. There are no tori. (Enlarged or redundant oral structures may cause oropharyngeal obstruction.)

Endoscopic nasopharyngoscopy (in the supine position). The nasopharynx is clear of any obstruction. The retropalatal airway space is narrow and has redundant soft tissue, and the space completely obliterates with Müller's maneuver (forced inspiratory effort against a closed mouth and nose). The retroglossal oropharynx and hypopharynx are narrow and partially obliterate (75%) with Müller's maneuver. Collapse of the lateral pharyngeal walls appears to contribute significantly to the airway collapse. There is no pathology of the endolarynx, and the vocal cords are functional.

IMAGING

The lateral cephalometric radiograph is the initial diagnostic study of choice, which can be taken in a relaxed position and with Müller's maneuver. Although it is a static two-dimensional representation of a dynamic three-dimensional space and is taken in an upright position on an awake patient, it is standardized, inexpensive, and readily available. It provides an excellent overview of the craniofacial skeleton to identify and quantify any skeletal deformities, including the position of the maxilla and mandible in relation to the cranial base, as well as soft tissue anatomy (see Chapter 8, the section on Orthognathic Surgery). The distance from the hyoid bone to the mandibular plane (normal is 11 to 19 mm), the posterior airway space (normal is 10 to 16 mm), the length of the soft palate (normal is 34 to 40 mm), and the thickness of the soft palate (normal is 6 to 10 mm) are important measurements in the work-up of OSAS. CT and MRI provide the most three-dimensional and volumetric information on the upper airway and surrounding soft tissues, but they are not very practical or cost-efficient.

In this patient, the lateral cephalometric radiograph showed a hypoplastic mandible causing a Class II skeletal discrepancy, a retropositioned pogonion, a posterior airway space of 6 mm, a long and thick soft palate, and a normal hyoid–to–mandibular plane distance.

LABS

No laboratory values are needed in the initial work-up of OSAS. Thyroid hormone or thyroid-stimulating hormone levels are routinely ordered at some sleep centers but may not be warranted. A preoperative CBC is required for patients undergoing surgical treatment (hemoglobin and hematocrit are commonly elevated in OSAS). A baseline arterial blood gas analysis is indicated in some individuals. Other laboratory values are ordered based on the patient's medical history.

An electrocardiogram is required for all patients with OSAS. OSAS is considered a cardiac risk factor. Hypertension and obesity are additional cardiac risk factors that are commonly seen in patients with OSAS.

In this patient, the CBC and electrocardiogram were within normal limits.

POLYSOMNOGRAPHY

Polysomnography ("sleep study") is the gold standard for diagnosing sleep-related breathing disorders. The electroencephalogram, electrocardiogram, electro-oculogram, electromyogram, heart rate, oxygen saturation, airflow, and respiratory efforts are monitored and recorded during sleep. The number of apneas (cessation of airflow lasting 10 or more seconds) and hypopneas (abnormal respirations lasting 10 or more seconds, with a 30% or more reduction in airflow and 4% or higher oxygen desaturation) are calculated. The episode of apnea is categorized as obstructive (no airflow despite inspiratory effort), central (no airflow and no inspiratory effort), or mixed (both central and obstructive component). The RDI, or apnea/hypopnea index (AHI), is the total number of apneic and hypopneic events divided by the total number of hours of sleep (i.e., the average number of apnea and hypopnea events per hour). The RDI is used to quantify the severity of OSA and to monitor the patient's response to treatment.

In this patient, the PSG showed an RDI of 51 (severe OSA). All episodes of apnea were obstructive in nature. The lowest oxygen saturation was 81%. There were no cardiac arrhythmias (prolonged hypoxemia can precipitate premature ventricular contractions or sinus bradycardia).

ASSESSMENT

A 46-year-old obese man with severe OSAS (also termed obstructive sleep apnea-hypopnea syndrome) due to obstruction at the level of oropharynx (retropalatal and retroglossal) and hypopharynx (type II obstruction)

OSA can be classified as mild, moderate, or severe based on the patient's RDI or AHI (Table 13-7), which are arbitrarily defined and therefore inconsistent in the literature. When OSA is associated with daytime somnolence, OSAS is diagnosed. Upper airway obstruction can occur at three levels (nasopharynx, oropharynx, and hypopharynx). Type I upper airway obstruction involves the oropharynx only. Type II involves both the oropharynx and hypopharynx. Type III involves only the hypopharynx.

TREATMENT

The treatment of OSAS first begins with a proper diagnosis along with recognition of the level or levels of upper airway obstruction and severity of the disease. Nonsurgical management, namely lifestyle changes, should be initiated immediately, regardless of the severity of disease or anticipated surgical plan. This includes weight loss therapy and cessation of alcohol use. Obesity is seen in 60% to 70% of patients with OSAS. It has been shown that a 10% weight loss improves the RDI by 26%, while a 10% weight gain worsens the RDI by 32%. Alcohol or any other sedatives can worsen the RDI

Table 13-7.	Classification of OSAS Based on RDI (AHI)*		
	Mild OSAS	**Moderate OSAS**	**Severe OSAS**
RDI (AHI)	5-15	15-30	>30

From Gottlieb DJ, Whitney CW, Bonekat WH, et al: Relation of sleepiness to respiratory disturbance index, *Am J Respir Crit Care Med* 159(2):502-507, 1999.
AHI, Apnea/hypopnea index; *OSAS,* obstructive sleep apnea syndrome; *RDI,* respiratory disturbance index.
*Because classification of OSAS is arbitrary, there are several variations in the literature. These are the most recent classification recommendations.

(longer and more frequent obstructions) in patients with OSAS or cause snorers to develop OSAS. Thus alcohol avoidance is recommended in all susceptible patients.

Other nonsurgical treatments include nasal continuous positive airway pressure (nCPAP), oral appliances, and modified sleep positions (RDI doubles when supine, compared with lateral decubitus position). nCPAP or bilevel CPAP (BiPAP) is titrated to pressures sufficient to eliminate upper airway obstruction by preventing soft tissue collapse. It is a highly effective treatment if the patient is able to tolerate the device (noncompliance is the major reason for failure of this modality). All patients should be given a test trial of nCPAP to determine if they will be able to tolerate its use. True long-term compliance is much lower than the self-reported compliance, and the overall acceptance rate is near 50%. Several Food and Drug Administration–approved mandibular repositioning or advancement appliances are available (the Herbst and Klearway appliances are the most popular). They work by positioning the mandible and tongue forward (50% to 100% of maximum protrusive movement as tolerated), which brings the attached soft tissue anteriorly, thereby opening the posterior airway space. On average, oral appliances reduce the RDI by 56%. The Herbst appliance has been reported to decrease the mean RDI from 48 to 12. The Klearway appliance was shown to improve the RDI to less than 15 in 80% of patients with moderate OSA and 61% of patients with severe OSA.

If nCPAP or an oral appliance is not tolerated by the patient, or if the oral appliance does not improve the patient's RDI to acceptable levels, surgical options should be considered. Tracheotomy was once considered the gold standard for OSA (100% effective), but it is no longer widely accepted except for very extreme cases. Site-specific or staged surgical reconstruction of the airway is now considered the standard of care. Nasal obstructions (deviated septum, inferior turbinate hypertrophy, internal nasal valve collapse, nasal polyps, or bony spurs) should be corrected in all patients, including those patients being managed nonsurgically. Nasal reconstruction may include a septoplasty, radiofrequency inferior turbinate reduction (somnoplasty), spreader grafts, or polypectomy. A variety of staged-reconstruction protocols have been developed and studied. There is no conclusive evidence on which surgical protocol is most effective.

The soft palate (retropalatal oropharynx) is addressed by surgical ablation or radiofrequency volumetric reduction (somnoplasty). Uvulopalatopharyngoplasty was popularized by ENT surgeons as an alternative to tracheotomy and was frequently and injudiciously recommended to most all patients. When uvulopalatopharyngoplasty was the sole surgical modality, success rates were less than 50%. Failures were attributed to base of tongue obstruction, which were not addressed with the uvulopalatopharyngoplasty. Others viewed the uvulopalatopharyngoplasty procedure as too radical with an unacceptable incidence of velopharyngeal insufficiency and hypernasality, therefore advocating the more conservative uvulopalatoplasty or uvulopalatal flap procedures. More

recently, soft palate pillar implants have been introduced to stiffen the soft palate, reducing the amount of snoring and improving sleep apnea.

The retrolingual oropharyneal and hypopharyneal airway space can be improved with procedures that advance the genioglossus muscle and hyoid bone. The anterior mandibular osteotomy (genial window osteotomy, preferred when pogonion is in normal position) or inferior sagittal osteotomy (sliding genioplasty, preferred when pogonion is retropositioned) advances the genioglossus and geniohyoid muscles. The hyoid bone can be further positioned superiorly and anteriorly with a hyoid myotomy and suspension (hyoid bone is suspended to the anterior mandible) or with a modified hyoid suspension technique (hyoid bone is secured to the thyroid cartilage). When uvulopalatopharyngoplasty or uvulopalatoplasty is combined with a genial tubercle advancement with or without hyoid suspension, substantially higher success rates are reported.

Maxillomandibular advancement has been shown to improve posterior airway space and increase lateral pharyngeal wall stability, thus preventing its tendency to collapse. Maxillomandibular advancement may be performed in various stages of surgical treatment, depending on the surgeon's preference and clinical indications. The maxillomandibular complex is typically advanced 10 mm. Adjunctive procedures can be performed based on site-specific principles (uvulopalatopharyngoplasty, genial advancement, hyoid suspension). Success rates vary in the literature. Waite and colleagues reported a 65% success rate (RDI less than 10) when maxillomandibular advancement was the sole treatment. Prinsell reported 100% success (RDI less than 10) in 50 consecutive patients when maxillomandibular advancement was combined with genial advancement.

In this patient, nCPAP trial was initiated, but the patient was unable to tolerate the device. He subsequently elected to receive surgical management consisting of an uvulopalatal flap procedure and advancement genioplasty (inferior sagittal osteotomy). A bilateral sagittal split osteotomy mandibular advancement, in conjunction with the uvulopalatoplasty and advancement genioplasty, would have been ideal, but the patient was not able to afford preoperative orthodontic therapy. His postoperative RDI was 20 with significant improvement in daytime somnolence. He was offered a modified hyoid suspension or maxillomandibular advancement as the second-stage surgery.

COMPLICATIONS

The morbidity and mortality of untreated OSAS far outweigh the individual complications of nonsurgical and surgical intervention. He and associates reported an 8-year survival rate of patients with an RDI greater than 20 to be 63%, whereas an RDI of less than 20 corresponded to an 8-year survival rate of 96%. Hypertension is seen in one to two thirds of all OSAS cases and is a major risk factor for coronary artery disease, congestive heart failure, and cerebrovascular accident. Untreated OSAS results in higher mortality rates from cardiovascular events. Untreated OSAS also increases the incidence of transient ischemic attacks and stroke and may have a stronger correlation than that with coronary artery disease. Studies have also shown that daytime somnolence associated with OSAS is a major cause of traffic-related accidents and death.

Complications are specific for individual procedures, which are beyond the scope of this section. Velopharyngeal insufficiency is a well-documented postoperative complication of uvulopalatopharyngoplasty. The risk of velopharyngeal insufficiency is greater when it is combined with maxillomandibular advancement. Li and colleagues report a less than 10% incidence of "mild" velopharyngeal insufficiency with simultaneous maxillary advancement and uvulopalatopharyngoplasty.

DISCUSSION

Various staged surgical protocols have been developed that combine different site-specific surgeries into two to three stages. Because OSAS typically involves more than one anatomical level or area of obstruction, a combined surgical approach is warranted in most cases. This was recognized due to the low success rate when OSAS was treated with uvulopalatopharyngoplasty alone. Riley and associates described a two-stage process to treat type II obstruction. Stage 1 consisted of uvulopalatopharyngoplasty, genial advancement, and hyoid suspension. When stage 1 surgery was considered a failure, maxillomandibular advancement was performed as stage 2 surgery. Riley and associates in 1990 reviewed 40 patients undergoing stage 2 surgery (maxillomandibular advancement) and found a 97% success rate. Lee and colleagues in 1999 used a three-stage surgical treatment for type II obstruction:

- **Stage 1.** Uvulopalatopharyngoplasty and genial advancement
- **Stage 2.** Maxillomandibular advancement
- **Stage 3.** Hyoid myotomy and suspension

In a review of 35 patients using the three-stage protocol, Lee and colleagues found a 69% success rate (RDI less than 20) after stage 1 treatment. The mean preoperative and postoperative RDIs were 53 and 19, respectively. Three patients underwent stage II surgery (maxillomandibular advancement), resulting in postoperative RDI of 10 or less in all three patients. Maxillomandibular advancement can also be used as an effective first line of treatment in moderate to severe cases of OSAS, as evidenced by Prinsell's review of 50 consecutive cases in 1999 with a reported 100% successful outcome.

Bibliography

Bond T: Evaluation and diagnosis of sleep-disordered breathing, *Oral Maxillofac Surg Clin N Am* 14:293-296, 2002.

He J, Kryger MH, Zorick FJ: Mortality and apnea index in obstructive sleep apnea: experience in 385 male patients, *Chest* 94:9-14, 1988.

Hendler BH, Costello BJ, Silverstein K, et al: A protocol for uvulopalatopharyngoplasty, mortise genioplasty, and maxillomandibular advancement in patients with obstructive sleep apnea: an analysis of 40 cases, *J Oral Maxillofac Surg* 59:892-897, 2001.

Hoekema A, deLange J, Stegenga B, et al: Oral appliances and maxillomandibular advancement surgery: an alternative treatment protocol for the obstructive sleep apnea-hypopnea syndrome, *J Oral Maxillofac Surg* 64:886-891, 2006.

Lee NR: Surgical evaluation for reconstruction of the upper airway, *Oral Maxillofac Surg Clin N Am* 14:351-357, 2002.

Lee NR, Givens CD, Wilson J, et al: Staged surgical treatment of obstructive sleep apnea syndrome: a review of 35 patients, *J Oral Maxillofac Surg* 57:382-385, 1999.

Li KK, Guilleminault C, Riley RW, et al: Obstructive sleep apnea and maxillomandibular advancement: an assessment of airway changes using radiographic and nasopharyngoscopic examinations, *J Oral Maxillofac Surg* 60:526-530, 2002.

Li KK, Powell N, Riley R: Radiofrequency thermal ablation therapy for obstructive sleep apnea, *Oral Maxillofac Surg Clin N Am* 14:359-363, 2002.

Li KK, Riley R, Powell N: Complications of obstructive sleep apnea surgery, *Oral Maxillofac Surg Clin N Am* 15:297-304, 2003.

Lowe AA: Principles of oral appliance therapy for the management of sleep disordered breathing, *Oral Maxillofac Surg Clin N Am* 14:305-317, 2002.

Moore KE, Esther MS: Current medical management of sleep-related breathing disorders, *Oral Maxillofac Surg Clin N Am* 14:297-304, 2002.

Prinsell JR: Maxillomandibular advancement surgery in a site-specific treatment approach for obstructive sleep apnea in 50 consecutive patients, *Chest* 116:1519-1529, 1999.

Riley RW, Powell NB, Guilleminault C: Maxillary, mandibular, and hyoid advancement for treatment of obstructive sleep apnea: a review of 40 patients, *J Oral Maxillofac Surg* 48:20-26, 1990.

Riley RW, Powell NB, Guilleminault C: Obstructive sleep apnea syndrome: a surgical protocol for dynamic upper airway reconstruction, *J Oral Maxillofac Surg* 51:742-747, 1993.

Schmitz JP, Bitoni DA, Lemke RR: Hyoid myotomy and suspension for obstructive sleep apnea syndrome, *J Oral Maxillofac Surg* 54:1339-1345, 1996.

Thornton WK, Roberts DH: Nonsurgical management of the obstructive sleep apnea patient, *J Oral Maxillofac Surg* 54:1103-1108, 1996.

Vorona RD, Ware JC: History and epidemiology of sleep-related breathing disorders, *Oral Maxillofac Surg Clin N Am* 14:273-283, 2002.

Waite PD, Wooten V, Lachner J, et al: Maxillomandibular advancement surgery in 23 patients with obstructive sleep apnea syndrome, *J Oral Maxillofac Surg* 47:1256-1261, 1989.

14 Medical Conditions

Shahrokh C. Bagheri, DMD, MD

This chapter addresses:
- Congestive Heart Failure
- Acquired Immunodeficiency Syndrome
- End-Stage Renal Disease
- Liver Disease
- von Willebrand Disease
- Oral Anticoagulation Therapy With Coumadin in Oral and Maxillofacial Surgery
- Alcohol Withdrawal Syndrome and Delirium Tremens
- Acute Asthmatic Attack
- Diabetes Mellitus
- Diabetic Ketoacidosis
- Acute Myocardial Infarction
- Hypertension

"Greater knowledge grants further humility"

Safe management of the oral and maxillofacial surgery patient requires an understanding of medial comorbidities that may complicate the perioperative or long-term outcome of procedures. Although it is not possible to describe the large array of medical conditions that may have surgical implication in oral and maxillofacial surgery, in this chapter we have selected 12 medical conditions that will be encountered in the routine practice of any surgical subspecialty.

When necessary, consultation with other medical or surgical subspecialties (for example, a cardiologist or a nephrologist) should be obtained to gain the adequate information for safe surgical treatment.

Congestive Heart Failure

David Verschueren, DMD, MD, and Shahrokh C. Bagheri, DMD, MD

CC

A 66-year-old (congestive heart failure [CHF] is predominantly a disease of the elderly) man with a previous history of heart failure presented to the emergency department after he was involved in a motor vehicle accident, complaining of shortness of breath and "broken bones in my face."

HPI

The patient was the unrestrained driver in a low-velocity head-on collision, sustaining injury to the face, with no reported loss of consciousness. He was brought to the emergency department via ambulance and upon presentation was found to be in moderate respiratory distress (most common presenting symptom of acute CHF exacerbation is dyspnea). The patient was admitted for multisystem trauma evaluation and possible CHF exacerbation. The oral and maxillofacial surgery service was consulted for the management of the facial trauma.

PMHX/PDHX/MEDICATIONS/ALLERGIES/SH/FH

The patient had a history of myocardial infarction 6 years earlier, with subsequent coronary artery bypass graft surgery without complications (documented previous coronary artery disease [CAD]). He also has a previous diagnosis of essential (idiopathic) hypertension, which is controlled by a single-drug regimen using hydrochlorothiazide (thiazide diuretic). He admits to poor compliance with his medications (risk factor for CHF exacerbation) and was previously diagnosed with CHF with a documented ejection fraction of 35% (ejection fraction is the percentage of blood that is ejected forward into the systemic circulation by the left ventricle with each contraction: normal is greater than 55%). He is taking lovastatin (HMG-CoA reductase inhibitor [cholesterol-lowering medication]) for hypercholesterolemia (risk factor for CAD). The patient has a 30 pack-year history of smoking (risk factor for CAD); he quit smoking after his myocardial infarction.

CAD involves varying degrees of impaired blood supply (oxygen) to the myocardium (causing ischemic heart disease), thereby rendering the heart at risk to ischemic events (angina, myocardial infarction) with potential functional impairment of the myocardium and subsequent systolic dysfunction. This systolic dysfunction (heart failure) will lead to backup of blood (congestion)—hence, the term "congestive heart failure." Risk factors for CHF include CAD (causes 50% to 75% of cases), pulmonary hypertension, valvular heart disease, pericardial disease, and cardiomyopathy (dilated or hypertrophic myocardium), or restrictive lung disease.

EXAMINATION

Advanced trauma life support primary survey. The results are negative except for moderate respiratory distress. The patient is immediately placed on supplemental oxygen with improvement of his work of breathing.

General. He is awake, alert, and oriented times three, with an increase in respiratory effort evidenced by use of accessory muscles of respiration.

Vital signs. His blood pressure is 110/75 mm Hg, heart rate 120 bpm (tachycardia), respirations 28 per minute (tachypnea), and temperature 37.1°C.

Maxillofacial. Examination is consistent with right zygomaticomaxillary complex fracture.

Cardiovascular. The examinations revealed regular rate and rhythm with normal S_1 sound (closure mitral and tricuspid valve) and S_2 sound (closure aortic and pulmonic valves). An S_3 sound is auscultated at the left sternal border at the fifth intercostal space (an S_3 sound is heard in early diastole and is secondary to rapid ventricular filling in a dilated cardiac chamber). The point of maximum impulse (generated by the left ventricle as it touches the inner chest wall during systole) is laterally displaced with a parasternal heave (elevation of the chest wall to the left of the sternum). The jugulovenous pressure is elevated at 15 cm (normal, less than 9 cm) with a positive hepatojugular reflex (distention of the jugular veins on application of pressure in the right upper abdominal quadrant). Hepatojugular reflex and elevated jugulovenous pressure are signs of venous congestion seen in association with right-sided heart failure secondary to the backup of venous return to the right side of the heart, with subsequent distention of the neck veins and hepatic congestion.

Pulmonary. Use of the accessory muscles of respiration (sternocleidomastoid, scalenes, pectoralis major and minor, and serratous anterior muscles). Dyspnea is exacerbated when assuming the supine position (orthopnea). Bilateral basilar rales (fluid in the alveolar spaces), with dullness to percussion (due to pleural effusions) in the lung bases (fluid accumulation in the lungs is secondary to left-sided heart failure).

Abdominal. The abdomen is nontender and nondistended, with hepatomegaly and the liver percussed at 10 cm below the costal margin (hepatic congestion due to right-sided heart failure).

Extremity. Lower extremities show 3+ pitting edema at the ankles (significant fluid in the extravascular compartments due to venous congestion causing capillary leakage; this is usually first noted in the lower extremities due to the added effect of gravity).

IMAGING

A chest radiograph is the minimum imaging modality for the evaluation of CHF exacerbation. This is valuable for the evaluation of pulmonary edema and infiltration and for the approximation of the heart size. Echocardiography (transthoracic or transesophageal) is also useful for the evaluation of ventricular and valvular function and determination of the ejection fraction. The earliest finding of left-sided heart failure on the chest radiograph is cephalization of the pulmonary vessels. Normally, the vessels in the lung bases are larger and more numerous than those in the lung apices. This is secondary to the effects of gravity and anatomically larger volume of the lungs at the base. With the progression of heart failure, the increased pressure is transmitted "backward" to the pulmonary veins and capillaries (hence, the term "backward failure"). The lung bases are affected first; therefore, blood is preferentially "shunted" to the upper or more cephalad lobes, giving the radiographic appearance of cephalization. If the pressure in the vessels continues to rise, the fluid in the interstitium will become radiographically evident as interstitial edema, bronchial wall thickening, and interlobular septa. The most noticeable are the Kerley B lines (B = bases). These are short thin perpendicular lines extending to the pleura at the lung bases on a chest radiograph.

Chest radiograph. Bilateral blunting of the costophrenic angles with pronounced infiltrates in the lower lobes is seen (consistent with bilateral pleural effusions and pulmonary edema).

Cephalization of the pulmonary vessels bilaterally. Increased cardiac silhouette (an increased cardiac silhouette, spanning over one third of the thoracic cavity on an anteroposterior film is indicative of an enlarged heart or dilated cardiomyopathy).

Transthoracic echocardiography (transesophageal echocardiography is a more accurate technique compared with transthoracic echocardiography, but it requires the insertion of a probe into the esophagus). Imaging shows dilated left ventricle consistent with dilated cardiomyopathy with decreased wall motion (systolic dysfunction) and mild mitral regurgitation. The pulmonic, aortic, and tricuspid valves are without stenosis or regurgitation. The ejection fraction is estimated at 25% (compromised ventricular function). No pericardial fluid and normal wall thickness are seen in all four chambers. Moderate elevation of the pulmonary artery pressure is evidenced.

CT (maxillofacial). CT reveals a displaced right zygomaticomaxillary complex fracture. A CT scan of the chest can also be used to further evaluate the pulmonary parenchyma and cardiac structures.

LABS

Brain natriuretic peptide level is 2000 pg/ml (normal, less than 100 pg/ml).

With CHF, increased pressure and workload on the heart trigger the myocardial cells to secrete natriuretic peptides. Atrial myocytes secrete increased amounts of atrial natriuretic peptide, and the ventricular myocytes secrete both atrial and brain natriuretic peptides in response to the high atrial and ventricular filling pressures. Both of these peptides work as a natriuretic, diuretic, and vasodilator agents and help reduce both preload and afterload. The plasma concentrations of both hormones are increased in patients with asymptomatic and symptomatic CHF.

Electrocardiogram

- **Rate.** Tachycardic at 120 bpm
- **Rhythm.** Regular; each P wave followed by a QRS; each QRS is preceded by a P wave; QRS complexes occurring at regular intervals
- **Axis.** Positive deflection in lead I; negative deflection in lead aVF (indicative of left-axis deviation secondary to left ventricular hypertrophy)
- **Intervals.** PR interval less than 0.20 second, or five small boxes on electrocardiogram paper (greater than five small boxes is consistent with atrioventricular node block), QRS less than 0.12 second, or three small boxes (greater than three small boxes indicates widened QRS), QT less than half the distance from QRS to QRS complex (normal)
- **Infarctions.** Q waves in leads V_1 through V_5 (hallmark of old myocardial infarction); no flipped T waves, ST-segment elevation or depression (signs of acute ischemic events)
- **Other.** Loss of precordial R-wave progression in leads V_1 through V_6 (suggestive of left ventricular hypertrophy/cardiomyopathy)

ASSESSMENT

A 66-year-old man status post motor vehicle accident with a previous history of heart disease now presenting with acute CHF exacerbation (Class IV heart failure) with subsequent pulmonary edema and a displaced right zygomaticomaxillary complex fracture

TREATMENT

Fluid retention in heart failure is initiated by the fall in cardiac output, leading to edema and decreased effective arterial volume, further leading to activation of the renin-angiotensin-aldosterone and sympathetic nervous systems and exacerbating fluid retention and volume overload.

The pharmacotherapy of heart failure is aimed at improving cardiac function (contractility and stroke volume) and reducing the workload of the heart (preload and afterload reduction). The Frank-Starling mechanism describes the relationship of cardiac output (stroke volume) to end-diastolic volume (pressure). With increasing end-diastolic volume, the myocardium compensates by increasing cardiac output. In CHF, the myocardium fails to respond to the increase in the end-diastolic volume, causing congestion of the circulation.

The cardiac glycosides, most commonly represented by digitalis, are positive inotropic agents that increase myocardial contractility and prolong the refractory period of the atrioventricular node. Diuretics, β-blockers, angiotensin-converting enzyme (ACE) inhibitors, and angiotensin receptor blockers are also used selectively or in combination for the treatment of heart failure. A review of data from the Prospective Randomized Study of Ventricular Failure and the Efficacy of Digoxin (PROVED) and Randomized Assessment of Digoxin on Inhibitors of Angiotensin-Converting Enzyme (RADIANCE) trials supports the use of combination therapy for initial management. Loop diuretics are usually introduced first for volume control (preload reduction). The goal is to improve the signs and symptoms of volume overload, such as dyspnea and peripheral edema. ACE inhibitors are typically initiated during or after the optimization of diuretic therapy (afterload reduction). β-Blockers can be used (if the patient is not bradycardic) once the patient is stable on ACE inhibitors. These are initiated at a low dose and titrated to effect. Digoxin is initiated in patients who continue to have symptoms of heart failure despite this regimen; it is also used for rate control in atrial fibrillation. Angiotensin receptor blockers are added to this regimen in patients with New York Heart Association (NYHA) functional Class II to III heart failure, while spironolactone or eplerenone (potassium-sparing diuretics) are used in patients with Class IV heart failure. Other treatment modalities may include hemodynamic monitoring, anticoagulation, pacemaker, mechanical circulatory support, and surgery (heart transplantation).

In this patient, the cardiology service was consulted and the patient was treated with Lasix (loop diuretic), lisinopril (ACE inhibitor), and labetolol (α/β-blocker). The patient became hemodynamically stable and his cardiovascular symptoms improved within 36 hours (decreased shortness of breath, orthopnea, and paroxysmal nocturnal dyspnea; resolution of peripheral edema and pleural effusions; and improved ejection fraction to 45%). Subsequently, the patient was cleared for surgery and was taken to the operating room for fixation of the right zygomaticomaxillary complex under general anesthesia.

COMPLICATIONS

Trauma patients commonly present with exacerbations of previous medical conditions due to the increased physiological stress of trauma. Particular attention should be given to the overall status of the patient and not just the maxillofacial region. It is often difficult to determine the etiology of trauma in relation to the preexisting medical conditions. An acute exacerbation of a preexisting medical condition could cause alterations in the mental or physical status, contributing to the traumatic episode. Similarly, the physiological stress and injury from trauma can accentuate a preexisting condition, complicating the management and outcome of trauma patients.

Complications of untreated CHF include death, cardiac arrhythmias, pulmonary edema, thromboembolic episodes, and peripheral edema resulting in skin breakdown.

DISCUSSION

Heart failure can result from any structural or functional cardiac disorder that impairs the ability of the heart to pump blood. It is characterized by specific symptoms, such as dyspnea, fatigue, fluid retention, and weight gain. There are several etiologies to heart failure including idiopathic, myocarditis/endocarditis (viral/bacterial infections), ischemic heart disease, infiltrative disease (amyloidosis, sarcoidosis), peripartum cardiomyopathy, hypertension, HIV infection, connective tissue disorders, substance abuse, and certain medications (Figure 14-1).

The classification systems used for the management of CHF are based on the severity, systolic versus diastolic dysfunction, and left-sided versus right-sided failure. Heart failure is classified by severity using the NYHA classification (most commonly used). This categorizes patients into one of four functional classes, depending on the degree of effort needed to elicit symptoms:
- **Class I.** Symptoms of heart failure only at levels that would limit normal individuals
- **Class II.** Symptoms of heart failure with ordinary exertion
- **Class III.** Symptoms of heart failure on less than ordinary exertion
- **Class IV.** Symptoms of heart failure at rest

Heart failure can be further broken down into stages to help guide treatment:
- **Stage A.** High risk for heart failure, without structural heart disease or symptoms
- **Stage B.** Heart disease with asymptomatic left ventricular dysfunction
- **Stage C.** Prior/current symptoms of heart failure
- **Stage D.** Advanced heart disease and severely symptomatic or refractory heart failure

When using the right or left designation as the etiology of heart failure, it is the symptomatology and physical examination findings that determines anatomical side of the failing heart. With right-sided heart failure, there is elevation of the jugulovenous pressure, peripheral edema, and hepatomegaly. In left-sided heart failure, fluid backs up in the lungs causing dyspnea, cough, pleural effusions, and rales. Sustained left-sided heart failure will eventually cause right-sided heart failure. Therefore, the most common cause of right-sided failure is left-sided failure.

Systolic versus diastolic heart failure designation involves determination of failure as a result of impaired contraction or inefficient relaxation. Systolic dysfunction is commonly measured by the ejection fraction, while diastolic dysfunction is

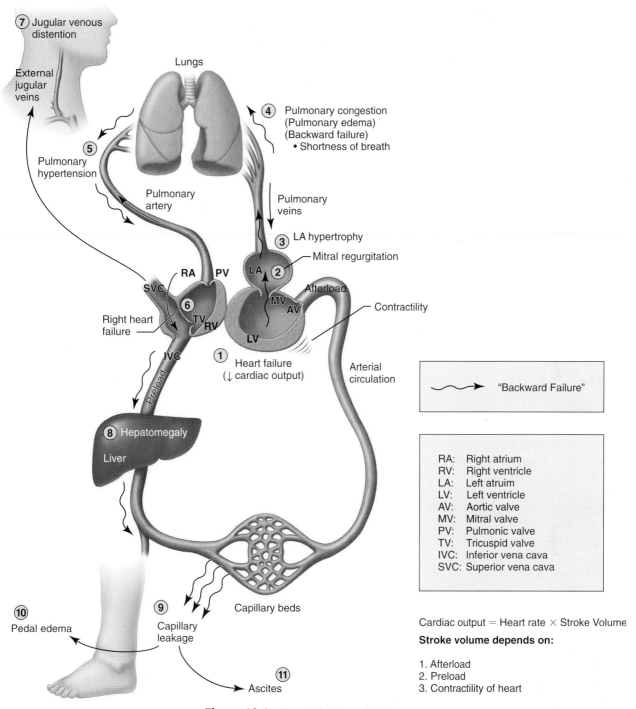

Figure 14-1 Congestive heart failure.

determined by estimation of the left ventricular end-diastolic volume (or pressure). Causes of diastolic dysfunction include myocardial hypertrophy, amyloid deposition, or cardiac tamponade. Systolic dysfunction is more common, but diastolic dysfunction is becoming increasingly recognized.

It is critical to recognize CHF early in the trauma patient. The unpredictable progression to multisystem failure can be devastating. A thorough physical examination and a high index of suspicion must be maintained to assess cardiac, pulmonary, and volume status.

Bibliography

Grady KL, Dracup K, Kennedy G, et al: Team management of patients with heart failure. A statement for healthcare professionals from the Cardiovascular Nursing Council of the American Heart Association, *Circulation* 102:2443, 2000.

Hunt SA, Baker DW, Chin MH, et al: ACC/AHA guidelines for the evaluation and management of chronic heart failure in the adult: executive summary. A report of the American College of Cardiology/American Heart Association Task Force on Practice Guidelines (Committee to Revise the 1995 Guidelines for the Evaluation and Management of Heart Failure) developed in collaboration with the International Society for Heart and Lung Transplantation endorsed by the Heart Failure Society of America, *J Am Coll Cardiol* 38:2101, 2001.

Knudsen CW, Omland T, Clopton P, et al: Diagnostic value of B-type natriuretic peptide and chest radiographic findings in patients with acute dyspnea, *Am J Med* 116:363, 2004.

Young JB, Gheorghiade M, Uretsky BF, et al: Superiority of "triple" drug therapy in heart failure: insights from the PROVED and RADIANCE trials. Prospective Randomized Study of Ventricular Function and Efficacy of Digoxin. Randomized assessment of digoxin and inhibitors of angiotensin-converting enzyme, *J Am Coll Cardiol* 32(3):686-692, 1998.

Acquired Immunodeficiency Syndrome

Mehran Mehrabi, Maj. USAF, DC, and Shahrokh C. Bagheri, DMD, MD

CC

A 46-year-old man who is seropositive for HIV is referred to your office complaining that, "I am having pain in my mouth, and I need my teeth out in order to get dentures."

HPI

The patient has been under routine dental care, but during a recent yearly checkup, he was found to have multiple mobile teeth (accelerated periodontal disease is seen with HIV infection). This sudden change in his oral health has coincided with a recent exacerbation of his HIV infection as measured by an increase in his viral load, decrease in his CD4 count, and onset of gastrointestinal and constitutional symptoms. He has had several previous hospital admissions. Currently, he complains of a foul-smelling mouth odor (halitosis), gingival pain, loosening teeth, gingival bleeding, and exposed roots. The onset of pain has contributed toward difficulty with hygiene and further accumulation of calculus.

PMHX/PDHX/MEDICATIONS/ALLERGIES/SH/FH

The patient tested positive for HIV 6 years ago. He believes to have acquired the virus through unprotected sexual contact. On his most recent hospital admission, his CD4 count was measured at 108 cells/dl; therefore, he was diagnosed with AIDS (CD4 count of less that 200 cells/dl is an AIDS-defining feature). His internist indicated that his recent episode of pneumonia was due to the recent decline in his CD4 count.

There are no particular preoperative criteria before maxillofacial surgery in patients with HIV infection or AIDS. However, each patient should be assessed for risks and benefits of surgery. Some of the common concerns in a surgical patient are the hemoglobin and platelet count. Despite popular belief, the lymphocyte count or viral load does not alter maxillofacial surgical intervention. Nonetheless, a patient with rapidly declining lymphocytes or rise in viral load should be reassessed before any surgical intervention.

EXAMINATION

General. The patient is a cooperative man with evidence of muscle wasting (cachexia) who appears anxious (generalized muscle wasting is seen with advancing AIDS).

Vital signs. His blood pressure is 121/79 mm Hg (hypotension), heart rate 90 bpm, respirations 14 per minute, temperature 37.8°C (with advanced AIDS, it is not uncommon to have a normal temperature despite the presence of an acute infection; this is due to the failure and/or deficiency of available white blood cells to mount an appropriate inflammatory response, which results in fever), and Sao_2 92% on room air (a recent history of pneumonia can result in a decrease in baseline oxygen saturation at room air).

Maxillofacial. There is no evidence of hair loss or patchy ulceration on the scalp (scalp ulceration may be seen in patients with disseminated fungal diseases such as cryptococcal infection. These ulcerations may also present in the oral cavity or peripheral extremities. A biopsy can be used to confirm the diagnosis. This finding can be used as a sign to evaluate other organs for fungal invasion). There is bilateral temporal wasting and prominent zygomatic arches. On examination of the neck, there is a soft dorsal hump (lipodystrophy may result either directly from HIV or as a side effect of antiretroviral therapy, particularly protease inhibitors). Other physical signs to investigate are seborrheic dermatitis (dandruff), vesicular rash with central umbilication in the forehead (molluscum contagiosum), and enlargement of the parotid glands (lymphoepithelial cyst).

Intraoral. The examination indicates poor oral hygiene and a fetid breath. There is a generalized inflammation of the maxillary and mandibular gingiva, exposed buccal bone, and 2+ teeth mobility. Gentle palpation of the gingival tissue results in bleeding and pain. There is no facial or intraoral fluctuance and no obvious swelling (in addition to HIV gingivitis and HIV periodontitis, the oral examination should concentrate on the presence of warts (human papillomavirus), oral neoplastic growth such as Kaposi sarcoma (human herpesvirus 8), hairy leukoplakia (Epstein-Barr virus), candidiasis, and other fungal infections. Aphthous ulcers, lymphoma, herpes, and cytomegalovirus ulcerations may be seen in patients with AIDS.

Chest. His chest is clear to auscultation (if the patient presents with crackles, a chest radiograph would be indicated).

Cardiovascular. Examination revealed regular rate and rhythm, S_1 and S_2, and no gallops, rubs, or murmurs (HIV virus may affect the heart and result in dilated cardiomyopathy, but this is not common).

IMAGING

A routine preoperative chest radiograph is not indicated unless the patient's history or clinical examination is suggestive of symptoms such as shortness of breath, decrease in oxygen saturation at room air, or a productive cough. A chest radiograph along with arterial blood gas analysis may be valuable.

In this patient, the panoramic radiograph demonstrates areas of moderate and severe vertical interproximal bone loss, consistent with severe to moderate periodontal disease.

LABS

During the perioperative evaluation of the HIV infection–positive patient, a complete blood count is valuable but should be used with caution. A rise in the white blood cell count may not be seen in response to physiological or inflammatory demands, as would be seen in the immune-competent individuals. The lymphocyte subset can be used to assess the susceptibility to opportunistic infections. The neutrophil count may be elevated with bacterial infections. The hemoglobin and hematocrit may be used to assess volume status (hemoglobin would be falsely elevated). Hemoglobin and platelet levels may be depleted, and subsequently patients may require packed red blood cell or platelet transfusions before major surgery.

Additional tests may be helpful depending on the extent of the surgical procedures or the presence of concurrent comorbidities associated with immune suppression. Arterial blood gas analysis is helpful when assessing the pulmonary status in a patient with active pneumonia. A basic metabolic panel may be used to evaluate intravascular fluid status in dehydrated and volume-depleted patients. Blood urea nitrogen–to–creatinine ratio of greater than 20 is suggestive of volume depletion. The coagulation factors are rarely depleted in HIV-infected patients, but HIV or other infections may predispose a patient to disseminated intravascular coagulation. Coagulation studies should be obtained as needed. Evaluation of hepatic function is also important. Although HIV may affect liver function directly, of more concern is a concurrent infection with hepatitis B or C virus (note that the route of transmission is similar for HIV and hepatitis B and C viruses).

ASSESSMENT

AIDS secondary to HIV infection, now complicated by acute necrotizing ulcerative periodontitis, requiring full mouth extraction

TREATMENT

There is some controversy regarding the optimal time to initiate treatment for patients who are seropositive for HIV. Most infectious disease specialists start pharmacotherapy when the CD4 count drops below 200 cells/mm^3. Current recommendations consist of a combination of a nucleoside reverse transcriptase inhibitor, a non–nucleoside reverse transcriptase inhibitor, and a protease inhibitor. This combination is commonly referred to as highly active antiretroviral therapy (HAART) (Tables 14-1 to 14-3).

When the patient presents with a CD4 count of less than 200 cells/mm^3, the treatment is trimethoprim-sulfamethoxa-

Table 14-1.	Nucleoside Reverse Transcriptase Inhibitors	

Nucleoside Reverse Transcriptase Inhibitor	Abbreviation	Side Effects
Retrovir	AZT	Anemia, neutropenia
Videx	DDI	Pancreatitis, PN
Hivid	DDC	Pancreatitis, PN
Zerit	D4T	Pancreatitis, PN
Epivir	3TC	Also used for HBV
Ziagen	ABC	Rash, death

PN, Peripheral neuropathy.

Table 14-2.	Nonnucleoside Reverse Transcriptase Inhibitors

Nonnucleoside Reverse Transcriptase Inhibitor	Side Effects
Nevirapine (Viramune)	Hepatotoxicity, hepatic necrosis during the first 4 weeks
Delavirdine (Rescriptor)	Rash and headache
Efavirenz (Sustiva)	Teratogenic, Steven-Johnson rash, hallucination and nightmare

Table 14-3.	Protease Inhibitors	

Protease Inhibitor	No. of Pills Consumed Daily	Common Side Effects
Indinovior (Crixivan)	6	Nephrolithiasis
Ritonavir (Norvir)	12	Weakness, loss of appetite, nausea and vomiting
Invirase/fortovase (Saqunavir)	9	Gastrointestinal disturbances
Nelfinavir (Viracept)	10	Gastrointestinal disturbances, most common being diarrhea
Amprenavir (Agenerase)	16	Severe rash
Lopinovir/ritonavir (Kaletra)	6	Hepatitis

zole for *Pneumocystis carinii* (now called *Pneumocystis jiroveci*) prophylaxis. At a CD4 count of less than 100 cells/mm^3, there is an increasingly susceptibility to toxoplasmosis infections. Because this is treated with the same medication, no additional prophylactic is needed. When the CD4 count drops to less than 50 cells/mm^3, there is a high risk of mycobacterium avium complex infection. This is empirically treated with clarithromycin or azithromycin (macrolide antibiotics). Viral infections such as herpes simplex virus are treated with famcyclovir or acyclovir (there is prophylactic treatment; patients are treated only in the face of infection). Some infections such as *Candida* species may present at a CD4 count of less than 500 cells/mm^3, but prophylactic treatment of fungal infections is not recommended.

The initial treatment of acute necrotizing ulcerative periodontitis consists of fluid resuscitation as needed, analgesics, and antibiotic therapy. With generalized severe periodontal disease, full mouth extraction is both definitive and curative. Patients with HIV infection are treated aggressively to prevent any odontogenic sources of infection, which can potentially cause severe complications in a patient with a declining immune system.

This patient underwent outpatient full mouth extraction under intravenous sedation. Following surgical treatment, the alveolar ridges healed without complications.

Immune suppression can be due to defects in various aspects of the immune system. Concerns and cautions are not the same when dealing with different defects of the immune system. For example, a patient who is neutropenic is more susceptible to bacterial infection, while T-lymphocyte deficiency increases susceptibility to fungal, viral, and parasitic infections.

In oral surgical procedures, there are more complications associated with neutropenia (sepsis, oral ulceration, periodontal disease) compared with lymphopenia. For the neutropenic patient, preoperative antibiotics are used to prevent sepsis. Postoperative antibiotics may also be used.

COMPLICATIONS

Patients affected by HIV infection may present with thrombocytopenia. This can be due to idiopathic thrombocytopenic purpura or thrombotic thrombocytopenic purpura. Idiopathic thrombocytopenic purpura is an autoimmune disorder, resulting from antibodies to glycoprotein platelet 2β3α receptors. This may present as an acute (mostly in children) or chronic (mostly in women) condition. The treatment consists of prednisone, intravenous immunoglobulin, splenectomy, azathioprine, or vincristine. Thrombotic thrombocytopenic purpura presents as a combination of five symptoms: renal failure, central nervous system abnormalities, fever, thrombocytopenia, and anemia. The exact etiology is not well understood. There is a similar syndrome known as hemolytic uremic syndrome that is caused by *Escherichia coli* O157:H7. In the presence of neurological symptoms, the diagnosis of thrombotic thrombocytopenic purpura is made; however, when renal failure is the prominent feature, it is usually due to hemolytic uremic syndrome. The treatment for thrombotic thrombocytopenic purpura is plasmaphoresis. There are other causes for both idiopathic thrombocytopenic purpura and thrombotic thrombocytopenic purpura as well. Idiopathic thrombocytopenic purpura may be caused by any viral infection, leukemia, lupus erythematosus, cirrhosis, antiphospholipid syndrome, and medications (quinine, heparin). Thrombotic thrombocytopenic purpura can be caused by cancer, bone marrow transplantation, pregnancy, and medication (ticlodipine, clopidogrel, cyclosporine, mitomycin, tacrolimus/FK-506, interferon-α).

The risk of postoperative infection in a patient with HIV infection or AIDS who undergoes maxillofacial surgery is controversial at best. While earlier studies showed an increased risk of infections in the HIV-infected population, this has not been confirmed by more recent studies. Most studies were conducted before the advent of HAART. There is a need for prospective evaluation for the risk of infections after various maxillofacial surgeries. Currently there are no recommendations regarding the presurgical or postsurgical care of a patient with HIV infection compared with healthy control patients.

DISCUSSION

Immune deficiency may be an inherited, acquired, or iatrogenic disorder. Inherited defects may result from quantitative or qualitative defects of the cells or cellular pathways involved in immunity (neutrophil, macrophages, complement, lymphocytes). Immune suppression is also seen with organ transplantation for prevention of host versus graft or graft versus host disease and in chemotherapy. Acquired immune deficiency is seen with conditions such as diabetes, leukemia, and AIDS.

AIDS was recognized in 1981 after multiple homosexual male patients were diagnosed with pneumocystis pneumonia and Kaposi sarcoma (more recently found to be also associated with human herpesvirus 8). Before 1981, pneumocystis pneumonia was commonly seen in cancer patients, and Kaposi sarcoma was endemic to Africa and the Mediterranean region. In 1984, HIV, a retrovirus belonging to the lenti virus family, was discovered concurrently by French and American scientists. The virus can be transmitted via exposure of body fluids through sexual contact, needle sharing, paraphernalia, or blood transfusions (horizontal transmission) or from mother to fetus (vertical transmission). Once in the bloodstream, HIV targets the lymphocytes and macrophages, which are the only cells with CD4$^+$ receptors. T cells with a CXCR4 chemokine coreceptor are called T tropic, and macrophages with CCR5 are called M tropic. The virus is unable to infect these cells in the absence of these coreceptors. Interaction of the CD4 receptor with the viral glycoprotein 120 changes its stereochemistry exposing glycoprotein 41, which binds to heparin sulfate within the membrane of the host cells, fusing the viral envelope with the cell membrane. Once genetic material enters the cell, a complementary DNA or coda is made from the original RNA by the enzyme reverse transcriptase. This complementary DNA joins the host DNA by using the enzyme integrase, forcing the cell to make necessary proteins to replicate the virus. Finally, the packaged virus leaves the host cell, using the cell membrane as viral envelope and subsequently infecting other cells.

After inoculation, a patient typically seroconverts in approximately 3 weeks, although the time period can range from 9 days to as long as 6 months. Routine laboratory testing for HIV before this date will result in a negative test. The patient may be asymptomatic or develop flu-like symptoms. The viral load rapidly rises and then falls during this period while the CD4 count rapidly drops before returning to nearly its original level. During the following years, if untreated,

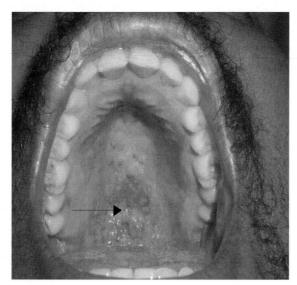

Figure 14-2 Cryptococcal infection of the palate in a patient with AIDS.

there is a steady decrease in the CD4 cell count, along with an increase in the viral load. In general, the viral load is a reflection of the speed of progression of AIDS, while the CD4 cell count is reflective of the current immune status and is used to evaluate susceptibility to opportunistic infections.

As of this writing, HIV has infected more than 1 million Americans. This population is increasing at the rate of 40,000 new infections each year. Among oral and maxillofacial surgery patients, the prevalence of HIV is estimated to be as high as 4.8% in certain demographic areas. Although HAART has resulted in a significant drop in opportunistic infections such as those presenting with oral manifestation, it has not eradicated these complications.

Oral manifestation of HIV may aid in diagnosis as well as prognosis of the disease. These lesions are seen in up to 30% to 80% of patients positive for HIV, and they may be infectious (bacterial, viral, fungal, and parasitic), neoplastic, or idiopathic. In a study published by Diz Dios and colleagues, there was a reduction of oral lesions from 74.2% to 28.5% following the use of HAART. However, in that study there was a significant drop in patient follow-up due to death or relocation. A study by Aguirre and associates evaluated 72 patients with various oral diseases. A significant improvement was seen in the prevalence of pseudomembranous candidiasis from 80% to 32% with the use of HAART. Only a small change was seen in acute necrotizing periodontitis. Tappuni and colleagues evaluated 284 patients infected with HIV and concluded that oral lesions are seen significantly less often in patients receiving monotherapy compared with patients receiving no therapy. Furthermore, the use of HAART resulted in a statistically significant reduction of lesions compared with the use of monotherapy.

The differential diagnosis of oral lesions seen with HIV may be divided into bacterial, viral, fungal, neoplastic, and idiopathic categories. Bacterial infections may present as acute necrotizing gingivitis or periodontitis. Viral infections such oral papillomas are caused by the human papillomavirus and are commonly seen. Fungal infections such as histoplasmosis or cryptococcosis can cause oral ulcerations (Figure 14-2). An example of intraoral neoplastic disease is Kaposi sarcoma, caused by the human herpesvirus 8, which is most commonly seen in homosexual males. Idiopathic xerostomia is commonly seen, resulting in cervical caries.

The surgical management of patients with HIV infection or AIDS requires an understanding of the pathophysiology, medications, and associated disease processes.

Bibliography

Aguirre JM, Echebrria MA, Ocina E: Reduction of HIV-associated oral lesion after highly active antiretroviral therapy, *Oral Surg Oral Med Oral Pathol Oral Radiol Endod* 88:114-115, 1999.

Carey JW, Dodson TB: Hospital course of HIV-positive patients with odontogenic infections, *Oral Surg Oral Pathol Oral Med Oral Radiol Endod* 91:23-27, 2001.

Depoala LG: Human immunodeficiency virus disease: natural history and management, *Oral Surg Oral Med Oral Pathol Oral Radiol Endod* 90:266-270, 2000.

Diz Dios P, Ocampo A, Miralles C, et al: Changing prevalence of human immunodeficiency virus-associated oral lesion, *Oral Surg Oral Med Oral Pathol Oral Radiol Endod* 90:403-404, 2000.

Dodson TB: HIV status and the risk of post-extraction complications, *J Dent Res* 76:1644-1652, 1997.

Dodson TB: Predictors of postextraction complications in HIV-positive patients, *Oral Surg Oral Med Oral Pathol Oral Radiol Endod* 84:474-479, 1997.

Dodson TB, Nguyen T, Kaban LB: Prevalence of HIV infection oral and maxillofacial surgery patients, *Oral Surg Oral Med Oral Pathol Oral Radiol Endod* 76:272-275, 1993.

Dodson TB, Perrott DH, Gongloff RK, et al: Human immunodeficiency virus serostatus and the risk of postextraction complications, *Int J Oral Maxillofac Surg* 23:100-103, 1994.

Frame PT: HIV disease in primary care, *Prim Care* 30:205-237, 2003.

Mehrabi M, Bagheri S, Leonard MK Jr, et al: Mucocutaneous manifestation of cryptococcal infection: report of a case and review of the literature, *J Oral Maxillofac Surg* 63:1543-1549, 2005.

Miller EJ Jr, Dodson TB: The risk of serious odontogenic infection in HIV-positive patients: a pilot study, *Oral Surg Oral Med Oral Pathol Oral Radiol Endod* 86:406-409, 1998.

Patton LL: Hematologic abnormalities among HIV-infected patients: associations of significance for dentistry, *Oral Surg Oral Med Oral Pathol Oral Radiol Endod* 88:561-567, 1999.

Ray N, Doms RW: HIV-1 coreceptors and their inhibitors, *Curr Top Microbiol Immunol* 303:97-120, 2006.

Schmidt B, Kearns G, Perrott D, et al: Infection following treatment of mandibular fractures in human immunodeficiency virus seropositive patients, *J Oral Maxillofac Surg* 53:1134-1139, 1995.

Sleasman JW, Goodenow MM: HIV-1 infection, *J Allergy Clin Immunol* 111:S582-S592, 2003.

Tappuni AR, Flemming JP: The effect of antiretroviral therapy on the prevalence of oral manifestations in HIV-infected patients: a UK study, *Oral Surg Oral Med Oral Pathol Oral Radiol Endod* 92:623-628, 2001.

End-Stage Renal Disease

Gary F. Bouloux, MD, DDS, MDSc, FRACDS, FRACDS(OMS), and Shahrokh C. Bagheri, DMD, MD

CC

A 68-year-old (age is a risk factor) African American (highest risk factor) woman with a history of end-stage renal disease presents with her third episode of acute pericoronitis in 18 months.

HPI

The patient has an impacted lower third molar that causes intermittent pain and has given rise to moderate right-sided facial swelling, fever, malaise, and anorexia.

PMHX/PDHX/MEDICATIONS/ALLERGIES/SH/FH

Her medical history is notable for poorly controlled diabetes mellitus, hypertension, hypercholesterolemia (all risk factors), and end-stage renal disease. Her dental history is significant for multiple extractions over the past 20 years. Medications include insulin, felodipine (calcium channel blocker), metoprolol (β-blocker), losartan (angiotensin receptor blocker), and furosamide (loop diuretic). She has a 28 pack-year smoking history (risk factor).

EXAMINATION

General. The patient is a mildly obese woman in mild distress secondary to pain.

Vital signs. Her blood pressure is 162/98 mm Hg, heart rate 104 bpm, respirations 18, and temperature 38.8°C.

Neurological. She is alert and oriented to place, time, and person.

Maxillofacial. There is fluctuant, tender, and erythematous right-sided facial swelling extending from the angle of the mandible to the right submandibular space. The floor of mouth and the oropharyngeal airway are normal. The right mandibular third molar (tooth No. 32) is noted to be impacted with swelling of the surrounding operculum. Right submandibular lymphadenopathy is noted.

Pulmonary. The chest is clear to auscultation bilaterally

Cardiovascular. She has a regular rate and rhythm with no murmurs, rubs, or gallops.

Extremity. There is no swelling, edema, or muscle weakness.

IMAGING

A panoramic radiograph reveals a mesioangular impacted right mandibular third molar with a pericoronal radiolucency. Renal osteodystrophy (secondary hyperparathyroidism) is evident as seen by a generalized "ground-glass" pattern of the bone, loss of lamina dura, and a maxillary unilocular radiolucency (osteitis fibrosa cystica). This is a result of decreased renal conversion of 25-hydroxycholecalciferol to 1,25-dihydroxycholecalciferol (active vitamin D). A decrease in active vitamin D results in reduced gastrointestinal adsorption of calcium with a corresponding increase in parathyroid hormone to augment serum calcium levels by increasing bone resorption.

LABS

Laboratory tests are ordered based on the severity and acuity of symptoms related to end-stage renal disease in conjunction with the patient's nephrologist/internist. Baseline complete blood count, metabolic panels, liver function tests, and coagulation studies are usually obtained.

The following laboratory study results were obtained for this patient:

- Complete blood count: white blood cells 14,000/µl, hemoglobin 9.2 g/dl, hematocrit 29.2%, platelets 265,000/µl
- Chemistry: sodium 145 mEq/L, potassium 5.6 mEq/L, bicarbonate 22 mEq/L, blood urea nitrogen 48 mg/dl, creatinine 3.9 mg/dl, glucose 167 mg/dl, calcium 7 mg/dl, phosphate 5.2 mg/dl
- Coagulation studies: prothrombin time 11 seconds, partial thromboplastin time 33 seconds, international normalized ratio 1.0
- Liver function tests: aspartate aminotransferase 42 U/L, alanine aminotransferase 33 U/L, γ-glutamyl transpeptidase 43 U/L, alkaline phosphate 34 U/L
- Urinalysis: 3+ proteinuria; no red blood cells, white blood cells, or casts

The laboratory findings are characteristic of end-stage renal disease. The hemoglobin and hematocrit are decreased secondary to the decreased production of erythropoietin by the kidneys. The elevated blood urea nitrogen and creatinine levels reflect the decreased glomerular filtration rate, which is also responsible for the elevated serum potassium. Proteinuria is a result of increased glomerular permeability. The decreased calcium is a result of decreased gastrointestinal absorption secondary to decreased renal production of active vitamin D.

ASSESSMENT

End-stage renal disease complicating management of an odontogenic abscess

TREATMENT

The management of a patient with end-stage renal disease is often complicated. Of particular concern is fluid status and electrolyte balance. Correction of metabolic and fluid abnormalities should be made in conjunction with the nephrologist before any surgical interventions. This may be accomplished by judicious hydration, careful electrolyte replacement, and medications. As renal disease progresses, either peritoneal dialysis or hemodialysis may become necessary. Hypertension is typically very difficult to adequately treat with medication alone, and invariably some degree of hypertension will need to be tolerated. Many medications, particularly antibiotics, will need to be appropriately dosed for the glomerular filtration rate or avoided altogether. All patients able to take oral nutrition should have a renal diet low in sodium, potassium, and protein. Patients receiving dialysis are best scheduled for surgery the day after dialysis (to optimize fluid and electrolyte balance) with a resumption of their usual dialysis the day after surgery. Because patients frequently are heparinized for dialysis, a minimum of 6 hours is prudent after cessation of heparin. Patients with successful renal transplants may be considered to have adequate renal function but are commonly receiving immunosuppressive drugs, including corticosteroids, placing them at increased risk for infections and adrenal insufficiency in the perioperative period.

The initial management of this febrile and anorexic patient included fluid resuscitation. Normal saline 1-L bolus was given followed by a maintenance rate of 125 ml/hr. Fluid resuscitation reduced the serum creatinine to 3.4 mg/dl, suggesting that some of the renal insufficiency was secondary to dehydration. The patient's elevated temperature was treated with acetaminophen (avoid nonsteroidal antiinflammatory drugs in end-stage renal disease as they decrease renal blood flow). While the degree of hyperkalemia was only mild, an electrocardiogram was performed to evaluate for loss of P waves, widened QRS complex, and peaked T waves (none of which were present). Kayexalate was given orally to lower the serum potassium level. The patient was begun on intravenous clindamycin. No dosing adjustment was needed as the clearance of this drug is largely hepatic. Preoperative pain control was achieved primarily with a scheduled hydrocodone/acetaminophen combination with morphine for breakthrough pain. Hydrocodone and morphine are metabolized hepatically via conjugation but their metabolites are renally excreted. The half-lives therefore tend to increase in end-stage renal disease and a reduction in frequency of administration (every 8 hours) was needed to avoid toxicity and excessive sedation.

Hyperglycemia was initially treated with sliding scale insulin. On the second day after admission, incision and drainage of the right submandibular abscess and removal of the right mandibular third molar were performed under a general anesthetic. The postoperative course was uneventful. The patient was placed on a renal diet (low protein) as soon as she was able to eat, and at that time her usual insulin regimen was begun.

COMPLICATIONS

The development of uremic syndrome due to end-stage renal disease (often when the glomerular filtration rate is less than 10 ml/min) is associated with a variety of symptoms. These symptoms are listed in Table 14-4 and herald the urgent need for dialysis.

This syndrome is due to the combined effects of the accumulation of various metabolites (not just urea). It is preferable that treatment be initiated before the onset of uremic syndrome (generally when the glomerular filtration rate approaches 15 ml/min).

The single most feared complication of end-stage renal disease is the development of acute renal failure on top of the underlying chronic renal insufficiency. Causes of acute renal failure can be divided into prerenal, renal, and postrenal. The most likely cause of prerenal failure is hypovolemia secondary to blood loss or dehydration, as in our case. Laboratory indices that suggest a prerenal source includes a blood urea nitrogen–to–creatinine ratio of greater than 20 and a fractional excretion of sodium of less than 1%. Furthermore, the rapid improvement in serum creatinine with fluid resuscitation is highly suggestive. Renal causes of acute renal failure include acute tubular necrosis, acute interstitial nephritis, and acute glomerulonephritis. Acute tubular necrosis may occur

Table 14-4.	Symptoms of Uremic Syndrome Due to End-Stage Renal Disease
System	**Symptoms**
Central nervous	Irritability, insomnia, lethargy, seizures, coma
Musculoskeletal	Weakness, gout, pseudogout, renal osteodystrophy
Hematological	Anemia, coagulopathy
Pulmonary	Noncardiogenic pulmonary edema, pneumonitis
Cerebrovascular	Pericarditis, arrhythmias, cardiomyopathy, atherosclerosis
Gastrointestinal	Nausea, vomiting, anorexia, gastrointestinal bleeding
Acid-base/volume	Hyperkalemia, volume overload (other electrolyte disturbances)
Endocrine	Hyperparathyroidism, hyperlipidemia, increased insulin resistance
Dermatological	Pruritus, skin discoloration (yellow)

secondary to either hypoperfusion or toxic agents such as myoglobinuria (rhabdomyolysis), contrast agents, drugs (aminoglycosides, amphotericin), crystals (acyclovir, sulfonamides), or uric acid (tumor lysis syndrome). The hallmark laboratory feature of acute tubular necrosis is muddy brown casts within the urine. Acute interstitial nephritis may occur with many drugs and is a potential concern in any patient with end-stage renal disease. Drugs that can cause acute interstitial nephritis include cephalosporins, β-lactams, penicillins, Bactrim (sulfamethoxazole-trimethoprim), diuretics, and nonsteroidal antiinflammatory drugs. The presence of eosinophils within the urine is highly suggestive. The last potential cause of acute renal failure is postrenal obstruction. This is usually secondary to urethral obstruction from calculi or prostatic hypertrophy. It can also occur temporarily after removal of a regular urethral Foley catheter in an otherwise healthy individual. A postrenal cause of acute renal failure that is distal to the ureteral orifices can be diagnosed with measurement of the postvoid residual. This is measured by having the patient void naturally and then placing a temporary catheter in the bladder to record the volume of remaining urine. A volume of less than 50 ml is considered normal.

Another common complication of end-stage renal disease is the failure to adjust medication dose. Most drugs are metabolized in the liver and ultimately excreted by the kidney. Many metabolites of hepatically metabolized drugs are themselves metabolically active to some degree. The net result is an increase in the half-life of many drugs. In the presence of end-stage renal disease, it is possible to develop drug toxicity from failing to adjust either the drug dose or, more important, the frequency of drug administration. Drugs that are primarily renally cleared are also likely to accumulate if not dosed appropriately and need to be adjusted accordingly. While many drugs are relatively nontoxic, failure to renally dose a drug can result in significant morbidity and mortality.

DISCUSSION

There are many causes of end-stage renal disease. Diabetes mellitus is a common cause and, as in our patient, may be complicated by uncontrolled hypertension and hypercholesterolemia. General management of the patient with end-stage renal disease includes a low-protein diet (less than 50 g/day), sodium restriction (less than 2 g/day), potassium restriction, fluid restriction, correction of hyperkalemia/hypokalemia, and either peritoneal or hemodialysis as required. The management of hyperkalemia requires an electrocardiogram (wide QRS, peaked T waves, loss of P waves), moderate intravenous hydration, kayexalate, and, in severe cases, dextrose and insulin. Hypokalemia is typically a result of excessive loop diuretic and requires oral or parenteral replacement. Furthermore, perioperative care may complicated by impaired drug excretion, corticosteroids or immunosuppressive drugs, hypertension, anemia, and arrhythmias related to hyperkalemia. Bleeding may also complicate end-stage renal disease as a result of uremia. Bleeding time is typically elevated due to platelet dysfunction and von Willebrand factor abnormalities. Uremia is best controlled through dialysis, while von Willebrand factor levels may be increased with 1-deamino-8-D-arginine vasopressin, cryoprecipitate, or fresh frozen plasma.

Bibliography

Barrierre SL, Jacobs RA: Clinical use of antimicrobials. In Katzung B, editor: *Basic and clinical pharmacology,* ed 6, Norwalk, CT, 1995, Appleton and Lange, pp 760-761.

Grant J: Nephrology. In Ferri F, editor: *The care of the medical patient,* ed 5, Philadelphia, 2001, Elsevier, pp 574-616.

Klag MJ, Whelton PK, Randall BL, et al: Blood pressure and end stage renal disease in men, *N Engl J Med* 334(1):13-18, 1995.

Ziccardi VB, et al: Management of the oral and maxillofacial surgery patient with end stage renal disease, *J Oral Maxillofacial Surg* 50(11):1207-1212, 1992.

Liver Disease

Gary F. Bouloux, MD, DDS, MDSc, FRACDS, FRACDS(OMS), and Shahrokh C. Bagheri, DMD, MD

CC

A 54-year-old white man presents to the emergency department complaining that, "I was hit in the face and my teeth do not meet right . . . it has not stopped bleeding."

HPI

The patient was punched in the face the day before admission while intoxicated with alcohol. He denies loss of consciousness but reports the progressive development of left facial swelling, pain, and difficulty eating (secondary to malocclusion). In addition, he describes persistent ooze from inside his mouth where he was hit (secondary to coagulopathy). He was subsequently diagnosed with a left mandibular angle fracture.

PMHX/PDHX/MEDICATIONS/ALLERGIES/SH/FH

The patient was diagnosed with alcoholic cirrhosis of the liver and associated portal hypertension 2 years ago. He has had several hospital admissions over the past year for worsening ascites (fluid in the abdomen) and one for upper gastrointestinal bleeding (secondary to esophageal varices). He has had no regular dental care. His current medications include furosamide (loop diuretic), spironolactone (potassium-sparing diuretic), and propranolol (nonselective β-blocker). He drinks two quarts of wine every other day.

EXAMINATION

General. Generalized muscle wasting (secondary to poor nutrition and protein catabolism) and lethargy (secondary to hepatic encephalopathy).

Vital signs. His blood pressure is 155/92 mm Hg (elevated blood pressure), heart rate 72 bpm, respirations 22 per minute (tachypnea), and temperature 36.2°C.

Neurological. The patient is alert and oriented times three (person, place, and time) but intermittently confused, with asterixis (flapping of hands with arms and palms fully extended; sign of hepatic encephalopathy).

Maxillofacial. Examination reveals scleral icterus (due to hyperbilirubinemia), fetor hepaticus (due to elevated serum ammonia level), enlarged parotid glands, and left mandibular angle swelling and ecchymosis.

Chest and pulmonary. There are bilateral crackles in the lung bases (fluid in the alveolar spaces), bilateral gynecomas-

tia (enlarged breasts secondary to testicular atrophy), and hair loss over the chest.

Cardiovascular. The patient has regular rate and rhythm, with no murmurs, gallops (S_3 or S_4), or rubs.

Abdominal. The abdomen is nontender and distended with shifting dullness (due to ascites) and splenomegaly (due to portal hypertension secondary to liver cirrhosis). The examination also reveals nodular hard hepatomegaly and caput medusa (tortuous periumbilical veins secondary to portal hypertension).

Extremity. There is bilateral lower extremity 1+ pitting edema (secondary to hypoalbuminemia), Dupuytren contracture in the right index and middle finger (flexion deformity of the fingers secondary to flexor tendon fibrosis), and palmar erythema.

Skin. Multiple small petechiae, spider angiomas, and testicular atrophy (all secondary to elevated estrogen levels) are present.

LABS

The laboratory test in the work-up of liver disease can be complex and crucial in the evaluation of the extent of liver damage and associated systemic involvement. Complete blood count generally shows a macrocytic anemia (mean corpuscular volume is greater than 100 μm^3) (secondary to vitamin B_{12} and folate deficiency) with thrombocytopenia (secondary to hypersplenism and increased sequestration). Elevated blood urea nitrogen and creatinine levels can be seen, especially if there is associated hepatorenal syndrome (HRS). Hypokalemia and hypomagnesemia are also common with malnutrition and need to be corrected. An elevated prothrombin time, partial thromboplastin time, and international normalized ratio are secondary to decreased synthesis of coagulation factors. Prothrombin time is often elevated first because of the shorter half-life of the vitamin K–dependent factor VII that is part of the extrinsic pathway measured best by the prothrombin time (even small decreases in factor VII will result in increased prothrombin time). Elevated liver function tests reflect hepatocellular dysfunction. Both aspartate aminotransferase and alanine aminotransferase levels are elevated, with the aspartate aminotransferase–alanine aminotransferase ratio usually greater than 2:1 in alcoholic hepatic damage. Elevated alkaline phosphatase and γ-glutamyl transpeptidase levels are also seen (reflecting cholestasis). High blood ammonia levels reflect the inability of the liver to covert ammonia to urea for excretion by the kidneys. Hypoalbuminemia is reflective of decreased albumin production in the liver. Finally, unconjugated hyperbilirubinemia (causing scleral icterus) is seen because of decreased bilirubin conjugation by the liver.

For this patient, the following laboratory tests were obtained:

- Complete blood count: white blood cells 4500/µl, hemoglobin 9.5 g/dl, hematocrit 30.1%, platelets 62,000/µl
- Chemistry: sodium 133 mEq/L, potassium 3.1 mEq/L, blood urea nitrogen 48 mg/dl, creatinine 1.8 mg/dl, glucose 172 mg/dl, magnesium 1.0 mg/dl, ammonia 67 mmol/L, albumin 2.2 mg/dl
- Coagulation studies: prothrombin time 20 seconds, partial thromboplastin time 43 seconds, international normalized ratio 1.9
- Liver function tests: aspartate aminotransferase 141 U/L, alanine aminotransferase 84 U/L, γ-glutamyl transpeptidase 45 U/L, alkaline phosphotase 51 U/L.

IMAGING

A panoramic radiograph reveals a fracture of the left mandibular angle.

For evaluation and diagnosis of liver cirrhosis, a CT-guided liver biopsy can be done as needed to demonstrate destruction of normal hepatic architecture with fibrotic changes, confirming the diagnosis of liver cirrhosis.

ASSESSMENT

Mandibular fracture complicated by hepatic dysfunction secondary to alcoholic cirrhosis

TREATMENT

Preoperative preparation of patients with severe liver disease is of paramount importance to prevent perioperative complications. Preoperative management includes the administration of thiamin 100 mg (to prevent Wernicke encephalopathy characterized by ophthalmoplegia, ataxia, and memory impairment), a nutritious diet, and multivitamins with folic acid and vitamin B$_{12}$ supplementation (excess alcohol consumption is often associated with nutritional deficiencies). Any coagulopathy needs to be addressed preoperatively (see Complications).

In this patient, the hypokalemia and hypomagnesemia were corrected with potassium chloride and magnesium sulfate infusions. Librium, a benzodiazepine, was given as a taper over 4 days to prevent life-threatening alcohol withdrawal. Due to the risk of aspiration (increased in alcoholics), the patient was also started on a proton pump inhibitor (decreases gastroesophageal reflux and the degree of chemical pneumonitis should aspiration occur). Due to the obvious respiratory distress as a result of the ascites, paracentesis (removal of peritoneal fluid) was performed; the removal of 4 L of fluid brought on an immediate reduction in the work of breathing and respiratory rate. The patient was started on

furosamide and spironolactone to reduce the severity and frequency of recurring ascites. The hepatic encephalopathy was treated with administration of lactulose (to decrease ammonia production by enteric bacteria). The coagulopathy was treated with 6 units of fresh frozen plasma (to overcome deficiencies of multiple coagulation factors) and 4 units of platelets (to increase the platelet numbers to greater than 100,000 cells/µl). Subsequently, the patient underwent open reduction with internal fixation of the fracture without complications.

COMPLICATIONS

Complications for patients with liver disease are inherently dependent on the degree of functional impairment of the liver and concomitant preoperative systemic conditions.

Patients tend to be protein depleted, fluid overloaded, vitamin deficient, and coagulopathic with electrolyte abnormalities and to have an impaired ability to metabolize medications.

Adjunctive enteral feeding (nasogastric or orogastric tube) may be necessary in the perioperative period to meet caloric needs, especially in the setting of oral and maxillofacial surgery where chewing may be difficult (e.g., intermaxillary fixation, swelling, pain). Parenteral nutrition may also be considered but only in the setting of compromised gastrointestinal function (if the gut works, use it). Caloric requirements should be calculated with consideration to reducing the protein/amino acid content to prevent exacerbation of any encephalopathy. The latter is thought to relate to the blood ammonia level, which can be further reduced with the use of lactulose. Malnutrition and impaired protein synthesis impair wound healing, which can present as increased wound breakdown and delayed healing.

Coagulopathy may be the result of decreased platelets from splenic sequestration (hypersplenism occurs secondary to portal hypertension, which is secondary to liver cirrhosis). Platelet transfusion is the only treatment for thrombocytopenia. Ideally, the patient should be transfused to a platelet number of greater than 100,000/µl.

Coagulopathy may also be the result of decreased hepatic synthesis of clotting proteins, as is often the case with end-stage liver disease, or it may be the result of decreased absorption of fat-soluble vitamins (vitamins A, D, E, and K) from the gastrointestinal tract. The latter is more common with cholestatic liver disease (decreased bile salts reduce the absorption of fat and fat-soluble vitamins). In this situation, vitamin K can be administered with an appropriate increase in the synthesis of vitamin K–dependent coagulation factors (factors II, VII, IX, and X). The end point for management is a substantial improvement in or normalization of the prothrombin time. When decreased hepatic synthesis of coagulation proteins is the result of intrinsic liver disease, transfusion with fresh frozen plasma is the treatment of choice. Care must be taken to avoid worsening of the total body fluid overload, which is typical of ascites and may precipitate pulmonary edema.

Liver failure may also be associated with hepatopulmonary syndrome, hepatorenal syndrome (with electrolyte disturbances), upper gastrointestinal bleeding, nonalcoholic steatohepatitis, and subacute bacterial peritonitis. In addition, most drugs are metabolized by the liver and as such may need to be dosed appropriately or avoided altogether. Drugs that are renally excreted are preferable to those that require hepatic metabolism. End-stage liver disease can be treated with liver transplantation, although most patients die from liver disease or are not eligible for transplantation. Transplant recipients have a functionally normal liver but are immunosuppressed to prevent graft rejection. This may result in an increase in both opportunistic and perioperative infections.

DISCUSSION

Liver disease can be the result of many insults. The most common causes are alcohol consumption and viral hepatitis. Hepatitis C is more common than hepatitis B, with an estimated 4 million cases in the United States. As many as 90% of these cases are chronic. Viral hepatitis also poses a risk for transmission to the surgeon and operating room staff from needle stick injury. Particular care should be taken to reduce this risk. The causes of liver dysfunction are many, but the consequences are often similar. Cirrhosis is the final common pathway of chronic inflammation and is irreversible. Alcoholic cirrhosis may coexist with alcoholic hepatitis. Liver dysfunction is associated with malnutrition, protein catabolism, poor wound healing, coagulopathy, portal hypertension, splenomegaly, ascites, portosystemic venous shunts (esophageal, periumbilical, retro-peritoneal and hemorrhoidal shunts), encephalopathy, and impaired drug metabolism and clearance. All these factors combine to make management of the patient with liver disease a challenging and difficult task.

Bibliography

Patel T: Surgery in the patient with liver disease, *Mayo Clin Proc* 74(6) 593-599, 1999.

Scully C, Cawson R: Hepatic disease. In *Medical problems in dentistry,* ed 2, Costa Mesa, CA, 1987, Wright Publishing, pp 197-224.

Wiklund RA: Preoperative preparation of patients with advanced liver disease, *Crit Care Med* 32(suppl):106-115, 2004.

von Willebrand Disease

Danielle Cunningham, DDS, and Shahrokh C. Bagheri, DMD, MD

CC

A 16-year-old girl is referred to your office for evaluation of an asymptomatic radiopaque mass of the maxilla consistent with a complex odontoma.

HPI

The lesion was identified on routine radiographic examination for an unerupted primary premolar. There was no history of pain, fever, swelling, or drainage from the area.

PMHX/PDHX/MEDICATIONS/ALLERGIES/SH/FH

The parents denied any significant PMHx. However, on further questioning, a history of prolonged bleeding, including heavy menstruation and several episodes of epistaxis without the need of hospitalization, were identified (positive history of abnormal bleeding). This was first noted after the loss of her mandibular primary incisors. Careful questioning also revealed a history of "easy" bruising on her extremities. The parents recall previous episodes of prolonged bleeding with other family members (von Willebrand disease [vWD] is an autosomal dominant disorder). The remaining history was negative.

EXAMINATION

General. The patient is a well-developed and well-nourished cooperative white girl in no apparent distress, whose height and weight are above the 50th percentile.

Maxillofacial. There is no notable facial swelling. During intranasal examination with a nasal speculum, slight epistaxis was noted. Intraoral examination reveals bilateral buccal mucosa ecchymosis (skin discoloration caused by the escape of blood into the tissues from ruptured blood vessels).

Chest, abdominal, and extremity. Multiple petechiae (pinpoint size hemorrhages of small capillaries often seen with quantitative and qualitative platelet dysfunction) are seen on the upper and lower extremities, abdomen, and chest.

IMAGING

Panoramic radiograph reveals a well-defined radiopacity of the right anterior maxilla with multiple teeth-like structures and an associated impacted first premolar (consistent with a compound odontoma). There are no routine imaging studies necessary to evaluate vWD unless there is a suspicion of internal hemorrhage, especially in the setting of trauma.

LABS

There are five laboratory tests used to screen for vWD (1) plasma von Willebrand factor (vWF) (ristocetin cofactor activity assay used to measure platelet aggregation), (2) plasma vWF antigen, (3) partial thromboplastin time, (4) factor VIII activity, and (5) bleeding time. The ristocetin cofactor activity assay is the "gold standard" for diagnosis of vWD; however, it is difficult to obtain an accurate level. The levels of vWF will rise during pregnancy, periods of stress, or hormone replacement therapy. Therefore patient anxiety may acutely elevate the levels of vWF despite a relative deficiency. A positive screening test and/or a high index of suspicion based on the clinical history may indicate further testing is necessary.

A vWF multimer and ristocetin-induced platelet aggregation can be used to confirm the diagnosis. These tests are also used to determine the subtype of vWD. An additional test that is gaining acceptance is the platelet function test, which is dependent on vWF and platelet function. This is used as a screening test for vWD due to its high specificity and sensitivity.

ASSESSMENT

Compound odontoma of the maxilla requiring removal complicated by vWD

TREATMENT

There are five modalities of treatment for vWD:
1. Desmopressin (1-desamino-8-D-arginine-vasopressin [DDAVP])
2. vWF replacement therapy (using cryoprecipitate)
3. Antifibrinolytic agents
4. Topical agents (thrombin or fibrin sealants)
5. Estrogen therapy in women with no contraindications

DDAVP is a synthetic analog of antidiuretic hormone, without vasopressor activity. It acts by increasing vWF and factor VIII levels, by indirectly stimulating the release of vWF from endothelial cells. DDAVP may be administered intravenously, intramuscularly, or intranasally. If given intravenously or intramuscularly for acute bleeding, the dose is 0.3 µg/kg (maximum, 20 µg). An increase in vWF and factor VIII levels is seen within 30 to 60 minutes, with a duration of approximately 6 to 12 hours. Intranasal administration has gained popularity in patients with less serious bleeding and for pre-medication before minor surgical procedures. The usual dose is 150 μg for children weighing less than 50 kg and 300 μg for larger children and adults. A test dose should be administered to observe the effects on vWF. DDAVP should not be administered to patients with type 2B vWD because it may worsen the disease (see Discussion). It also does not seem to be as efficacious in patients with severe bleeding disorders and type 3 disease, probably secondary to the lack of stored vWF.

Replacement therapy with vWF would appear to be the "gold standard" for treatment. However, for cryoprecipitate (which contains factor VIII) to contain viable vWF, it cannot be pasteurized, only screened. Therefore, cryoprecipitate is the only choice for patients with type 2B or 3, because these patients cannot be treated with DDAVP (see later). For significant bleeding, the goal of replacement therapy is to maintain the activity of factor VIII and vWF between 50% and 100% for 3 to 10 days.

Fibrinolytic therapy using tranexamic acid (Amicar) can also be used. This prevents the lysis of the blood clots and can be especially useful for bleeding from the mucous membranes. This class of drugs may be given orally or intravenously. With oral administration, it must be given three or four times over a 24-hour period (secondary to their short half-life) for a period of 3 to 7 days. Topical agents such as Gelfoam (absorbable sponge made from gelatin) and Surgicel (oxidized regenerated cellulose) soaked in topical thrombin can also be used for local hemostasis.

In several studies, estrogen was found to increase the levels of vWF in women taking oral contraceptives and hormone replacement therapy. However, no long-term studies have looked at the risk:benefit ratio for hormone replacement therapy in vWD.

Treatment is determined by clinical findings and the extent of hemorrhage. There are no good laboratory tests that correspond with the severity of the disease. vWF is not a reliable marker of the severity because this value can be artificially elevated in certain physiological states such as stress or pregnancy. Therefore a past history of bleeding is an important clue toward the severity of the disease and determination of optimal therapy.

In this case, the patient was referred to a hematologist for preoperative consultation and evaluation. Subsequently, the patient had a normal ristocetin activity and platelet levels. The hematologist recommended premedication with 150 μg of DDAVP and postoperatively with four doses of Amicar for 24 hours. The patient was subsequently sedated in the office, and the odontoma was removed. Surgicel was placed in the defect and sutured with resorbable sutures. Hemostasis was observed in the office before discharge. At 1-week follow-up, the patient denied any complications and was healing appropriately.

COMPLICATIONS

The most obvious complication of vWD is persistent hemorrhage. If persistent after extractions, Surgicel, topical thrombin, direct pressure, and DDAVP may be used, unless contraindicated. In the setting of acute bleeding, cryoprecipitate is the treatment of choice. Cryoprecipitate can be used to treat all types of vWD. (Cryoprecipitate contains factors VIII and XIII, vWF, fibrinogen, and fibronectin. It can be stored at −18°C for up to 1 year.)

Each treatment regimen has various side effects. DDAVP may cause vasodilation, headache, hypotension, or hypertension (which is usually mild). More serious complications of DDAVP include tachyphylaxis (rapid development of immunity to a drug) and significant hyponatremia and seizures secondary to water retention. Therefore DDAVP is usually limited to once-daily dosing along with water restriction and careful monitoring of serum sodium levels.

Replacement with cryoprecipitate carries an increased risk of transmission of blood-borne pathogens secondary to the inability to adequately pasteurize the extract. Fortunately, with the advent of more sensitive blood testing, the risk of transmission is low.

Prolonged use of antifibrinolytic therapy carries the risk of thrombosis. Hypercoagulable patients need to be carefully evaluated. Topical agents are generally safe but are costly and can only be used as a local measure. Certain preparations of topical thrombin may contain bovine factor V and with broad exposure could precipitate the formation of antibodies to this factor that cross-reacts with human factor V, aggravating hemorrhage.

DISCUSSION

vWD is the most common inherited bleeding disorder, affecting approximately 1% of the population. Most patients do not seek medical attention and are only diagnosed on the basis of unexplained heavy bleeding (e.g., during menstruation) or easy bruising. This disorder is characterized by a mutation in the vWF itself or in the amount of vWF produced. This factor is responsible for primary hemostasis by aiding platelet aggregation and adherence to the endothelial lining, as well as serving as a carrier protein for factor VIII. The half-life of factor VIII is significantly shortened when not bound to vWF.

There are three subtypes of inherited vWD. Types 1 and 2 are autosomal dominant, with type 1 being the most common form of the disease (approximately 70%). Type 1 is a quantitative deficiency in vWF itself. Symptoms range from mild to moderately severe. It is possible that the deficiency may be from abnormally fast clearance of the protein or inadequate production.

Type 2, which is usually autosomal dominant, is a qualitative abnormality of vWF. Type 2 is then subdivided into four subtypes: 2A, 2B, 2M, and 2N. The classification is based on where the mutation occurs on the vWF itself.

Type 2B (approximately 5%) contains the defect on the platelet binding site itself, which actually increases binding of platelets to vWF. This in turn takes platelets out of circulation, causing thrombocytopenia. It is imperative to determine this subtype, especially if treatment is to be instituted, because treatment with DDAVP may actually exacerbate the condition. DDAVP causes an increase in the release of vWF, subsequently causing an increase binding of platelets to vWF and removing more platelets from circulation and worsening the thrombocytopenia.

Type 2N (N is for Normandy, where it was first described) is an autosomal recessive disorder that is very rare. The defect affects the ability of vWF to bind to factor VIII, but the ability to bind with factor VII remains normal. Therefore platelet function remains normal (as well as the quantity of available vWF), but factor VIII levels are greatly reduced. Because this subtype is recessive, a second mutated allele must also be inherited for symptoms to develop. It can be difficult to distinguish this subtype from factor VIII deficiency (hemophilia), because in both conditions the patients have low levels of factor VIII. Type 2N should be considered when a patient presents with a family history of autosomal penetrance (seen in both males and females, not sex-linked, Mendelian genetics) rather than X-linked.

Type 3 is very rare (approximately 1:1 million) and is characterized by a complete absence of or very low levels of vWF, which results from different genetic defects, including nonsense, missense, and frameshift mutations. These patients have severe bleeding and at first may be diagnosed as having factor VIII deficiency before vWF testing is obtained.

vWD may also be acquired with various disease states, usually autoimmune conditions such as systemic lupus erythematosus. Other mechanisms include decreased synthesis, proteolysis, binding to tumor cells, and increased clearance of vWF.

Bibliography

Aledort LM: Treatment of von Willebrand's disease, *Mayo Clin Proc* 66:841, 1991.

Chang AC, Rick ME, Ross Pierce L, et al: Summary of a workshop on potency and dosage of von Willebrand factor concentrates, *Hemophilia* 4(suppl 3):1, 1998.

Federici AB, Berntorp E, Lee CA, et al: A standard trial infusion with desmopressin is always required before factor VIII/von Willebrand factor concentrates in severe type 1 and 2 von Willebrand disease: results of a multicenter European study [abstract], *Thromb Haemost* suppl:795, 1999.

Lethagen S, Harris AS, Sjorin E, et al: Intranasal and intravenous administration of desmopressin: effect on factor VIII/vWF, pharmacokinetics and reproducibility, *Thromb Haemost* 58:1033, 1987.

Mannucci PM: Treatment of von Willebrand's disease, *N Engl J Med* 351:683, 2004.

Mazurier C, Dieval J, Jorieux SK, et al: New von Willebrand factor (vWF) defect in a patient with factor VIII deficiency but with normal levels and multimeric patterns of both plasma and platelet vWF. Characterization of abnormal vwF/ FVIII interaction, *Blood* 75:20, 1990.

McKeown LP, Connaghan G, Wilson O, et al: 1-Desamino-8-arginine-vasopressin corrects the hemostatic defects in type 2B von Willebrand's disease, *Am J Hematol* 51:158, 1996.

Moffat EH, Giddings JC, Bloom AL: The effect of desamino-D-arginine vasopressin (DDAVP) and naloxone infusions on factor VIII and possible endothelial cell (EC) related activities, *Br J Haematol* 57:651, 1984.

Posan E, McBane RD, Grill DE, et al: Comparison of PFA-100 testing and bleeding time for detecting platelet hypofunction and von Willebrand disease in clinical practice, *Thromb Haemost* 90:483, 2003.

Ratnoff OD, Saito H: Bleeding in von Willebrand's disease, *N Engl J Med* 290:1089, 1974.

Rodeghiero F, Castaman G, Dini E: Epidemiological inverstigation of the prevalence of von Willebrand's disease, *Blood* 69:454, 1987.

Shepherd LL, Hutchinson RJ, Worden EK, et al: Hyponatremia and seizures after intravenous administration of desmopressin acetate for surgical hemostasis, *J Pediatr* 114:470, 1989.

Sutor AH: DDAVP is not a panacea for children with bleeding disorders, *Br J Haematol* 108:217, 2000.

Wagner DD: Cell biology of von Willebrand factor, *Annu Rev Cell Biol* 6:217, 1990.

Oral Anticoagulation Therapy With Coumadin in Oral and Maxillofacial Surgery

Gary F. Bouloux, MD, DDS, MDSc, FRACDS, FRACDS(OMS), and Shahrokh C. Bagheri, DMD, MD

CC

A 54-year-old woman is referred to your clinic for removal of multiple teeth before partial denture construction.

HPI

The patient has multiple carious teeth that are nonrestorable. She is planning to have a new maxillary partial denture constructed after the removal of the teeth. She does not complain of any pain or swelling. She has not previously seen a dentist for 8 years and has not had any extractions other than her wisdom teeth 35 years earlier.

PMHX/PDHX/MEDICATIONS/ALLERGIES/SH/FH

Her past medical history is remarkable for paroxysmal atrial fibrillation and multiple transient ischemic attacks in her late 40s and a subsequent cerebrovascular accident at age 49. As a result of the cerebrovascular accident, she has significant left leg weakness. She has a 30 pack-year history of smoking, elevated serum cholesterol and triglycerides, and hypertension (all are additional risk factors for cerebrovascular accident). Her current medications include warfarin (Coumadin), atorvastatin (HMG CoA reductase inhibitor), hydrochlorothiazide (diuretic), and felodipine (calcium channel blocker). She has no known drug allergies.

EXAMINATION

General. The patient is a cooperative woman in no acute distress.

Vital signs. Her blood pressure is 130/84 mm Hg, heart rate 66 bpm, respirations 12 per minute, and temperature 36°C.

Intraoral. There are multiple carious teeth and root fragments.

Neurological. Weakness (3/5) of left lower extremity with brisk knee and ankle reflexes (upper motor neuron injury secondary to cerebrovascular accident). There are no other focal neurological signs.

Extremity. Mild atrophy of the left lower extremity (disuse atrophy) is seen.

Skin. Multiple bruises are noted on the upper and lower extremities (secondary to anticoagulation therapy).

LABS

Prothrombin time is used to measure the adequacy of the extrinsic and common pathway of clotting mechanisms. Specifically, it measures the clotting ability of factors I (fibrinogen), II (prothrombin), V, VII, and X. Deficiencies of these clotting factors prolong prothrombin time (normal range, 11 to 13 seconds). However, most laboratories report prothrombin time results that have been adjusted to the international normalized ratio, using the international sensitivity index for the particular thromboplastin and instrument combinations used to perform the test. The normal value is designated as 1.0. Coumadin therapy affects the function of factors II, VII, IX, and X. Factor VII has the shortest half-life and therefore is the most important factor in determining the functioning of the extrinsic pathway.

For this patient, the following laboratory test results were observed:

- Complete blood count: white blood cells 4000/μl, hemoglobin 12.4 g/dl, platelets 365/μl hematocrit.
- Coagulation studies: prothrombin time 48 seconds, partial thromboplastin time 33 seconds, international normalized ratio 3.2.
- Bleeding time is a test of platelet function and is not indicated in this patient.

IMAGING

Panoramic radiograph reveals multiple maxillary carious teeth and several root fragments.

ASSESSMENT

Multiple carious teeth and root fragments requiring surgical extractions in a patient on anticoagulation therapy with Coumadin for prevention of thromboembolic disease

TREATMENT

Given the potential for paroxysmal atrial fibrillation and therefore the risk of further thromboembolic events, it was decided to continue her Coumadin in this patient in the perioperative period. Her regular dose of Coumadin was, however, reduced with consultation with the primary care physician to lower the international normalized ratio to below 2.5 (to

382

reduce the likelihood of excessive perioperative bleeding) while maintaining a satisfactory level of anticoagulation. Under general anesthesia, multiple teeth were removed using small atraumatic mucoperiosteal flaps and minimal bone removal. Any soft tissue bleeding was controlled with electrocautery. The extraction sockets were then packed with hemostatic bovine collagen (Avitene), and the wounds were closed carefully with slowly resorbing Vicryl (polyglactin) horizontal mattress sutures. The wounds were carefully inspected before terminating the procedure. The patient was given a 5% transexamic acid mouthwash to be used four times a day and for 1 day postoperatively. The patient continued to take her Coumadin throughout the hospital admission. A soft diet and avoidance of strenuous activity were recommended for the first postoperative week.

COMPLICATIONS

Postoperative bleeding can complicate any surgical procedure. While this may be secondary to inadequate wound hemostasis, postoperative wound breakdown, or infection, it may also be the result of systemic coagulopathy, as in our patient. When postoperative bleeding does occur, a rapid assessment of the severity of the bleeding must be made. When the bleeding is severe, the patient must be admitted to hospital for fluid resuscitation, typed and cross-matched, and transfused if the hemoglobin and hematocrit are sufficiently low or the patient is symptomatic. After initial stabilization, attention must be directed at stopping the bleeding. Local measures can aid in hemostasis. However, in coagulopathic patients (as in this case), local measures may not suffice and a systemic approach to the control of hemorrhage may be necessary. Platelets, fresh frozen plasma, and cryoprecipitate can all be given depending on the etiology. Bleeding secondary to therapeutic Coumadin can be treated with vitamin K, although it usually takes 12 to 24 hours for any significant reversal of the anticoagulation to occur. Bleeding secondary to unfractionated heparin can be treated with protamine sulfate with immediate reversal of the anticoagulation. Bleeding secondary to thrombasthenia (dysfunctional platelets but normal numbers) may be hereditary (Glanzmann thrombasthenia or Bernard-Soulier syndrome) or, more commonly, due to aspirin or Clopidogrel (platelet adenosine diphosphate receptor inhibitor). The only immediate therapy available is platelet transfusion. Bleeding may also be secondary to vWD. This is one of the more common hereditary hematological disorders (in addition to hemophilia A). Deficiency of vWF may be treated with DDAVP if mild or fresh frozen plasma, cryoprecipitate, or factor VIII concentrate if severe (see section on von Willebrand Disease). Hemophilia A and B are hematological disorders characterized by deficiencies of factors VIII and IX, respectively, and they can be readily treated with recombinant factor replacement. The need to replace these factors is largely dependent on the baseline factor level and the planned surgical procedure.

Necrosis of the skin is a rare complication of oral anticoagulation with Coumadin. The lesions can present as ecchymosis followed by a large bullae containing deep red fluid. This does not appear to be dose related. The etiology of Coumadin-related skin necrosis is unclear, although it presents histologically as vasculitis and thrombosis. This may be a result of a transient prothrombotic state that occurs with the initiation of Coumadin therapy. This is thought to be the result of reduced levels of functional proteins C and S. Proteins C and S have shorter half-lives than do factors II, VII, IX, and X and therefore are theoretically the first proteins of the coagulation cascade to be affected by the initiation of Coumadin therapy. The diagnosis of skin necrosis mandates cessation of Coumadin therapy and replacement with unfractionated or low-molecular-weight heparin.

Coumadin is also a drug with a narrow therapeutic window that has many important interactions with other medications. Many other drugs inadvertently increase the level of anticoagulation by displacing Coumadin from albumin (it is 99% bound to albumin). Furthermore, Coumadin is metabolized by the liver, and other drugs may either induce or suppress hepatic enzymes with resultant alterations in the level of anticoagulation. All medications that are to be administered to a patient on Coumadin should be reviewed for possible drug interactions.

DISCUSSION

The coumarin anticoagulants (warfarin and dicumarol) are potent anticoagulants that inhibit the cofactor function of vitamin K. Factors II, VII, IX, and X and proteins C and S are all dependent on vitamin K for their synthesis by the liver. Coumadin treatment results in the inhibition of the enzyme vitamin K epoxide reductase, which is required to maintain vitamin K in the reduced state needed for functional coagulation protein synthesis. Proteins C and S are required for fibrinolysis, and the production of nonfunctional proteins usually results in a minimal and clinically insignificant prothrombotic state. Factors II, VII, IX, and X are required for thrombosis and clot formation, and the production of nonfunctional proteins results in a state of anticoagulation that is clinically significant.

When surgery is planned, the simplest way to manage patients on Coumadin is to continue it before the surgical procedure. Simple extractions and minor oral surgery can usually be completed while on Coumadin without complication using local measures provided that the international normalized ratio is less than about 2.5. Local measures include minimizing surgical trauma, primary closure, and use of hemostatic material such as bone wax, oxidized cellulose, or bovine collagen. Antifibrinolytics such as ε-aminocaproic acid and transexamic acid stabilize the formed blood clot by helping to reduce the natural process of fibrinolysis. Transexamic acid mouthwash has the advantage of being applied as a 5% topical mouthwash and is without systemic effect. More involved surgery will require the same local measures but, in addition, the patient will have to be switched to another anticoagulant or anticoagulation will have to be discontinued.

Table 14-5.   Patients at Risk for Thromboembolism

Thromboembolic Events Risk	Condition	Action
Low	Atrial fibrillation Deep venous thrombosis (DVT) without high-risk features	Stop Coumadin several days before procedure and resume Coumadin on the day of surgery.
Intermediate	Atrial fibrillation and age >65 years with diabetes mellitus Coronary artery disease or hypertension Prosthetic heart valves DVT >3 months without high-risk features	Stop Coumadin several days before surgery, use low-molecular-weight heparin (LMWH) perioperatively subcutaneously (hold LMWH on day of surgery) and resume Coumadin on the day of surgery.
High	Atrial fibrillation with heart failure Multiple prosthetic heart valves DVT >3 months with high-risk features such as malignancy Known thrombophilic state	Stop Coumadin several days before surgery, use unfractionated heparin perioperatively intravenously (hold unfractionated heparin 6 hours before procedure) and resume Coumadin on the day of surgery.

Initially, patients are stratified according to the risk of thromboembolism (Table 14-5).

Bibliography

Dunn A, Turpie A: Perioperative management of patients receiving oral anticoagulants: a systematic review, *Arch Intern Med* 163(8):901-908, 2003.

Handin R: Disorders of the platelet and vessel wall. In Isselbacher K, et al, editors: *Harrison's principles of internal medicine,* ed 13, New York, 1994, McGraw-Hill, pp 1800-1803.

Syed J: Peri-procedural thromboprophylaxis in patients receiving chronic anticoagulation therapy, *Am Heart J* 147:3-15, 2004.

Tiede D, et al: Modern management of prosthetic valve anticoagulation, *Mayo Clin Proc* 73:665-680, 1998.

Alcohol Withdrawal Syndrome and Delirium Tremens

Fariba Farhidvash, MD, and Chris Jo, DMD

CC

A 35-year-old Caucasian man presents to the emergency department stating that, "I was hit in the face and I think that my jaw is broken" (alcoholism is 2.5 times more prevalent in males).

HPI

The patient was involved in a bar fight several hours earlier and was hit in the face with a fist by another man, resulting in a displaced left mandibular angle fracture (confirmed with a panoramic radiograph). On arrival to the emergency department, he appeared intoxicated with a strong scent of alcohol from his breath; however, he was alert and oriented times three (person, place, and time) and denied any loss of consciousness. He was admitted to the oral and maxillofacial surgery service in preparation for open reduction with internal fixation of his mandibular fracture. The admitting resident did not include delirium tremens precautions in his admission orders, because the patient denied any history of excessive alcohol use or abuse or previous withdrawal symptoms (patients frequently describe the tremulousness, agitation, and/or anxiety of alcohol withdrawal as the "shakes"). The patient had an uneventful first night, but his operation was postponed due to operating room availability. On the second hospital day, early symptoms of alcohol withdrawal (agitation, anxiety, tremulousness, nausea and vomiting) were noted. Later that evening, the patient wandered the halls of the ward, mumbling to himself and unable to sleep (insomnia). He became progressively more agitated, exhibiting aggressive behavior toward the nursing staff. You are called to evaluate the patient in the middle of the night and find him trembling in his bed, hollering incoherent sentences at the television and yelling that there are spiders in the room (visual hallucinations). He is uncooperative to examination and does not respond to questioning. Detailed questioning of the available family members reveals that the patient had been a heavy drinker for several years and had been on a binge for the past several days.

PMHX/PDHX/MEDICATIONS/ALLERGIES/SH/FH

The patient drinks at least a six-pack of beer and a half-pint of gin a day (alcohol dependence/addiction). His last drink was two nights ago, just before being assaulted.

The Diagnostic and Statistical Manual of Mental Disorders, Fourth Edition (DSM-IV) has a set of diagnostic criteria for alcohol abuse and dependence that is beyond the scope of this section. In summary, alcohol abuse manifests as the recurrent use of alcohol despite negative consequences that cause disruptions at home or work, affecting one's health, or involving the law. Alcohol dependence is based on the compulsion to drink despite adverse consequences and is not related to the amount or frequency of drinking.

The CAGE questionnaire is a simple verbal test composed of four questions that can be quickly administered to identify patients at risk for alcoholism (Box 14-1). Patients with two affirmative answers are seven times more likely to be alcohol dependent. The sensitivity of the CAGE questionnaire is 75% to 90% in most studies. Other questionnaires that are used are the AUDIT and TWEAK questionnaires.

EXAMINATION

General. The patient is extremely agitated, sweating, and shaking restlessly in bed (signs of sympathetic overdrive).

Vital signs. His blood pressure is 180/90 mm Hg (hypertensive), heart rate 130 bpm (tachycardia), respirations 22 per minute (tachypnea), and temperature 37.8°C (rules out fever as the cause of altered mental status).

Neurological. The patient is awake but extremely agitated and is not oriented to place, time or situation. His speech is slurred, his pupils are dilated (mydriasis secondary to sympathetic overdrive) but equal and reactive to light (dilated pupils that are not reactive may indicated intracranial injury and elevated intracranial pressures), extraocular eye movements are intact, and his face is symmetrical (facial asymmetry during animation may indicate an upper or lower motor neuron lesion of cranial nerve VII). He is uncooperative with the motor and sensory examination but is moving all extremities well and is very tremulous (the grossly normal strength examination in the face and extremities makes a focal cerebral lesion unlikely).

Reflexes: Findings reveal +2/4 in all extremities, and the toes are downgoing bilaterally (upgoing toes is an abnormal finding in the adult patient and is termed a Babinski sign). A nonfocal motor examination with downgoing toes is supportive of the absence of a focal upper motor neuron lesion.

Maxillofacial. The examination is consistent with a left mandibular angle fracture.

Cardiovascular. The patient is tachycardic with no murmurs, gallops, or rubs (chronic alcoholics may have significant cardiac comorbidities).

Abdominal. He has a soft, nontender, slightly enlarged liver (hepatomegaly due to chronic alcohol consumption) and

Box 14-1.	The CAGE Questionnaire

The **CAGE** questions are:

C Have you ever felt the need to *cut down* on drinking?
A Have you ever been *annoyed* with criticism about your drinking?
G Have you ever felt *guilty* about something you did while drinking?
E Have you ever had a morning *eye-opener* to get you going or to treat withdrawal symptoms?

From Ewing JA: Detecting alcoholism: the CAGE questionaire, *JAMA* 252:1905-1907, 1984.

no ascites (intraperitoneal serous fluid or ascites would be seen in advanced hepatic dysfunction).

IMAGING

Imaging studies for evaluating the trauma patient with altered mental status should include a noncontrast head CT scan. Altered mental status can be due to acute drug or alcohol intoxication, electrolyte disturbances, hypoxia, sepsis, or metabolic derangements commonly seen with alcohol withdrawal syndrome. Altered mental status can also be an early or late manifestation of closed head injury. Any acute changes in mental status warrants a head CT to rule out an undetected or blossoming intracranial injury.

For this patient, an initial head CT was not ordered upon admission due to the absence of focal neurological signs or loss of consciousness. Although this patient is most likely experiencing alcohol withdrawal syndrome and delirium tremens, a head CT was ordered after the onset of his altered mental status to evaluate for closed head injury. The head CT was normal.

Plain radiographic studies of the mandible confirmed the diagnosis of a left mandibular angle fracture.

LABS

During the initial evaluation of an intoxicated trauma patient with maxillofacial injuries, a blood alcohol level and urine drug screen, in conjunction with a head CT, are recommended to account for altered or decreased mental status. Liver function tests are indicated for patients with liver cirrhosis (including aspartate aminotransferase, alanine aminotransferase, albumin, bilirubin, prothrombin time, partial thromboplastin time, and international normalized ratio), to evaluate for possible coagulopathies in the surgical patient. A complete blood count (including platelets) is warranted, because anemia (particularly macrocytic) and thrombocytopenia (due to liver dysfunction) are commonly seen in alcoholics. A complete metabolic panel is mandatory to rule out electrolyte derangements as the source of altered mental status and to monitor the electrolyte abnormalities associated with chronic alcohol abuse and malnutrition (such as hypomagnesemia). A baseline electrocardiogram is recommended, especially in the older population, because cardiac disorders are commonly associated with alcohol consumption.

This patient presented with an initial blood alcohol level of 250 mg/dl (legal intoxication level is 0.08%, or 80 mg/dl, in most states) and a negative urine drug screen. Aspartate aminotransferase and alanine aminotransferase were 110 U/L and 50 U/L, respectively (aspartate aminotransferase and alanine aminotransferase are typically double or triple the normal values in patients who are chronic alcoholics). His hemoglobin was 11 g/dl, hematocrit 34%, and mean corpuscular volume 110 μm^3 (macrocytic anemia due to malnutrition and likely vitamin deficiency, such as B_{12}). The electrocardiogram showed sinus tachycardia, and the remainder of the laboratory values were within normal limits.

ASSESSMENT

A 35-year-old man with a left mandible fracture now complicated by alcohol withdrawal syndrome and delirium tremens, presenting with altered mental status and agitation (hyperexcitable state)

Alcohol withdrawal syndrome and delirium tremens describe a spectrum of symptoms observed after a relative or absolute withdrawal from alcohol in susceptible individuals (especially those who are chronic consumers of large amounts of alcohol). The physiological mechanisms of alcohol withdrawal are based on the inhibitory γ-aminobutyric acid (GABA) and excitatory (glutamate) neurotransmitters of the brain. Alcohol increases the effects of GABA on the $GABA_A$ receptor, thus increasing its inhibitory effects. Also, it inhibits the excitatory effects of glutamate at the *N*-methyl-D-aspartate (NMDA) receptor, thereby decreasing neuronal excitability. During alcohol withdrawal, a state of hyperexcitability and autonomic dysfunction becomes apparent (hypermetabolic state).

TREATMENT

Identification of patients who are at risk for developing alcohol withdrawal syndrome or delirium tremens is the most important step for prevention of these two conditions. Patients with a recent (several days) history of significant alcohol consumption (chronic or binge drinkers) are at risk for alcohol withdrawal syndrome and delirium tremens. Older patients with other medical comorbidities are at a greater risk. On hospitalization, patients will not have access to alcohol and may develop a range of signs and symptoms consistent with alcohol withdrawal syndrome and delirium tremens (some hospital facilities have alcoholic beverages available for delirium tremens prevention).

Preventive measures should be taken to reduce the risk of developing alcohol withdrawal syndrome and delirium tremens. Benzodiazepines are the first-line agents for treatment and prevention—they are used either as needed or on a fixed schedule to prevent the development of the symptoms, based on the patient's history and the severity of symptoms. Scheduled dosing is recommended for patients considered to be at moderate or high risk; this also allows for a smoother withdrawal. With scheduled dosing of medications, doses high enough to relieve symptoms are given over the first 24 to 48 hours and slowly weaned by about 20% a day over the next 3 to 5 days. Longer-acting benzodiazepines such as diazepam (Valium) starting at 5 to 10 mg PO/IV/IM every 6 to 8 hours or chlordiazepoxide (Librium) starting at 25 to 100 mg PO/IV/IM every 4 to 6 hours may be used to reduce rebound effects and significantly decrease withdrawal symptoms. Shorter-acting benzodiazepines include lorazepam (Ativan) at 1 to 4 mg PO/IV/IM every 4 to 8 hours and orazepam (Serax) starting with 15 to 30 mg PO every 6 to 8 hours may be used in patients with significant comorbidities such as liver failure with associated decreased hepatic metabolism. Nonpharmacological measures include maintaining a calm, tranquil environment and a nonconfrontational interaction to help decrease anxiety. Patients presenting with symptoms of anxiety, tremulousness, and agitation after recent cessation of alcohol use should be treated promptly (with longer-acting benzodiazepines).

Intravenous fluids, replacement of electrolytes (such as magnesium), folic acid, and intravenous thiamine (given before administration of glucose to prevent the development of Wernicke's encephalopathy) are essential to rehydrate the patient and correct any possible vitamin deficiencies. Standard "delirium tremens precautions/prophylaxis" orders include thiamine 100 mg IM/IV daily, folate 1 mg PO/IV daily, multivitamins PO/IV, magnesium sulfate 1 g IM/IV daily, and benzodiazepines as needed or scheduled as discussed earlier.

With the onset of full-blown delirium tremens, the patient should be admitted to the intensive care unit, with administration of scheduled benzodiazepines to ameliorate delirium symptoms and decrease the incidence of seizures. For the autonomic symptoms, (such as tachycardia and hypertension), antihypertensive medications may become necessary. β-Blockers may be used to treat tachycardia and hypertension, but caution should be used because they may precipitate delirium. Clonidine (central α-agonist) may also be used to treat autonomic symptoms without any adverse effects on mental status. If withdrawal symptoms are severe and refractory despite benzodiazepine use, the patient may require endotracheal intubation for airway protection and administration of a general anesthetic such as a propofol (propofol has been shown to be effective in refractory delirium tremens). Usual supportive care is included throughout delirium tremens (which may include four-point restraints).

The differential diagnosis of altered mental status can be extensive, particularly in the absence of an appropriate history and examination. Broad categories include toxic (drug overdose or toxicity), metabolic (hypoglycemia, hepatic encephalopathy, or uremia), infectious (systemic or central nervous system), inflammatory (demyelinating disease or central nervous system vasculitis), vascular (large vessel infarction or intracranial hemorrhage), traumatic etiologies (increased intracranial pressure secondary to closed head injury), hypoxemia and/or hypercarbia, electrolyte abnormalities, or acute

psychotic episodes secondary to underlying psychiatric disorders. The differential diagnosis should be categorically narrowed to the most likely etiology given the clinical setting. Head imaging to rule out traumatic brain injuries, vascular accidents (such as intracranial hemorrhage), infectious processes (such as cerebral abscesses), or other cerebral lesions should be obtained early. If an infectious etiology involving the central nervous system is suspected, a lumbar puncture (after checking prothrombin time, partial thromboplastin time, and international normalized ratio) is essential to rule out meningitis or encephalitis. Urine and/or serum toxicology screens can rule out drug or alcohol abuse. A complete metabolic panel, including liver function tests, calcium, magnesium, ammonia, and thyroid function tests, can help identify certain metabolic derangements. Urinalysis and blood cultures should be obtained in cases of suspected urinary or hematogenous infectious processes contributing to mental status changes. In the obtunded patient, subclinical seizure activity should be considered. This can be evaluated using an electroencephalogram.

For this patient, failure to identify the patient's risk factors and poor communication among staff members contributed to the lack of preventative measures for alcohol withdrawal syndrome and delirium tremens. On the onset of symptoms of delirium tremens, scheduled lorazepam 2 mg IV and chlordiazepoxide 50 mg IV every 4 hours was initiated, followed by replacement of fluids, electrolytes, and multivitamins. The patient's condition progressively improved over the course of the day, with resolution of the tachycardia and normalization of the blood pressure. Librium was continued on a scheduled basis for the next 2 days and subsequently slowly tapered at 25 mg PO every 4 hours on day 3, followed by 10 mg PO every 4 hours on day 4 to prevent benzodiazepine withdrawal. Clonidine was not used because the patient's autonomic dysfunction normalized. The patient underwent open reduction with internal fixation of his mandible fracture without complications (closed reduction is frequently not well tolerated by patients who are poorly compliant). The patient was counseled about the importance of drinking cessation and the long-term effects of heavy alcohol use and was assisted to obtain help via support groups such as Alcoholics Anonymous or from professional counselors (psychiatrists or psychologists), with the help of the hospital social worker.

COMPLICATIONS

Inherent to the diagnosis of delirium tremens is the autonomic instability (fluctuating blood pressure, heart, and respiratory rates) that is life threatening if not appropriately managed. Withdrawal seizures rarely require aggressive antiepileptic pharmacological interventions (benzodiazepines are usually sufficient). Rarely, the seizure may become prolonged, leading to status epilepticus, a neurological emergency characterized by continuous seizures (clinical or subclinical) lasting longer than 5 minutes or multiple seizures with a 30-minute period in which the patient does not return to baseline between seizures. This may lead to permanent cerebral damage or if not managed aggressively. The mortality rate of untreated alcohol withdrawal syndrome and delirium tremens is about 15%, mostly secondary to cardiovascular and respiratory collapse.

DISCUSSION

Alcohol withdrawal syndrome and delirium tremens characterize the spectrum of symptoms observed after a relative or absolute withdrawal from alcohol, especially with chronic use. Delirium primarily involves alterations of attention and is characterized by a fluctuating course, difficulty with concentration, and altered mental status. Tremens refers to the tremors seen in patients with delirium tremens. Most patients who stop alcohol use acutely do not develop withdrawal symptoms or simply experience minor symptoms that do not require medical attention. Clinically significant alcohol withdrawal symptoms occur in about 25% of patients. Untreated, 10% of these patients will progress to more severe symptoms such as seizures. Delirium tremens is the last stage of alcohol withdrawal, which occurs in 5% of patients undergoing withdrawal symptoms, with a mortality rate of 5% to 15% when untreated.

The physiological mechanism of alcohol withdrawal is based on the inhibitory and excitatory neurotransmitters of the brain. Alcohol increases the effects of the $GABA_A$ receptor by increasing its inhibitory effects. In contrast, glutamate (excitatory neurotransmitter that acts on the NMDA receptor) is inhibited, thereby decreasing neuronal excitability. The presence of alcohol has an inhibitory effect by enhancing $GABA_A$ and depressing the NMDA receptor. On withdrawal of alcohol, there is an abrupt cessation of the neuronal inhibition and a subsequent state of hyperexcitability.

There are multiple stages of withdrawal based on the chronology of symptoms occurring after the cessation of alcohol use. These stages, from least to most severe, include acute intoxication, alcohol withdrawal, withdrawal seizures, and delirium tremens. Withdrawal may be apparent as early as 6 hours after the last drink but may last up to 12 to 24 hours and symptoms include agitation, anxiety, tremulousness, insomnia, and hallucinations (visual, auditory, or tactile) with a clear sensorium (the patient is aware that he or she is hallucinating). Withdrawal seizures, which have a 2% to 5% incidence in alcohol withdrawal syndrome and delirium tremens, typically occur approximately 48 hours after cessation of alcohol use and present as generalized tonic-clonic seizures. Delirium tremens peaks at 48 to 72 hours after the last drink. The patient may present with delirium, diaphoresis, or fever, but the key feature of delirium tremens is autonomic instability.

Wernicke-Korsakoff syndrome encompasses two different syndromes associated with chronic alcohol use and severe malnutrition. Wernicke's encephalopathy is primarily a clinical diagnosis with the classic triad of encephalopathy, ophthalmoplegia, and ataxia. Confusion is usually of a subacute to chronic nature and is characterized by inattention, memory loss, and apathy. Ophthalmoplegia (weakness or paralysis of one or more of the extraocular muscles) mostly involves the lateral recti but may also involve any of the extraocular muscles. Nystagmus (rhythmic, oscillation of the eyes) is commonly present in the lateral and/or vertical gaze. Ataxia is the unsteady, clumsy motion of the extremities and, more common, the trunk. Untreated, Wernicke's encephalopathy has a mortality rate of 10% to 20%. It is treated by the administration of thiamine 50 to 100 mg IV once a day (should be given before glucose, because glucose will further deplete thiamine and accelerate the development of Wernicke's encephalopathy). Korsakoff syndrome primarily involves memory impairment without significant deficits of other cognitive functions such as attention or social behavior. This is also characterized by both anterograde and retrograde amnesia along with confabulation, in which the patient's recall is distorted in relation to reality (a prominent feature). This is also treated by thiamine, but the prognosis is less favorable.

Bibliography

Bayard M, Mcintyre J, Hill K, et al: Alcohol withdrawal syndrome, *Am Fam Phys* 69:1443-1450, 2004.

Bradley W, Daroff R, Fenichel G, et al: *Neurol Clin Pract* 2:1503-1505, 2000.

Critical care aspects of alcohol abuse, *South Med J* 98:372-381, 2005.

Maimon WN, Davis LF: Management of acute alcohol withdrawal, *J Oral Maxillofac Surg* 40:361-366, 1982.

Morris PR, Mosby EL, Ferguson BL: Alcohol withdrawal syndrome: current management strategies for the surgery patient, *J Oral Maxillofac Surg* 55:1452-1455, 1997.

Acute Asthmatic Attack

Joyce T. Lee, DDS, MD, and Shahrokh C. Bagheri, DMD, MD

CC

A 17-year-old boy with a history of asthma is referred to your office for evaluation of symptomatic partially impacted third molars.

Asthma is seen in about 3% to 5% of the population and can occur in any age group; however, it is particularly common in children and young adults and is the most common chronic disease in this age group.

HPI

The patient is a high school student with a history of pain and recurrent episodes of pericoronitis to his mandibular third molars. He is referred by his general dentist for evaluation and treatment.

PMHX/PDHX/MEDICATIONS/ALLERGIES/SH/FH

The patient has a history of asthma diagnosed at age 8. He relates that his asthmatic episodes are usually exacerbated by exercise and seasonal allergies (other common triggers to asthma exacerbation include cold weather, tobacco smoke, recent upper respiratory infection, and certain medications including nonsteroidal antiinflammatory drugs). He has had two previous visits to the local emergency department secondary to acute episodes that did not readily respond to his albuterol (β_2-agonist) inhaler and required intravenous methylprednisolone (systemic corticosteroid), nebulized albuterol, and ipratropium (anticholinergic bronchodilator). The episodes resolved without the need for endotracheal intubation (a history of emergency department visits and endotracheal intubation both correlate with the severity of asthma. The most powerful predictive feature in the history that reveals the potential of a severe life-threatening exacerbation is any history of prior intubation and mechanical ventilation). The patient does not have a history of status asthmaticus (asthmatic episode that is refractory to treatment). His last asthma attack was approximately 1 month earlier (the frequency of attacks is an indicator of the control of this patient's asthma). His current medications include an albuterol metered-dose inhaler used as needed and 10 mg montelukast sodium daily (leukotriene receptor antagonist). He routinely monitors his status by using a peak flowmeter (patients use this device to monitor changes in his or her forced expiratory volume in 1 second [FEV_1]; see later). The patient states that he smokes occasionally (cigarette smoke is an airway irritant that may precipitate bronchospasm). He also has a history of allergic rhinitis (hay fever) and eczema. There is a positive history of asthma in several of his family members (in patients with an allergic component to their asthma, there frequently is a strong family history of asthma or other allergies. Genetic factors may play a role in the pathogenesis of asthma. However, it is important to mention that not all asthmatic patients have allergies and that the association between asthma and allergies is not entirely clear).

EXAMINATION

General. The patient is a well-developed and well-nourished boy in no apparent distress.

Vital signs. Vital signs are stable with normotensive blood pressure (pulsus paradoxus is a clinical sign of severe asthma exacerbation defined by an inspiratory fall in systolic blood pressure of greater than 15 mm Hg).

Maxillofacial. The patient has partially erupted impacted third molars. The tongue is normal in size. He has a Class I skeletal and dental relationship. The maximal interincisal opening is 45 mm. The uvula, soft, and hard palates are easily visualized, and bilateral tonsils are within normal limits in size and recessed within the tonsillar crypts (Mallampati Class I). The thyromental distance is greater than four finger-widths (evaluation of the airway is important especially in patients who may require advanced airway interventions).

Cardiovascular. The patient has regular rate and rhythm with no murmurs, gallops (S_3 or S_4), or rubs (patients with asthma can have other comorbidities such as chronic obstructive pulmonary disease, which may produce "splitting" of the second heart sound with an accentuated pulmonic component).

Chest. The chest is bilaterally clear to auscultation (the major symptoms during an acute asthmatic attack are cough, dyspnea, expiratory wheezing, and chest tightness. Wheezing is not pathopneumonic with asthma and merely reflects airflow obstruction through a narrow airway).

LABS

No studies are indicated in the routine care of a well-controlled patient with asthma. However, poorly controlled patients are often referred for pulmonary function testing. The most objective and relevant test to measure the degree of airway obstruction in asthmatic patients is the FEV_1 and the peak expiratory flow. In well-controlled patients, the FEV_1 should represent 80% of the forced vital capacity (in comparing obstructive versus restrictive pulmonary diseases, the

389

vital capacity and FEV_1 are decreased in both; however, there is an increase in both the functional residual capacity and residual volume in obstructive diseases, whereas both functional residual capacity and residual volume are decreased in restrictive lung diseases).

IMAGING

The panoramic radiograph is significant for partial bony impacted third molars.

Chest radiographs are not indicated in asymptomatic patients with a history of asthma and are not particularly helpful other than ruling out other diseases. During acute asthmatic exacerbations, the chest radiograph may reveal hyperinflation of the lung fields (flattened diaphragm) and decreased vascular markings.

ASSESSMENT

An American Society of Anesthesiologists (ASA) Class II patient with four impacted third molars who is planned for extractions under intravenous sedation anesthesia (ASA II is defined as a patient with a mild systemic disease that is well controlled and poses no limitations in daily activities)

TREATMENT

After reviewing the risks, benefits, and alternatives, the patient elected to have his third molars removed under intravenous general anesthesia the next day. The patient was instructed to record his peak flow the morning of the surgery and to bring his albuterol metered-dose inhaler with spacer to the office (spacers are devices used to increase the effectiveness of medication delivery).

The patient's lungs were clear to auscultation bilaterally (due to the episodic nature of this disease, pulmonary auscultation should be conducted routinely before surgery). After the patient was prepared for surgery, he self-administered three puffs of albuterol (90 μg per puff) using his spacer. Intravenous general anesthesia was achieved with midazolam 5 mg, fentanyl 50 μg, and propofol titrated to effect (propofol is the preferred general aesthetic agent in the asthmatic patient because there is a higher incidence of wheezing during anesthesia induction with intravenous methohexitol [Brevital] compared with propofol). On removal of the last third molar, the patient became diaphoretic, agitated, tachycardic at 140 bpm, and tachypneic with shallow breaths at 25 bpm (tracheal tugging, use of accessory muscles of respiration, and intercostal retractions are other signs of severe asthmatic exacerbation). The surgical sites were packed, the oropharynx was suctioned out, and the tongue was retracted as the airway was repositioned and supported. The patient's condition continued to deteriorate with a progressive decline in oxygen saturation as measured by the pulse oximeter. Inspiratory suprasternal retractions revealed the obstructive nature of the patient's condition. The diagnosis of an acute asthmatic attack

was made. Two puffs of albuterol were given, as well as two puffs of ipratropium bromide, while the vital signs were monitored closely. Supplemental 100% oxygen was delivered via a full face mask. Minutes later, the patient begins to show worsening signs of dyspnea, chest tightness, and cyanosis with further drop of the pulse oximeter reading to below 85%. The emergency medical services system was activated, and 0.5 mg of a 1:1000 solution of epinephrine was injected subcutaneously. An attempt to mask ventilate with 100% O_2 revealed airway resistance and chest tightness. Positive pressure ventilation with bag-mask technique was unsuccessful despite airway repositioning. A 10-mg dose of intravenous succinylcholine was given, and the patient's anesthesia was deepened with 50 mg ketamine IV (ketamine is a dissociative agent with potent bronchodilatory effects. Causes of bronchospasm often attribute to light anesthesia and hence ketamine is a valuable drug to consider). The patient's airway soon became easier to ventilate with the bag-mask technique with 100% oxygen at flow rate of 12 L/min (consideration should be given to administration of diphenhydramine 50 mg IV in cases of suspected allergic response; 20 mg of dexamethasone IV can also be used to reduce the inflammatory response). He responded with a gradual rising of the pulse oximeter reading, diminished chest wall rigidity, and an improvement in air exchange and compliance. His vital signs normalized with the exception of a persistent tachycardia (one of residual side effects of repeated doses of sympathomimetics is tachycardia). On arrival of the emergency medical services personnel, the patient was transported to the hospital for further observation of his acute asthmatic event.

COMPLICATIONS

Complications arising in patients with asthma range from mild wheezing and dyspnea to severe bronchospasm, hypoxia, and death. Bronchospasm is a life-threatening emergency that must be treated as soon as it is recognized. In the office setting, it is important to alert emergency medical services as soon as possible because conditions may deteriorate rapidly. The incidence of bronchospasm is low in well-controlled patients undergoing outpatient intravenous general anesthesia.

Bronchospasm is the acute manifestation of asthma. This results in increased airway resistance causing a decreased ratio of FEV_1 to forced vital capacity (Figure 14-3). Signs and symptoms of bronchospasm include dyspnea, stridor, wheezing, mucus secretion, and hypoxia. Initial treatment should include 100% oxygen and an inhaled β_2-agonist. β_2-Agonists relax the smooth muscle in bronchial walls and produce bronchodilation.

The astute clinician should also look for causes of the asthma exacerbation such as undiagnosed latex allergies or medication allergies. Urticaria, pruritus, and facial edema are findings consistent with allergic reactions that may produce bronchospasm. If this is suspected, diphenhydramine and corticosteroids should be administered intravenously. Administration of epinephrine may be indicated in patients experiencing bronchospasm refractory to inhaled β_2-agonists. One milligram injected subcutaneously is the most common dose and route of administration.

Theophylline and aminophylline (a phosphodiesterase inhibitor) produce bronchodilation and has been previously considered in the management of bronchospasm. (Aminophylline was once used with caution because it has a narrow therapeutic index and may produce arrhythmias.) In recent years, multiple clinical trials have shown that aminophylline and theophylline not only result in no further bronchodilation but also increase toxicity; hence, this category of drugs has since fallen out of the treatment protocol. If bronchospasm persists and the patient is hypoxic, intubation is indicated. It is important to realize that intubation does not protect against or treat the bronchospasm. However, it will facilitate ventilation of the narrowed airways and allow effective delivery of nebulized medications. If mechanical ventilation is used after intubation, it is important to be mindful that asthma is an obstructive airway disease and that overzealous high pressure or flow on inspiration can cause barotrauma, resulting in either a pneumothorax or tension pneumothorax.

DISCUSSION

Asthma is a common chronic respiratory condition that can present with acute exacerbations. It afflicts children as well as adults and is highly variable in severity, response to treatment, and clinical presentation. It is a form of obstructive airway disease characterized by acute and reversible increase in airway resistance. Recent evidence suggests that asthma does produce changes in the respiratory epithelium. The prevalence of asthma is 5% in the adult and 10% in the pediatric populations. There is evidence that this is increasing in the United States, especially in urban pediatric populations. The various types of asthma are categorized according to the underlying etiology of the exacerbation. These may include atopic or IgE mediated, exercise induced, occupational, infectious, or aspirin induced. Although the mediators that produce an acute asthmatic attack vary, the resulting physiological responses are similar for all types of asthma. Because airway resistance is inversely related to the diameter of the bronchial lumen, pediatric patients are predisposed to rapid decompensation during bronchospasm (Figure 14-4).

Perioperative management of patients with asthma is primarily based on risk stratification. Successful management of asthma requires active patient and physician partnership. Patients must understand the pathophysiology of their disease and need for medication compliance and have the ability to monitor the current status of their disease state. Many emergency visits in asthmatics are attributed to patients not understanding their disease. Elective surgery is contraindicated in asthmatic patients who are not well controlled. Patients should be asked about their medication regimens, understanding of

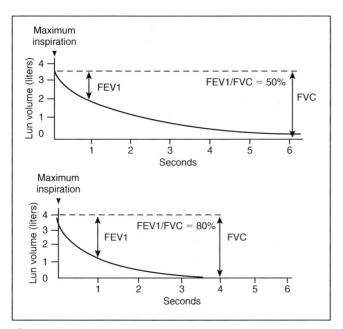

Figure 14-3 Forced vital capacity in a patient with an airway obstruction (**A**) and in a normal individual (**B**).

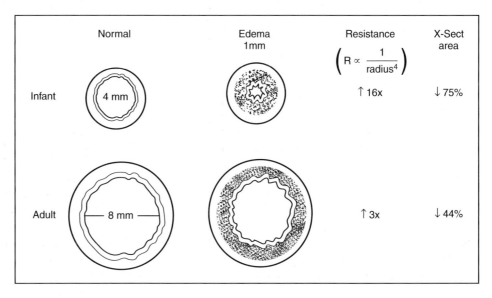

Figure 14-4 Airway resistance in the infant and an adult patient.

medication delivery, and use of peak flowmeters. Patients who are not optimized should be referred to their primary care physician for evaluation before elective surgery.

Intraoperative management of asthmatic patients should place emphasis on adequate oxygenation, avoiding excessive airway stimulation through the use of throat packs and suctioning. A pretracheal stethoscope can be recommended for auscultation monitoring. In patients who are intubated, decreased tidal volumes and increased end-tidal carbon dioxide may indicate bronchospasm. During extubation, minimal stimulation of the airway is advised. "Deep" extubation may be prudent to avoid excessive excitement from the emerging patient because it may generate enormous negative pressure, resulting in acute pulmonary edema. Administration of a dose of intravenous lidocaine before extubation will also decrease airway stimulation. Despite these precautions, some patients with asthma will experience bronchospasm during their surgical course. Management of an acute asthmatic exacerbation should consist of early detection and intervention. Bronchospasm is a potentially life-threatening emergency that must be treated. Treatment should consist of assessment of vital signs, supplemental oxygen, inhaled β_2-agonists, injectable sympathomimetics, corticosteroids, and ventilatory support if indicated.

Bibliography

Bone RC: Goals of asthma management. A step-care approach, *Chest* 109:1056, 1996.

Currie GP: Recent developments in asthma management, *Br Med J* 330:585, 2005.

DiGiulio GA, Kercsmar CM, Krug SE, et al: Hospital treatment of asthma: lack of benefit from theophylline given in addition to nebulized albuterol and intravenously administered corticosteroid, *J Pediatr* 122:464, 1993.

Ezekiel MR: *Handbook of anesthesiology,* Laguna Hills, CA, 2004, CCS Publishing.

Fanta CH, Rossing TH, McFadden ER Jr: Glucocorticoids in acute asthma. A critical controlled trial, *Am J Med* 74:845, 1983.

Hurford WE: *Clinical anesthesia procedures of the Massachusetts General Hospital,* ed 5, Philadelphia, 1998, Lippincott-Raven.

Newman KB, Milne S, Hamilton C, et al: A comparison of albuterol administered by meter-dose inhaler and spacer with albuterol by nebulizer in adults presenting to an urban emergency department with acute asthma, *Chest* 121:1036, 2002.

Owen CL: New directions in asthma management, *Am J Nurs* 3:99, 1999.

Pizov R, Brown RH, Weiss YS, et al: Wheezing during induction of general anesthesia in patients with and without asthma, *Anesthesiology* 82(5)1111, 1995.

Rea HH, Scragg R, Jackson R, et al: A case-controlled study of deaths from asthma, *Thorax* 41:833, 1986.

Rodrigo GJ, Rodrigo C: The role anticholinergics in acute asthma treatment: an evidence based evaluation, *Chest* 121:1977, 2002.

Rodrigo GJ, Rodrigo C, Hall JB: Acute asthma in adults: a review, *Chest* 125:1081, 2004.

Rossing TH, Fanta CH, Goldstein DH, et al: Emergency therapy of asthma: comparison of the acute effects of parenterol and inhaled sympathomimetics and infused theophylline, *Am Rev Respir Dis* 122:365, 1980.

Diabetes Mellitus

Mehran Mehrabi, Maj. USAF, DC, and Shahrokh C. Bagheri, DMD, MD

CC

A 18-year-old man with history of type 1 diabetes mellitus presents to the oral and maxillofacial surgery clinic complaining that, "my wisdom teeth are hurting."

HPI

For the past week, the patient has had mild, progressively exacerbating lower jaw pain that is worse with function. He denies any history of fever, swelling, or facial erythema. There is no history of trauma. He explains that his blood sugar has been well controlled (poorly controlled blood glucose would predispose to the development of an infection).

PMHX/PDHX/MEDICATIONS/ALLERGIES/SH/FH

The patient was diagnosed with type 1 diabetes mellitus at age 10 and has been taking insulin for the past 8 years. He is currently being followed by his family practitioner. His medications include glargine (Lantus [long-acting synthetic insulin that provides a steady concentration of insulin]) once a day and preprandial lispro (Humalog [short-acting insulin]) three times a day. He has no prior surgeries but had been hospitalized for hypoglycemia twice during the previous year (previous episodes of hypoglycemia are a risk factor for future episodes). He reports his blood glucose has been between 80 and 160 mg/dl during the prior week as measured with his home Accu-Chek device (ideal preprandial blood glucose is between 80 and 120 mg/dl).

There is no family history of diabetes mellitus (type 1 diabetes mellitus has a strong association with *HLA-DR3, DR4,* and *DQ* alleles; however, a family history is often lacking. A positive family history is often seen with type 2 diabetes mellitus).

EXAMINATION

General. The patient is a thin, calm, and cooperative man (unlike patients with type 2 diabetes, those with type 1 are frequently thin and/or cachetic).

Vital signs. His vital signs are stable and he is afebrile.

Maxillofacial. There is no facial edema, erythema, or induration. The patient is able to open his mouth without restriction (no signs of acute infection).

Intraoral. Examination is consistent with bilateral pericoronitis of the left and right mandibular third molars (teeth Nos. 17 and 32, respectively). The right and left maxillary third molars (teeth Nos. 1 and 16, respectively) are in traumatic occlusion with the associated operculum of the mandibular third molars. The remainder of the dentition is free of caries or periodontal disease.

IMAGING

For the surgical management of patients with diabetes mellitus, the need for adjunctive imaging studies is dictated by the clinical findings, and suspicion of sources of infection or pathology. Nonodontogenic sources of infection should be considered in all patients.

The panoramic radiograph of this patient showed partial bony impacted left and right mandibular third molars. The right and left maxillary third molars were supraerupted, with no other radiographic signs of pathology.

LABS

For the routine work-up of a patient with well-controlled diabetes mellitus, no routine preoperative laboratory testing is necessary for minor oral surgical procedures, except for a preoperative blood glucose, especially in the poorly controlled patient. Hypoglycemia should be treated with oral or intravenous glucose (dextrose) as needed, and hyperglycemia may need to be treated with an insulin preparation. Elective surgical procedures should be delayed in the face of excessively abnormal blood glucose readings. Patients with infectious processes that require surgical intervention should be treated promptly, because infections are frequently the precipitating cause of the glycemic abnormality.

An effective objective tool to assess patient compliance and long-term hyperglycemic status is measurement of the glycosylated hemoglobin (Hb_{A1c}) level. Prolonged elevation of serum blood glucose causes glycosylation of hemoglobin within red blood cells. Because the life expectancy of red blood cells is 120 days, Hb_{A1c} gives an estimate of glycemic control during the past 90 to 120 days. An Hb_{A1c} greater than 5% is consistent with diabetes, and a value of greater than 7% is indicative of poor glycemic control. Therefore, Hb_{A1c} directly correlate with poor glycemic control for the previous 3 to 4 months. For patients undergoing major surgery, a complete metabolic panel and blood count should also be obtained.

For this patient, the serum Hb_{A1c} level was at 6.5%, and the serum blood glucose was 125 mg/dl.

ASSESSMENT

Pericoronitis of partially impacted left and right mandibular third molars, exacerbated by traumatic occlusion of right and left maxillary third molars, in a patient with well-controlled type 1 diabetes mellitus

TREATMENT

Pharmacological management of diabetes mellitus consists of oral hypoglycemic agents (type II), insulin and insulin analogs (types I, II, and IV), and insulin pumps (type I). Oral hypoglycemic agents decrease plasma glucose by various mechanisms. Sulfonylureas (glypizide, glyburide) and glitinides (repaglinide, nateglinide) stimulate the production of insulin by the pancreas. Glucophage (metformin) decreases hepatic glucose production by inhibiting gluconeogenesis and glycogenolysis. Alpha-glycosidase inhibitors (acorbose), which are rarely used due to the high incidence of flatulence and abdominal discomfort, prevent carbohydrate absorption from the intestinal tract. Table 14-6 provides a summary of some currently available insulin preparations.

Current insulin formulations in the United States are biosynthetic, generated from human DNA since 1983. The "old-fashioned" insulin produced by mashing pork or beef pancreas was introduced in 1920s. In July 2005, the manufacturing company announced discontinuation of animal-based insulin production. However, animal-based insulin continues to be available in other countries.

The perioperative management of patients with diabetes is variable, depending on the type of diabetes, underlying pathologies, and severity and extent of the anticipated procedure. An understanding of the acute and chronic complications of diabetes, along with a preemptive strategy, provides a successful outcome. The operation should be scheduled early in the morning. Generally, oral hypoglycemic agents are stopped the day before surgery. Short-acting insulin medications should be avoided on the morning of surgery to prevent dangerous hypoglycemia. For short ambulatory procedures, long-acting insulin preparations such as glargine may be continued. For major procedures requiring hospital admission, cessation of the long-acting insulin 1 to 2 days before surgery and administration of a short-acting insulin may be advocated.

When discussing diabetes, the term "treatment" was not advocated because the underlying disease was not altered with any of these medications. In 2000, new clinical trials on islet cell transplantation have had promising results. Multiple cadaveric islets were prepared and transplanted in recipient patient's liver. In the same year, a study by Shapiro and associates consisting of seven patients resulted in 100% success rate with total independence from exogenous insulin.

This patient was scheduled for extraction of the left and right mandibular and maxillary third molars using intravenous sedation. The patient was instructed to take nothing by mouth after midnight and was scheduled for an early morning appointment. He was instructed to continue taking glargine but to withhold lispro insulin in the morning.

On the morning of surgery, the patient appeared to be jittery and nervous. His skin was slightly clammy, and his palms were sweaty (sympathetic response to hypoglycemia). He was found to be tachycardic with heart rate of 120 bpm and a blood pressure of 120/80 mm Hg. On placement of the intravenous catheter, the patient became less responsive (neurological effect of hypoglycemia). Based on the patient's history and clinical observations, the diagnosis of hypoglycemia was made and 1 ampule of 50% (25 g) dextrose was administered. A simultaneous Accu-Chek reading confirmed a blood glucose level of 55 mg/dl (hypoglycemia). Within minutes, the patient became more responsive and the heart rate decreased to 80 bpm. Retrospectively, it was found that the patient had misunderstood the preoperative instructions and, while he had refrained from breakfast in the morning, he had continued his routine insulin injections just before arriving to the office. The surgery was completed without any perioperative complications.

COMPLICATIONS

The complications of diabetes mellitus can be divided into acute and chronic categories. Acute complications primarily include diabetic ketoacidosis (discussed later in this chapter), nonketotic hyperosmolar syndrome, and hypoglycemia. Chronic complications are predominantly related to the long-term effects of hyperglycemia on the vasculature and can be divided into microvascular (retinopathy, nephropathy, neuropathy) and macrovascular disease (accelerated atherosclerosis, coronary artery disease, myocardial infarction).

Table 14-6. Some Commonly Available Insulin Preparations			
Preparation	**Onset**	**Peak Effect (hr)**	**Duration of Action (hr)**
Lispro (Humalog)	5 min-0.25 hr	0.5-1	2-4
Novolog	5 min-0.25 hr	0.5-1	2-4
Regular insulin (Humulin R, Novolin R)	0.5 hr	2-5	8-12
NPH (Humulin N, Novolin N)	1-2.5 hrs	8-14	16-24
Lente	1-2.5 hrs	8-12	16-24
Protamine zinc (Ultralente)	4-6 hrs	10-18	>32
Glargine (Lantus)	2-3 hrs	7-12	24-48

The symptoms of hypoglycemia may be confused with those of cerebrovascular events, vasovagal syndrome, or a variety of disorders considered in the differential diagnosis of a delirious patient (hypoxia, infection, metabolic abnormalities, myocardial infarction, and medication overdose and withdrawal). Hypoglycemia is defined as a blood glucose level of less than 60 mg/dl. The symptoms may be divided into those that are neurological and those that are secondary to increased adrenergic (sympathetic) outflow. Neurological symptoms consist of visual disturbances, paresthesias, lethargy, irritability, delirium, confusion, seizures, and coma. The adrenergic symptoms consist of nausea, anxiety, weakness, sweating, and tremors. In a previously undiagnosed patient, the differential diagnosis should include primary or secondary hyperinsulinemia (insulinoma). Other important considerations include sepsis, malnutrition, and liver failure. The most common reason for hypoglycemia in a diabetic patient is insulin mismanagement. Patients with renal failure are more prone to hypoglycemia because a small fraction of gluconeogenesis is conducted by the kidneys. Treatment of hypoglycemia in an awake patient consists of oral glucose administration (such as orange juice). If the patient has intravenous access, dextrose 10% or 50% in water ($D_{10}W$ or $D_{50}W$) is acceptable. In the unconscious patient with no intravenous access, 1 mg of glucagon IM/SC can be administered. Diazoxide, octeriotide, and hydrocortisone are other alternatives. Diabetic ketoacidosis and nonketotic hyperosmolar coma are discussed elsewhere in this book. It is important to treat any suspicion of hypoglycemia rapidly, because hyperglycemia in a misdiagnosed patient does not have any immediate emergent complications; however, untreated undiagnosed hypoglycemia may be devastating.

It is commonly known that patients with diabetes mellitus are more susceptible to infections. However, these patients are not necessarily more prone to infection but, rather, once infected, they do not respond as effectively compared with healthy individuals. It is thought that various steps in neutrophil function are altered, including leukocyte adherence, chemotaxis, and phagocytosis. The antioxidants, which are involved in the bactericidal activity, may also be altered. The defects in neutrophil function are at least partially reversible by strict glycemic control (blood glucose between 80 and 110 mg/dl). However, it is hypothesized that the pathophysiology of the immunological defects in diabetes mellitus is not exclusively related to glycemic control.

DISCUSSION

Diabetes mellitus is a prevalent and destructive endocrine disorder that may affect any organ in the body. More than 216 million people are affected worldwide, with approximately 16 million affected in the United States. It is the leading cause of blindness, nontraumatic leg amputation, and end-stage renal disease. It is also implicated as a risk factor in cardiac, cerebral, and vascular disease processes. The most common type, non–ketone-induced diabetes mellitus, is on the rise, correlating with the increased incidence of obesity in the United States. Mokdad and colleagues in 2001 randomly selected a cohort of 200,000 adult patients and observed the prevalence of diabetes to be 7.9%, an increase from 7.3% in 2000. The prevalence of obesity defined as a body mass index greater than 30 kg/m^2 was 20.9%, an increase of 5.6% from the previous year.

Insulin is an anabolic hormone produced by the beta cells of the pancreas. Its production is stimulated by elevated blood glucose, causing the subsequent effects of glucose uptake by cells, promotion of triglyceride synthesis and storage, inhibition of ketogenesis, and activation of various enzymes (such as glycogen synthase, HMG-CoA reductase, lipid lipases), while inhibiting catabolic pathways such as gluconeogenesis and ketogenesis (Figure 14-5). The counterregulatory hormones are cortisol, epinephrine, growth hormone, and glycogen. The hyperglycemia seen in diabetes is not only due to the lack of insulin butalso due to the imbalance between insulin and its counterregulatory hormones.

Diabetes is a disorder resulting from deficiency or defects in insulin action. The pathophysiology is related to defects in the production (type 1 diabetes, juvenile-onset diabetes, ketoacidosis-prone diabetics), defects at the site of action (type 2 diabetes, adult-onset diabetes, non–ketoacidosis-prone diabetics), as a part of another disease (type 3 or secondary diabetes including a wide variety of diseases such as Cushing disease, hemochromatosis, cystic fibrosis), or gestational diabetes (type 4).

Symptoms of diabetes, although unique, are variable in onset of presentation based on the type of diabetes. Type 1 diabetes mellitus commonly presents with acute symptoms, whereas type 2 diabetes mellitus may go undiagnosed for many years. Presenting symptoms of type 3 diabetes are variable, based on the primary disease. Type 4 diabetics usually present at 24 to 28 weeks of gestation. Symptoms, regardless of diabetic subtype, consist of polyuria, weight loss, increased appetite, fatigue, blurred vision, and thirst. The initial diagnosis is often made due to symptoms arising from oral or vaginal candidiasis and diabetic ketoacidosis.

The diagnosis of diabetes mellitus is based on objective blood tests, distinguishing between three categories of patients:
1. Patients with diabetes mellitus
2. Patients with impaired fasting glucose
3. Patients with normal glucose metabolism

Patients with impaired fasting glucose are more prone than is the general population to develop diabetes. Diabetes is diagnosed when fasting blood glucose is greater than 126 mg/dl, a random blood glucose is greater than 200 mg/dl, or a 2-hour postprandial blood glucose is greater than 200 mg/dl after consumption of an oral glucose load of 75 g.

Diabetes is a costly disease that until recently had only symptomatic treatment. A patient's compliance with daily injections and diabetic diets is frequently difficult to control, especially in the unmotivated patient. Islet cell transplantation for type 1 diabetes shows promise, providing an alternative with the potential for more definitive treatment.

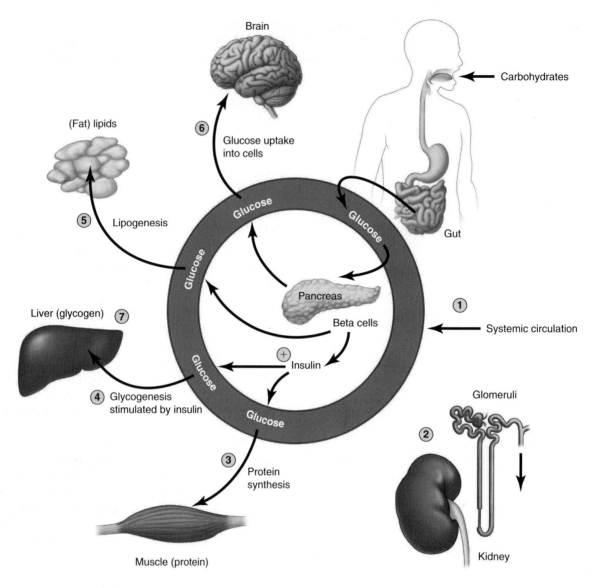

Figure 14-5   The actions of insulin.

In the absence of insulin:

1. Blood glucose increases
2. Glucose spills out into the urine (osmotic diuresis causing dehydration)
3. Decreased protein synthesis (catabolism)
4. Increased gluconeogenesis and decreased glycogenesis further increasing plasma glucose
5. Lipid breakdown (lipolysis)
6. The brain cells cannot uptake glucose, and instead use ketones
7. Increased ketones (ketogenesis) causes ketoacidosis

Bibliography

Joshi N, Caputo GM, Weitekamp MR, et al: Infections in patients with diabetes mellitus, *N Engl J Med* 341:1906-1912, 1999.

Marks JB: Perioperative management of diabetes, *Am Fam Physician* 67:93-100, 2003.

Mayfield J: Diagnosis and classification of diabetes mellitus: new criteria, *Am Fam Physician* 58:1355-1362, 1998.

Mokdad AH, Ford ES, Bowman BA, et al: Prevalence of obesity, diabetes and obesity related health risk factors, *JAMA* 298:76-79, 2003.

Rehman J, Mohammed K: Perioperative management of diabetic patients, *Curr Surg* 60:607-611, 2003.

Robertson PR: Islet transplantation as a treatment for diabetes: a work in progress, *N Engl J Med* 350:694-705, 2004.

Shapiro AMJ, Lakey JRT, Ryan EA, et al: Islet transplantation in seven patients with type 1 diabetes mellitus using a glucocorticoid-free immunosuppressive regimen, *N Engl J Med* 343:230-238, 2000.

Diabetic Ketoacidosis

Mehran Mehrabi, Maj. USAF, DC, and Shahrokh C. Bagheri, DMD, MD

CC

A 17-year-old diabetic female patient presents to the oral and maxillofacial surgery clinic 5 days after extraction of her four third molars complaining of "nausea and vomiting."

HPI

The patient reports a history of poor oral intake and frequent emesis (vomiting) for the past 3 days. She has been feeling progressively more fatigued with general malaise (secondary to dehydration). Because she has not been able to eat or drink regularly, she decided to discontinue all her insulin injections (lack of insulin is the key etiology in the development of diabetic ketoacidosis).

She also complains of blurry vision (secondary to volume depletion), vague abdominal pain (metabolic acidosis will result in gastric distention and blockage), cramping of her extremities (secondary to hypokalemia and dehydration commonly associated with diabetic ketoacidosis), an elevated temperature (secondary to development of infection and dehydration), and swelling of the left mandible that has progressively exacerbated over the past 48 hours. She reported an increase in the frequency of urination (polyuria) in the first few postoperative days but has not voided for the past day (initial osmotic diuresis causing dehydration). At first, her mother was not concerned with a developing infection because her mouth actually smelled "fruity" (acetone breath odor secondary to elevated plasma ketones). She became anxious when her daughter appeared progressively sleepy (stupor and coma can be caused by rapid increases in blood osmolarity causing water to be drawn out of the central nervous system, resulting in cellular dehydration and changes in consciousness). The on-call surgeon was contacted the night earlier and attributed the nausea and vomiting to excessive narcotic intake. The swelling was assessed via telephone to appropriately correspond to postsurgical edema. She was prescribed promethazine and advised to see the treating surgeon the next day (any suspicion of diabetic ketoacidosis should prompt evaluation in the emergency department as soon as possible. Unrecognized diabetic ketoacidosis can be deleterious).

PMHX/PDHX/MEDICATIONS/ALLERGIES/SH/FH

The patient had diabetes mellitus type 1 diagnosed at age 14. She takes regular insulin (short-acting insulin) and NPH (intermediate-acting insulin) twice a day under the care of an endocrinologist. She denies the use of alcohol, tobacco, and recreational drugs.

EXAMINATION

General. The patient is an intermittently nonresponsive girl who does not follow commands (altered mental status). She is breathing without obstruction, but it is deep and slow (Kussmaul breathing).

Vital signs. Her blood pressure is 101/50 mm Hg (hypotension), heart rate 114 bpm (tachycardia), respirations 8 per minute, and temperature 38.8°C (afebrile).

Orthostatics. On going from the supine to the standing position, the heart rate increases to 140 bpm, and blood pressure decreased to 80/40 mm Hg (a rise in heart rate to greater than 30 and/or a decrease in systolic blood pressure to greater than 20 or diastolic blood pressure greater than 10 is an indication of severe volume depletion).

Maxillofacial. The patient has significant tenderness (dolor), edema (tumor), and erythema (rubor) of the left lower face. Her face is warm (calor) to touch (cardinal signs of inflammation). Fluctuance is palpated over the angle of the mandible. She is unable to open her mouth more than 10 mm (trismus, suggestive of masticator space infection). The patient is able to maintain her secretions (drooling would be indicative of significant oropharyngeal swelling or dysphagia).

Intraoral. Examination reveals purulence around the extraction socket of the left mandibular third molar, with surrounding gingival edema and erythema. The floor of the mouth is soft and not raised. There is moderate swelling of the left lateral pharyngeal wall with slight deviation of the uvula (indicative of left lateral pharyngeal spread of infection).

Cardiovascular. The patient has sinus tachycardia with intermittent pause correlating to premature ventricular contractions (electrolyte abnormalities such as hyperkalemia will result in abnormal heart rhythms).

Pulmonary. His chest is bilaterally clear to auscultation with deep breathing.

Abdominal. The abdomen demonstrates generalized pain on palpation but is otherwise nontender and nondistended.

IMAGING

A panoramic radiograph and a CT scan of the head and neck may be indicated to evaluate the spread of infection in the parapharyngeal and masticator spaces and for evaluation of the airway. In patients with compromised renal function as determined by an elevated creatinine level, contrast CT is contraindicated. Noncontrast CT, although less valuable at demonstrating soft tissue spread of infection, can still be of value.

LABS

A full set of laboratory studies (complete blood count, electrolytes, and urinalysis) is essential in the management of diabetic ketoacidosis. The following laboratory study results were obtained for this patient:

- Hemogram: white blood cell count of 18.2 cells/µl with a differential of 70% neutrophils, 20% bands, 8% lymphocytes, 1% monocytes, and 1% eosinophils (elevated neutrophil count is indicative of acute inflammation); hemoglobin and hematocrit of 15 mg/dl and 45 %, respectively (volume depletion will result in overestimation of hemoglobin and hematocrit); platelet count within normal limits
- Basic metabolic panel: Na^+ of 150 mEq/dl (elevated secondary to dehydration), K^+ of 6.5 mEq/dl (elevated secondary to acidosis causing transcellular shift of K^+ into the extracellular space in exchange for H^+ ions), Cl^- of 95 mEq/dl (normal chloride is consistent with an anion gap metabolic acidosis), bicarbonate of 10 mEq/dl (a low bicarbonate is indicative of metabolic acidosis), blood urea nitrogen of 60 mEq/dl, creatinine of 3.0 mEq/dl (blood urea nitrogen and creatinine are both elevated secondary to decreased intravascular volume: prerenal azotemia), glucose of 550 mg/dl (primarily secondary to the lack of insulin)
- Arterial blood gas analysis: pH of 7.01, Pco_2 of 25 mm Hg, Po_2 of 90 mm Hg on Fio_2 of 40%(a pH of 7.01 is a strong acidemia. These findings, along with a low Pco_2, are indicative of metabolic acidosis with respiratory compensation)
- Urine analysis: positive ketones, +3 glucosuria (the proximal convoluted tubules ability to reabsorb glucose is maximized at a blood glucose of 180 to 200 mg/dl after which glucose is spilled into urine, causing osmotic diuresis); +2 proteinuria (glomeruli damage in diabetic nephropathy will result in protein wasting and nephrotic syndrome; microproteinurea is an indicative of diabetic nephropathy and may be avoided or delayed by daily intake of ACE inhibitors)
- Urine dipstick test: +4 for nitroprusside (indicative of acetoacetate and acetone [ketones] in the urine)

Electrocardiogram

The electrocardiogram shows widened QRS and peaked T waves (secondary to hyperkalemia) and occasional premature ventricular contractions.

ASSESSMENT

Diabetic ketoacidosis secondary to parapharyngeal and masticator space infection (infection is the leading cause of diabetic ketoacidosis)

TREATMENT

Treatment generally begins with the assessment of the ABCs—airway, breathing, and circulation. Intravenous fluid (start with normal saline and subsequently switch to $D_5^{1}/_2NS$ [5% dextrose in 0.45% normal saline]) is the first line of treatment. This will address dehydration and decrease the plasma glucose by dilution. Any indication of cardiac instability (peak T waves, wide QRS, and premature ventricular contractions) due to hyperkalemia should be treated first with calcium gluconate. This is followed by an intravenous insulin drip to gradually decrease serum glucose, as well as osmolarity (osmoles of solute per liter of solution). The difference between the measured osmolarity and calculated osmolarity (2Na + glucose/18 + blood urea nitrogen/2.8 + ethanol/4.6) is called the osmolal gap; this would be elevated due to the high ketones or other anions (which are unmeasured anions and therefore the cause of an anion gap metabolic acidosis). A rapid reduction in osmolarity will result in cerebral edema and should be avoided. The combination of hydration and insulin will decrease potassium. Urine output is carefully monitored for evaluation of fluid status. With correction of acidosis, the serum potassium may precipitously decrease, requiring careful monitoring and supplementation (insulin causes transfer of hydrogen ions from the extracellular space to the intracellular space). Other electrolytes to consider are magnesium and phosphate, both which may need to be replenished. Patients commonly have deficiencies of the B-complex vitamins (due to malnutrition), particularly thiamine, which should be corrected. Bicarbonate is rarely recommended for the treatment of acidosis (high risk for development of cerebral edema). It is generally reserved for patients with a pH less than 7.0.

This patient was admitted to the hospital and started on intravenous normal saline. Calcium gluconate was administered to maintain cardiac stability. The patient was started on a regular insulin drip with frequent blood glucose checks to adjust the dose. The potassium level was evaluated intermittently and supplemented as needed. When the blood glucose was measured below 200 mg/dl, dextrose supplementation was used to prevent dangerous hypoglycemia. The insulin drip was continued until resolution of the metabolic acidosis. The patient was empirically started on ampicillin-sulbactam (combination of β-lactam and β-lactamase inhibitor) and was taken to the operating room for surgical drainage of the infection. The intravenous fluid was changed to $D_5^{1}/_2NS$ when the patient was deemed hemodynamically stable. Urine output improved, metabolic acidosis and pseudohyperkalemia (elevated plasma potassium despite total body depletion secondary to shift of potassium from the intracellular space due to high H^+ concentration) resolved, and the patient was transferred to the ward. An American Diabetic Association 1800-kcal diet was initiated. The patient remained afebrile, with normalization of his white blood cell count, electrolytes, and urine analysis. He was subsequently discharged to home care on a 10-day regimen of amoxicillin with clavulinic acid.

COMPLICATIONS

Complications of diabetes can be divided into acute and chronic. The acute complications include hypoglycemia (see the section on Diabetes Mellitus earlier in this chapter), diabetic ketoacidosis, and the hyperosmolar hyperglycemic syndrome. Chronic complications include microvascular and macrovascular disease. Patients with diabetic ketoacidosis generally present with metabolic acidosis with blood glucose below 500 mg/dl, whereas patients with nonketotic hyperglycemia coma present with a blood glucose level of over 1000 mg/dl with no acidosis. The pathophysiology of both disorders is related to the physiological response to stress. Infection (which is the most common cause of diabetic ketoacidosis), trauma, ischemia (cerebrovascular accident, myocardial infarction), or volume depletion can induce signals to increase catecholamines, cortisol, growth hormone, and glucagon (insulin counterregulatory hormones that increase gluconeogenesis) and cause an imbalance of glucose metabolism. These stress hormones increase blood glucose and osmolarity while decreasing cellular insulin. The lack of insulin results in ketone production by the liver and the development of an anion gap metabolic acidosis. Diabetic ketoacidosis also presents with nausea, vomiting, abdominal pain, polyurea, polydipsia, weight loss, diplopia, delirium, or coma. Objective laboratory studies reveal a metabolic acidosis, pseudohyperkalemia, glucosuria, and both serum and urine β-hydroxybuterate and acetoacetate (ketones). Due to the rapid onset of acidosis and good renal clearance in the younger patient population with type 1 diabetes, the blood glucose level rarely exceeds 800 mg/dl.

Diabetic ketoacidosis is the most commonly observed acute complication of type 1 diabetes. Patients with type 2 diabetes may also develop diabetic ketoacidosis, but this is not common. The second most common cause of diabetic ketoacidosis is patient noncompliance with insulin.

As demonstrated by the Diabetes Control Clinical Trial (DCCT) strict glycemic control is the single most important factor in preventing and/or delaying the long-term complications of diabetes. However, patients will also need appropriate blood pressure and serum cholesterol management to reduce the associated cardiovascular risk factors. ACE inhibitors are particularly beneficial in diabetic persons—not only for blood pressure control but also for their ability to delay diabetic nephropathy. Patients may also benefit from cholesterol-lowering medications such as the HMG CoA reductase inhibitors to achieve low-density lipoprotein levels of less than 110 mg/dl. Yearly ophthalmological examinations should be conducted for early diagnosis and management of diabetic retinopathy. Routine foot care is essential for the detection of foot ulcers secondary to diabetic peripheral neuropathy. A low-fat diet, exercise, and weight loss have been show, to decrease the severity of insulin resistance in type 2 diabetes.

DISCUSSION

The diagnosis of diabetic ketoacidosis is based on history, clinical examination, and laboratory findings. The work-up should included serum glucose and electrolytes, anion gap, blood urea nitrogen, creatinine, urine analysis including ketones, electrocardiogram, complete blood count, arterial blood gas, Hb_{A1c} levels, and any tests required to determine the underlying cause.

The differential diagnosis of a patient with ketosis also includes alcoholism and starvation, but only diabetic ketoacidosis presents with hyperglycemia. The excess anions (ketones) in diabetic ketoacidosis cause an anion gap metabolic acidosis (gap acidosis) (discussed in Diabetes Mellitus). The differential diagnosis includes methanol toxicity, uremia, diabetic ketoacidosis, paraldehyde ingestion, isoniazide toxicity, Isopropyl alcohol toxicity, lactic acidosis, ethylene glycol toxicity, and salicylate toxicity. However, only diabetic ketoacidosis will produce hyperglycemia. The symptoms of diabetic ketoacidosis can arise rapidly (within 24 hours), manifesting as polyurea, polyphagia, polydipsia, weakness and fatigue, as well as nausea and vomiting, along with vague abdominal pain. Mental status may range from normal to profound coma. As dehydration becomes pronounced, the hypovolumic polyurea will not be as prominent.

Acidosis will result in a shift of potassium ions from the intracellular to the extracellular compartments. This causes elevation of the plasma potassium concentration. However, with the glucose-driven osmotic diuresis, potassium is excreted by the kidneys, causing depletion of total body potassium despite elevated plasma levels. Hence, the term pseudohyperkalemia (seen in over one third of patients with diabetic ketoacidosis). With the correction of acidosis, the extracellular potassium shifts back to the intracellular space, causing significant lowering of plasma potassium. The plasma potassium needs to be repleted as the acidosis is corrected to avoid life-threatening hypokalemia.

Another acute complication of diabetes is hyperosmolar hyperglycemic syndrome, which has a less insidious onset compared with diabetic ketoacidosis. It generally begins with mild hyperglycemia, which is compensated by glycosourea. As hyperglycemia worsens, osmotic diuresis will waste more glucose through urine. If the patient maintains adequate hydration, the kidneys will continue to excrete the excess glucose. As the patient becomes confused or incapacitated, oral hydration decreases, and the kidneys' ability to excrete glucose is diminished, exacerbating hyperglycemia and causing the mental status changes. During treatment, the plasma glucose level should be reduced no faster than 75 to 100 mg/dl/hr. A more rapid decline could cause brain edema.

Chronic complications of diabetes consist of microvascular and macrovascular disease. Microvascular disease, including nephropathy, neuropathy, and retinopathy, is seen in both forms of diabetes. Type 2 diabetes is the leading cause of end-stage renal disease. The earliest sign of renal failure is microalbuminuria (greater than 50 mg/day); however, a routine urine dipstick will not be positive at this level. Frank proteinuria (nephrotic syndrome) may occur up to 15 years after the initial diagnosis of diabetes. Tight glycemic control, blood pressure control, and a diet low in protein may delay the onset of renal disease. Diabetic retinopathy is the leading cause of blindness. Retinopathy may manifest as either ischemic or proliferative (more severe). Following the onset of proliferative retinopathy, blindness will occur in about 5 years. Some preventive modalities with the use of a laser are available. Diabetic neuropathy has a broad range of presentations but can be categorized into three:

1. Distal sensory polyneuropathy resulting in decreased vibratory and other sensory stimuli; can result in minor trauma to the feet that may go unnoticed for significant periods of time
2. Diabetic mononeuropathy presents as neuropathy of a large peripheral nerve such as the radial or ulnar nerves or a cranial nerve (most commonly cranial nerves VI or VII)
3. Autonomic neuropathy, which can be responsible for silent ischemia (see the section on Acute Myocardial Infarction), diabetic gastroparesis, neurogenic bladder, and erectile dysfunction

The macrovascular diseases present due to the increased risk factors for CAD seen in diabetes secondary to accelerated atherosclerosis from elevated triglycerides and hypercholesterolemia (and low high-density lipoprotein). The nephropathy along with other microvascular diseases predisposes to hypertension. Neuropathy and autonomic dysfunction may result in an unusual presentation of myocardial infarction (silent myocardial infarction), causing a delay in diagnosis and treatment.

Bibliography

Abramson E, Arky R: Diabetic acidosis with initial hypokalemia, *JAMA* 196:401-403, 1966.

Adrogue HJ, Lederer ED, Suski WN, et al: Determinants of plasma potassium levels in diabetic ketoacidosis, *Medicine* 65:163-172, 1986.

Adrogue HJ, Madias N: Management of life-threatening acid-base disorder: first of two parts, *N Engl J Med* 338:26-34, 1998.

Chiasson J, Aris-jilwan N, Belanger R, et al: Diagnosis and treatment of diabetic ketoacidosis and hyperglycemic hyperosmolar state, *CMAJ* 168:859-866, 2003.

Fulop M, Tannenbaum H, Dreyer N: Ketotic hyperosmolar coma, *Lancet* 2:635-639, 1973.

Jerums G, MacIsaac RJ: Treatment of microalbuminuria in patients with type 2 diabetes mellitus, *Treat Endocrinol* 1:163-73, 2002.

Kitabchi AE, Umpierrez GE, Murphy MB, et al: Hyperglycemic crises in patients with diabetes mellitus, *Diabetes Care* 26(suppl 1):S109-S117, 2003.

Kreisberg RA: Diabetic ketoacidosis: new concepts and trends in pathogenesis and treatment, *Ann Intern Med* 88:681-695, 1978.

Matz R: Management of the hyperosmolar hyperglycemic syndrome, *Am Fam Physician* 60:1468-1476, 1999.

Narins RG, Cohen JJ: Bicarbonate therapy for organic acidosis: the case for its continued use, *Ann Intern Med* 106:615, 1987.

Page MM, Alberti KG, Greenwood R, et al: Treatment of diabetic coma with continuous low-dose insulin infusion, *Br Med J* 2:687-660, 1974.

Trachtenbarg DE: Diabetic ketoacidosis, *Am Fam Physician* 71:1705-1714, 2005.

Umpierrez G, Greire AX: Abdominal pain in patients with hyperglycemic crisis, *J Crit Care* 17:63-67, 2002.

Acute Myocardial Infarction

Joyce T. Lee, DDS, MD, and Shahrokh C. Bagheri, DMD, MD

CC

A 57-year-old man with a history of hypertension, coronary artery disease, and hypercholesterolemia is referred to your office for evaluation of a biopsy-proved mandibular dentigerous cyst.

Perioperative cardiovascular risk assessment includes recognition of the following risk factors: advanced age, sedentary lifestyle, male gender, tobacco use, a history of previous myocardial infarction or pathological Q waves seen on an electrocardiogram, hypertension, diabetes mellitus (particularly type 1), hypercholesterolemia, history of cerebrovascular accidents, a positive family history of heart disease, and morbid obesity (risk factors are categorized into major, intermediate, and minor).

HPI

The patient is diagnosed with a small dentigerous cyst of the posterior mandible.

The preoperative assessment for patients includes inquiry into the patient's ability to perform daily activities that reflect the status of cardiopulmonary function. This includes any history of dyspnea (shortness of breath) on walking up a flight of stairs, orthopnea (inability to sleep or lie prone without becoming short of breath), paroxysmal nocturnal dyspnea (spontaneous shortness of breath during sleep periods), history of pedal edema, and a sedentary lifestyle. Unstable or unexplained symptoms and recent significant health events are good indicators for additional preoperative questioning and testing.

Risk assessment is not exclusive for patients with known cardiac disease because a significant number of patients have undiagnosed CAD. The guidelines published by the American College of Cardiology/American Heart Association outline the algorithm for cardiovascular risk assessment for individuals at risk for noncardiac surgery.

PMHX/PDHX/MEDICATIONS/ALLERGIES/SH/FH

The patient has a history of hypertension, angina, CAD, and hypercholesterolemia (risk factors for myocardial infarction) for which he has been on medications for the past 15 years (there are three types of angina: stable angina, unstable angina, and Prinzmetal angina). He denies any history of previous myocardial infarction, cerebrovascular accidents, or any recent hospitalizations (the American Heart Association recommends deferring any elective surgery within 6 months

of an acute myocardial infarction [AMI]). His last physical examination was 1 year ago, at which time several minor adjustments were made to his medications. His past surgical history includes an appendectomy and cholecystectomy under general anesthesia without any perioperative complications (a positive history of adverse events to anesthesia is significant in assessing future risk of surgery under general anesthesia). His medications include amlodipine (calcium channel blocker), furosemide (loop diuretic), K-Dur (potassium chloride), Atorvastatin (cholesterol-lowering medication: HMG-CoA reductase inhibitor), and nitroglycerin (vasodilator) tablets as necessary for angina. He has smoked one pack per day for the past 20 years and admits to a sedentary lifestyle but has no symptoms of depression (depression is a common comorbid condition in patients with CAD and a well-documented risk factor for recurrent cardiac events and mortality). His family history is significant for his father who died from a massive AMI at the age of 50 (risk factor).

EXAMINATION

General. The patient is a moderately obese man in no distress.

Vitals. Vital signs are normal except for a baseline blood pressure of 155/88 mm Hg (moderate hypertension).

Maxillofacial. There is minimal expansion of the buccal cortex of the left posterior mandible.

Cardiovascular.

1. Inspection: The chest wall appears normal. The point of maximum impulse is located at the normal position along the midclavicular line at the fifth intercostal space (lateralization of the point of maximum impulse would be indicative of ventricular hypertrophy).

2. Auscultation: No audible bruits are heard using the bell of the stethoscope. This portion of the examination includes auscultation for bruits at the neck (carotid), mid abdomen (aorta), and lateral abdomen (renal). Audible bruits would be indicative of atherosclerotic plaques suggestive of systemic atherosclerosis.

   Auscultation of the heart reveals a regular rate and rhythm, no murmurs, normal S_1 and S_2 (splitting of S_2 is considered pathological) with no S_3 or S_4 noted (S_3 is caused by left ventricular volume overloading or dilation, whereas S_4 is caused by poor compliance and stiffness of the left ventricles. S_3 is seen with heart failure).

3. Jugular venous pressure: This is within normal limits at 3 cm above the sternal angle. Jugular venous distention is

a sign of venous hypertension most commonly secondary to right-sided heart failure.

4. Peripheral pulses and extremities: Findings are 2+ distal upper and lower extremities. Peripheral pulses are inspected for symmetry and strength (pulsus alternans denotes an alternating strong and weak pulse, signifying heart failure). There is no edema of the extremities (sign of heart failure) or clubbing of the nail beds (seen with chronic pulmonary disease).

5. Fundoscopic: Examination reveals bilateral retinal plaques (secondary to atherosclerosis) and arteriovenous nicking (secondary to hypertension). Examination of the retina is an important part of a complete cardiovascular examination because it allows direct visualization of the microvasculature.

Pulmonary. The chest is bilaterally clear to auscultation. With left-sided heart failure, blood backs into the pulmonary circulation and causes "congestion" and fluid leaking out of the pulmonary capillaries into the interstitium, leading to pulmonary edema ("wet lungs"), which would be detected as rales or crackles on auscultation of the lungs.

IMAGING

Other than a panoramic radiograph, no other routine radiographic imaging studies are indicated for excision of a cyst under intravenous sedation. A preoperative chest radiograph may be obtained in select patients based on the history and physical examination findings.

The panoramic radiograph demonstrates a 2 × 2-cm unilocular radiolucency of the posterior mandible consistent with a dentigerous cyst.

LABS

The preoperative laboratory tests for the evaluation of a patient with significant cardiovascular disease should be done in conjunction with the treating cardiologist.

Ejection fraction is the percentage of the stroke volume that is expelled from the left ventricle with systole and can be estimated using echocardiography. Although this is not routinely ordered, it is the most pertinent preoperative test in terms of assessing a patient's cardiac function. A normal ejection fraction ranges between 55% and 70%.

A variety of stress tests in conjunction with electrocardiographic monitoring may also be performed to further stratify cardiac function in higher-risk patients. The cardiovascular system is tested, or "stressed," by physical activity as the patient walks on a treadmill or pharmacologically using sympathomimetic agents (such as Persantine or dobutamine) in an attempt to test for myocardial ischemia. Determination of cardiac tolerance and risk stratification is based on symptoms and the present electrocardiographic findings such as flipped T waves or ST-segment depression or elevation.

Echocardiography is another diagnostic test that may be performed either transesophageally (more accurate) or transthoracically to assess cardiac structural abnormalities such myocardial wall motion and dynamic valvular function. Several physiological parameters such as degree of valvular insufficiency or stenosis, ejection fraction, and stroke volume can be estimated from echocardiography. Cardiac catheterization is the "gold standard" test for evaluation of cardiac function. However, this is not routinely recommended for preoperative assessment given the invasive nature of this procedure.

Evaluation of blood cholesterol levels is also important for assessment of future risks of cardiovascular events. The American Heart Association recommends targeting high-density lipoprotein cholesterol to over 45 mg/dl while limiting low-density lipoproteins to below 120 mg/dl. However, the target low-density lipoprotein level may vary depending on the patient's comorbidities.

For this patient, his most recent testing was done at his last physical examination several months ago. A cardiac stress test revealed an ejection fraction of 60%. His total cholesterol was 250 mg/dl, high-density lipoprotein 27 mg/dl, low-density lipoprotein 175 mg/dl, and total plasma triglyceride 375 mg/dl. The basic metabolic profile was within normal limits (levels of potassium must be monitored in the hypertensive person on diuretics). A treadmill cardiac stress test did not reveal any signs of myocardial ischemia at a target heart rate of 90%.

His 12-lead electrocardiogram revealed no abnormalities. Electrocardiography is an invaluable tool in providing information on cardiac conduction, vascular resistance, chamber enlargement, electrolyte disturbances, drug toxicities, myocardial ischemia, infarction, and pulmonary emboli. Elevation of the ST segment is strongly suspicious of myocardial injury, whereas ST depression is suggestive of myocardial ischemia.

ASSESSMENT

A 57-year-old man with a history of heart disease, hypertension, and hypercholesterolemia, requiring outpatient removal of a dentigerous cyst under intravenous sedation anesthesia

The treating cardiologist was contacted for perioperative risk assessment for an elective low risk surgery, and he stratified the patient as low risk for surgery with no specific recommendations. A medical clearance for surgery serves to assess the patient's risk of morbidity and mortality in the perioperative period. There is insufficient evidence to support the use of β-blockers for patients undergoing low-risk procedures; however, they are frequently used for intermediate- and high-risk patients.

TREATMENT

After discussion of the risks, benefits, and alternatives, the patient elected to proceed with the procedure. He was instructed to withhold all his morning medications with the exception of his blood pressure pills, which are to be taken with a small sip of water. The patient was also counseled on the benefits of tobacco cessation and dietary and exercise habits.

Surgery was carried out with the patient monitored using the ASA I standards for outpatient procedures (ASA I monitoring includes electrocardiogram, blood pressure, heart rate, and pulse oximeter monitoring). Intravenous anesthesia was planned using a combination of Versed and Fentanyl. Five minutes into the procedure, the electrocardiogram shows multiple unifocal premature ventricular contractions at the rate about 10/min. The patient's oxygen saturation declined from 98% on room air to 92% with 4 L/min oxygen flow via a nasal cannula. His oxygen flow was increased to 8 L/min with improvement of the oxygen saturation to 97%. The patient then suddenly became noticeably agitated, tachypneic with shallow breaths, and tachycardic with a heart rate of 135 bpm (agitation can be a sign of hypoxia). The procedure was aborted, and all intravenous anesthetics were halted. His blood pressure now measured at 90/45 mm Hg (hypotension). His condition continued to deteriorate with ST-segment elevation and multifocal premature ventricular contractions on the electrocardiogram. He remained tachycardic with persistent hypotension. The patient is now emerging from anesthesia and complains of chest tightness while putting his fist over this chest (a positive Levine sign is when the patient places his or his hand over the sternal region due to the dull, aching, squeezing discomfort from an AMI). A diagnosis of AMI was suspected and the emergency medical services system was immediately activated. The emergency medical services personnel arrived within minutes and transported the patient to a local hospital.

A suspected AMI should be managed with use of the American Heart Association adult advanced cardiovascular life support (ACLS) algorithm for ischemic chest pain. Immediate treatment should include administration of supplemental oxygen (to increase oxygen delivery), along with 160 to 325 mg of aspirin (to inhibit platelet function and clot propagation). Sublingual nitroglycerin (vasodilator) is administered to increase coronary blood flow, which would reduce cardiac ischemia and therefore pain. If chest pain is not resolved, morphine should be administered intravenously. The mnemonic MONA (morphine, oxygen, nitroglycerin, and aspirin) outlines this treatment. Simultaneous to these measures, vital signs and oxygen saturation should be monitored. Intravenous access should to be initiated immediately for access to drug delivery. A 12-lead electrocardiogram, serum cardiac markers, serum electrolytes and coagulation studies, and a portable chest radiograph should be obtained as soon as possible. The decision to treat the patient with pharmacological agents (such as heparin, glycoprotein IIb/IIIa receptor inhibitors, intravenous nitroglycerin, or β-blockers) is determined by the electrocardiogram findings along with the continuous clinical assessment. Rapid assessment by trained personnel to determine the need for cardiac catheterization (percutaneous coronary intervention), subsequent coronary artery bypass graft surgery, or fibrinolytic therapy for revascularization is essential.

COMPLICATIONS

The most feared complication of an AMI is sudden death (most commonly due to ventricular fibrillation or myocardial rupture). The immediate- and long-term sequelae of an AMI is related to the extent and location of the necrotic myocardial tissue. Subsequent inflammatory and electrical conduction abnormalities that lead to mechanical dysfunction of the heart can be variable in both chronology and severity.

Cardiac arrhythmias are commonly seen during an AMI. Infarction of specialized myocardial tissue such as the sino-atrial node, atrioventricular node, or bundle branches can lead to a variety of arrhythmias and conduction blocks. Ventricular fibrillation is a nonperfusing rhythm that needs to be rapidly identified and treated via the ACLS protocol.

Impaired myocardial function can cause failure of the heart to adequately pump blood into the systemic circulation, with subsequent congestion of blood into the pulmonary circulation, resulting in CHF (see Congestive Heart Failure earlier in this chapter). AMI may also lead to *cardiogenic shock,* which is defined as tissue hypoperfusion secondary to heart failure resulting in decreased cardiac output and hypotension.

Ischemia or necrosis of specific anatomical locations may result in mechanical dysfunctions such as rupture of the papillary muscles, ventricular septal perforation, or rupture of the ventricular free wall and subsequent cardiac tamponade (usually resulting in death). Other long-term complications include pericarditis (inflammation of the pericardium) and thromboembolic events originating within the cardiac chamber secondary to endothelial injury, stasis of blood, and turbulent flow.

DISCUSSION

The prevalence of cardiovascular diseases in the United States is between 20% and 25%, accounting for nearly 40% of fatalities from all causes. It is estimated that cardiac deaths and myocardial infarction occur in 0.2% (50,000 deaths) of all cases of surgery under general anesthesia annually. As the baby boomer population ages and the number of patients undergoing elective surgery increases, perioperative cardiovascular evaluation should be performed meticulously in patients at risk.

The etiologies of myocardial infarction span a broad range of pathological processes including atherosclerosis with thromboembolic events, vascular syndromes, coronary aneurysms, primary and drug-induced coronary spasms (cocaine), severe conditions of oxygen demand (aortic stenosis), and hyperviscosity states (polycythemia vera). Signs and symptoms of AMI are not always evident. Approximately 20% of patients who sustained AMI are asymptomatic with retrospective positive electrocardiographic findings. This is particularly significant in the diabetic patient, who may not experience painful symptoms due to underlying peripheral neuropathy.

Recent studies have provided evidence that the use of β-blockers reduces the morbidity and mortality in patients with heart failure due to left ventricular systolic dysfunction. By reducing the sympathetic drive and hence workload to the myocardium, β-blockers have been shown to reduce the rate of reinfarction and recurrent ischemia. In addition, ACE inhibitors have recently been proven to increase survival in patients with AMI.

With progressive ischemia and subsequent myocardial infarction, the electrocardiographic findings include T-wave inversions (ischemia), ST-segment elevation (suggestive of acute myocardial infarct), ST-segment depression (nontransmural infarct or ischemia), and the development of Q waves (indicative of myocardial infarction). The leads in which these changes occur correspond to the area of cardiac injury. On a 12-lead electrocardiogram, leads V_1 through V_6 are designated as the precordial chest leads and leads I, II, III, aVL, aVR, and aVF are the limb leads. An inferior infarct commonly presents with abnormalities in leads II, II, and aVF, while findings on leads V_1 through V_6 represent injury to the anterior wall.

Cardiac enzymes are plasma diagnostic markers released during myocardial necrosis. Based on the onset of injury, concentration, and metabolic half-life of the enzymes released, myocardial cell necrosis can be confirmed. In addition, the approximate time of infarction can be predicted. Several enzymes are used, including creatine kinase, creatine phosphokinase, creatine kinase–myocardial band, myoglobin, lactate dehydrogenase, aspartate aminotransferase, and troponin I or T. Creatine kinase, creatine phosphokinase, myoglobin, and lactate dehydrogenase are not specific to myocardial tissue and can be elevated from other etiologies, The creatine kinase–myocardial band enzymes can also be found in skeletal muscles and are not as cardiac specific for myocardial tissue as initially expected. Troponins T and I are currently the markers of choice for determining acute cardiac injury because they have absolute cardiac specificity and are much more sensitive than the creatine kinase–myocardial

band enzyme. Troponin levels can be detected as soon as 12 hours postinjury and remain elevated until 10 to 12 days later. Myocardial muscle creatinine kinase isozymes typically peak at 24 hours with a return to normal range in the 48- to 72-hour period. Other enzymes changes include elevation of aspartate aminotransferase at a 48-hour period with a return to normal in 4 to 5 days, and lactate dehydrogenase that typically peaks at day 5 with a return to normal by days 7 to 10.

In summary, in the event of an AMI in the office setting, early detection of symptoms is critical. Defibrillation for indicated arrhythmias, symptomatic management with morphine, oxygen, nitroglycerin, and aspirin are essential and must be provided swiftly. Current antithrombolytic therapy and/or cardiac catheterization in the hospital setting can significantly increase patient survival.

Bibliography

ACC/AHA guideline update for perioperative cardiovascular evaluation for noncardiac surgery: executive summary: a report of the American College of Cardiology/American Heart Association Task Force on Practice Guidelines (Committee to Update the 1996 Guidelines on Perioperative Cardiovascular Evaluation for Noncardiac Surgery), *J Am Coll Cardiol* 39:542-553, 2002.

Andreoli TE, Carpenter CC, Griggs RC, et al: *Cecil's essentials of medicine,* ed 5, Philadelphia, 2003, WB Saunders.

Crawford MH: *Current diagnosis and treatment in cardiology,* ed 2, New York, 2006, McGraw-Hill.

Cummins RO: *ACLS provider manuel,* Dallas, 2004, American Heart Association.

Farrell MH, Foody JM, Krumholz HM: Beta-blockers in heart failure: clinical applications, *JAMA* 287:890-897, 2002.

Fuster V, Alexander RW, O'Rourke RA, et al: *Hurst's the heart,* ed 11, Philadelphia, 2006, McGraw-Hill.

Huffman JC, Smith FA, Blais MA, et al: Recognition and treatment of depression and anxiety in patients with acute myocardial infarction, *Am J Cardiol* 98:319-324, 2006.

Lillly LS: *Pathophysiology of heart disease,* ed 3, Philadelphia, 2002, Lippincott Williams and Wilkins.

Hypertension

Mehran Mehrabi, Maj. USAF, DC, and Chris Jo, DMD

CC

A 40-year-old African American man presents to the office complaining that, "my wisdom teeth are hurting" (essential hypertension is most commonly diagnosed during the third to fifth decades of life and has a higher prevalence in African American males).

HPI

The patient complains of a 2-week history of bilateral posterior mandibular pain associated with his lower third molars. He initially self-treated himself with ibuprofen, which provided temporary relief. On triage of the patient, his blood pressure is elevated, which he attributes to the dental pain. He states that he has never seen a primary care physician and denies any history of hypertension. He denies headache, dizziness, blurred vision, chest pain, lower extremity edema, and shortness of breath (signs of potential end organ damage).

PMHX/PDHX/MEDICATIONS/ALLERGIES/SH/FH

The patient describes himself as "healthy as a horse" (hypertension is an asymptomatic disease) but physically out of shape due to lack of exercise. He does not take any medications at this time. He smokes one pack of cigarettes daily and has consumed two alcoholic beverages daily for the last 10 years (smoking, alcohol, and sedentary lifestyle increase the risk of hypertension and CAD). He is single and his typical diet consists of fast foods (a diet high in sodium, saturated fat, and simple sugars). His family history is significant for sudden death of his father at the age of 44 secondary to heart attack (family history of myocardial infarction is significant when paternal age is less than 45 and maternal age is less than 55). His father also was known to be a diabetic for the last 6 years (family history of diabetes and CAD are nonpreventable risk factors, whereas obesity, smoking, and excessive alcohol consumption are preventable risk factors for cardiovascular disease).

EXAMINATION

General. The patient is alert and oriented, calm, and cooperative and follows command well. He appears to be in no apparent distress. He weighs 240 pounds and is 5 feet 7 inches tall (a body mass index of 37.6 kg/m^2 consistent with class II obesity).

Vital signs. His blood pressure is 185/104 mm Hg in the right arm sitting and 181/101 mm Hg in the left arm sitting (while an interarm blood pressure difference of about 10 mm Hg may be normal, a greater difference may be consistent with aortic dissection), heart rate 80 bpm, respirations 16 per minute, temperature 37.4°C, and visual analog scale for pain at 2 of 10 (severe pain may cause an acute increase in blood pressure).

Maxillofacial. There is no facial edema, erythema, or induration. Neck examination is benign with no evidence of masses or lymphadenopathy. The jugular venous distention is undetectable (a jugular venous pressure greater than 3 cm or a measured central venous pressure greater than 8 is consistent with right ventricular failure. The most common cause of right ventricular failure is left ventricular failure).

Intraoral. Examination is consistent with pericoronitis associated with partial bony impacted lower third molars.

Fundoscopic. Examination demonstrates arteriovenous nicking and an arteriolar light reflex ("copper wiring"), with no evidence of retinal necrosis or disc edema. Fundoscopic examination provides a direct examination of vasculature. The retinal vessels share similar pathophysiology as cerebral and coronary blood vessels. The initial changes seen with hypertension include vasoconstriction followed by hyaline degeneration. As blood pressure increases, one may see the arterial narrowing (atrioventricular nicking) and arteriolar light reflex (copper wiring). In uncontrolled hypertension, there is a breakdown of the blood–retina barrier and presentation of hemorrhage and areas of infarction (cotton-wool spots).

Cardiovascular. There are no carotid, femoral, or renal bruits present (indicative of peripheral vascular disease). On palpation of the heart, the apical impulse is palpated at the fifth intercostal space and the midclavicular line (normal position). It is enlarged at 4 cm (normal is 2 to 3 cm), sustained and strong in intensity (indicative of ventricular hypertrophy). On auscultation, there is an S_1 (first heart sound) and S_2 (second heart sound) as well as S_4 gallop (pathological heart sound during late diastolic period produced by atrium pushing on inelastic myocardium), just before S_1 (S_3, which may present in patients with CHF that may be secondary to uncontrolled hypertension, is heard shortly after an S_2). The rhythm is regular (irregularly irregular rhythm can be due to atrial fibrillation caused by hypertension). There is no murmur or rub on auscultation. Peripheral pulses are bounding, with rapid upstroke and 2+ intensity, and synchronous with appropriate amplitude (delayed femoral pulse compared with radial is consistent with coarctation, a congenital cause of hypertension).

Pulmonary. The chest is clear to auscultation bilaterally. There are no crackles or wheezing (cardiogenic wheeze is produced by pulmonary edema in acute CHF).

Abdomen. The patient is obese and has no evidence of surgical scars or striae (present in hypercortisolism secondary to adrenal tumor, pituitary tumor, or paraneoplastic syndromes). Bowl sounds are present on auscultation. The abdomen is soft and nontender to palpation. The kidneys are nonpalpable (persons with enlarged kidneys, such as seen in polycystic kidney disease, may present with hypertension). The liver is 10 cm at the midclavicular line (normal is 10 to 12 cm). The aorta is palpable and is not enlarged (if enlarged, would be suggestive of an acute abdominal aneurysm).

IMAGING

The panoramic radiograph is the study of choice when evaluating third molars. In the setting of controlled hypertension, no additional radiographs are required for minor surgical procedures. On evaluation of hypertensive urgency or emergency at the emergency department, additional studies are required and may include a chest radiograph (to evaluate for cardiogenic pulmonary edema and cardiomegaly), electrocardiogram (to rule out AMI), and/or head CT (to rule out intracerebral hemorrhage), based on clinical history and findings a preoperative electrocardiogram is warranted for patients undergoing general anesthesia with risk factors for cardiovascular disease (hypertension, diabetes, smoking, hypercholesterolemia, and age above 45 in males and 55 in females).

LABS

Laboratory studies are obtained based on the patient's medical history. For the patient with hypertension who presents for minor surgical procedures, no laboratory studies are indicated. Several laboratory parameters may measured by the primary care physician or preoperatively to detect secondary causes of hypertension: plasma sodium (rennin-producing tumors, renal disease), potassium (renal or adrenal disease), creatinine (renal disease), urine vanillylmandelic acid (pheochromocytoma), serum cortisol, or thyroid-stimulating hormone, which are all markers of potential causes of secondary hypertension. An astute clinician uses the patient's history and physical examination to develop a differential diagnosis.

Radiographic, laboratory, and other tests are used to assess the validity of specific diagnoses.

ASSESSMENT

Partial bony impacted lower third molars with pericoronitis complicated by elevated blood pressure

The diagnosis of hypertension requires additional blood pressure readings. If these readings are confirmed in subsequent evaluations, the patient would classify as having stage II hypertension.

According to the seventh report of the Joint National Committee on Prevention, Detection, Evaluation, and Treatment of High Blood Pressure (JNC-7), a normal systolic blood pressure is less than 120 mm Hg and a normal diastolic blood pressure is less than 80 mm Hg. The blood pressure may be considered normal, prehypertensive, stage I hypertension, or stage II hypertension (Table 14-7). The effects on the end organs such as heart, brain, kidney, or eyes are in a linear relationship.

TREATMENT

Management of the hypertensive patient begins with an accurate diagnosis. Blood pressure is determined by cardiac output (stroke volume multiplied by heart rate) and total peripheral resistance. It is measured with the patient in a sitting position with the arm at the level of the heart. Patients should avoid smoking and caffeine 30 minutes and 1 hour, respectively, before a blood pressure reading is made. Note that a large cuff will produce an erroneously low reading, and a small cuff will produce an erroneously high blood pressure. The blood pressure can be measured in both arms. A difference greater than 10 mm Hg may be suggestive of aortic dissection. The most common site for measurement of blood pressure is the brachial artery. The cuff is applied to the arm. It is tightened as the radial pulse is palpated, and the pressure is raised until it is 30 mm Hg above where the radial pulse disappears. This technique will ensure that an auscultatory gap (a period of silence as the blood pressure cuff pressure decreases) will not result in an erroneously low reading. Measurements are repeated two or three times in different settings before the diagnosis of hypertension is made.

A blood pressure reading should be obtained before surgical procedures, even in the absence of symptoms or a positive medical history. Contraindications to surgery in a hypertensive patient are not based on actual blood pressure but rather

Table 14-7.	Classification of Blood Pressure for Adults			
Blood Pressure	Normal (mm Hg)	Prehypertension (mm Hg)	Stage I Hypertension (mm Hg)	Stage II Hypertension (mm Hg)
Systolic	<120	120-139	140-159	>160
Diastolic	<80	80-89	90-99	>100

based on clinical judgment in assessing risks and benefits of surgical or nonsurgical interventions. Elective procedures should be deferred with a sudden unexplained rise in blood pressure. When a hypertensive patient presents with symptoms of hypertensive emergency (diplopia, dizziness, headaches, shortness of breath, sudden leg swelling, chest pain), elective surgery is deferred, and the patient should be referred to the emergency department for further work-up and management.

Consultation with the primary care physician is valuable when possible, but may not always be feasible. If there is no surgical emergency, temporary analgesia may be achieved with long-acting local anesthesia and analgesic medications. When treating an urgent surgical problem in a hypertensive patient, one may choose local anesthesia office sedation, or hospital-based general anesthesia depending on the clinician's training and comfort, location of practice, and facility's monitoring capability.

When patients with a history of hypertension present for office intravenous sedation, they should continue with their daily antihypertensive medications. Abrupt withdrawal of certain antihypertensive medications such as clonidine or β-blockers may result in hypertensive urgencies (rebound hypertension). General anesthetic medications that may result in hypertension such as ketamine (sympathomimetic effects) should be avoided or used cautiously. Local anesthetics with vasoconstrictors should be used cautiously and sparingly. Most dental literature recommends limiting epinephrine to 0.04 mg in patients with cardiovascular disease; however, this is a subject of controversy. A recent report, published by the Agency for Healthcare Research and Quality, evaluated the use of local anesthesia for dental extractions with and without epinephrine in hypertensive and normotensive individuals. The difference in systolic blood pressure and heart rate when using epinephrine versus no epinephrine was 4 mm Hg and 6 bpm, respectively, in hypertensive patients when using up to 2 carpules (1.8 ml each) of anesthetic agents.

The cause of intraoperative hypertensive episodes needs to be rapidly assessed and appropriately managed. Hypertension may be due to hypoxia, hypercarbia, anxiety, pain, full bladder, prior medications, or idiopathic (primary hypertension). Common intravenous antihypertensives used in ambulatory surgery are β-blockers and hydralazine. β-Blockers such as esmolol (short acting) and labetalol (longer acting) decrease blood pressure and heart rate, while hydralazine will decrease blood pressure with concurrent reflex tachycardia. It is extremely important not to treat numbers but evaluate the patient as a whole: the patient's age and past medical history and family history (age, race, family history of hypertension), social history (cocaine, methamphetamine, methoxymethyl methamphetamine abuse), initial blood pressure (baseline), type of procedure, medications used (ketamine), respiratory rate (pain), heart rate, and temperature (malignant hyperthermia) should be considered.

During general anesthesia, patients on hypertensive medications may also be susceptible to episodes of hypotension. Propofol administered as a bolus can lower the systolic blood pressure up to 30 mm Hg, which can be exaggerated in patients with hypertension. Inhalation general anesthetics may also precipitously lower mean arterial pressures (due to vasodilation). Hypotension most commonly responds well to bolus fluid administration. If the patient is not responsive to conservative fluid treatment, a vasopressor agent may be required. The choice in vasopressor agent depends on both the blood pressure and heart rate. In the hypotensive and bradycardic patient, vasogenic stimulators that cause a reflex bradycardia should be avoided (phenylephrine). Ephedrine should be used for the hypotensive and bradycardic patient unresponsive to intravenous fluid bolus and a decreased the level of anesthesia. Phenylephrine is ideal for the hypotensive and tachycardic patients.

Patients (particularly elderly) who are admitted to the hospital are at an increased risk of hypotension than hypertension. This may be due to hospitals' low sodium diet, concurrent medications, narcotic use, or lack of physical activity. Therefore, hypertensive medications such as diuretics, ACE inhibitors, angiotensin receptor blockers, α-blockers, or calcium channel blockers should be prescribed when the blood pressure is elevated. β-Blockers should be continued not only for their cardioprotective effect but also for possible rebound tachycardia (perioperative administration of β-blockers has been shown to decrease anesthetic complications). Rebound hypertension also is commonly seen with clonidine, but this medication is now rarely used. When patients are discharged from the hospital or office, they should continue their prior antihypertensive medication regimen.

This patient was started on penicillin, analgesic medications, and chlorhexidine mouthwash. He was referred to his primary care physician for evaluation and management of his blood pressure. Three subsequent blood pressure readings in the physician office, as well as automatic blood pressure monitor at the local pharmacy, reflected a systolic blood pressure of 175 to 185 mm Hg and a diastolic blood pressure of 95 to 105 mm Hg. The patient was instructed to restrict sodium and alcohol intake, to quit smoking, and to start aerobic exercises. However, the patient remained hypertensive at 150/90 mm Hg. He was subsequently placed on hydrochlorothiazide (diuretics are considered first-line therapy). At follow-up, his blood pressure was 130/82 mm Hg. After his blood pressure was stabilized, the patient was scheduled for surgical extraction of the lower third molars using intravenous sedation. He was instructed to continue his hydrochlorothiazide (antihypertensive medications should be continued in the perioperative period). His blood pressure remained stable throughout the procedure.

COMPLICATIONS

Hypertensive urgency is hypertension with a blood pressure above 210/120 mm Hg in an asymptomatic patient. Patients are admitted to the emergency department, and the blood pressure is gradually lowered with oral medications (oral sublingual nifedepine, felodipine, captopril and furosemide). The blood pressure should not be abruptly reduced to less than 160/110 mm Hg, due to the risk of cerebral and myocardial hypoperfusion.

Hypertensive emergency is hypertension with evidence of end organ damage (brain, heart, kidneys, eyes) such as retinal hemorrhages and exudates, papilledema, renal failure (malignant nephrosclerosis), neurological symptoms (headache, weakness, or neurosensory deficit), and cardiac symptoms such as chest pain. Intravenous medications such as nitroprusside (0.25 to 0.5 µg/kg/min up to 8 to 10 µg/kg/min), Nicardipine (5 to 15 mg/hr) or labetalol (0.5 to 2 mg/min) may be used to control blood pressure. Note that nitroprusside may result in cyanide toxicity, which may be treated with sodium thiosulfate. Nonintravenous routes such as oral, nasal, or transcutaneous can be used, but they are not as titratable. A rapid decline in blood pressure can be as harmful as a rapid rise. Close monitoring of vital sign is more critical than the route of administration.

Chronic complications of hypertension include CAD, CHF, cerebrovascular accident, renal disease, ophthalmological disease, and others. Treatment of hypertension significantly reduces the risk of CAD, myocardial infarction, heart failure, and cerebrovascular accidents.

Antihypertensive medications can cause various side effects or complications, including orthostatic hypotension (especially in the elderly population), resulting in syncope and ground-level falls.

DISCUSSION

Hypertension is a frequently referred to as a "silent killer" and is a common disorder. In the United States, it is most prevalent among African Americans followed by Hispanics and whites. The incidence of hypertension increases with age and excess body weight. Other risk factors include genetics (hypertension is twice more common when one or both parents have hypertension), alcohol consumption, tobacco use, and male gender. Other factors such as salt intake or type A personality has not been shown to be risk factors for the development of hypertension. However, a low-salt diet decreases blood pressure in hypertensive patients, whereas a high-salt diet makes hypertension more resistant to therapy.

Hypertension may be divided into primary or essential (95%) and secondary (5%) categories. Although secondary hypertension is less common, diagnosis is important because frequently a cure rather than treatment is possible. Essential (idiopathic) hypertension is generally diagnosed before age 30 or after the age 50, whereas secondary hypertension is most commonly identified between ages 30 and 50. Secondary hypertension tends to be more severe and less susceptible to routine treatment used for essential hypertension.

Secondary hypertension includes a variety of hormonal or structural defects. Elevation of steroid levels (primary adrenal tumor, secondary pituitary tumor, or tertiary paraneoplastic syndrome), calcium (hyperparathyroidism), and hypothyroidism (and hyperthyroid crisis) are common hormonal etiologies. The structural defect such as coarctation of the aorta or renal artery stenosis and intracranial hypertension may also cause systemic hypertension.

Treatment should be considered when two or three consecutive blood pressure readings are found to be above 140/80 mm Hg. Conservative treatment such as weight reduction, low-salt (sodium) diet, aerobic exercises, and secession of alcohol and tobacco products can be beneficial in preventing medical therapy. Two landmark studies evaluated the effect of diet on hypertension.

In the Treatment of Mild Hypertension Study (TOMHS), 902 patients with diastolic blood pressure of 90 to 100 mm Hg underwent a sodium and alcohol restriction, weight reduction and increase physical activity with improvement of systolic and diastolic blood pressures of 8.6 mm Hg compared with the placebo group. The Dietary Approach to Stop Hypertension (DASH) consisted of 459 hypertensive patients with blood pressures less than 160/90 mg Hg who were placed on a diet consisting of fruits and vegetables and low saturated fats. Blood pressure was reduced by 5.5/3.0 mm Hg in normotensive patients and by 11.4/5.5 mm Hg in hypertensive patients. This was followed by DASH/low-sodium trial illustrating an additive affect. The blood pressure reduction with a low-sodium diet works independent of a healthy diet low in saturated fats and high in fruits and vegetables.

Various studies such as the Medical Research Council (MRC) trial (showing the cardioprotective effect of β-blockers over thiazide diuretics in patients with CAD), Captopril Prevention Project (CAPPP study, showing the benefits of ACE inhibitors in diabetics), U.K. Prospective Diabetes Study, STOP Hypertension Trial, Heart Outcomes Prevention Evaluation (HOPE), Losartan Intervention for Endpoint Reduction (LIFE), and Australian National Blood Pressure (ANBP) studies have examined various initial therapies.

The JNC-7 recommendations are based on the Antihypertensive and Lipid-Lowering Treatment to Prevent Heart Attack Trial (ALL HAT). This study was a randomized examination of 45,000 patients with hypertension and one other risk factor such as left ventricular hypertrophy, diabetes, cerebrovascular accident, etc. The current recommendation is for initiating a low-dose hydrochlorothiazide (a sodium potassium channel blocker at the distal tubule of kidneys) as first-line antihypertensive therapy (higher doses may produce hypokalemia, hypertriglyceridemia, hyperglycemia, and gout).

A β-blocker may be a better choice in patients with CAD due to its post–myocardial infarction cardioprotective effect. Also, it may be the drug of choice in patients with migraine-type headaches, glaucoma, angina pectoris, essential tremor, and resting tachycardia. Sudden cessation of this medication can produce a withdraw reaction and should be avoided. ACE inhibitors prevent the formation of angiotensin II as well as aldosterone. They are commonly considered as the initial therapy in diabetic patients with microproteinuria and may benefit in post–myocardial infarction cardioprotection comparable to that of β-blockers. ACE inhibitors are contraindicated in patients who develop angioneurotic edema, hyperkalemia, and, rarely, neutropenia following its administration. A dry cough is a side effect of ACE inhibitors most likely due to the buildup of bradykinins and is best treated by changing to another class of medication. Angiotensin receptor blockers are an alternative to ACE inhibitors in certain patients.

Calcium channel blockers are potent vasodilators; in general, they are not recommended for initial therapy. Their use in patients with CHF increases mortality. They also exacerbate the reflux in patients known to have gastroesophageal reflux disorder. The α-blockers such as prazosin, doxazosin, and terazosin are not first-line medications. They produce syncope, headache, and weakness. They may be indicated in patients with benign prostatic hypertrophy. Antihypertensive medications considered safe during pregnancy include methyldopa and hydralazine, which generally are not considered in nonpregnant patients.

Other antihypertensive medications such as clonidine (central α_2-agonist), trimethaphan (ganglionic blocker), and phentalamine and pheynoxybenzamine (competitive and noncompetitive α_1- and α_2-blockers) are rarely used except for specific indications.

Hypertension is a common asymptomatic disease; if not treated, it may result in various end organ injuries. CAD, CHF, cerebrovascular accidents, end-stage renal disease, retinal disease, and peripheral vascular disease are examples of complications. A dental office is more frequently visited than a primary care physician's office for "otherwise healthy" individuals and may be the first place that a patient's blood pressure is evaluated. Nonpharmacological therapy such as weight reduction, diet modification, exercise, and alcohol and tobacco cessation is an inexpensive and effective way of reducing blood pressure with few side effects. When pharmacological therapy is indicated, a compromise should be made regarding the most acceptable side effects in order to prevent complications and achieve patient compliance.

Bibliography

Bursztyn M: Blood pressure difference between arms, *Arch Intern Med* 157:818, 1997.

Cardiovascular Effects of Epinephrine in Hypertensive Dental Patients. Summary, Evidence Report/Technology Assessment Number 48. AHRQ Publication Number 02-E005, March 2002. Agency for Healthcare Research and Quality, Rockville, MD. http://www.ahrq.gov/clinic/epcsums/ephypsum.htm. Accessed June 14, 2006.

Chobanian AV, Bakris GL, Black HR, et al: The Seventh Report of the Joint National Committee on Prevention, Detection, Evaluation, and Treatment of High Blood Pressure: the JNC 7 report, *JAMA* 289:2560-2572, 2003.

Dahlof B, Devereux RB, Kjeldsen SE, et al: Cardiovascular morbidity and mortality in the Losartan Intervention For Endpoint reduction in hypertension study (LIFE): a randomized trial against atenolol, *Lancet* 359:995-1003, 2002.

Hansson L, Lindholm LH, Niskanen L, et al: Effect of angiotensin-converting-enzyme inhibition compared with conventional therapy on cardiovascular morbidity and mortality in hypertension: the Captopril Prevention Project (CAPPP) randomized trial, *Lancet* 353:611-616, 1999.

Heart Outcomes Prevention Evaluation Study Investigators: Effects of ramipril on cardiovascular and microvascular outcomes in people with diabetes mellitus: results of the HOPE study and MICRO-HOPE substudy, *Lancet* 22;355(9200):253-259, 2000.

Miall WE: Beta-blockers vs. thiazides in the treatment of hypertension: a review of the experience of the large national trials, *J Cardiovasc Pharmacol* 16(suppl 5):S58-S63, 1990.

Neaton JD, Grimm RH Jr, Prineas RJ, et al: Treatment of Mild Hypertension Study. Final results. Treatment of Mild Hypertension Study Research Group, *JAMA* 270:713-724, 1993.

Neutel JM, Smith DH, Wallin D, et al: A comparison of intravenous nicardipine and sodium nitroprusside in the immediate treatment of severe hypertension, *Am J Hypertens* 7:623, 1994.

Sacks FM, Svetkey LP, Vollmer WM, et al: Effects on blood pressure of reduced dietary sodium and the Dietary Approaches to Stop Hypertension (DASH) diet. DASH-Sodium Collaborative Research Group, *N Engl J Med* 344:3-10, 2001.

Schulz V: Clinical pharmacokinetics of nitroprusside, cyanide, thiosulphate and thiocyanate, *Clin Pharmacokinet* 9:239, 1984.

Vaughan CJ, Delanty N: Hypertensive emergencies, *Lancet* 356:411, 2000.

Appendix A: Abbreviations

AAOMS	American Association of Oral and Maxillofacial Surgeons
ABC	airway-breathing-circulation
AC	activated charcoal
ACC	acinic cell carcinoma
ACE	angiotensin-converting enzyme
ACLS	advanced cardiac life support
AdCC	adenoid cystic carcinoma
ADR	adverse drug reaction
AHA	American Heart Association
AHG	acute herpetic gingivostomatitis
AHI	apnea-hypopnea index
AIDS	acquired immunodeficiency syndrome
ALT	alanine aminotransferase
AMI	acute myocardial infarction
AMPLE	allergies–medications–past medical history/pregnancy–last meal–environment/events surrounding trauma
ANB	A point–nasion–B point (angle)
ANS	anterior nasal spine
ANUP	acute necrotizing ulcerative periodontitis
ARB	angiotensin receptor blockers
ARF	acute renal failure
AS	Apert syndrome
ASA	American Society Of Anesthesiology
ASP	acute suppurative parotitis
AST	asparate aminotransferase
ATLS	advanced trauma life support
ATN	acute tubular necrosis
AVPU	awake–responds to voice–responds to pain–unresponsive
AWS	alcohol withdrawal syndrome
BAL	blood alcohol level
BMI	body mass index
BMP	basic metabolic panel
BP	blood pressure
bpm	beats per minute
BRONJ	bisphosphonate related osteonecrosis of the jaws
BUN	blood urea and nitrogen
C	centigrade
CAD	coronary artery disease
CAD-CAMC	computer-assisted design — computer-assisted manufacturing
CBC	complete blood count
CC	chief complaint
CPP	cerebral perfusion pressure
CHF	congestive heart failure
CHI	closed head injury
CL	cleft lip
CLP	cleft lip and palate
CMP	complete metabolic panel
CMV	cytomegalovirus
CN	cranial nerve
CNS	central nervous system
Co	condylion
COPD	chronic obstructive pulmonary disease
CP	cleft palate
CRI	chronic renal insufficiency
CRP	chronic recurrent parotitis
CSF	cerebrospinal fluid
CT	computed tomography
CTX	c-telopeptide
CVA	cerebrovascular accident
CVS	cardiovascular system
CXR	chest x-ray
$D5_{1/2}NS$	5% dextrose in half normal saline
DC	dentigerous cyst
DDAVP	1-desamino-8-D-arginine vasopressin
DKA	diabetic ketoacidosis
DT	delerium tremens
DVT	deep venous thrombosis
EBV	Epstein-Barr virus
ED	emergency department
EEG	electroencephalogram
EF	ejection fraction
EKG	electrocardiogram
ELISA	enzyme-linked immunosorbent assay
EMG	electromyogram
EMS	emergency medical services
EOG	electro-oculogram
ESRD	end-stage renal disease
FDG	fluorodeoxyglucose
FE_{Na}	fractional excretion of sodium
FEV_1	forced expiratory volume in 1 second
FH	family history
FH	Frankfurt horizontal
FIO_2	fraction of inspired percent oxygen concentration
FISS	Facial Injury Severity Scale
FNA	fine needle aspiration
GCS	Glasgow Coma Scale
GFR	glomerular filtration rate
GGT	γ-glutamyl transpeptidase
GI	gastrointestinal

HAART	highly active antiretroviral therapy		NSP	nonsuppurative parotitis
HDL	high-density lipoprotein		NT/ND	nontender nondistended
HF	heart failure			
HFM	hemifacial microsomia		OD	right eye (ocular dexter)
HIV	human immunodeficiency virus		OG	orogastric
HPI	history of present illness		OKC	odontogenic keratocyst
HR	heart rate		OMFS	oral and maxillofacial surgery
hr	hours		ONJ	osteonecrosis of the jaws
HRT	hormone replacement therapy		OR	operating room
HSV	herpes simplex virus		ORIF	open reduction with internal fixation
HUS	hemolytic uremic syndrome		ORN	osteoradionecrosis
			OS	left eye (ocular sinister)
I&D	incision and drainage		OSA	obstructive sleep apnea
IAN	inferior alveolar nerve		OSAS	obstructive sleep apnea syndrome
ICD	intercanthal distance			
ICP	intracranial pressure		PAS	posterior airway space
ICU	intensive care unit		PCP	primary care physician
IM	intramuscular		PDHx	past dental history
IMF	intermaxillary fixation		PERRLA	pupils are equal, round, and reactive to
INR	international normalized ratio			light and accommodation
ITP	idiopathic thrombocytopenic purpura		PET	positron emission tomography
IV	intravenous		Pg	pogonion
			PMHx	past medical history
JVD	jugular venous distention		PND	paroxysmal nocturnal dyspnea
			PNI	perineural invasion
KOH	potassium hydroxide		PO	by mouth (Greek)
KS	Kaposi's sarcoma		POBHx	past obstetric history
			PRN	as needed (Greek)
LAD	lymphadenopathy		PRP	platelet-rich plasma
LDH	lactate dehydrogenase		PSG	polysomnograph
LDL	low-density lipoprotein		PT	prothrombin time
LFM	lowering the floor of the mouth		PTT	partial thromboplastin time
LN	lingual nerve		PVC	premature ventricular contraction
LOC	loss of consciousness		PVL	proliferative verrucous leukoplakia
MAP	mean arterial pressure		q8 h	every 8 hours
Me	menton			
MECa	mucoepidermoid carcinoma		RDI	respiratory distress index
mEq/L	milliequivalents per liter		RFFF	radial forearm free flap
mg	milligram		RR	respirations
MI	myocardial infarction		RRR	regular rate and rhythm
MIO	maximal interincisal opening			
MMA	maxillomandibular advancement		SAH	subarachnoid hemorrhage
MP	mandibular plane		Sao$_2$	oxygen saturation
MRI	magnetic resonance imaging		SCCa	squamous cell carcinoma
MRSA	methicillin-resistant *Staphylococcus aureus*		SH	social history
			SMAS	superficial musculoaponeurotic system
MVA	motor vehicle accident		SMV	submentovertex
MVC	motor vehicle collision		SNA	sella–nasion–A point (angle)
			SNB	sella–nasion–B point (angle)
NAC	*N*-acetylcystine		STAT	immediate (Latin)
NAD	no apparent distress		STSG	split-thickness skin graft
NG	nasogastric			
NOE	nasal orbital ethmoid		T	temperature
NPO	nothing by mouth (Greek)		TMD	temporomandibular dysfunction
NSAID	nonsteroidal antiinflammatory drug		TMJ	temporomandibular joint
NSC	nonsyndromic craniosynostosis		TTP	thrombotic thrombocytopenic purpura

UA	urinalysis
UDS	urine drug screen
UPP	uvulopalatoplasty
UPPP	uvulopalatopharyngoplasty
V_1	first division of the trigeminal nerve
V_2	second division of the trigeminal nerve
V_3	third division of the trigeminal nerve
VA	visual acuity
VAS	visual analog scale
VC	verrucous carcinoma
VPI	velopharyngeal incompetence

VSS AF	vital signs stable and afebrile
vWF	von Willebrand factor
WBC	white blood cell
WD/WN	well-developed and well-nourished
WNL	within normal limits
ZF	zygomaticofrontal
ZM	zygomaticomaxillary
ZMC	zygomaticomaxillary complex
ZS	zygomaticosphenoid
ZT	zygomaticotemporal

Appendix B: Normal Laboratory Test References for Adults

Type of Test	Test Result (Normal)
Blood	
acid phosphatate	0.11-0.60 U/L
AIDS serology	no evidence of HIV antigen or antibodies
AIDS T-lymphocyte marker (CD4 count)	total CD4 count >1,000 cells/mm^3
alanine aminotransferase (ALT)	8-20 U/L (elderly and infants higher than adults)
alkaline phosphatase (ALP)	42-128 U/L
ammonia level	15-110 µg/dl
aspartate aminotransferase (AST)	8-20 U/L (females slightly lower than males)
bilirubin, total	0.1-1.0 mg/dl
bilirubin, indirect	0.2-0.8 mg/dl
bilirubin, direct	0.1-1.3 mg/dl
bleeding time (BT)	1-9 min (Ivy method) (critical value >12 min)
blood culture and sensitivity	negative
blood gas	
pH	7.35-7.45
Pco$_2$	35-45 mm Hg
HCO$_3^-$	21-28 mEq/L
Po$_2$	80-100 mm Hg
O$_2$ saturation	95-100%
calcium	9.0-10.5 mg/dl
chloride	90-110 mEq/L
cholesterol	<200 mg/dl
complete blood count	see individual components (white blood cells, hemoglobin, hematocrit, platelets)
C-reactive protein	<0.8 mg/dl
creatine phosphokinase (CPK)	male 12-50 U/ml; female 10-55 U/ml
creatinine	male 0.6-1.2 mg/dl; female 0.5-1.1 mg/dl
D-dimer test	negative (no D-dimer fragments)
erythrocyte sedimentation rate (ESR)	male: ≤15 mm/hr, female ≤20 mm/hr
ethanol (blood alcohol level)	none
ferritin	male 12-300 ng/dl, female 10-50 ng/dl
γ-glutamyl transpeptidase (GGT)	8-38 U/L
glucose	70-105 mg/dl (also depends on fasting status)
glycosylated hemoglobin (A1c)	4-8%
hematocrit	male 42-52%, female 37-47%
hemoglobin	male 14-18 g/dl, female 12-16 g/dl
human chorionic gonadotropin (pregnancy test)	negative, unless pregnancy or pathology
lactate dehydrogenase	45-90 U/L
magnesium	1.2-2.0 mEq/L
myoglobin	0.85 ng/ml
osmolality	285-295 mOsm/kg
oximetry (pulse oximetry)	>95%
partial thromboplastin time (PTT)	30-40 sec
phosphorus	3.0-4.5 mg/dl
platelet count	150,000-400,000/mm^3
potassium	3.5-5.0 mEq/L
prealbumin	15-36 mg/dl
protein	6.4-8.3 g/dl
albumin	3.5-5.0 g/dl
prothrombin time (PT)	11.0-12.5 sec

red blood cell (RBC) count	male 4.7-6.1 million/mm^3, female 4.2-5.4 million/mm^3
reticulocyte count	0.5-2%
sodium	136-145 mEq/L
thyroid-stimulating hormone	2-10 µU/ml
blood urea nitrogen (BUN)	10-20 mg/dl
uric acid	male 2.1-8.5 mg/dl, female 2.0-6.6 mg/dl
white blood cell (WBC) count and differential count	
white blood cells	5,000-10,000/mm^3
neutrophils	55-70%
lynphocytes	20-40%
monocytes	2-8%
eosinophils	1-4%
basophils	0.5-1.0%

Urine

bilirubin	no bilirubin in urine
calcium, urine (24 hr)	vary with diet; normal diet 100-300 mg/day
chloride, urine (24 hr)	110-250 mEq/day
osmolality	12-14-hour fluid restriction: >850 mOsm/kg H_2O
potassium (24 hr)	25-120 mEq/L/day
sodium (24 hr)	40-220 mEq/L/day (varies greatly with dietary intake)
urinalysis (UA)	
appearance	clear
color	amber yellow
odor	aromatic
pH	4.6-8.0 (average, 6.0)
protein	none or ≤8 mg/dl
specific gravity	1.005-1.030
leukocyte esterase	negative
nitrites	negative
ketones	negative
crystals	negative
casts	none present
glucose	negative (<0.5 g/day)
white blood cells	0-4 cells/low-power field
white blood cell casts	negative
red blood cells	≤2/low-power field
red blood cell casts	none
vanillylmandelic acid	2-7 mg/24 hr

Index

Note: Page numbers followed by "f" refer to illustrations, page numbers followed by "t" refer to tables; page numbers followed by "b" refer to boxes

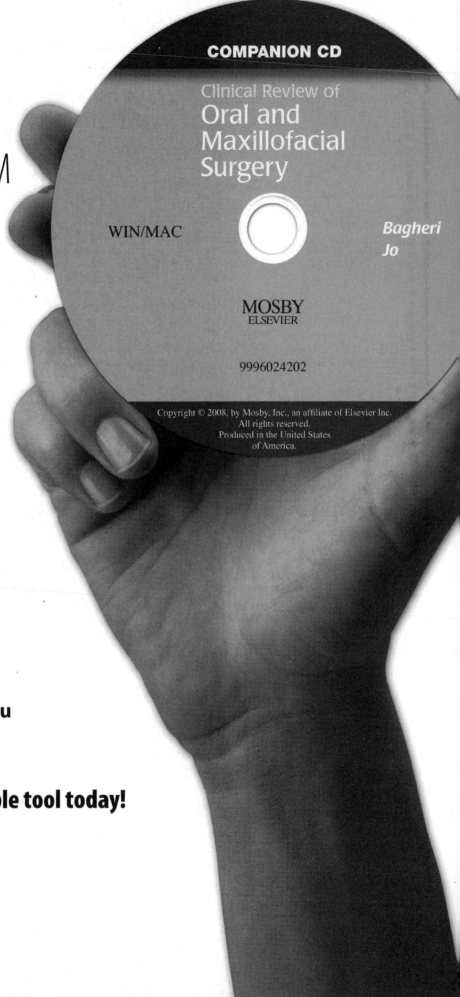